Atlas of Vaginal Reconstructive Surgery

Shlomo Raz

Atlas of Vaginal Reconstructive Surgery

Springer

Shlomo Raz
UCLA School of Medicine
Division of Pelvic Medicine
and Reconstructive Surgery
Los Angeles, CA
USA

Videos to this book can be accessed at http://link.springer.com/book/10.1007/978-1-4939-2941-2

ISBN 978-1-4939-2940-5 ISBN 978-1-4939-2941-2 (eBook)
DOI 10.1007/978-1-4939-2941-2

Library of Congress Control Number: 2015949702

Springer New York Heidelberg Dordrecht London

Printed on acid-free paper

Springer Science+Business Media LLC New York is part of Springer Science+Business Media (www.springer.com)

To my patients who have trusted me throughout the years

To my colleagues who continue to share with me and inspire me

To my residents and fellows who constantly challenge me and are the main motivation behind this atlas

To my family who have supported me so much throughout my entire career

Preface

> In writing for this book the lives of Alexander the king, and of Caesar, the conqueror of Pompey, I have before me such an abundance of materials that I shall make no other preface but to beg my readers not to complain of me if I do not relate all their celebrated exploits or even any one in full detail, but in most instances abridge the story. —Plutarch (A.D. 46–120)
>
> Student: Dr. Einstein, aren't these the same questions as last year's [physics] final exam? Dr. Einstein: Yes; but this year the answers are different. —Albert Einstein

This edition of the *Atlas of Vaginal Reconstructive Surgery* is the third I have published in the past 23 years (1992, 2002). New procedures, improvements in standard techniques, and entirely new methodologies have inspired me to write this edition. The basic premise is to provide the reader with a practical book that instructs, guides, reminds, and warns about the performance of vaginal pelvic surgery.

My intent was not to write a textbook that details every vaginal surgical procedure available, compares techniques, or discusses the literature on outcomes. Instead, this atlas is a practical guide to vaginal reconstructive surgery that reflects my own personal experience and knowledge accumulated in my research and surgical performance of more than 18,000 vaginal reconstructive procedures. This book also derives from my 30 years of experience teaching pelvic surgery to residents and fellows at the hospital of the UCLA School of Medicine. It is geared toward urology and gynecology residents with an interest in vaginal reconstructive surgery, to fellows training in Female Pelvic Medicine and Reconstructive Surgery, and to urologists and gynecologists with an interest in the field.

Again, this atlas is in no way an exhaustive account of every possible vaginal surgery that can be performed, but rather a description of particular procedures that I employ on a daily basis and that have been useful and successful in my personal practice.

The field of Female Pelvic Medicine and Reconstructive Surgery has advanced tremendously over the past 20 years, combining specialists and techniques from urology with those from obstetrics and gynecology. The creation of fellowship programs and a board-certifiable subspecialty in Female Pelvic Medicine and Reconstructive Surgery has further supported this advance. This interaction between the subspecialties has significantly improved the treatment of women with pelvic floor disorders. While laparoscopic and robotic surgery have developed to provide less invasive abdominal approaches, vaginal surgery remains a large component of the pelvic reconstructive procedures, and many pelvic conditions are better treated using a vaginal approach.

One significant concern in pelvic reconstructive surgery is that anatomy is not always correlated to function. On the one hand, a poor anatomical outcome can be minimally symptomatic, while, on the other, excellent anatomical reconstruction may be accompanied by poor functional results—exemplifying the dichotomy "feels good, looks bad" or "feels bad, looks good." Surgical outcomes should be measured by patient satisfaction and the absence of complications and de novo symptoms, separate from anatomical results.

Since 1990, the use of mesh for the treatment of stress incontinence has been common. Many modifications such as retropubic, obturator, and single-incision procedures have since been developed. After the initial success of mesh in the treatment of stress incontinence, surgeons and manufacturers expanded the use of mesh to treat vaginal prolapse. It took more than 10 years and several US Food and Drug Administration (FDA) notifications to realize the potential complications of mesh surgery for prolapse. Some of these complications are very significant and render patients permanently disabled, in chronic pain, or unable to have sexual relations, all resulting from a relatively simple elective surgery.

After performing more than 1600 stress incontinence and prolapse procedures using mesh (without using trocars or kits), I have abandoned its use and moved to only native tissue repairs. Aside from the FDA warning concerning potential complications arising from the use of mesh, we found that a not insignificant number of our patients develop late complications (even 5 and 10 years after the surgery). Thus, we have abandoned the use of mesh. This atlas does not include any prolapse surgery using mesh. The reader will find only the original description of the distal urethral polypropylene sling (DUPS) using mesh.

Atlas Structure

The text has been organized to be as useful as possible to the practicing vaginal surgeon. Each section is a tightly focused description of my preferred method of performing specific operations including hints and fine points that have proven of value in my own experience. As all surgeons know, there are many hints and tricks that we as surgeons have learned to ensure the success of a procedure, to help us avoid pitfalls, and to minimize the risk of complications.

This book is organized in nine chapters. The introduction discusses the anatomy of pelvic support and pathophysiology of stress incontinence. Further chapters cover surgery for incontinence, prolapse, urethral diverticula, vaginal fistula, reconstruction (including anal sphincter, neourethra, and closure of bladder neck), and surgery for urethral obstruction and for vaginal cysts and masses. The last chapter deals with complications of vaginal surgery.

Each surgical chapter covers a succinct summary of diagnosis, indications for surgery, and the surgical procedure itself. For each procedure, sequential operative photographs, drawings, and a short caption guide the reader through the steps used. References have been deliberately kept to a minimum at the end of each chapter and provide a guide for further reading.

I will consider this book a success if it inspires readers to generate ideas and solutions far beyond any that we have included in this book. If this book helps you improve outcomes of vaginal reconstructive surgery and search for continual improvement, it will have more than fulfilled its mission. I take full responsibility for any omissions or errors and if insufficient importance has been ascribed to any subject.

My gratitude to Lee Klein, Senior Editor at Springer, for all efforts and dedication to make this book a reality. Also my appreciation to the illustrators, in particular Wendy Vetter and her team. Their talents and skills add immeasurably to the book's usefulness.

A special thank you to Dr. Judy Choi for her diligent work on editing the surgical movies that are part of this book.

Semper investigans nun quam perficiens
Always searching, never quite achieving perfection

Los Angeles, CA Shlomo Raz, MD

Contents

1 The Anatomy of Pelvic Support ... 1
2 Surgery for Stress Incontinence ... 27
3 Surgical Repair of Anterior Vaginal Wall Prolapse ... 77
4 Excision of Urethral Diverticula ... 147
5 Transvaginal Repair of Fistulae ... 161
6 Reconstructive Surgery ... 211
7 Bladder Outlet Obstruction ... 237
8 Vaginal Cysts and Masses ... 261
9 Complications of Vaginal Surgery ... 285
Index ... 323

Contributor

Judy M. Choi Division of Pelvic Medicine and Reconstructive Surgery, UCLA School of Medicine, Los Angeles, CA90095, USA

The Anatomy of Pelvic Support

1

Clinicians involved in the care of women should possess a clear conceptual understanding of the anatomy and pathophysiology of pelvic support in order to effectively evaluate and treat disorders of pelvic floor relaxation. This chapter provides a basic review of the anatomy and musculofascial support of major pelvic structures and discusses their importance in clinically significant disorders of pelvic prolapse.

Clinical, urodynamic, radiological, and endoscopic evaluations, as well as operative experience on over 16,000 cases of pelvic reconstruction, have led us to a different understanding of the surgical anatomy and pathophysiology of female stress incontinence and vaginal support. Previously in our work, we recognized the difficulties in the interpretation of anatomic dissections obtained from whole-mount and step sections of the cadaver female pelvis. We found most valuable the use of static and dynamic MR images of the female pelvis and the surgical dissection and exposure of the retropubic and bladder neck area in patients with known pelvic prolapse or stress incontinence, as well as in women with normal control. Our findings support a simplified conceptual understanding of the anatomy of stress incontinence and pelvic support, allowing more rational treatment of these common disorders.

Conceptually, we can divide the vaginal canal into three compartments that have a distinct anatomical structure:

- The anterior compartment, including the urethra, bladder neck, and bladder
- The superior compartment, including the uterus and the cul-de-sac after hysterectomy
- The posterior compartment, including the rectum, the anal canal, the levator plate, the perineum, and the pelvic musculature

These three compartments have strong functional and anatomical interactions. For example, the function and support of the anterior compartment depend on intact posterior and superior compartments. Stress incontinence is in general only one of the manifestations of anterior vaginal wall relaxation, which very often coexists with other anatomical defects. If the superior or posterior compartments are deficient and are not repaired simultaneously with the anterior repair, the posterior and superior defect will be accentuated, and the repair of the anterior vaginal wall may not be long-lasting.

The anatomy of pelvic support comprises a number of elements:

- The bones
- The fascial support
- The muscles
- The nerves
- The vessels
- The pelvic organs
  - The urethra
  - The bladder
  - The uterus–vaginal vault
  - The rectum
  - The anal canal
  - The perineum

S. Raz, *Atlas of Vaginal Reconstructive Surgery*, DOI 10.1007/978-1-4939-2941-2_1

1.1 Pelvic Bones and Ligaments

The bony pelvis is the framework from which all pelvic structures ultimately draw support. The pubis and the ischium are the segments of the skeletal structure most important for pelvic support (Fig. 1.1). Some of the ligaments or condensed connective tissue important in pelvic support and function that will be discussed in this chapter include the sacrospinous ligament, the sacrotuberous ligament, the sacrouterine ligaments, the cardinal ligaments, the obturator membrane, the pubocervical fascia, and the prerectal and pararectal fascia (Figs. 1.2 and 1.3).

1.1.1 Sacrospinous Ligament

The sacrospinous ligament (SPL) extends from the ischial spine to the medial aspect of the sacrum. It is a strong triangular stricture covered by the coccygeus muscle. It can be considered the tendon of the coccygeus muscle. It is an important reference point for many vaginal procedures because of its distinct consistency and location, allowing the surgeon to guide the placement of sutures or needles in its proximity. Above the sacrospinous ligament is the piriformis muscle and the lumbosacral plexus where the origin of the sciatic nerve is located. The pudendal pedicle enters the sciatic foramen posterior to the lateral margin of the SP ligament under the ischial spine.

1.1.2 Sacrotuberous Ligament

The sacrotuberous ligament (STL) is a fan-shaped ligament of the posterior pelvis arising from the posterior sacrum to the ischial tuberosity. It primarily comprises collagen fibers and is strong enough to support the sacrum and prevent it from moving from its position under the body weight. It is a ligament of the sacroiliac joint, which is connected to the sacrum. Though it is not directly involved in pelvic floor relaxation or incontinence, it can lead to pelvic pain in patients with significant trauma of the pelvic structures.

1.1.3 Obturator Membrane

The obturator membrane is a strong, fibrous membrane that spans the obturator foramen. It is perforated superiorly, creating a passage where the obturator vessels and nerves cross to the medial compartment of the thigh. It provides an attachment surface for the internal and external obturator muscles. Obturator sling procedures cross the adductor muscles and the obturator internus and externus muscles. Single-incision slings rely on the placement of anchors through the obturator internus muscle and the obturator membrane.

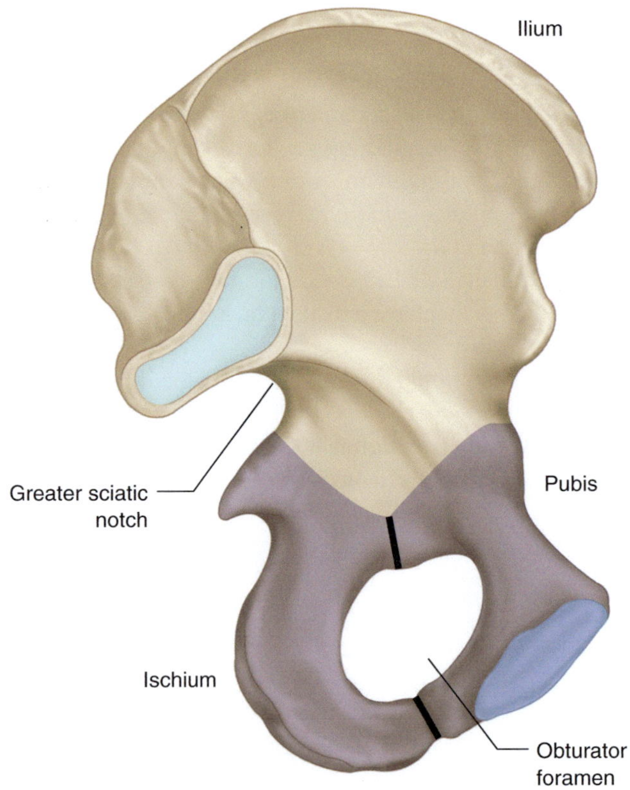

Fig. 1.1 Osseous structures supporting the pelvic organs include the pubic bone and ischium. The fusion of these two forms the obturator foramen, where the obturator membrane and muscles are inserted

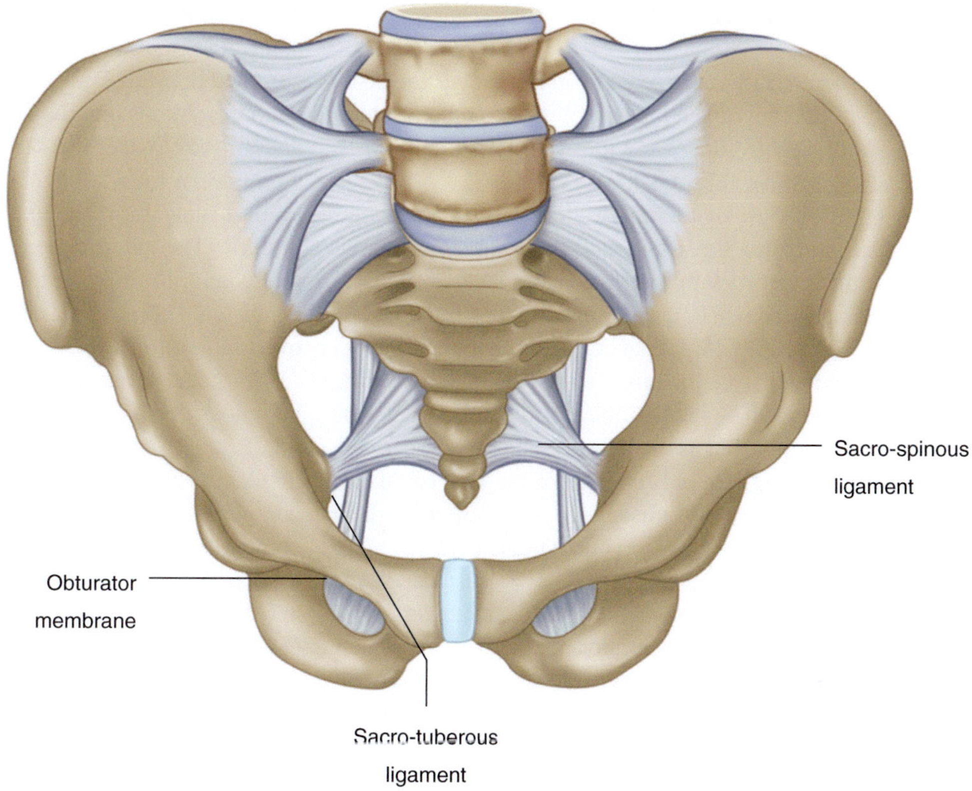

Fig. 1.2 The obturator membrane completely fills the obturator foramen except at its superior lateral aspect, where the obturator vessels and nerves emerge from the pelvis. The sacrospinous ligaments extend from the sacrum to the ischial spine, providing support and a very important landmark in pelvic surgery, which is easily palpated during vaginal surgery. Any procedure should avoid placement of sutures above the ligaments, where the piriformis muscle and lumbosacral nerve plexus are located

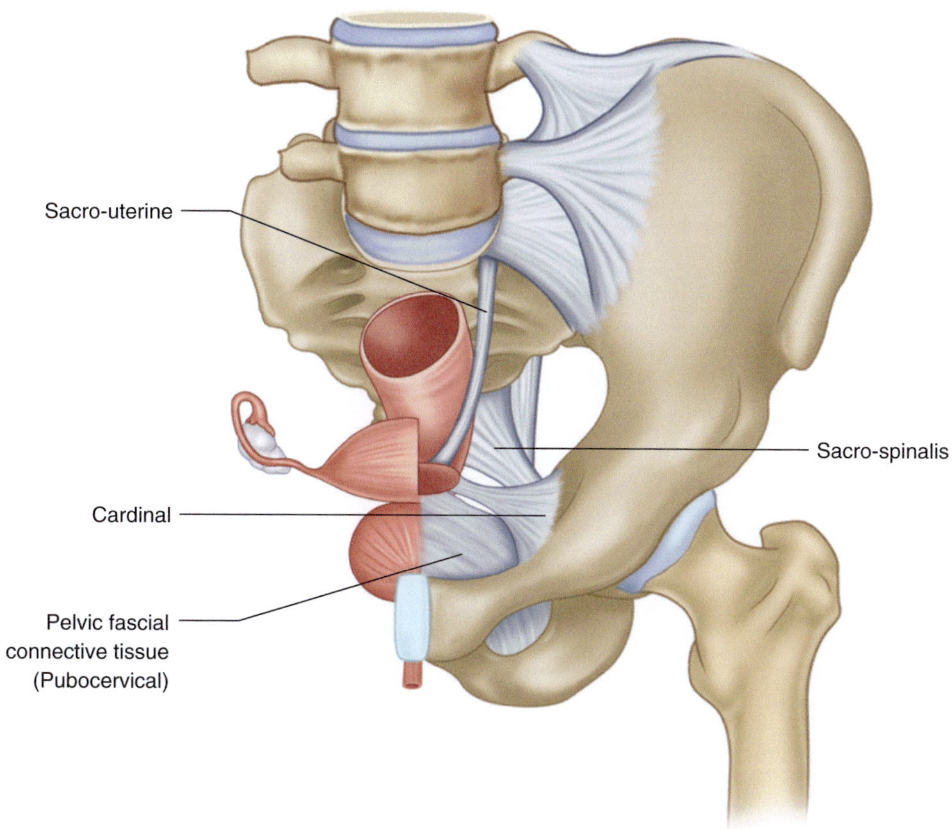

Fig. 1.3 Fascial structures important for pelvic support include the sacrouterine–cardinal complex, supporting the uterus and vaginal cuff, and the fascial connective tissue, supporting the pelvic viscera to the levator muscle (arcus tendineus fascia pelvis)

1.2 Pelvic Musculature

The pelvic bones and fascia (ligaments) make up the scaffolding, but the pelvic and perineal musculature, which attaches to this scaffolding, provides the floor upon which the pelvic organs rest (Fig. 1.4).

In a superior view of the pelvic floor, several muscular and fascial structures are seen: the piriformis, the internal obturator, the levator (with two main components, iliococcygeus and pubococcygeus), and the coccygeus muscle. The levator ani, comprising the pubococcygeus and iliococcygeus, can be viewed as the major inferior support of the urethra, vagina, and rectum. The medial fibers of the pubococcygeus muscles are also referred as the puborectalis muscle because of its role in the support and function of the anal canal and distal vagina. The levator muscle is a broad, thin sheet extending from the pelvic portion of the pubic bone lateral to the symphysis anteriorly and to the inner surface of the ischial spine posteriorly. Between these points it takes origin by the "arcuate line" of the obturator fascia (arcus tendineus levator ani). From these origins, the fibers extend back medially to unite with the fibers from the opposite side. In the anterior segment, the fibers fail to meet, forming a gap that is completed by the urogenital diaphragm. It is through this U-shaped hiatus that the vagina, rectum, and urethra exit the abdominal cavity. Fibers of the pubococcygeus muscle send a number of muscle fingers into these structures. Around the urethra, they form the extramural skeletal sphincter of the urethra. The fibers fuse posterior, lateral, and anterior to the rectum, forming part of the perineal support and the anal sphincter. The proximal half of the vagina lies horizontally over the levator plate.

Thus, the levator ani holds the intrapelvic organs like a hammock, providing support as well as stabilization during increases in intra-abdominal pressure (Fig. 1.5). Further dissection of this muscle, however, would indicate a more complex anatomy than this simple description suggests. In comparison with other skeletal muscles of the body, the levator has a much greater concentration of connective tissue, and fibers arising anteriorly condense into tough bands that engage in support of the pelvic viscera directly. After multiple deliveries, the relatively narrow levator hiatus opens widely.

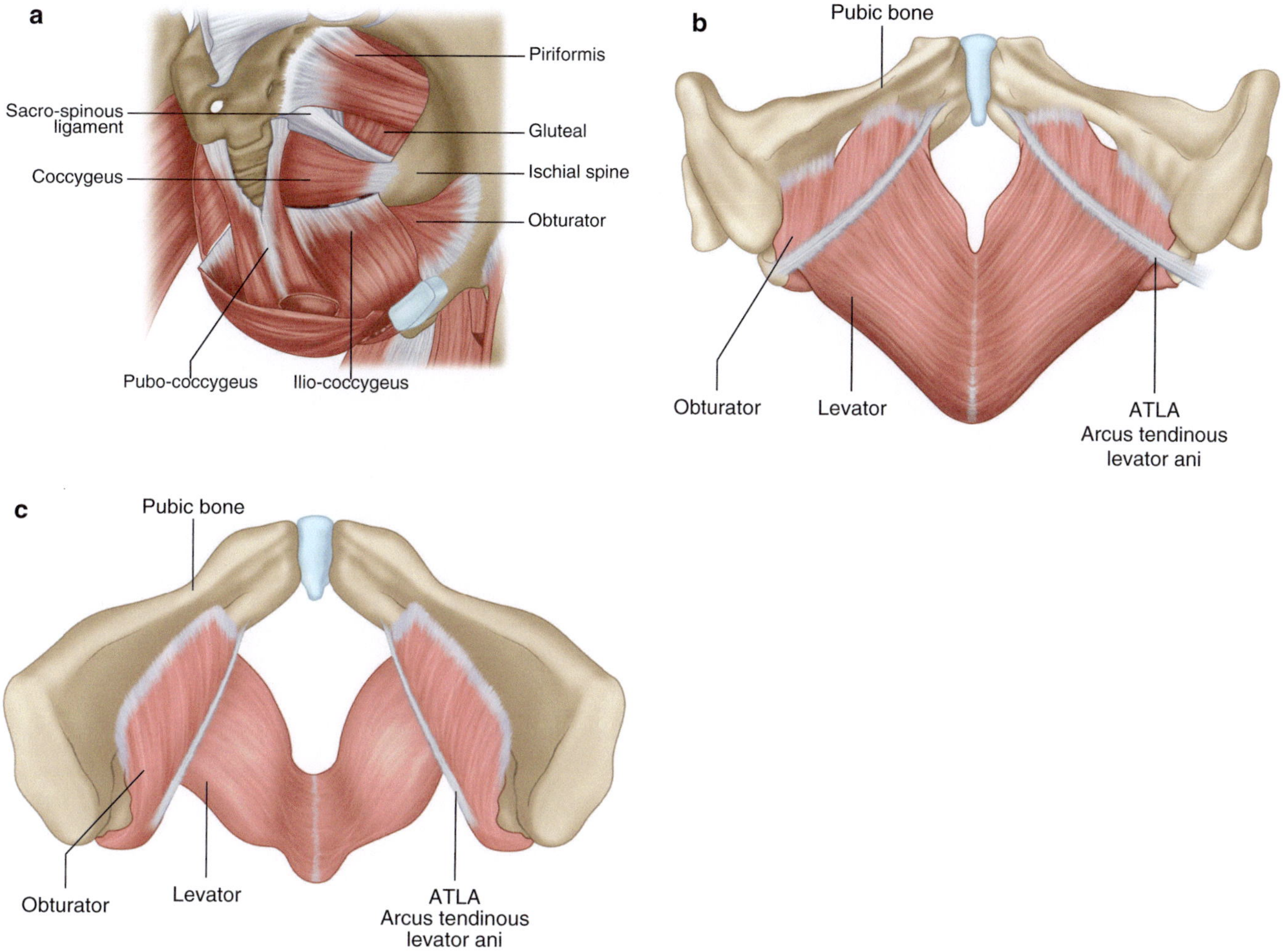

Fig. 1.4 Pelvic musculature and its relationship to the ischial spine and the sacrospinous ligament. The piriformis and gluteal muscles are seen in the space above the sacrospinous ligament. The iliococcygeus muscle inserts into the ischial spine and the obturator fascia (arcus tendineus levator ani) while attaching to the coccyx and anococcygeal raphe. The pubococcygeus inserts at the back of the pubis and the anterior arcus tendineus levator ani, extending toward the sacrococcyx. The pubovaginalis and puborectalis are not distinct muscles; rather, they are the medial segments of the pubococcygeus surrounding the vagina and rectum. (**a**) Three-dimensional MRI reconstruction of the pelvis in a young, nulliparous woman. The levator is inserted at the obturator fascia and the levator hiatus is relatively narrow. (**b**) A similar reconstruction in a patient with multiple deliveries shows the levator detached from the insertion at the obturator fascia, with widening of the levator hiatus. (**c**) Axial cut of a T2 MRI image of the pelvis showing the distribution of the pelvic musculature at the level of the trigone. The internal and external obturator are seen and the attachment of the levator musculature to the inner aspect of the obturator internus (arcus tendineus levator ani)

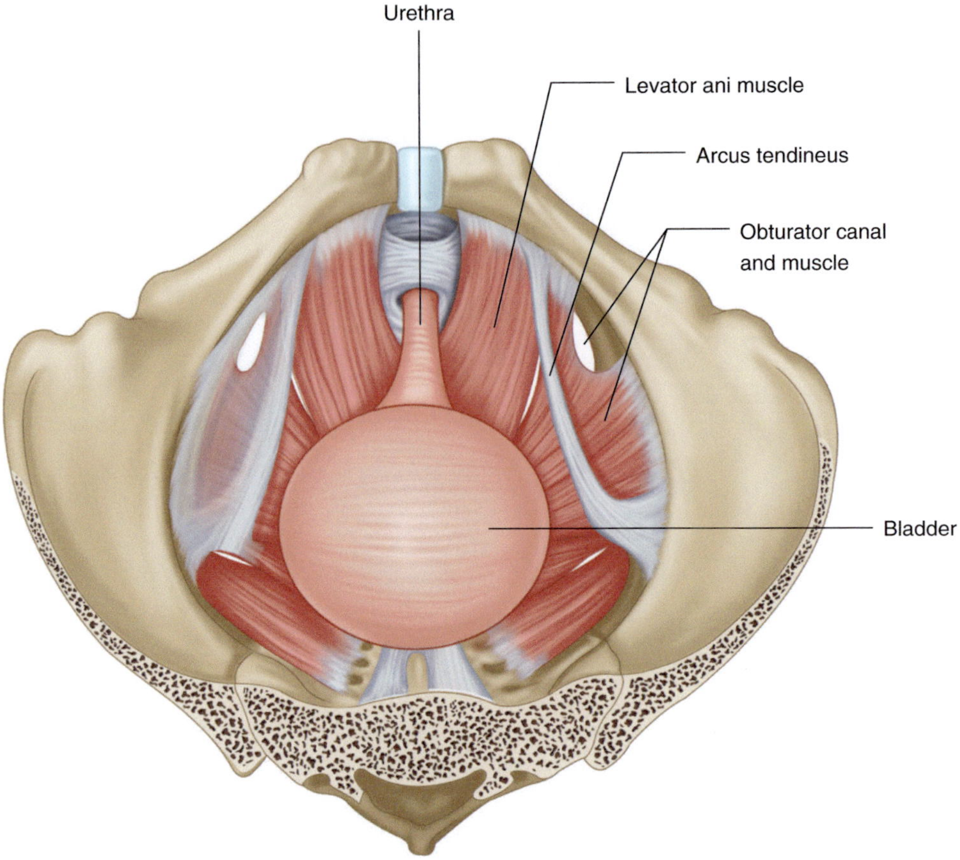

Fig. 1.5 Diagram of the pelvic support, depicting the bladder, the obturator muscle and foramen, and the arcus tendineus where the levators are inserting

1.3 Perineal Anatomy

The perineal anatomy adds further support to the pelvic structures (Fig. 1.6). The pubococcygeus muscle is open in the midline creating a hiatus through which the rectum, vagina, and urethra pass. Superficial to the pubococcygeus and iliococcygeus and covering the anterior segment of the levator hiatus is the perineal membrane, which attaches to the inner side of the pubic bone, joins the contralateral side at the central tendon of the perineum, and extends proximal into the posterior vagina for 2–3 cm, where the levator muscles are attached.

A line drawn between the ischial tuberosities divides the perineum into anterior urogenital and posterior anal triangles. The urogenital triangle in the female is divided in half longitudinally by the clitoris, urethra, and vaginal vestibule. The ischiocavernosus muscles cover the two clitoral crura as they attach to the ischia of the pubis. The bulbocavernosus muscles run on each side of the vestibule beneath the labia, between the clitoris anteriorly and the perineal body posteriorly. There are also two paired, superficial transverse perinei muscles, which run on each side of the perineal body to the ischial tuberosities laterally.

In the center of the anal triangle of the perineum is the anal canal. The muscle fibers of the superficial anal sphincter enclose the anus as they run between the anococcygeal ligament and the perineal body. The deep anal sphincter fibers completely encircle the anal canal and fuse superiorly with inferomedial fibers of the levator ani (pubococcygeus/puborectalis).

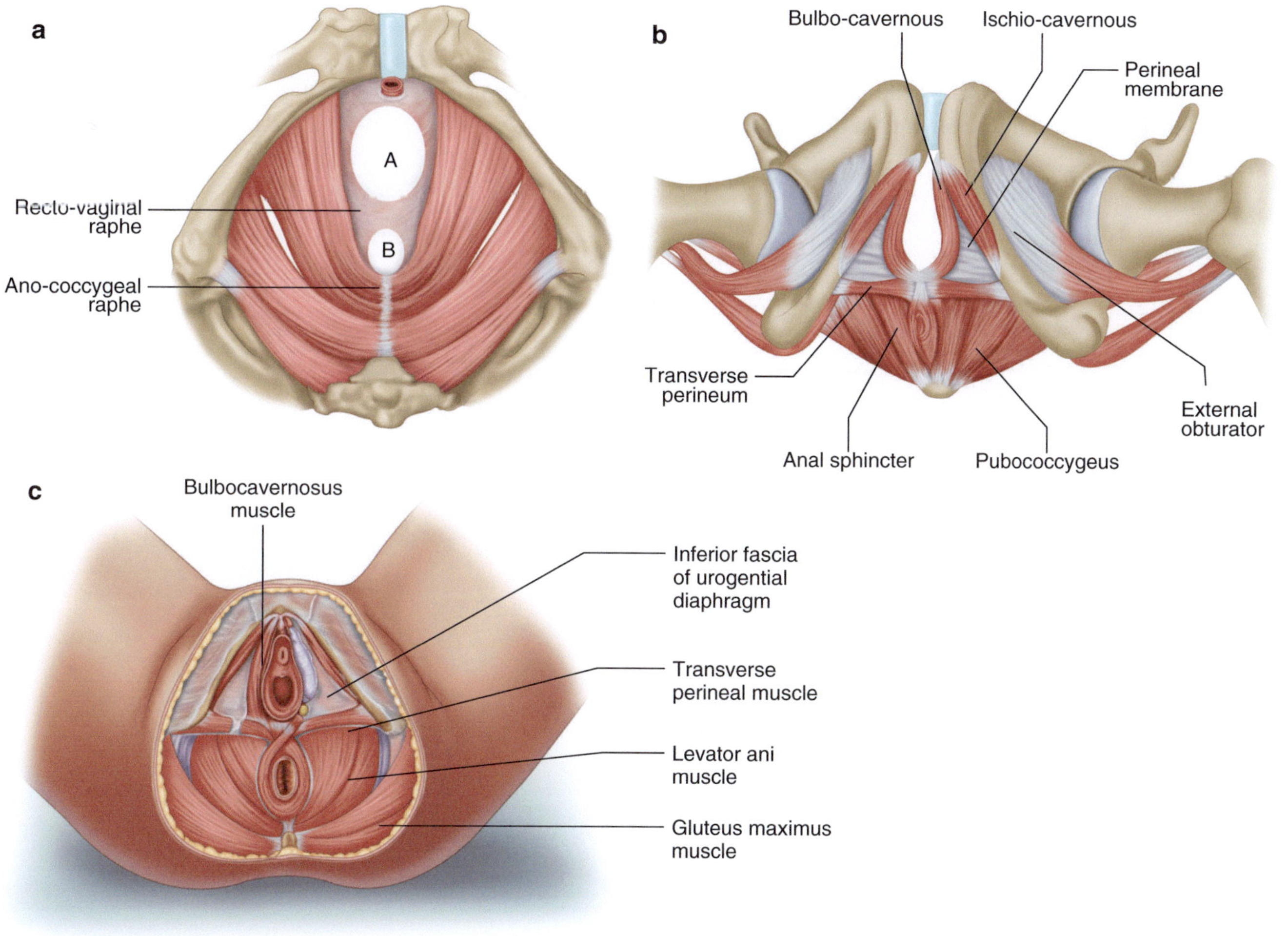

Fig. 1.6 (**a**) Superior view of the pelvis to show the pelvic musculature to include the piriformis, the coccygeus, the iliococcygeus, and pubococcygeus muscles. Through the genital hiatus the urethra, the bladder (*A*) and the rectum (*B*) cross the pelvic floor. The iliococcygeus inserts in a condensation of the internal obturator (arcus tendineus levator ani). (**b**) Diagram of the pelvic musculature depicting the levator hiatus, where the urethra, the vagina (*A*), and the rectum (*B*) are traversing from the pelvis. Extensions of the levator surround the organs as they cross the levator hiatus. Posterior to the rectum is the anococcygeal raphe. Between the rectum and vagina, the rectovaginal raphe provides the first line of support to the perineum and central tendon. Some fibers surround the urethral hiatus. (**c**) Diagram of an inferior view of the pelvic floor including the transverse perineum, the anal canal, the perineal membrane (inferior fascia of the urogenital diaphragm), the levator and the central tendon of the perineum

1.4 Support of Pelvic Organs

The vagina, bladder, urethra, and rectum are covered by connective tissue that supports the organs to the lateral pelvic wall musculature and fascia (arcus tendineus fascia pelvis) (Figs. 1.7, 1.8, and 1.9).

At the level of the urethra and the bladder, the pelvic connective tissue splits into a vaginal side (periurethral and perivesical fascia) and an abdominal side (endopelvic fascia) providing lateral support to the urethra, bladder neck, and the bladder, to the arcus tendineus fascia pelvis. The vaginal side of this connective tissue covering the urethra and bladder is called the pubocervical fascia, extending from the pubic bone to the arcus tendineus fascia pelvis laterally to the cervix and its supporting structures.

Similarly, the rectum is enclosed by connective tissue that attaches to the lateral pelvic wall. The prerectal and pararectal fasciae are only parts of this connective tissue; they are not defined ligaments.

Because surgical procedures are done in specific areas of the vaginal wall, depending on the anatomical location, we can define areas of specialization of the supporting connective tissue. As mentioned, these structures are not tendons or fascia, and they are not separate structures but rather are in continuity with the other areas of support. The separation into specific areas is artificial but helps in the understanding of the surgical anatomy, the exposure, and the use of these structures to reconstruct pelvic defects.

At the level of the bladder, the vaginal side of the pubocervical fascia is called perivesical fascia. It covers the anterior bladder wall and joins laterally to the posteriorly located endopelvic fascia to form the vesicopelvic ligament responsible for bladder support. At the level of the cervix and uterus, two areas of strong connective tissue anchor the cervix to the lateral pelvic wall (cardinal or lateral ligaments), and the sacrouterine ligaments anchor it to the sacrum and fascia of the coccygeus and levator fascia.

Again, we feel that all these ligaments are not distinct anatomical structures but are only part of the concentration of connective tissue responsible for pelvic organ support.

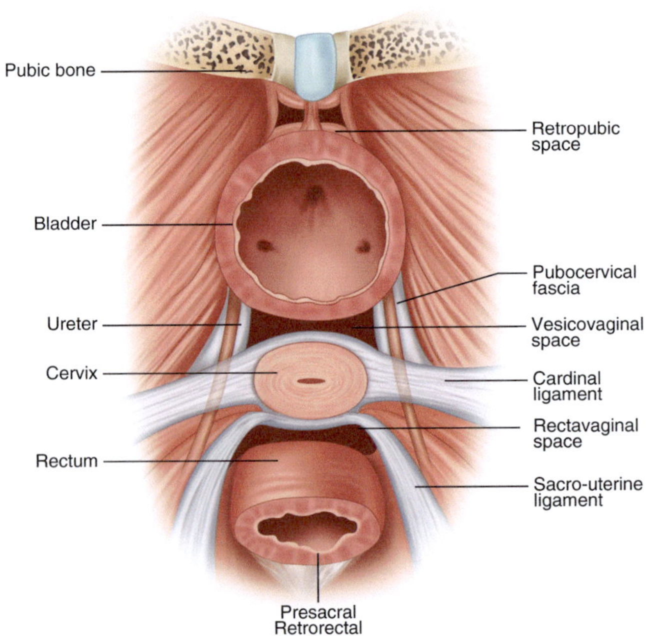

Fig. 1.7 Diagrammatic superior view of the pelvic organs, supporting fascia, and the spaces in between, including the presacral, rectovaginal, vesicovaginal, and retropubic spaces

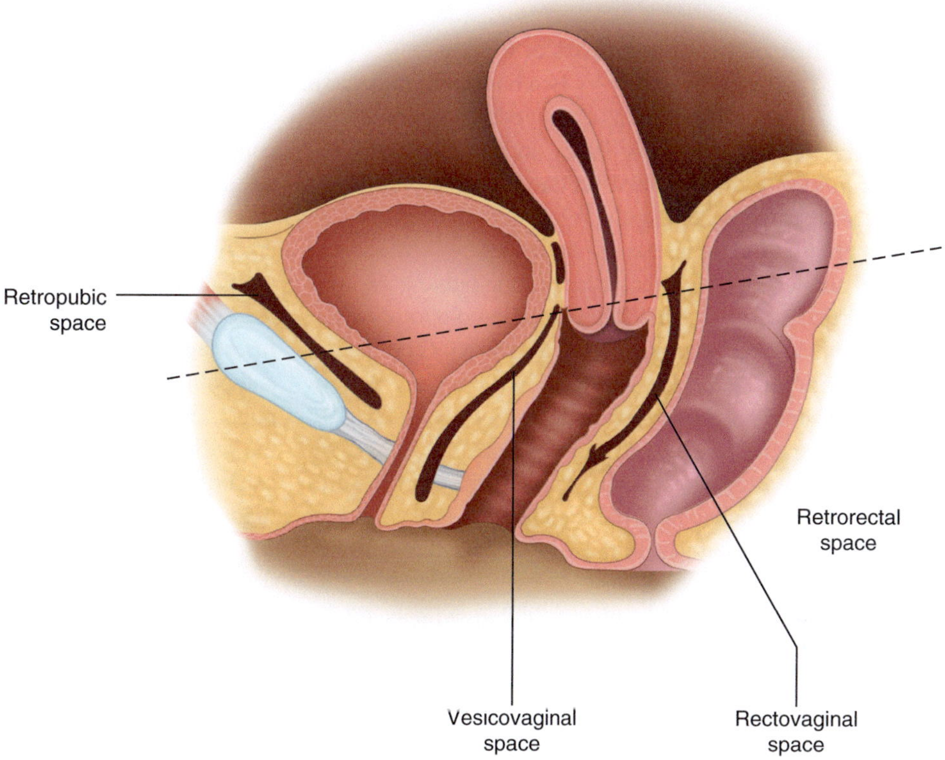

Fig. 1.8 Sagittal view of the pelvic organs depicting the retropubic, vesicovaginal, rectovaginal, and retrorectal spaces. It is in these spaces that the connective tissue supporting the pelvic organs to the lateral pelvic wall (levator) is present

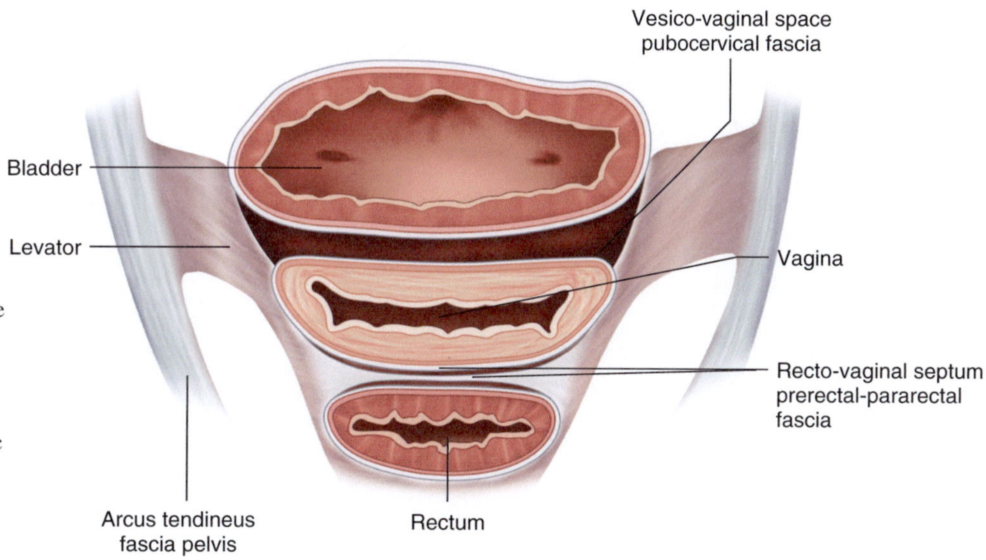

Fig. 1.9 Conceptual diagram of pelvic organ support. The connective tissues present in the retropubic space (endopelvic fascia), vesicovaginal space (pubocervical fascia), and prerectal space (prerectal fascia) surround the pelvic organs. They fuse laterally to insert into the levator fascia (arcus tendineus fascia pelvis)

1.4.1 Urethral Support

1.4.1.1 Pubourethral Ligaments or Fascia

The urethra is supported mainly by two bands of connective tissue: the pubourethral ligaments, connecting the urethra to the inferior rami of the pubic bone, and the urethropelvic fascia, connecting the proximal urethra to the lateral pelvic wall (arcus tendineus fascia pelvis).

The pubourethral ligaments are the best described and can be found connecting the inner surface of the pubic bone with the midurethra (Fig. 1.10a). They are homologous to the puboprostatic ligaments in men. They are the only connection of the urethra to the pubic bone (Fig. 1.10b). They help to support and stabilize the urethra and anterior vaginal wall to the inferior aspect of the pubic bone. Weakness in these ligaments permits posterior and inferior displacement of the urethra but does not contribute significant support to the bladder neck (Fig. 1.10c). Just distal to these ligaments, the extramural skeletal muscle fibers are located.

As described above, the pubourethral ligaments divide the urethra into three areas: a proximal third, including the bladder neck and intra-abdominal urethra; the midurethra, including the pubourethral ligament and the extramural skeletal musculature; and the distal third, which is only a conduit for the urine, without function with regard to continence. The proximal third of the urethra is responsible for passive continence; the midurethra is responsible for passive and active continence and acts as an important defense mechanism against sudden increases in abdominal pressures when the proximal urethra is incompetent. This is the thickest part of the urethra and corresponds to the area of highest concentration of skeletal musculature and the area of highest urethral pressure.

How are these ligaments or fascia seen in surgery? When entering the retropubic space during vaginal surgery, we create a window by detaching the urethropelvic ligament from the arcus tendineus fascia pelvis of the levator muscle (Fig. 1.10d). Inserting a finger into the retropubic space at the same spot and pointing the finger in an anterior direction, we can feel the pubourethral ligaments as they attach to the inferior rami of the pubic bone. Another view of the pubourethral ligaments can be seen during the suprameatal approach to the urethra for bladder neck closure or urethrolysis (Fig. 1.10e, f). Dynamic MRI can also demonstrate the function of the ligaments as the urethra rotates with strain, with the point of fixation on the inferior ramus of the pubic bone. In patients with pelvic floor relaxation, the attachment of the urethra to the inferior pubic bone is weakened, increasing the distance from the pubic bone to the urethra and therefore facilitating the downward and inferior rotation of the urethra. This anatomical change may affect the compensatory mechanism of the urethra during changes in abdominal pressure.

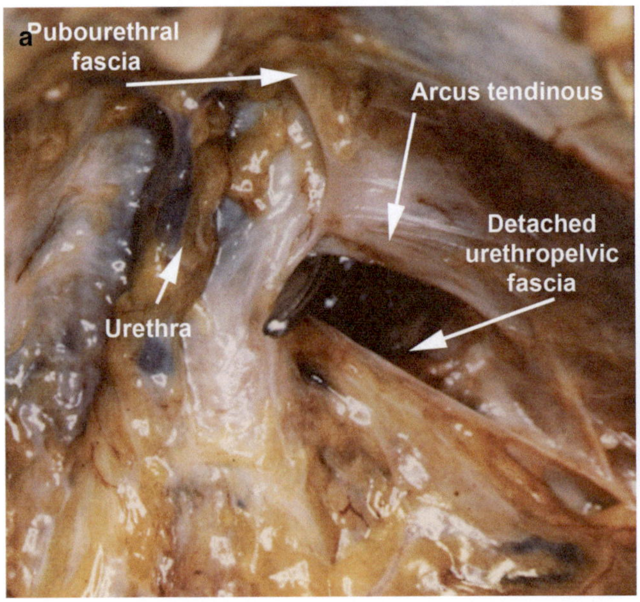

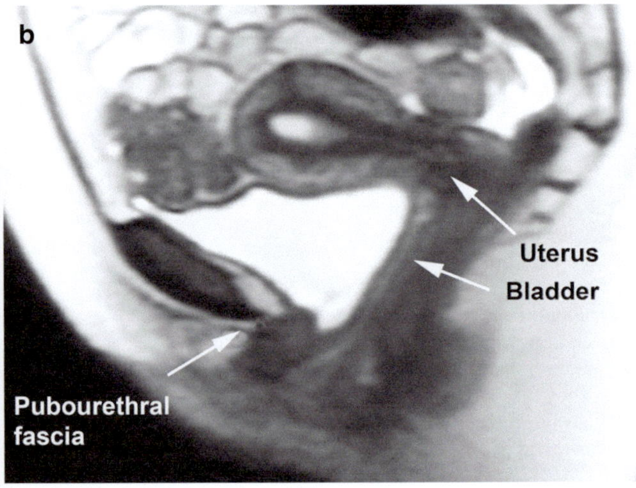

Fig. 1.10 (**a**) Cadaveric dissection. After penetration of the urethropelvic fascia, the retropubic space is exposed, revealing the arcus tendineus, the detached urethropelvic fascia, and the pubourethral fascia. (**b**) Sagittal midline pelvic MRI showing the attachments of the urethra to the inferior rami of the pubis. The pubourethral fascia is the only attachment of the urethra to the pubic bone. (**c**) Sagittal midline pelvic MRI during straining in a patient with stress incontinence and mild cystocele. The urethra shows downward rotation and separation from the inferior ramus of the pubic bone. (**d**) After entering the retropubic space and detaching the urethropelvic fascia from the arcus tendineus, just superior and medial is where the pubourethral fascia can be found, which supports the midurethra to the inferior ramus of the pubic bone. (**e**) Suprameatal incision exposing the anterior distal urethra. The retropubic space will be entered to detach the pubourethral fascia. (**f**) The retropubic space was entered anterior to the urethra, detaching the pubourethral fascia from the inferior ramus of the pubic bone

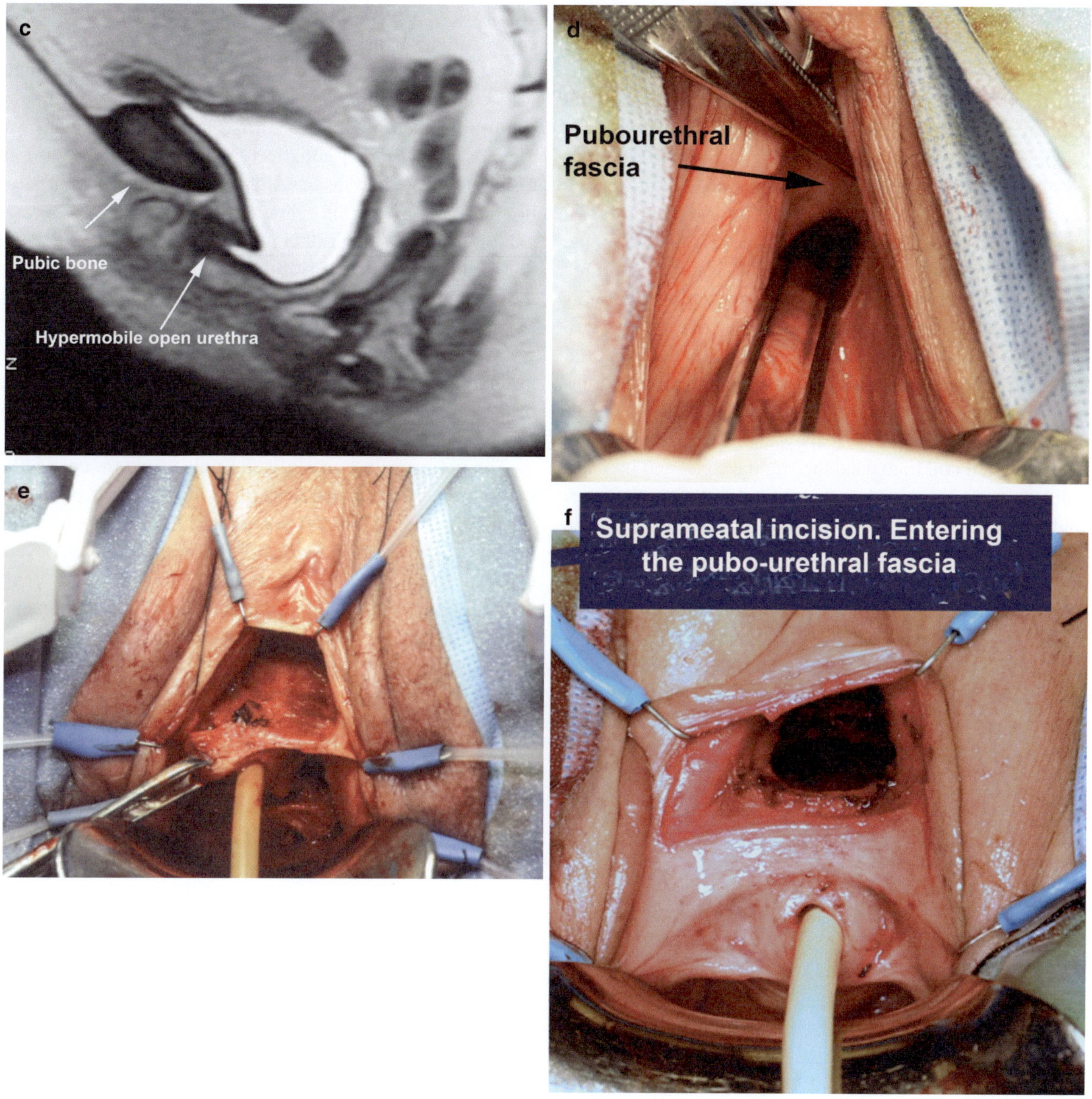

Fig. 1.10 (continued)

1.4.1.2 The Urethropelvic Fascia

The urethropelvic fascia is a name that we use to describe another "specialized" group of fibers of functional significance to stress incontinence, which support the urethra and bladder neck to the lateral pelvic wall (arcus tendineus fascia pelvis). This fascia is not a separate structure but rather an area of the condensed connective tissue around the pelvic viscera in charge of urethral support. The endopelvic fascia covers the abdominal side of the pelvic viscera, including the bladder neck and urethra; on the vaginal side, the urethra is covered by the periurethral fascia. The periurethral fascia is simply the area of the pubocervical fascia covering the urethra. Both the endopelvic and periurethral fasciae are fused laterally to support the proximal urethra to the arcus tendineus fascia pelvis of the levator muscle. MRI studies and surgical dissections help to clarify the anatomy of this structure. Using a vaginal coil to expand the vaginal canal and increase resolution, we can appreciate that the sphincteric unit is surrounded by the periurethral and endopelvic fasciae attaching lateral to the levator muscle (Fig. 1.11a, b). During stress incontinence surgery, we incise the lateral vaginal wall and enter the retropubic space by detaching the urethropelvic fascia from the arcus tendineus. Again, it is important to appreciate that the pubourethral and urethropelvic ligaments are not separate structures but merely an area of continuous connective tissue supporting the pelvic viscera and joined to the levator musculature.

The dissection of the vaginal wall from the urethra is avascular, and no distinct plane or space is encountered. Rather, the vagina and urethra are lightly fused so that the vaginal wall conforms to the shape of this periurethral fascia and follows its anatomy. In the normal female, the vaginal wall ascends laterally and superiorly and attaches very loosely to the urethropelvic fascia at its anchor to the lateral pelvic floor, thereby giving the characteristic "H" shape of the vaginal lumen in cross-sectional imaging (periurethral sulcus).

During vaginal surgery for incontinence, we often enter the retropubic space by dissection over the periurethral fascia by perforating the attachment of the ligaments (endopelvic and periurethral) to the lateral pelvic wall. With a finger in the retropubic space, we can anchor and feel the strength of the attachments and use this structure in the surgical correction of stress incontinence (Fig. 1.11c, d).

The urethropelvic fascia is the only structure connecting the urethra to the levator muscle. In the young, it provides a strong and elastic support connecting the bladder neck and urethra to the lateral pelvic wall. Contraction of the levator or obturator muscles will increase the tensile forces of the urethropelvic ligaments, improving seal and continence. Weakness of the levator plate and/or the urethropelvic fascia (owing to detachment or elongation of the urethropelvic ligaments) will facilitate urethral and bladder neck hypermobility, reducing the functional efficiency of the proximal urethra (Fig. 1.11e).

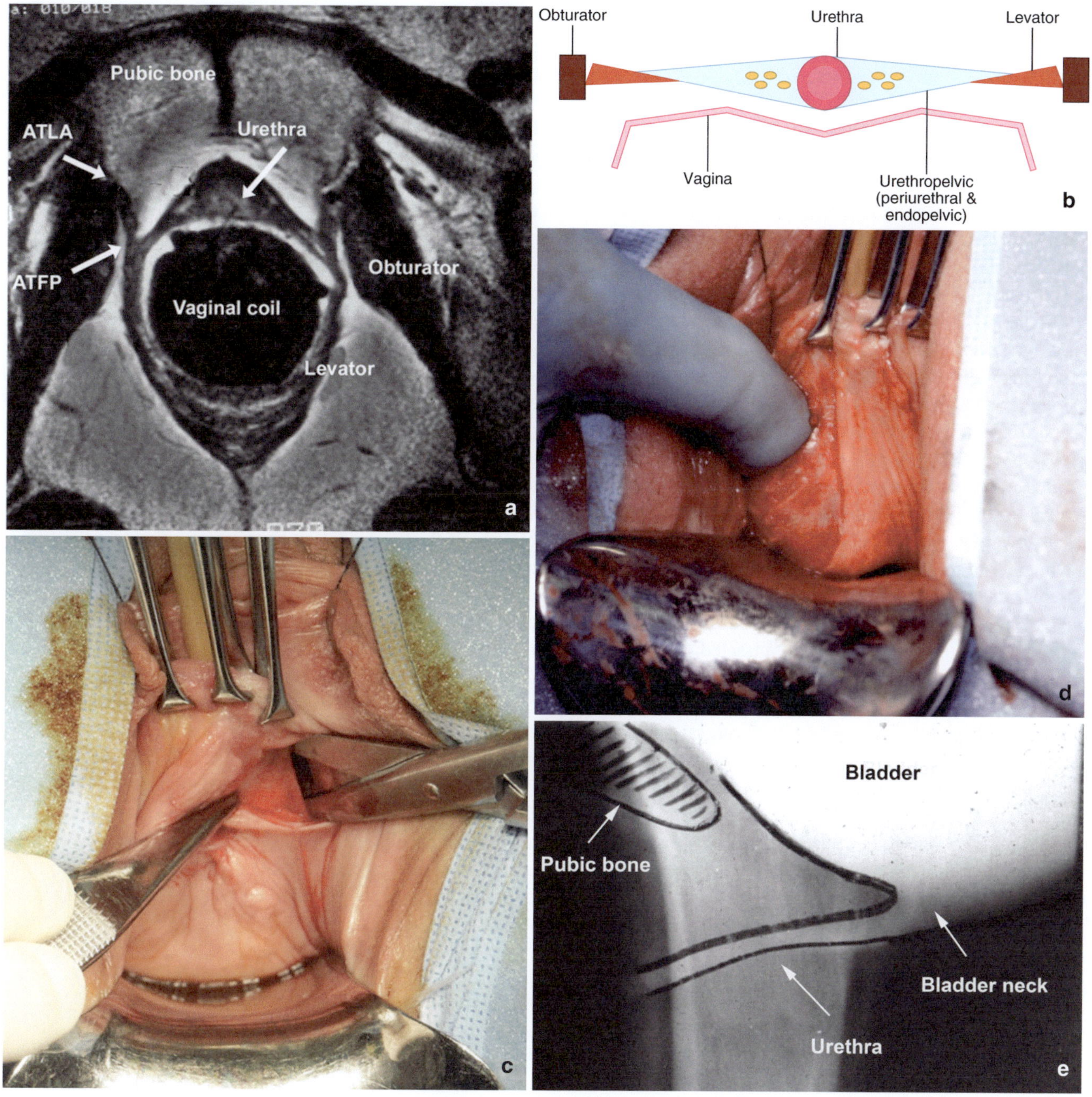

Fig. 1.11 (**a**) T2 MRI image of the urethra. Using a vaginal coil, the vaginal distension allows us to see the urethra supported like two wings laterally to the levator muscle. The levator inserts on a condensation of the obturator muscle. ATFP, arcus tendineus fascia pelvis; ATLA, arcus tendineus levator ani. (**b**) Diagram of the urethropelvic fascia, composed of a vaginal side (periurethral fascia) and an abdominal side (endopelvic fascia), both fusing laterally to support the urethra to the levator fascia (ATFP). (**c**) During stress incontinence surgery, dissection over the periurethral fascia allows detachment of the urethropelvic fascia from the arcus tendineus fascia pelvis. (**d**) With a finger in the retropubic space, the urethropelvic ligament is palpated and elevated. (**e**) Lateral cystogram in a patient with stress incontinence. During straining, the urethra is moved away from its normal close proximity to the inferior rami of the symphysis into a low position, owing to weakness of the pubourethral and urethropelvic fascia. Most patients with this anatomic defect do not lose urine unless there is an intrinsic sphincter defect

1.4.2 Bladder Support: The Vesicopelvic Fascia or Ligaments

Bladder support is very similar and only a continuation of the urethral support. "Vesicopelvic ligaments" is a name that we use to describe the trapezoid structure responsible for connecting the bladder to the lateral pelvic wall (Fig. 1.12a). It is not a separate structure but rather another specialization of the levator fascia responsible for bladder support. The endopelvic fascia covers the abdominal side of the bladder, and the perivesical fascia covers the vaginal side. Both fuse laterally to support the bladder to the arcus tendineus fascia pelvis (Fig. 1.12b).

During vaginal surgery, if a vertical incision is made in the anterior vaginal wall from the urethra to the cervix, the fascia from the pubic bone to the cervix (commonly known as the pubocervical fascia) is exposed. The segment of pubocervical fascia covering the bladder area is called the perivesical fascia. Surgical dissection around the perivesical fascia toward the lateral pelvic wall reveals the attachment of the bladder to the levator fascia (arcus tendineus). By entering this attachment, we enter the paravesical space. The margins of the vesicopelvic fascia can be seen as they are detached from the arcus tendineus, retracted, or used in surgical repair of bladder prolapse (Fig. 1.12c, d).

Trauma of delivery, hysterectomy, aging of the tissues, hormonal deficiency, and pelvic floor relaxation may produce three types of abnormalities of bladder support: a central defect, a lateral (paravaginal) defect, and a transverse–proximal defect (Fig. 1.12e). A combination of the three types is common. In central defects, the bladder is herniated in the midline, through the attenuated perivesical fascia, but the lateral support of the bladder is preserved (Fig. 1.13a, b). In patients with lateral defects, the attachment of the bladder to the lateral pelvic wall is defective, resulting in a sliding displacement of the bladder wall (Fig. 1.13c). With transverse defects, the pubocervical fascia is separated from its attachment to the cervix, producing a proximal descent of the bladder. The etiology of cystocele is complex and can include factors like levator musculature damage, denervation, elongation, or detachment of the fascial structures from their lateral anchors to the lateral pelvic wall. The presence of significant lateral and transverse cystocele is intimately related to vaginal vault support, and the outcome of surgery for significant cystocele depends to a great extent on the outcome of vaginal vault support.

Static and dynamic MRI and cystourethrogram have helped to define better the anatomy of anterior vaginal wall prolapse. As will be discussed later, the most common abnormality is a combination in which the lateral and central supports of the bladder are damaged, together with hypermobility of the urethra and bladder neck. The frequency of this combination has a great impact on the surgical correction of cystocele. We believe that if surgery is performed, most patients should have repair of all the anterior vaginal wall defects (unless contraindicated). Merely repairing the central defect without repairing the urethral defect and the lateral bladder defect can result in a significant rate of cystocele recurrence and the continuation or appearance of de novo stress incontinence. Abdominal surgeries such as Burch colposuspension or paravaginal suspension can correct only the lateral defect, and they are not indicated in the repair of cystocele with a significant central defect. Sacrocolpopexy can effectively repair vault prolapse and reduce the cystocele, but it will not correct urethral hypermobility or a significant central defect.

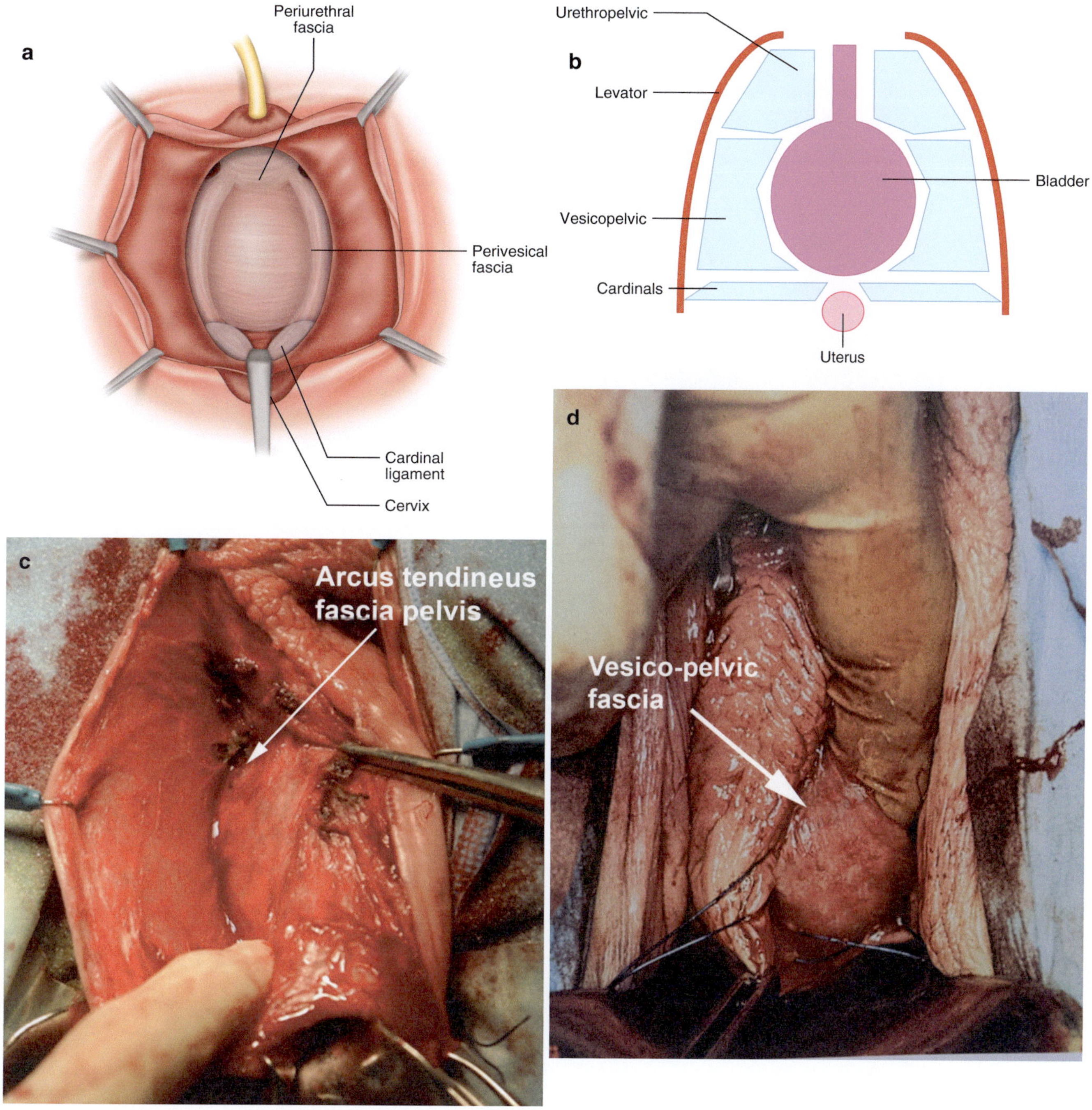

Fig. 1.12 (**a**) Diagram of the anterior vaginal wall after a vertical incision is made. The pubocervical fascia extends from the pubic bone to the cervix. The area of fascia around the urethra is called periurethral, and the area around the bladder is called perivesical fascia. (**b**) Diagram depicting the open anterior vaginal wall. The envelope of connective tissue around the urethra attaches to the levator fascia via the urethropelvic fascia (combination of periurethral and endopelvic). The envelope of connective tissue around the bladder attaches to the lateral pelvic wall via the vesicopelvic fascia (combination of perivesical and endopelvic). (**c**) Surgical dissection around the perivesical fascia during a cystocele repair shows the lateral attachments of the bladder to the lateral pelvic wall (arcus tendineus fascia pelvis). (**d**) After a lateral incision of the anterior vaginal wall, the perivesical fascia was entered, detaching the bladder from the arcus tendineus. The margins of the vesicopelvic fascia (a combination of perivesical and endopelvic) are palpated and retracted. (**e**) Most patients with significant anterior vaginal wall prolapse present with a combination of urethral hypermobility, central and lateral defects, and vault prolapse. Successful repair of this condition requires support of the vaginal cuff and urethral support as well as the repair of the lateral and central defects

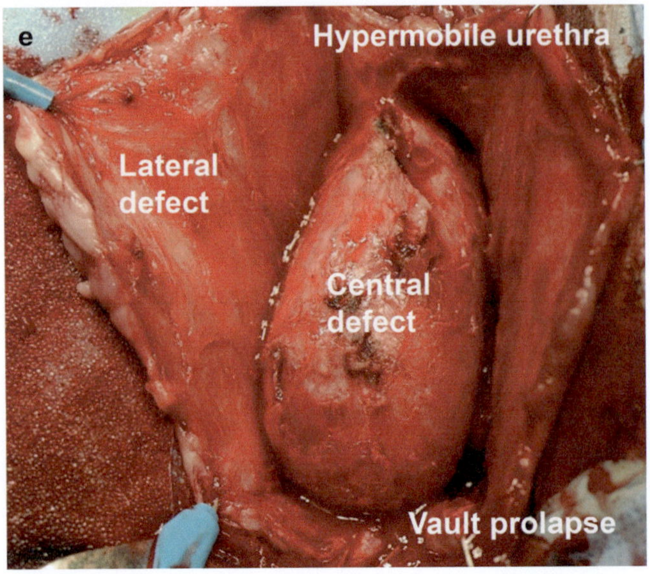

Fig. 1.12 (continued)

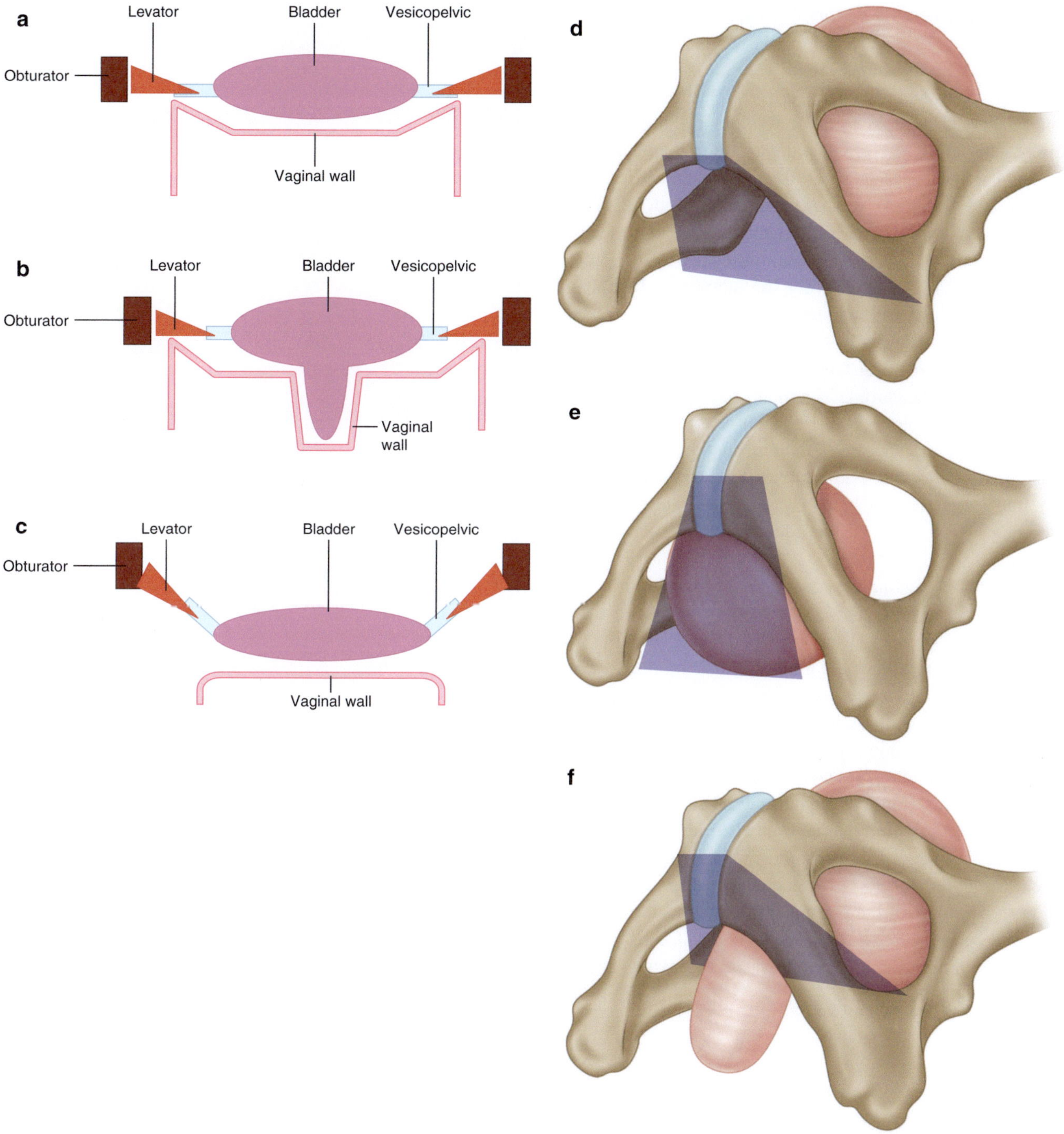

Fig. 1.13 (**a**) Diagram of the trapezoid supporting the anterior vaginal wall, associated distally to the urethral support, laterally to the arcus tendineus fascia pelvis, and posteriorly to the same supporting structures of the uterus and vaginal cuff (cardinal–sacrouterine complex). (**b**) Diagram depicting a central defect cystocele. The lateral support is present, but weakness of the perivesical fascia allows the bladder to prolapse centrally. (**c**) Diagram depicting a lateral defect cystocele, in which the lateral support of the bladder to the arcus tendineus is elongated or detached. (**d**) The anterior vaginal wall support is a trapezoid with the lateral walls at the arcus tendineus fascia pelvis, the distal support is similar to the urethra, and the proximal support is the same as the ureters and the vault (sacrouterine–cardinal complex). (**e**) In a lateral defect, the lateral attachment of the anterior vaginal wall is sliding downward owing to detached or elongated vesicopelvic fascia. (**f**) In a central defect, the lateral attachment is maintained, while the bladder is prolapsed through a central defect of the pubocervical fascia

1.4.3 Uterine and Vaginal Vault Support

The sacrouterine ligaments provide the most important support to the uterus and the vaginal cuff (*see* Fig. 1.3). The ligaments anchor the cervix to the anterolateral margins of the sacrum and pelvic fascia. They are strong in young women, but with aging, menopause, and multiple deliveries, they may become detached, attenuated, and elongated, leading to uterine or vault prolapse. The ligaments are important in vaginal reconstructive surgery, as vault suspension procedures are aimed to substitute for the attenuated ligaments. The total length of the ligaments is approximately 12 cm, with a distal attachment to the posterior lateral cervix and proximal vagina for a distance of 2–3 cm, where the ligaments fuse with the cardinal ligaments to form the cardinal–sacrouterine complex. The ligament curves around the rectum toward the sacrum, attaching at the S3 level with extensions toward S2. The superior anchor point is wide from the sacral foramina medially to the sacroiliac joint extending to the fascia of the coccygeus and sacrospinous ligaments.

The cardinal ligaments, also called Mackenrodt's ligaments, are thick, triangular concentrations of pelvic fascia containing the uterine arteries, which originate from the pelvic fascia in the region of the greater sciatic foramina. They insert into the lateral aspects of a ring of fascia encircling the uterine cervix and isthmus, and into the adjacent vaginal wall as well, providing major uterine and apical vaginal support. The cardinal ligaments fuse posteriorly with the sacrouterine ligaments and insert into the posterolateral aspect of the pericervical fascial ring and lateral vaginal fornices (Fig. 1.14). Further uterine support is provided by the broad ligaments, which are more superiorly located and covered by anterior and posterior folds of the peritoneum; they attach the lateral walls of the uterine body to the pelvic sidewall. They contain the fallopian tubes, the round and ovarian ligaments, and the uterine and ovarian vessels.

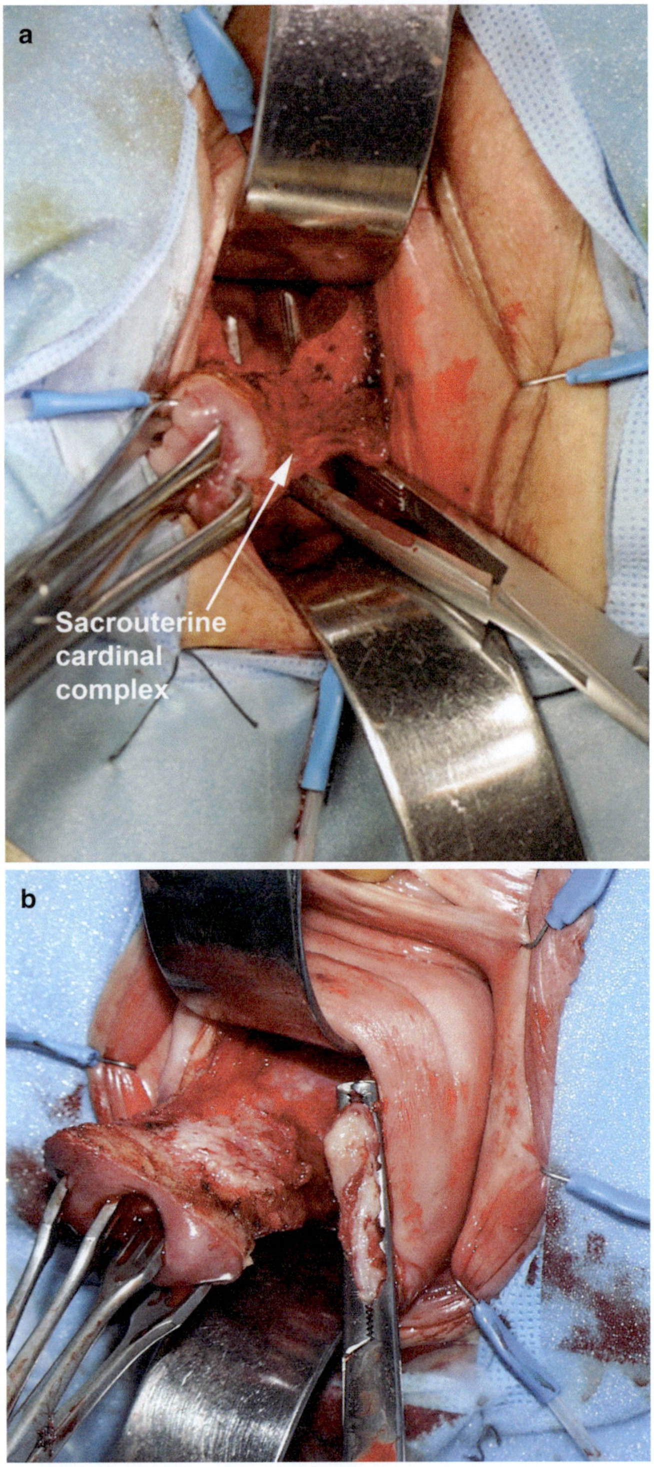

Fig. 1.14 (**a**) During vaginal hysterectomy, a curved clamp is inserted to isolate the sacrouterine–cardinal complex. (**b**) The cardinal–sacrouterine complex has been transected and separated from the uterus. A clamp is holding the ligaments

1.4.4 Support of the Posterior Vaginal Wall and Rectum

A complex fascial and muscular arrangement provides support to the posterior vagina and rectum, as connective tissue covers the anterior rectal wall (prerectal fascia) and the posterior rectal wall (anterior sacral fascia); they are fused laterally to attach to the levator muscle (arcus tendineus fascia pelvis).

When a woman with normal support is in the erect position, the posterior vaginal wall has a curvature (banana shape) with two distinct portions: proximal and distal. The proximal vagina forms a posterior angle of approximately 110° with the vertical line (Fig. 1.15a, b). The point of angulation indicates the point where the vagina crosses the pelvic floor musculature (pubococcygeus–puborectalis) (Fig. 1.15c). The proximal third of the vagina is in a horizontal plane resting over this levator plate. The distal vagina is in a more straight-up position, forming a 45° angle with the vertical line. This angle reflects the degree of support of the levators and the urogenital diaphragm pulling forward the distal vagina. Restoration of this anatomy is important in posterior vaginal wall reconstruction.

In patients with pelvic floor relaxation, the normal anatomy of the posterior vagina is lost. The levator plate descends (becoming convex instead of horizontal) (Fig. 1.16b), the levator hiatus enlarges, and the normal distal vaginal angulation of 110° disappears. The distal half of the vagina is no longer 45° from the vertical. The vagina is now rotated downward and posteriorly and is no longer in a high, supported horizontal position. Herniation of the rectum (rectocele) may ensue. MRI again can help in understanding the anatomical changes observed in patients with pelvic floor relaxation.

In patients with damage to the vaginal outlet (the perineal or urogenital diaphragm), the introitus is wider, and the distance between the urethra and posterior fourchette is increased (*see* Fig. 1.15). Different degrees of perineal tear may be seen, from minimal tears with only a small separation of the perineum to a severe degree in which the perineal structures have disappeared and the posterior vaginal wall reaches the anterior rectal wall.

As is the case with anterior vaginal wall defects, combined defects of posterior vaginal support at both the level of the pelvic floor and the perineum often occur, particularly in cases of severe prolapse. Three defects are generally present: weakness of the prerectal fascia covering the rectovaginal septum, widening of the levator hiatus and perineal membrane, and laxity of the perineal musculature. To provide normal introital size and improved posterior vaginal support, corrective surgery of the posterior vaginal wall should address all the defects: correction of the rectocele by reinforcement of the attenuated prerectal and pararectal fasciae, repair of the defect of the levator muscles by reapproximation of the widened perineal membrane, restoration of the horizontal supporting plate for the proximal vagina, and repair of the fascia and musculature of the perineum, when defective.

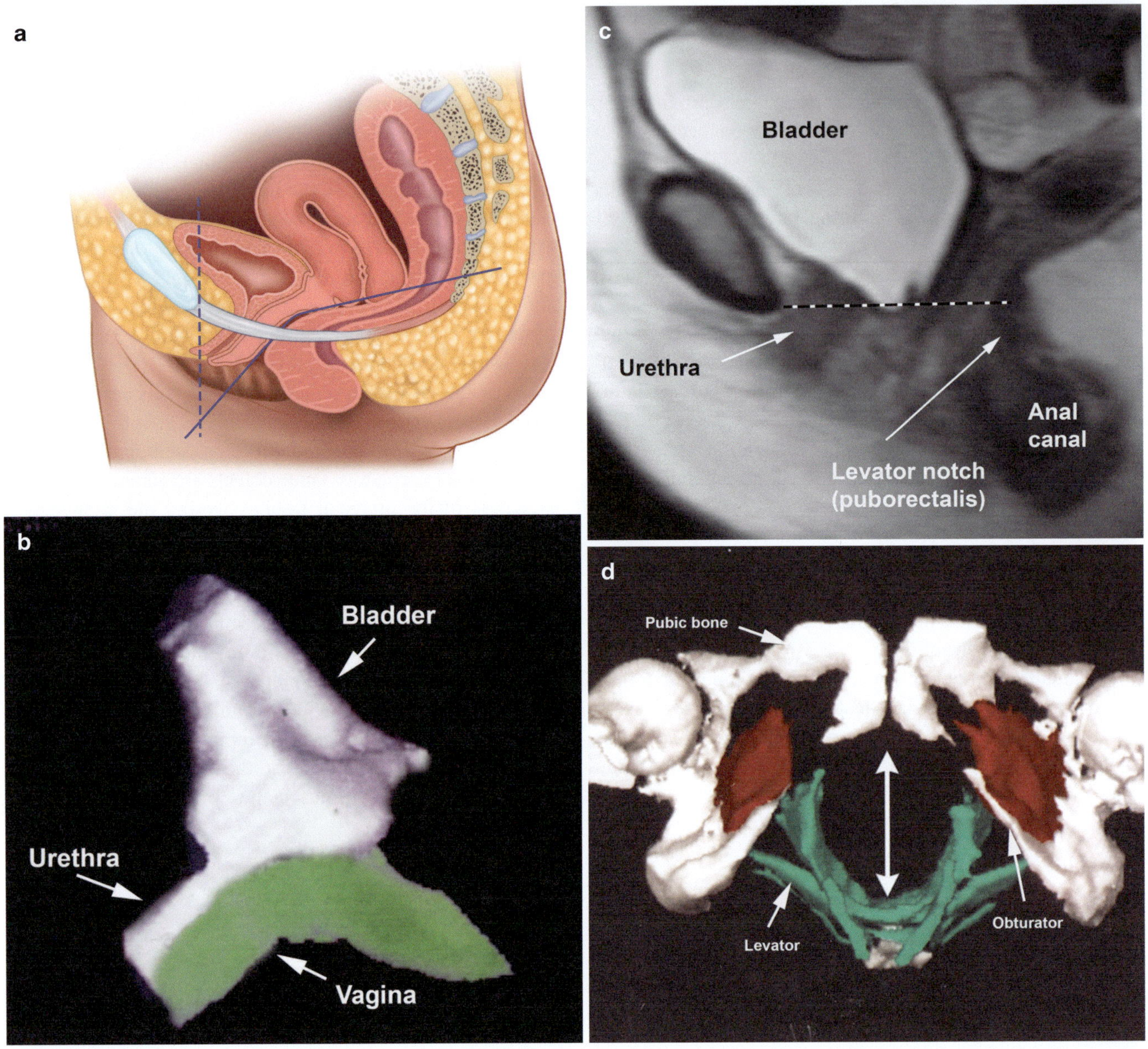

Fig. 1.15 (**a**) Diagram of pelvic organ support. The distal third of the vagina is at a 45° angle to the vertical line, even as the proximal vagina is in an almost horizontal plane (110° with the vertical line). The angulation or levator notch is the point of insertion of the pubococcygeus and puborectalis muscles, which pull the vaginal canal and rectum toward the pubic bone. (**b**) Three-dimensional MRI reconstruction of the vagina showing the elevation of the distal third at the point of insertion of the puborectalis. (**c**) Sagittal MRI of a patient without prolapse showing the urethra, the bladder, the anal canal, and the indentation (levator notch) where the puborectalis (part of the pubococcygeus) is inserted. During voluntary or reflect contraction, the levator pulls the vagina and rectum anteriorly toward the pubic bone. During voluntary relaxation, the distance increases and the levator descends. The distance between the inferior rami of the symphysis and the levator notch defines the size of the levator hiatus, usually 5–6 cm. (**d**) Three-dimensional reconstruction of the levator plate showing a wide levator hiatus in a patient with multiple deliveries and significant pelvic floor relaxation. (**e**) Sagittal MRI of a patient with posterior vaginal prolapse. The vaginal axis and the levator muscle are more vertical, the rectum protrudes from the vaginal canal, and there is disappearance of the levator notch. The distance between the anal canal and the inferior rami of the pubic bone is increased, confirming the widening of the levator hiatus

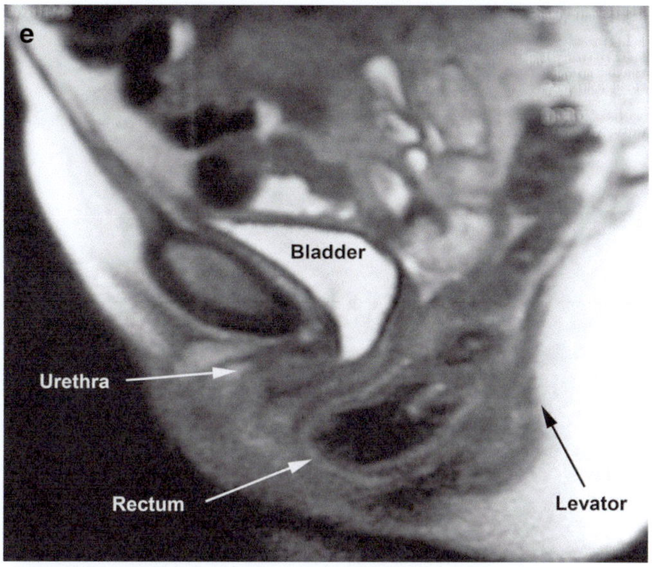

Fig. 1.15 (continued)

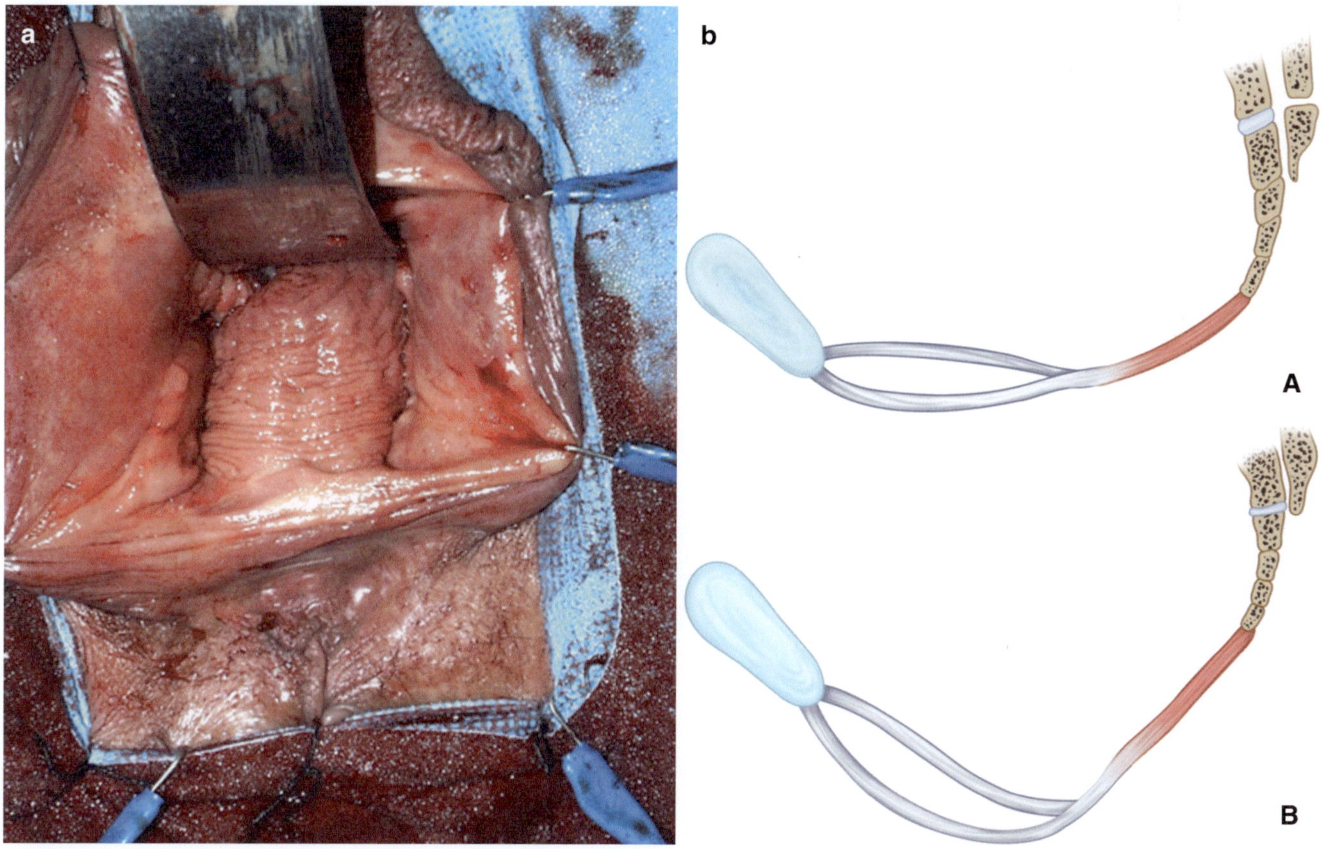

Fig. 1.16 (**a**) Exposure of the posterior vaginal wall in a patient with a large rectocele and widening of the levator hiatus. (**b**) Diagram depicting the anatomy of pelvic floor relaxation. The levator plate descends, losing its horizontal axis, and the levator hiatus widens. (**c**) The perineal membrane joins in the midline at the perineum and extends several centimeters inside the vaginal canal. The levators (pubococcygeus) attach to the perineal membrane. (**d**) Damage to the perineal membrane widens the perineum and the distal vagina. Approximation of the perineal membrane to the midline will narrow the levator hiatus and correct in great part the perineal defect. (**e**) The perineal membrane covers the puborectalis, pubococcygeus, and iliococcygeus muscles. It inserts in the inferior rami of the ischiopubic arch, joining the contralateral side in the central tendon of the perineum, leaving a hiatus for the vaginal canal. The ischiocavernosus muscles cover the crura of the clitoris, and the bulbocavernosus muscles cover the fibro-fatty issue of the labia. The transverse perineum inserts laterally in the ischial tuberosity and medially joins the bulbocavernosus muscle and external anal sphincter to form the central tendon of the perineum

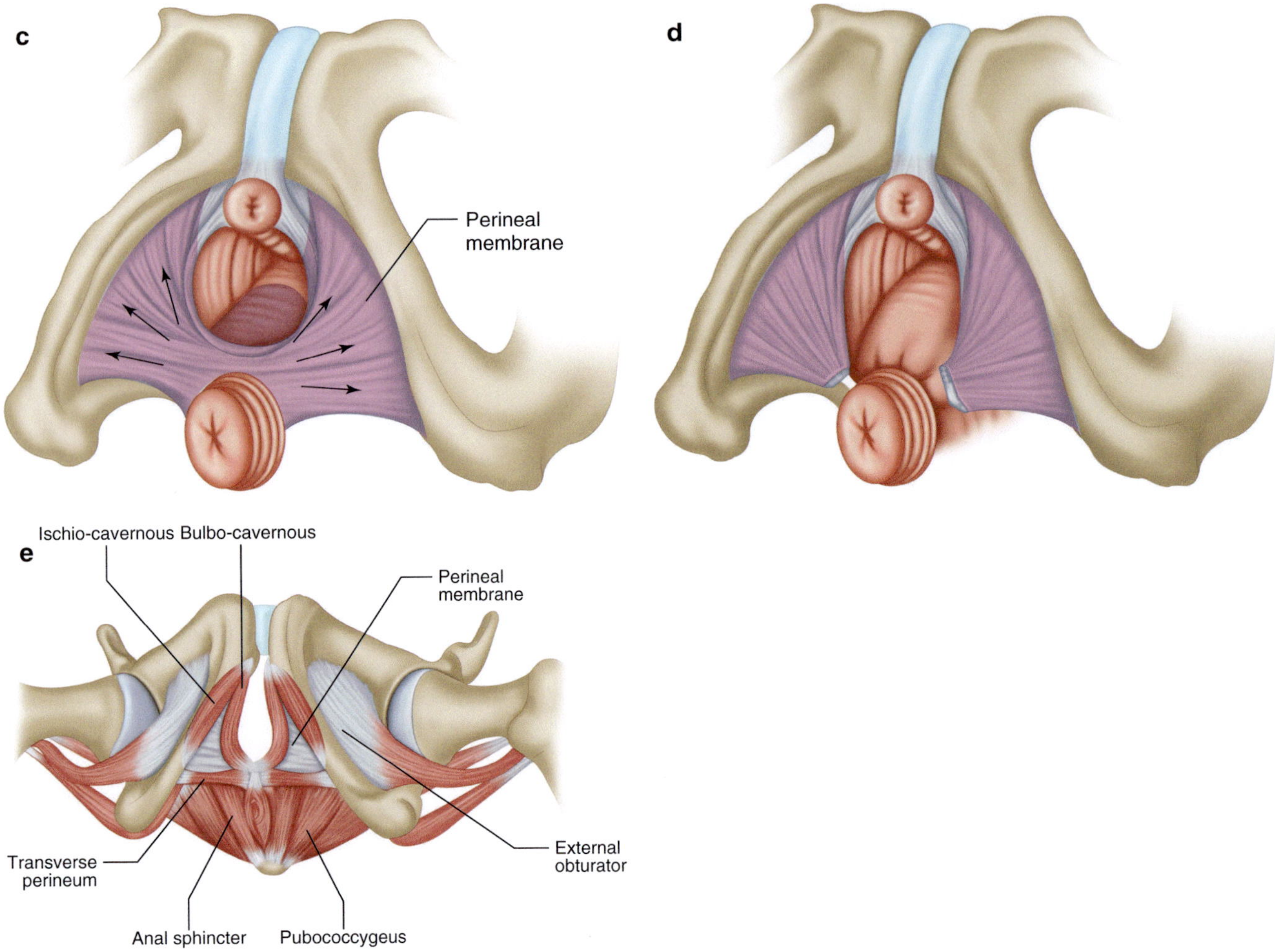

Fig. 1.16 (continued)

1.5 Innervation and Vascular Supply to the Pelvis

Figures 1.17, 1.18, and 1.19 show diagrams of the vascular supply and innervation of the pelvis and perineum, providing greater understanding of the anatomy of the pelvis.

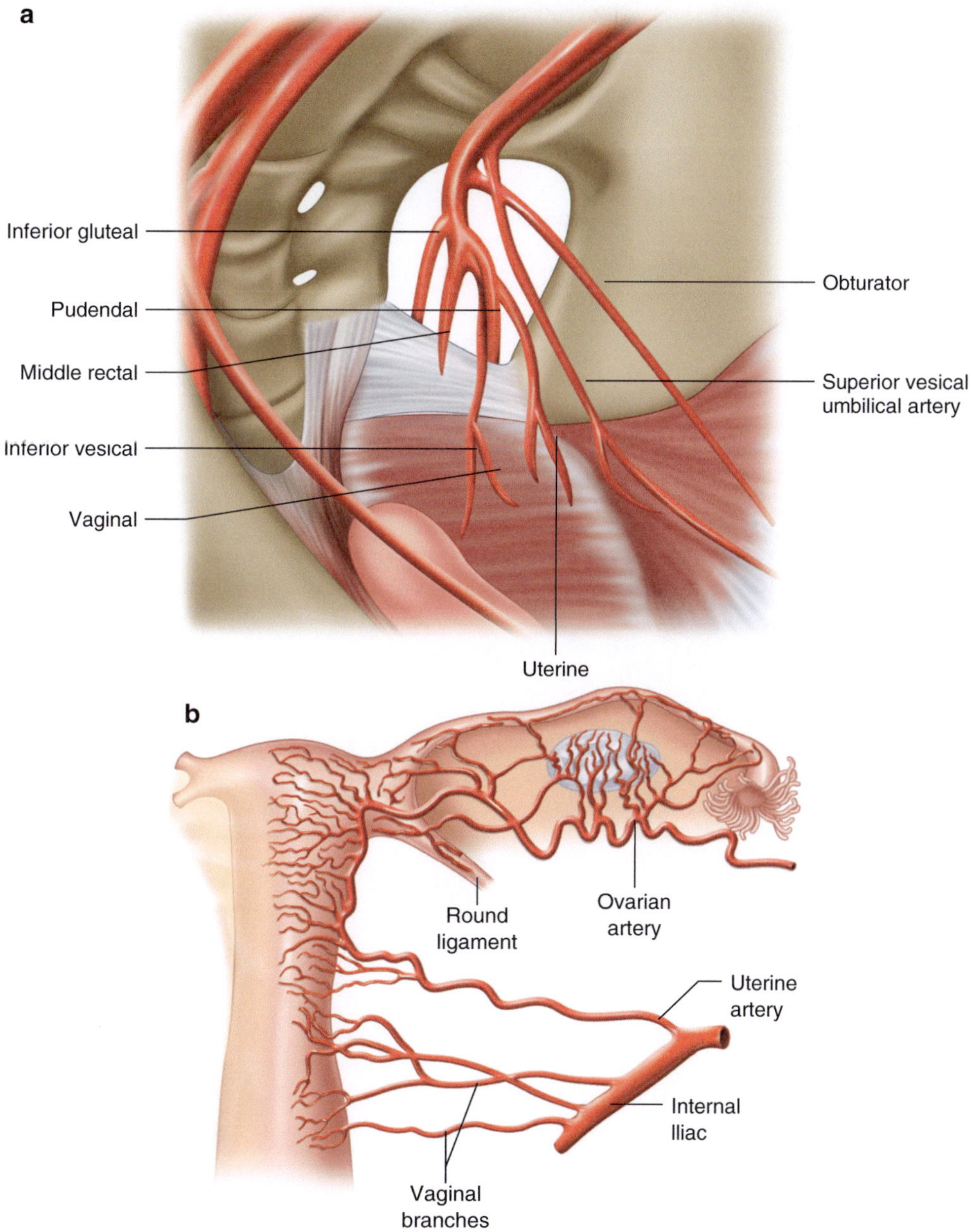

Fig. 1.17 (**a**) The internal iliac artery provides vascular supply to the pelvic organs, particularly from its anterior branch. The pudendal and inferior gluteal arteries run posterior to the sacrospinous ligaments. The other branches are the umbilical, superior vesical, uterine, inferior vesical, vaginal, and middle rectal arteries. (**b**) From the internal iliac artery, the vaginal and uterine arteries provide blood supply to the vagina and uterus through multiple small arterial branches. They anastomose to the ovarian artery, a branch from the anterior aorta

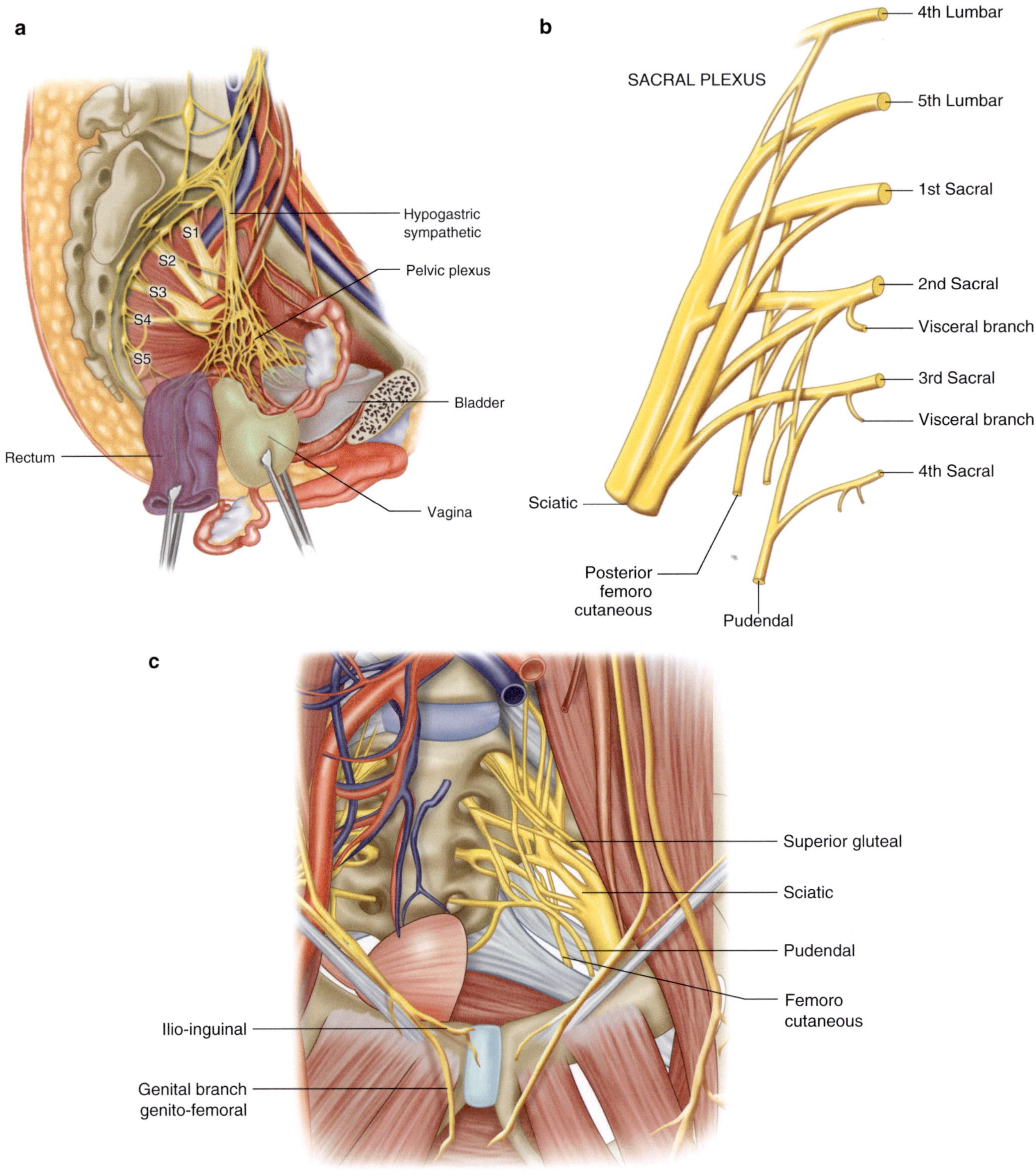

Fig. 1.18 (**a**) The hypogastric sympathetic plexus descends around the aorta and major pelvic vessels, joining the visceral branches of the sacral root (S2, S3, S4) to form the pelvic plexus lateral to the uterus and rectum. The pelvic plexus provides visceral (sympathetic and parasympathetic) innervation to the bladder, vagina, uterus, and rectum. (**b**) The sacral plexus originates from the sacral roots S2, S3, and S4, with anterior branches providing somatic and sensory fibers to the skin and muscular structures of the pelvis. Visceral branches of the sacral roots join the sympathetic hypogastric (T9–L1) forming the pelvic plexus. (**c**) From the sacral plexus, the pudendal nerve provides visceral and somatic innervation to most of the pelvic muscles and viscera (Adapted from Online Atlas: Visible Body). The femoral cutaneous nerve emerges behind the sciatic notch to provide genital branches to the posterior perineum and inferior labia. The ilioinguinal nerve provides innervation to the suprapubic area and superior labia. The genital branch of the genitofemoral nerve provides innervation to the labial area. The pudendal nerve provides somatic (motor and sensory) innervation to the pelvic musculature and skin structures of the perineum

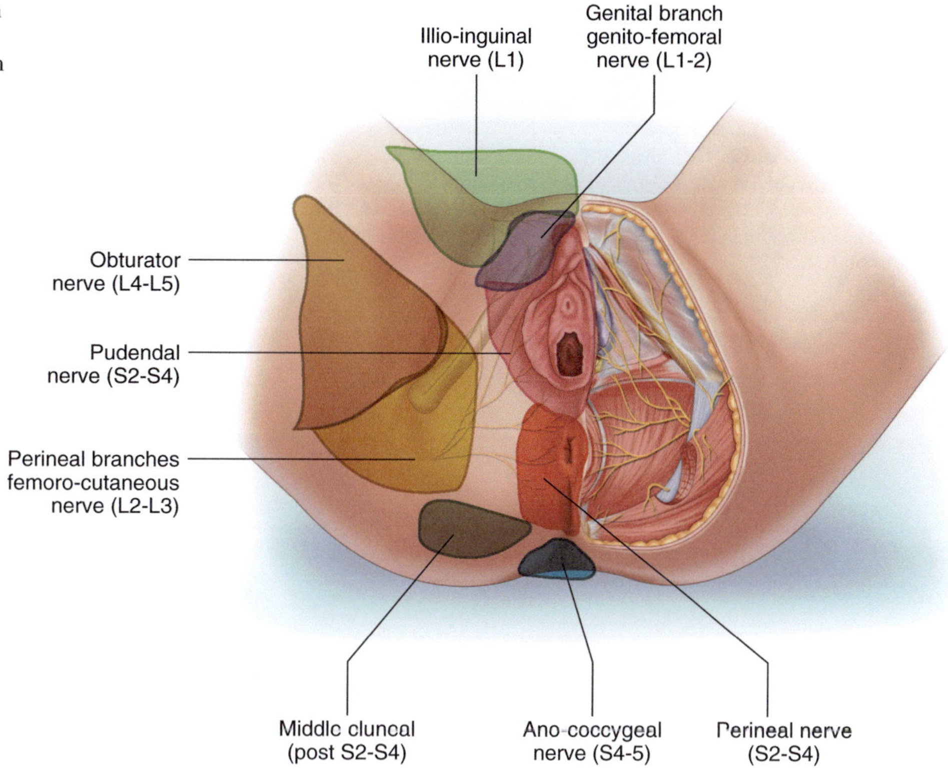

Fig. 1.19 Diagram of the perineum showing the approximate areas of sensory innervation originating from the different pelvic nerves

Suggested Reading

Ashton-Miller JA, DeLancey JO. Functional anatomy of the female pelvic floor. Ann N Y Acad Sci. 2007;1101:266–96.

Hsu Y, DeLancey JO. Functional anatomy and pathophysiology of pelvic organ prolapse. In: Raz S, Rodriguez L, editors. Female urology. 3rd ed. Philadelphia: Saunders-Elsevier Publishers; 2008. p. 542–5.

Maternal anatomy. In: Cunningham F, Leveno KJ, Bloom SL, Spong CY, Dashe JS, Hoffman BL, Casey BM, Sheffield JS, editors. Williams obstetrics. 24th ed. New York: McGraw-Hill; 2013.

Netter F. Reproductive system, Ciba collection of medical illustrations, vol. 2. Summit: Ciba-Geigy Corp., Medical Education Division; 1965.

Ramanah R, Berger MB, Parratte BM, DeLancey JO. Anatomy and histology of apical support: a literature review concerning cardinal and uterosacral ligaments. Int Urogynecol J. 2012;23(11):1483–94.

Visible body. 3D human anatomy. Argosy Publishing; 2014. http://visiblebody.com

2 Surgery for Stress Incontinence

2.1 Mechanisms of Normal Continence

Stress urinary incontinence—the involuntary loss of urine through the intact urethra as a result of a sudden increase in intra-abdominal pressure—creates a social problem to the patient. It is the end result of a deficient urinary control system in which the intra-abdominal pressure exceeds the resistance produced by the urethral closure mechanisms. Normal continence in the female results from the delicate balance of several forces, including closing forces of the urethra, a critical functional and anatomical urethral length, the ability of the pelvic floor and the urethra to increase urethral resistance at the time of stress, and the proper anatomical location of the sphincteric unit. We like to organize these factors in what we call the UCLA theory of female continence, in which the U signifies the urethral changes that occur during stress, the C represents the closing function of the urethra, the L is its functional and anatomical length, and A stands for anatomy. These factors are briefly described below.

2.1.1 Closure Forces of the Urethra: The Sphincteric Unit

The urethra is a short elastic tube (3–4 cm long) with a complex anatomical and functional structure. While the woman is resting, walking, or straining, it normally provides a leakproof closure, but during voiding it funnels and opens to permit complete bladder emptying (Fig. 2.1a, b).

The histological structure of the urethra can be seen as a thin, fibromuscular envelope filled with spongy tissue and infolded epithelium surrounded by smooth and skeletal muscle (Fig. 2.1c–e). We can describe three distinct structures: the mucosal sphincter (epithelium and spongy tissue), the smooth muscle and fibroelastic envelope, and the outer skeletal muscular sphincter.

The urethral mucosa is seen as a multilayer, infolded epithelium that meshes like interlocking fingers, to provide an efficient urethral seal. Under the mucosa is a rich, vascular cushion of spongy tissue. This combination, which we call the mucosal urethral sphincter, has a great degree of plasticity and easily deforms under minimal external pressures, providing an efficient seal. The urethra can conform around any inserted object (such as ureteric catheters) while still remaining leakproof. The epithelium and the spongy tissue are under hormonal control, and estrogen deprivation will lead to atrophy of the mucosa, flattening of the epithelium, atrophy of the spongy tissue, and a deficient urethral seal. Trauma of surgery, radiation, neurological conditions, atherosclerosis, and age-related changes may lead to further atrophy of the mucosal sphincter. As in a faucet, a good washer will provide a reliable seal with minimal pressure, but a faucet with a deficient washer will leak. Increasing outside pressure by tightening the faucet will not prevent leakage if the washer is defective. There is no correlation between urethral pressures and continence. Continence depends on the presence of adequate urethral resistance against increases in bladder pressure, and it is clear that the mucosal sphincter plays a very important role in achieving a complete urethral seal.

Around the urethral mucosa is a thin, fibromuscular envelope composed of elastic tissue, smooth muscle, and intrinsic slow-twitch skeletal musculature. This layer compresses the mucosal sphincter, enhancing the urethral resistance. Paralysis, trauma, surgery, radiation, or estrogen deficiency may alter the function of this envelope, inducing a decrease in urethral continence. Autonomic fibers from the sacral spine (S2–S4) and thoracic spine (T9–L1) control the smooth musculature.

Electronic supplementary material The online version of this chapter (doi:10.1007/978-1-4939-2941-2_2) contains supplementary material, which is available to authorized users.

S. Raz, *Atlas of Vaginal Reconstructive Surgery*, DOI 10.1007/978-1-4939-2941-2_2

The third component of the sphincteric unit with important function in continence is the intramural and extramural skeletal musculature. The extrinsic skeletal musculature is mainly composed of fast-twitch fibers responding to voluntary and involuntary reflexes. Involuntary contraction of the pelvic floor during exercise or a sudden change in abdominal pressures is a protective reflex to prevent incontinence. Another involuntary reflex provides basic tone to the skeletal musculature. The skeletal musculature plays an important role in female continence by its effect on the basic sphincter tone and the reflex and voluntary activity of the sphincter during stress.

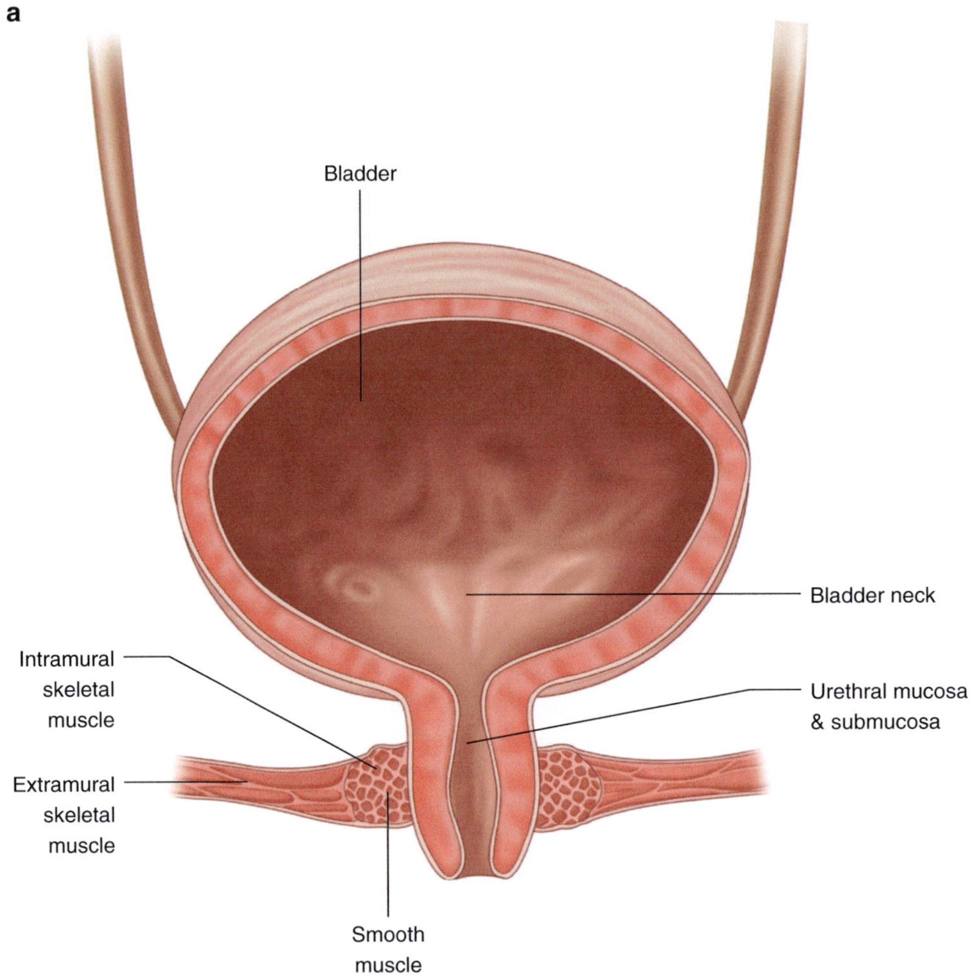

Fig. 2.1 (**a**) Diagram of the lower urinary tract showing the bladder, the bladder neck, and the urethra. The urethra is composed by the inner layer of the mucosa and submucosa, the smooth muscle, and the skeletal musculature (intramural and extramural). (**b**) Diagram of the sphincteric unit. The bladder neck is the primary mechanism of continence. Longitudinal and circular fibers of the trigone and detrusor muscle provide urethral closure during rest and the ability to open and funnel during micturition. The mucosal and submucosal layers extend along the urethral lumen containing a rich vascular plexus very important for urethral coaptation and continence. (**c**) Histology of the urethral wall showing the infolded urethral mucosa with a rich submucosal vascular plexus. Surrounding the inner layer is the smooth muscle and the intrinsic skeletal fibers. (**d**) Axial T2 MRI view of the midurethral area showing the dark fibromuscular envelope enclosing the inner mucosa and submucosal vascular plexus of the urethra. (**e**) Using a vaginal coil a longitudinal image of the urethral wall and mucosal and submucosal layers are seen with clarity. The urethra is not a muscular tube; rather it is an internal mucosal layer with a rich vascular plexus compressed by the outer muscular layer

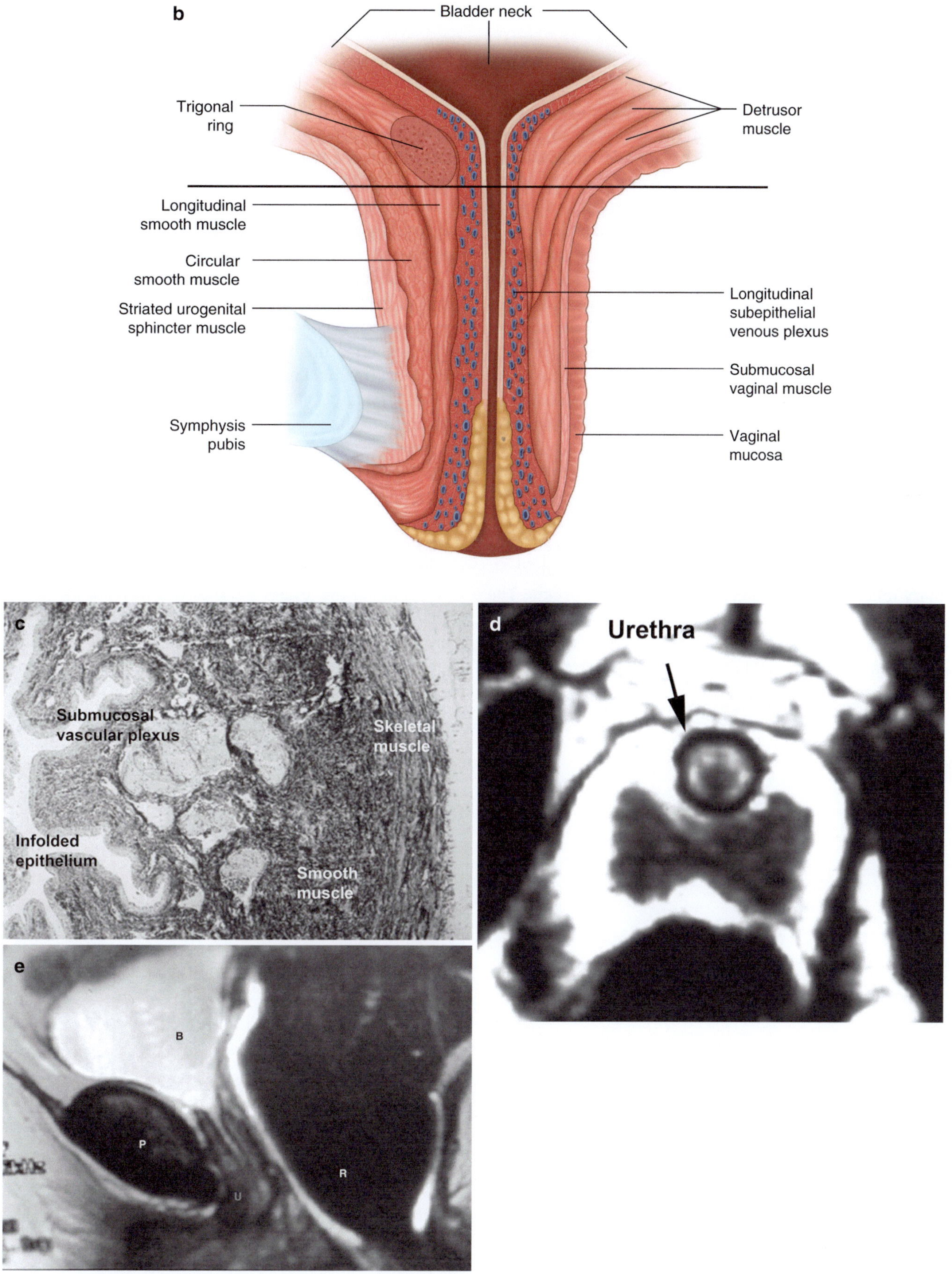

Fig. 2.1 (continued)

2.1.2 Urethral Length

The distance between the bladder neck and the external urethral meatus represents the anatomical length. The urethra can be divided into three segments: proximal, midurethral, and distal. The proximal urethra, the first level of female continence, comprises the bladder neck and intra-abdominal urethra; it is only 1½–2 cm long. A woman will remain continent if the midurethral and distal urethral functions remain intact, even if the proximal urethra and bladder neck are excised (as during total cystectomy), incised (as after a transurethral incision of the bladder neck), or reconfigured (as after Y–V plasty). With fluoroscopy during video urodynamic studies in the standing position, we can observe that the level of continence is at the bladder neck in most women who have normal continence, but in 20–30 % of these women, the bladder neck may be incompetent, confirming that the midurethral segment is the most important secondary area of continence. The midurethral segment is responsible for continence when the bladder neck is incompetent. The pubourethral ligament supports the urethra to the inferior rami of the symphysis. The midurethral area is where the reflex or voluntary contraction to sudden changes of intra-abdominal pressures and the voluntary and involuntary relaxation of the urethra during voiding occurs. The distal centimeter of the urethra does not have sphincteric function and acts as a mere conduit to direct the urinary stream outside the vaginal canal. It can be excised without affecting continence.

2.1.3 Anatomical Support

The anatomical support of the urethra was described in Chap. 1. Following are further details on the impact of the anatomical support for urethral continence.

The urethra is supported by three structures: the close attachment to the vaginal wall and the pubourethral and urethropelvic fasciae or ligaments (Fig. 2.2a).

The urethra moves together with the anterior vaginal wall and is tightly attached to the vaginal wall. Changes in vaginal support will affect urethral support and function (Fig. 2.2b).

The pubourethral fascia attaches the urethra to the inferior ramus of the pubic bone; it is the only connection of the urethra to the pubic bone (Fig. 2.3a, b). During strain, the normally supported urethra rotates a small amount under the pubic bone (minimal mobility), but in patients with deficient pubourethral fascia, the distance of the urethra from the inferior ramus of the symphysis is increased during strain, and the urethra is allowed to rotate considerably under the pubic bone (Fig. 2.3c–e).

The urethropelvic fascia comprises the endopelvic and periurethral fascia attaching the urethra to the lateral pelvic wall, the levator muscle, and the arcus tendineus fascia pelvis. It is the only connection of the urethra to the levator. Contraction of the levator muscles will increase the tension of the urethropelvic fascia, stabilizing the urethra and increasing urethral resistance. Weakened urethropelvic fascia leads to urethral hypermobility and deficient compensatory response of the urethra during stress (Fig. 2.4a–e).

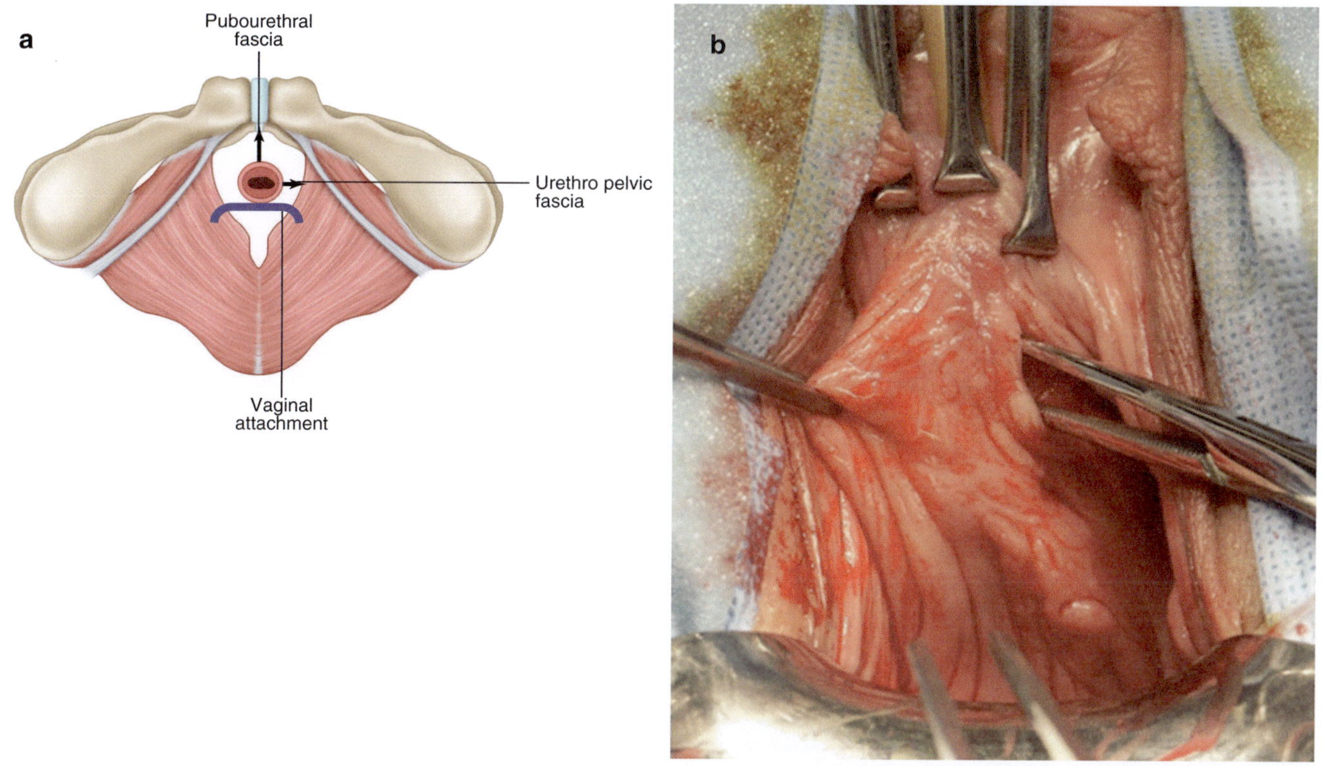

Fig. 2.2 (**a**) Diagram of the structures involved in urethral support. The superior support is provided by the pubourethral fascia, the lateral support by the urethropelvic fascia, and the inferior support by the intimate attachment to the urethra to the vaginal wall. (**b**) Dissection of the anterior vaginal wall shows the lack of a defined cleavage plane between the vaginal and urethral wall. The urethra moves together with the anterior vaginal wall

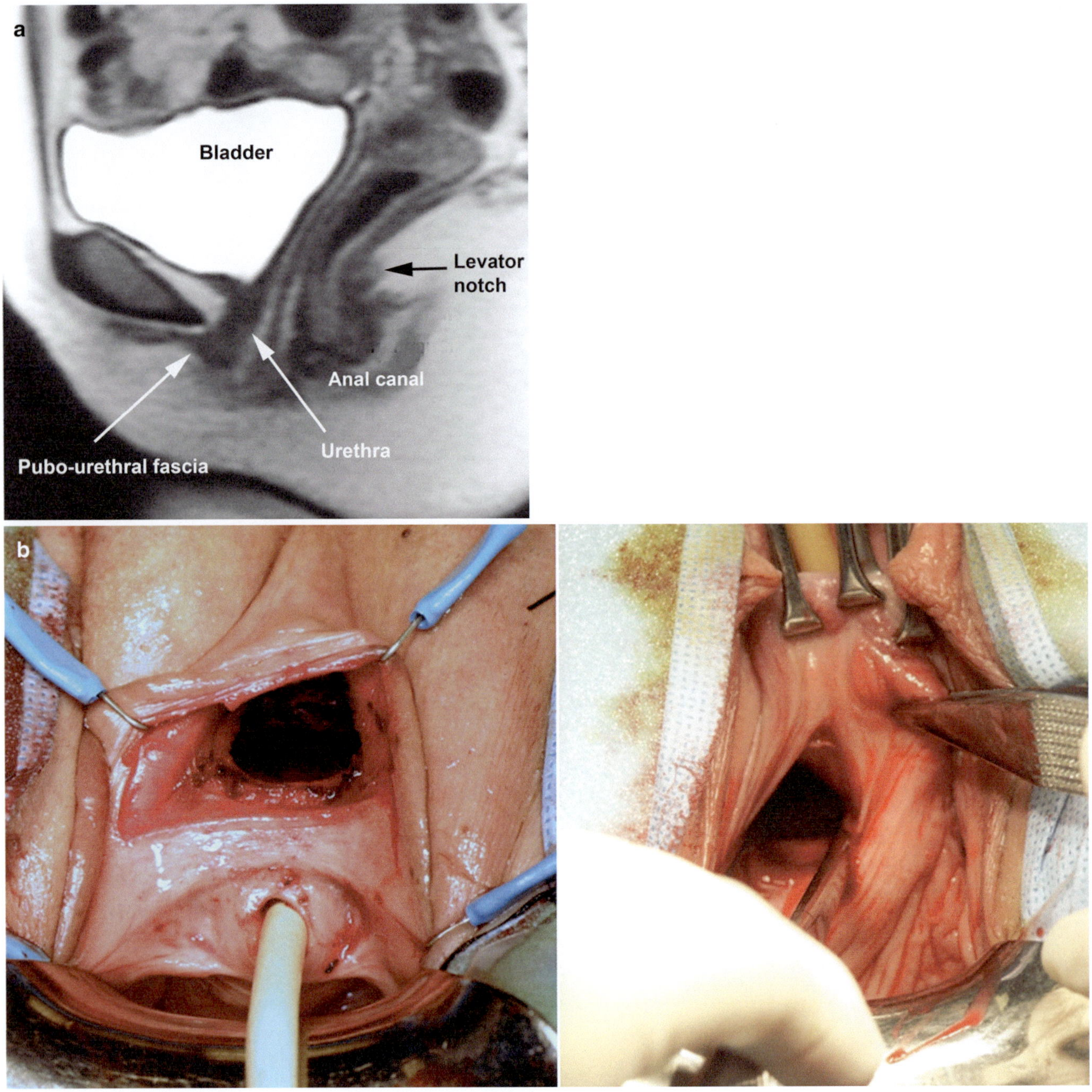

Fig. 2.3 (**a**) A suprameatal incision was made and the distal anterior aspect of the urethra is seen. Pubourethral fascia is detached from the inferior rami of the pubic bone. The urethropelvic fascia supports the urethra to the inferior rami of the pubic bone. (**b**) A lateral distal vaginal incision was made and the retropubic space is entered. The forceps separates the urethropelvic fascia from the arcus tendineus fascia pelvis. At the superior aspect of the incision we can see the pubourethral fascia. Inserting a finger into the retropubic space and pointing it toward allow us to palpate the pubourethral fascia under the pubic symphysis. (**c**) Lateral T2 MRI image of the pelvis with strain showing the downward rotation of the urethra under the inferior rami of the pubic bone. The pubourethral fascia is the only connection of the urethra to the inferior aspect of the pubic bone. (**d**) Lateral T2 image of the pelvis under strain in a patient with stress incontinence. The urethra further rotates under the pubic bone and funneling of the bladder neck is seen

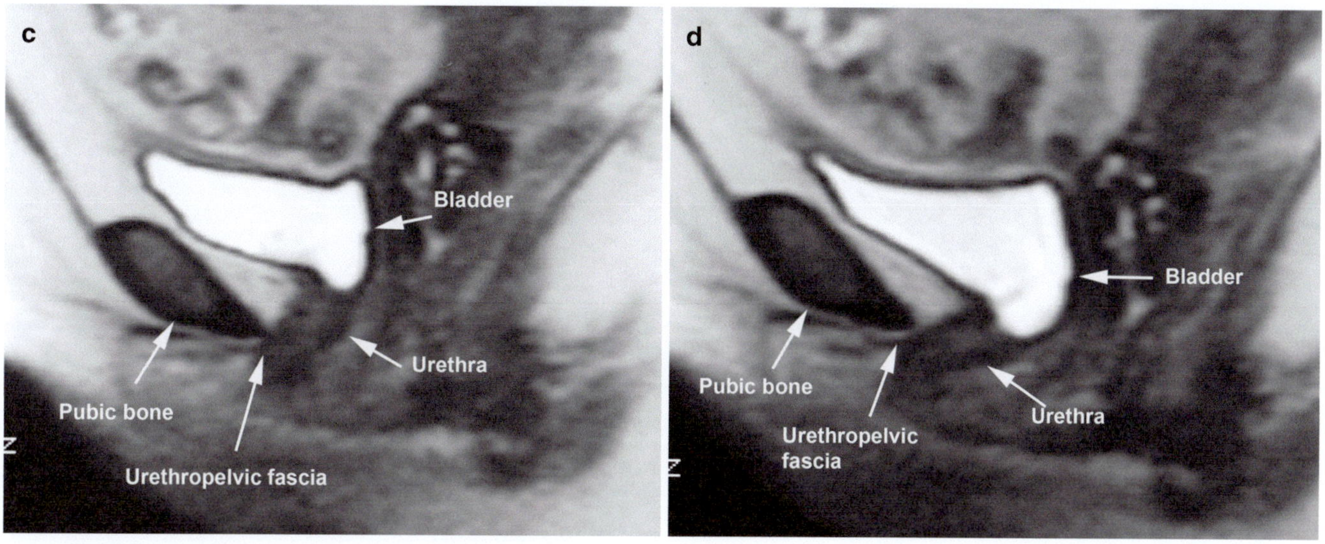

Fig. 2.3 (continued)

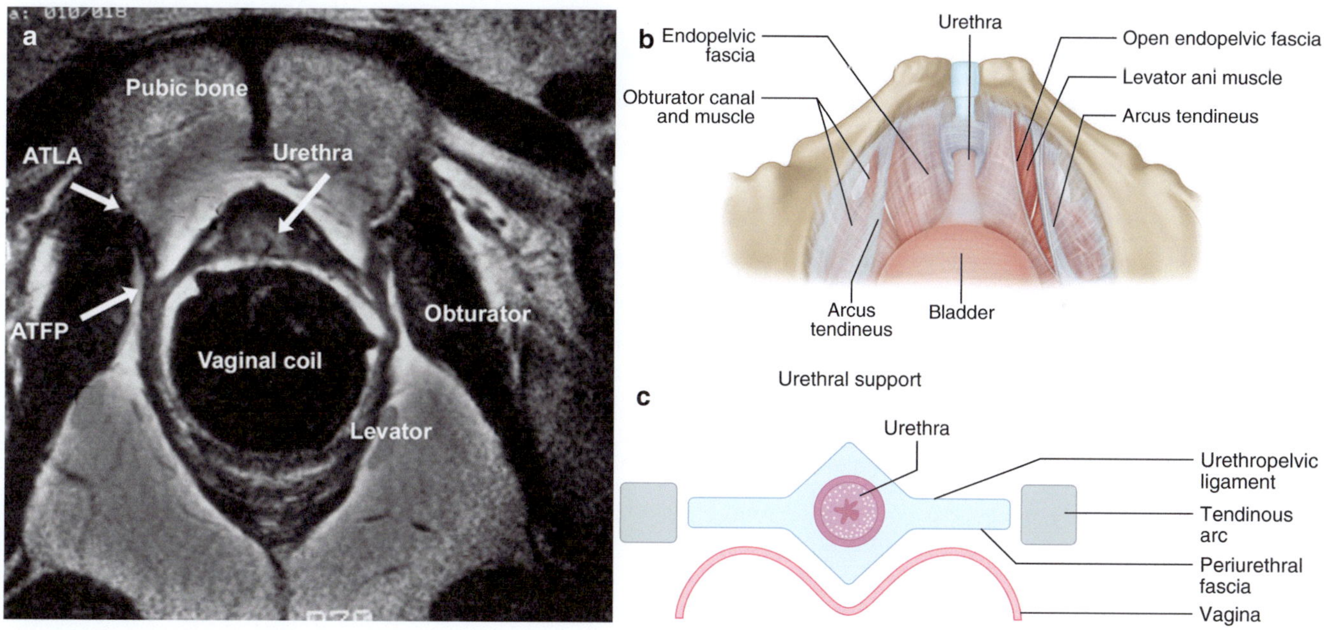

Fig. 2.4 (**a**) T2 MRI image of the urethra. Using a vaginal coil, the vaginal distension allows us to see the urethra supported like two wings laterally to the levator muscle. The urethropelvic fascia is composed by the periurethral fascia in the vaginal side and the endopelvic fascia in the abdominal side. The levator inserts on a condensation of the obturator muscle. ATFP, arcus tendineus fascia pelvis; ATLA, arcus tendineus levator ani. (**b**) Diagram of the abdominal view of the bladder support and urethra. The endopelvic fascia (the abdominal segment of the urethropelvic fascia) inserts laterally into the levator muscle (arcus tendineus fascia pelvis) inferior to the arcus tendineus levator ani. (**c**) Diagram of the lateral urethral support. The urethropelvic fascia is composed by the endopelvic and periurethral fascia. Both cover the sphincteric unit extending laterally to insert into the levator musculature (arcus tendineus fascia pelvis). The urethropelvic fascia is the only structure connecting the urethra to the lateral pelvic wall. (**d**) Diagram of the deficient urethropelvic fascia. The fascia can be attenuated or detached from the lateral levator musculature producing proximal urethral mobility and descent of the sphincteric unit. Poor levator function or relaxation will produce a similar effect. (**e**) During surgery a lateral incision of the anterior vaginal wall was performed, and the retropubic space was entered with scissors exposing the lateral margin of the urethropelvic fascia that was detached from the arcus tendineus fascia pelvis

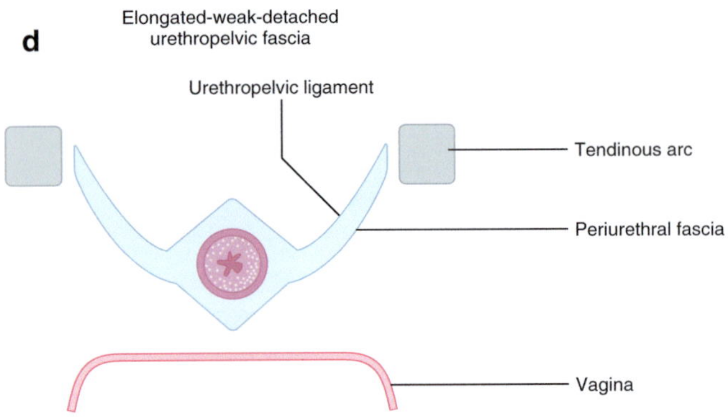

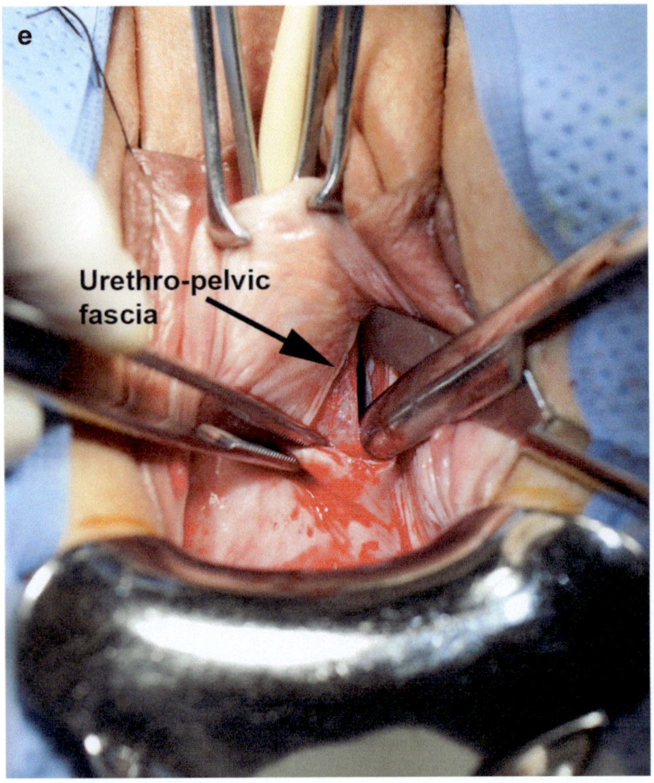

Fig. 2.4 (continued)

2.1.4 Urethral Changes During Stress: Compensatory Mechanisms

Sudden changes in intra-abdominal pressure have a marked effect on urethral function. Three changes seem to be of primary importance: (1) the backboard effect of urethral support, (2) the valvular effect at the bladder neck, and (3) the voluntary and reflex contraction of the pelvic floor.

The proximal urethra is an intra-abdominal structure, so any sudden increase of pressures will lead to a concomitant increase in urethral resistance and closure in the proximal urethra. A poorly supported urethra in a low, dependent position will mechanically tend to funnel and open during sudden increases of abdominal pressure (Fig. 2.5a). A properly supported urethra will respond to sudden changes in abdominal pressures with an increased urethral resistance as it is compressed against a strong posterior support (backboard effect); surgeries like a sling prevent the downward rotation of the urethra and create and hammock against which the urethra can be compressed during a sudden increase in abdominal pressure. A midurethral sling should support the urethra, increasing urethral resistance without direct increase in urethral pressures.

The normally supported urethra is superior to the bladder base and trigone creating an angulation of 90° with the bladder neck. This anatomical relation produces a valvular effect at the bladder neck. Sudden increases of abdominal pressure will increase this valvular effect in a well-supported urethra, protecting against incontinence. After a successful Burch colposuspension for stress incontinence, we very often can reproduce stress incontinence by elevating the bladder base in patients who were perfectly cured by the operation. This valvular effect also plays a significant role in the appearance of outlet obstruction in patients who undergo anti-incontinence procedures and had a cystocele before surgery or later develop a secondary cystocele.

The skeletal musculature has fast-twitch fibers providing a rapid pelvic floor response to acute events and slow-twitch fibers responsible for the basic skeletal muscle tone. In the resting state, the basic tone of the skeletal musculature increases with bladder filling. During sudden changes of intra-abdominal pressures, a reflex response of the fast-twitch fibers increases urethral closure and resistance. In patients with pelvic floor relaxation due to trauma of delivery, neuropathy of the pudendal nerve, hormonal changes, age, or multiple surgeries, this compensatory mechanism fails. The urethral resistance will not increase with changes in abdominal pressure, so a tendency for stress incontinence will ensue.

The skeletal musculature has a direct and indirect impact on urethral function. The only attachment of the urethra to the levator muscle is the urethropelvic ligaments. Voluntary or involuntary (cough reflex) contraction of the levators tenses the urethropelvic ligaments, providing support and increasing resistance. Elongated or detached urethropelvic ligaments or poor levator function will result in poor urethral compensation during sudden changes in abdominal pressures (Fig. 2.5). The extramural fibers of the urethra are poorly defined and may play a compensatory role in continence and urethral compensation. The intramural skeletal musculature surrounds the urethra. With aging, there is progressive denervation, atrophy, and loss of neuronal mass, further impacting urethral closure.

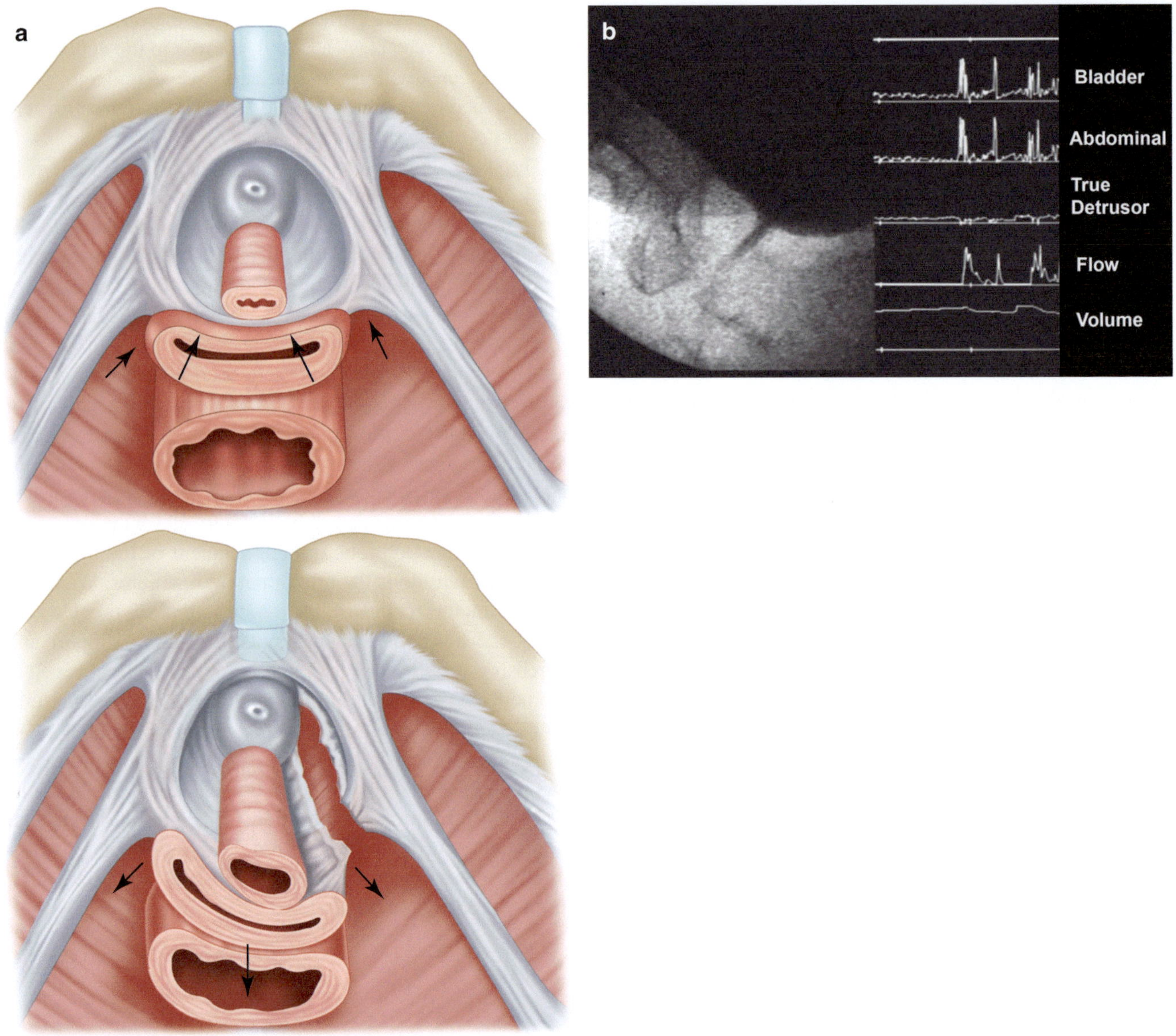

Fig. 2.5 (**a**) Diagram of the lateral support of the sphincteric unit. During sudden increase of abdominal pressure, there is a compensatory contraction of the levators (stress reflex). Levator contraction will increase the tensile forces of the urethropelvic fascia producing an increase of urethral resistance and protecting the urethra against leakage. Voluntary contraction of the levator as in pelvic floor exercises will have a similar effect. (**b**) When the urethropelvic fascia is detached or attenuated or the levator function is deficient, increase of abdominal pressures will not produce the reflex increase in urethral resistance that occurs in normal supported patients. Pelvic exercise in patients with significant deficient levator musculature will not produce any effect on urethral resistance or improve continence (**c**). Videourodynamic images of a patient with stress incontinence showing loss of urine per urethra (flow) in a patient with sudden changes of abdominal and vesical pressures without a change in the true detrusor pressures. Loss of urine during stress may or may not be associated with urethral mobility. Stress incontinence occurs due to a deficient sphincteric urine with a loss of the normal compensatory mechanism during stress

2.2 Clinical Correlates

Normally, anatomical support of the bladder neck and proximal urethra allows for thorough transmission of intra-abdominal pressure increases to this area of continence. Together with an intact sphincteric unit, with its coapting mucosal surface, and the reflex pelvic contraction at the time of cough or strain, a leakproof sphincter is achieved. Failure of one of the components of this delicate balance will not invariably produce stress incontinence because of the compensatory effect of the other factors. This effect also may explain the phenomenon whereby many patients with urethral hypermobility can be totally asymptomatic; only a small percentage of these patients have stress incontinence (Fig. 2.6). Although obstetric trauma and the resulting anatomical displacements tend to occur when the woman is in her 20s or 30s, symptomatic stress incontinence is found mainly around menopause, suggesting that hormonal changes (atrophy of urethral tissue) superimposed on the anatomical defect facilitate the loss of urine during stress. Stress incontinence seems therefore to occur as a result of a failure of compensatory mechanisms when one factor such as anatomy is abnormal. There is no doubt that the underlying anatomy is of great importance, as stress urinary incontinence is corrected by a surgery that usually also corrects the anatomy. But it is important to remember that anatomical defects alone are not causing stress incontinence; they are only one of the factors in a complex mechanism of pelvic floor relaxation. The actual anatomic basis of these pathophysiologic concepts is an area of both confusion and controversy, yet it is only through a clear conceptual understanding of the anatomy involved that rational treatment can be given.

We can now make a clinical correlate between the different anatomical defects of the anterior vaginal wall. We must highlight the importance of the insertion of the urethropelvic ligament to the lateral pelvic wall (arcus tendineus fascia pelvis). It is the only connection of the urethra to the levator muscle. The urethra is seen supported to the lateral pelvic wall and enclosed like a sandwich (between endopelvic and periurethral fasciae) by this fascial extension with both strength and elasticity, so as to rise and fall with changes in intra-abdominal pressure and with contraction or relaxation of the levator musculature.

As mentioned above, the pubourethral ligaments divide the urethra into three areas of continence: the intrapelvic, intra-abdominal proximal third (1.5 cm in length); a mid third, which includes the pubourethral ligaments; and a distal third, which serves only as a conduit for urine, without continence activity. Passive continence (resting involuntary control of continence) depends on the integrity, coaptation, and support of the proximal third of the urethra, but this area can be incised or excised, and the patient can remain continent because the mid third will take over as a secondary mechanism for passive continence. In some patients with significant stress urinary incontinence, the bladder neck is open and incompetent; in these cases, the midurethra is responsible for passive continence.

In a woman with normal continence, a complex compensatory mechanism is standing by to improve the seal effect of the urethra during any stress such as coughing, straining, or walking. The midurethral complex is not only a secondary mechanism for passive continence but is the area most responsible for active continence (voluntary control of urine by contraction of pelvic musculature). The area just distal to the pubourethral ligaments is outside the realm of the intra-abdominal forces, and it is the area of "high pressures" when urethral pressure studies are performed. There seems to be no relationship between urethral pressure and continence or incontinence. Urethral pressures are not changed after incontinence is cured or improved by a sling procedure or injection of a bulking agent. Voluntary contraction of the skeletal pelvic musculature is able to stop the urinary stream during voiding and increase urethral resistance during increases in abdominal pressure. During cough, strain, or any other sudden increase of abdominal pressures, there is a reflex involuntary contraction of the pelvic floor that increases urethra resistance and protects against any loss of urine. With age, multiple deliveries, and pelvic floor relaxation, the levator function becomes deficient, diminishing the reflex and voluntary activity of the pelvic floor as a protective mechanism against incontinence.

Other factors also participate to protect the urethra against involuntary loss of urine. A mild posterior bladder rotation against a well-supported urethra will increase the valvular effect of the bladder neck. In fact, many patients cured by a bladder suspension or sling procedure can have incontinence demonstrated by elevation of the bladder base at the time of strain. Voluntary or reflex contraction of the levator and obturator muscles will increase tension on the urethropelvic ligaments, thereby elevating and compressing the proximal urethra. Direct transmission of intra-abdominal forces to a well-supported proximal urethra will increase its closing mechanism. This backboard effect explains the curative effects of the sling procedures in which a hammock is created against which the urethra can be compressed during changes in abdominal pressure.

Pelvic floor relaxation and weakening of the urethropelvic and pubourethral ligaments will produce posterior and downward rotation of the proximal urethra and bladder neck. The compensatory mechanisms and the improved seal of the proximal urethra against sudden changes in abdominal pressures are impaired. Urethral hypermobility will transfer the bladder neck area to a dependent position in the pelvis, where sudden increases in intra-abdominal pressures will facilitate its funneling and opening, as the valvular effect is lost. A weak levator will not efficiently increase resistance during stress. The intra-abdominal forces are not transmitted efficiently to the proximal urethra. Nevertheless, a hypermobile urethra alone will not lead to incontinence unless the intrinsic sphincter function is impaired (urethral seal) (Fig. 2.7).

Surgical transfer of the proximal urethra to a more supported position will restore some of the urethral compensatory mechanisms against sudden changes in abdominal pressures (Fig. 2.8). Sling procedures provide dynamic support of the urethra without increasing urethra pressures (Fig. 2.9).

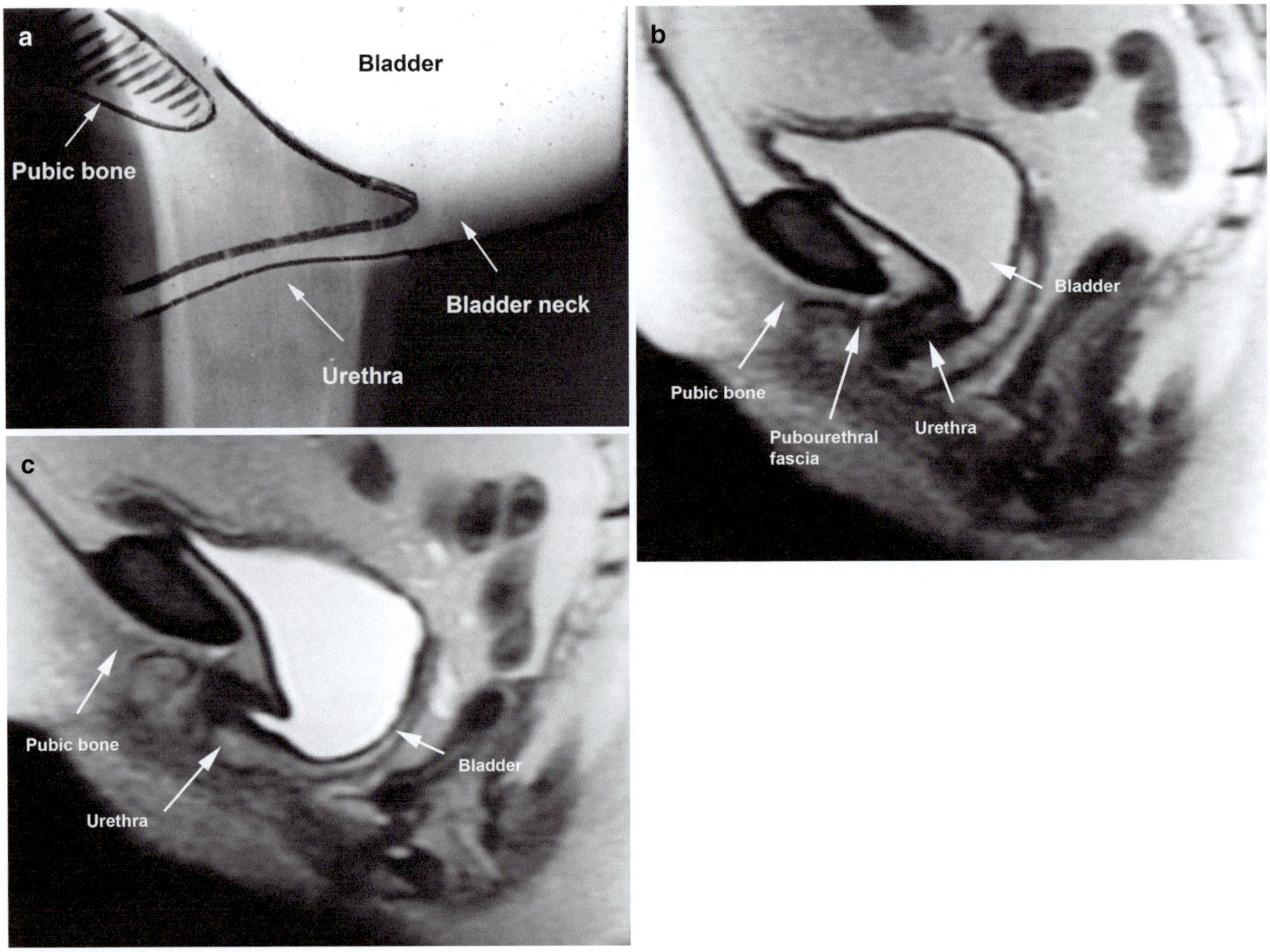

Fig. 2.6 (**a**) Lateral cystogram in a patient with significant urethral mobility. During straining, the urethra is moved away from its normal close proximity to the inferior ramus of the symphysis into a low position, owing to weakness of the pubourethral and urethropelvic fascia. Most patients with this anatomical defect do not lose urine unless there is an intrinsic sphincter defect. (**b**) Lateral T2 MRI of the pelvis in a patient with stress incontinence. In the relax films, the urethra is seen in a low position, still in close proximity to the inferior rami of the pubic bone (pubourethral fascia). (**c**) During strain there is downward rotation of the urethra under the inferior rami of the pubic bone, descent and funneling of the bladder neck, and an open urethra

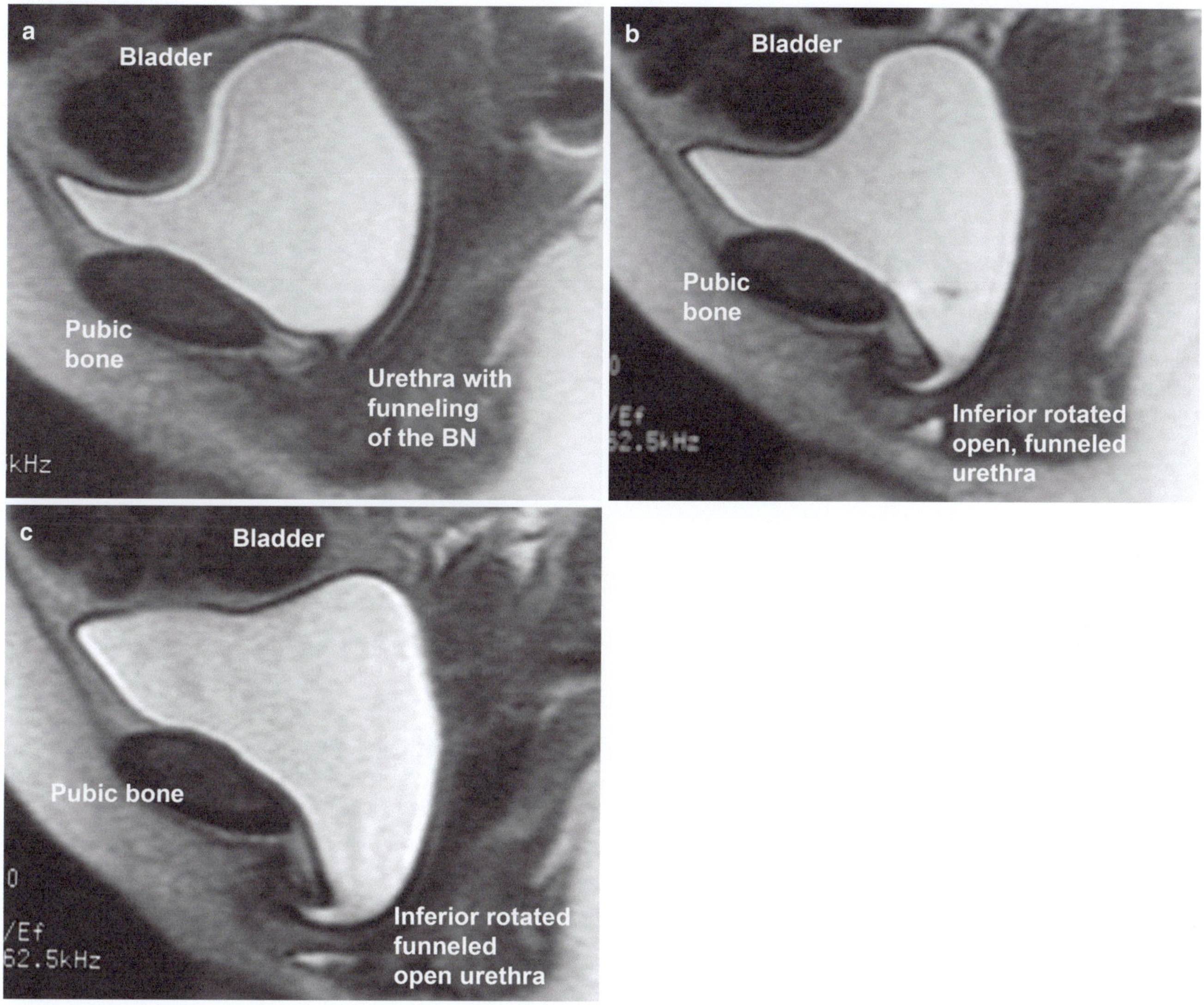

Fig. 2.7 (**a**) Lateral cystogram in a patient with stress incontinence. In the relax position, the bladder neck is at the level of the inferior rami of the pubic bone appearing to be incompetent (funneled). (**b**) With strain there is downward rotational descent of the urethra with further funneling of the bladder neck. (**c**) With further strain the urethra and bladder neck are totally open. It is now inferior to the pubic bone and the distance of the urethra to the inferior pubic bone has increased (weakness of pubo-urethral fascia). The urethra is open and the patient is leaking urine

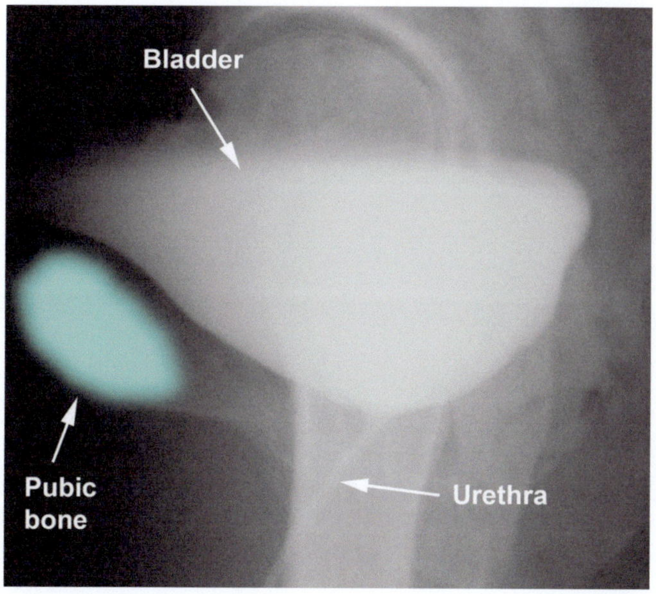

Fig. 2.8 Lateral cystogram in a patient after a successful sling procedure. Sling procedures prevent the sequence of funneling and downward rotation of the urethra. It is not only an anatomical correction that occurs after a sling but an important functional change. Slings allow proper transmission of abdominal pressures during strain. They create a hammock under the urethra (without compression) so increase abdominal pressures can increase urethral resistance during stress. The normal compensatory mechanism of the urethra is restored including the increase of urethral resistance by the levator contraction. The urethral elevation above the bladder level may also create a valvular effect improving continence (Burch procedure)

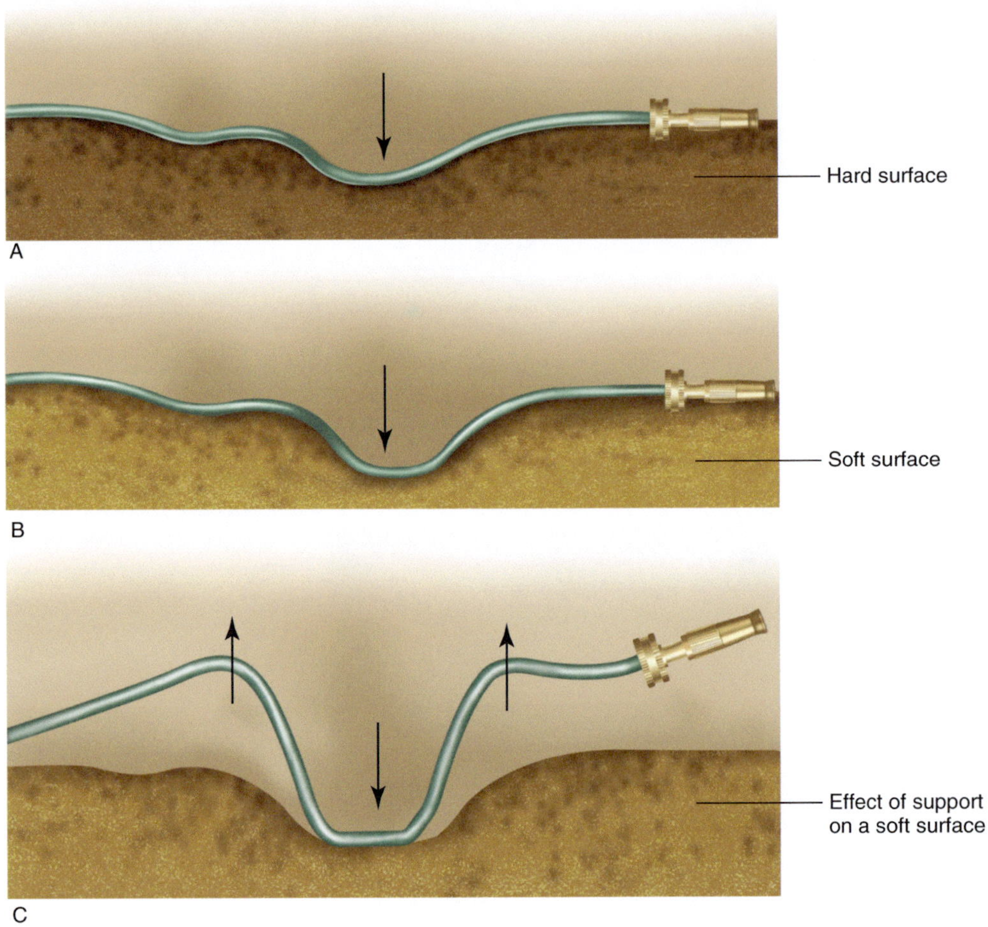

Fig. 2.9 Diagram to explain the impact of suburethral support on urethral function. Support alone can improve continence without direct impact on urethral pressures. (**a**) If a garden hose is placed under a strong surface, minimal superior compression is required to prevent the stream of water. (**b**) If the surface under the garden hose is soft and giving, higher forces are required to stop the stream of water. (**c**) If the garden hose is elevated without any direct compression, less superior pressure will be required to interrupt the flow of water

2.3 Surgical Correlates

Armed with this better understanding of the anatomy of stress incontinence, what surgical correlates can be drawn? First of all, a clinician who has a conceptual picture of the structures involved in support of the bladder neck and proximal urethra gains a better understanding of what actually occurs when surgical therapy is used. The various types of sling or suspension procedures provide dynamic support to the bladder neck and urethra, an increase in urethra resistance, and improved urethral coaptation without creation of an obstruction or urethral compression. In suspension procedures (like Burch or bladder neck suspensions), the vaginal wall is the supporting structure of the urethra; it does not have a suburethral component. Sling procedures have a suburethral component. The importance of this suburethral segment is unclear, as the incision of this suburethral segment of a sling after obstruction usually does not result in recurrence of the stress incontinence. These procedures increase urethral resistance during changes in abdominal pressure by a combination of factors: by creating a hammock against which the urethra is compressed, by allowing better transmission of intra-abdominal pressures, by allowing better compensation of urethral function during stress, or by creating a valvular effect.

As one gains a clearer view of the anatomy, it becomes apparent which structures are important for urethral support and, perhaps more importantly, where and how urethral surgery should be performed to avoid complications. The anatomical placement of sutures or sling material has a major impact on the eventual outcome. When performing a sling or vaginal suspension, placing the sutures or the sling material too close to the urethral wall creates a danger of obstruction and iatrogenic urethral damage. When a sling is done proximal to the bladder neck, there will be no impact on the continence mechanism. A sling procedure that is too tight or penetrates deeply into the periurethral fascia can result in urethral obstruction or erosion. Using translabial ultrasound and studying the final location of midurethral slings, we have found that 50 % are actually not in the midurethra. Urethral location of the mesh appears to have no impact on the clinical outcome of the surgery.

2.4 Treatment of Stress Incontinence

The remainder of this chapter describes various procedures in the treatment of stress incontinence. All the procedures in this section share similar indications, preoperative and postoperative care, and complications. The techniques given represent our own surgical technique. Even as most procedures for the treatment of stress incontinence are done with the mesh, we have nearly abandoned the use of the mesh for treatment of incontinence and pelvic prolapse. Though these days most patients request surgery without some elect to have these procedures and take the risk of short- and long-term mesh complications like pain or extrusion. We describe only one surgery using mesh: a sling procedure (distal urethral polypropylene sling) for simple stress incontinence. We now perform the spiral sling using autologous fascia.

2.4.1 Indications for Surgery

Indications for surgery are mainly stress incontinence or mixed incontinence with a primary component of stress. The degree of incontinence, prior surgeries or radiation, the quality of the vaginal tissues, and medical comorbidities are all factors dictating the type of surgery. For the patient with mild stress incontinence, a well-performed bladder neck suspension will produce a good outcome, but for the patient with multiple failed surgeries, severe incontinence, or incontinence after mesh removal, we will prefer an autologous fascial sling or spiral sling.

2.5 Bladder Neck Suspension (Raz Procedure)

2.5.1 Indications

The bladder neck suspension procedure was designed for the treatment of mild to moderate stress incontinence. The concept is to create a vaginal wall sling. It is not indicated for the patient with multiple failed surgeries and severe incontinence with minimal activity, for the patient after radiation, or in patients with a fixed open urethra. The bladder neck suspension (BNS) is similar to the Burch procedure but is performed transvaginally. The surgery aims at creating a hammock that supports the urethra during changes in intra-abdominal pressure while preventing urethral displacement and allowing proper transmission of abdominal pressures to the urethra and increase in urethral resistance during stress (hammock effect). The anatomical structures involved in the bladder neck suspension include the vaginal wall (excluding the epithelium), the periurethral and perivesical fascia at the level of the bladder neck and urethra, and the urethropelvic fascia that attaches the urethra to the levator muscles (arcus tendineus).

The clinical presentation of stress incontinence depends on the degree of severity of the urethral incompetence. Stress incontinence can manifest as only activity related, or it can be combined with urinary urgency. A history of prior failed surgical procedures, urethral trauma, or irradiation should be noted since a bladder neck suspension is not indicated on these patients. The patient may complain of urinary leakage during straining maneuvers in both the upright and supine positions. On physical examination, different degrees of anterior vaginal wall prolapse can be demonstrated, and stress incontinence can be confirmed during coughing or straining with the patient in the supine or standing position, with leakage demonstrated only at the time of stress. Cystourethroscopy can demonstrate a funneled bladder neck during straining that returns to normal when the stress is relieved. Important preoperative considerations include the degree of anterior vaginal wall prolapse (minimal, moderate, or severe), the degree of incontinence (minimal, moderate, or severe), and other anatomical abnormalities that require concomitant repair, such as uterine prolapse, enterocele, or cystocele.

2.5.2 Preoperative Considerations

A severely shortened and deformed urethra is a contraindication to a vaginal sling procedure. Urethral reconstruction, elongation procedures, and a fascial sling procedure may be better choices in these cases. Another contraindication is senile atrophic vaginitis, as the vaginal wall may not have sufficient integrity and tensile strength to be used as a sling. If recognized early, this problem can be circumvented with the preoperative administration of vaginal estrogen. Radiation or the patients with severe sphincteric damage after mesh removal are not candidates to the procedure.

2.5.3 Surgical Technique

The patient is placed in the dorsal lithotomy position. The lower abdomen and vagina are prepped and draped in a sterile fashion. A Foley catheter is inserted, and the bladder is emptied. A weighted vaginal speculum and a ring retractor with hooks are placed. One dose of prophylactic antibiotics is given.

Figure 2.10 illustrates the anterior vaginal wall, in which two oblique incisions are made in the distal vaginal area.

Figure 2.11 depicts the lateral dissection of the vaginal wall over the perivesical fascia to enter the retropubic space. The urethropelvic fascia is detached from the arcus tendineus of the levator muscle, and a window is made in the retropubic space. Any adhesions in the retropubic space are freed using sharp and blunt dissection.

A finger in the retropubic space exposes the lateral edge of the urethropelvic fascia that was detached from the arcus tendineus. This fascia is the only connection of the urethra to the levator muscle (Fig. 2.12).

Figure 2.13 demonstrates the placement of the suspension sutures. These sutures incorporate the periurethral fascia at the level of the mid- and proximal urethra and the perivesical fascia at the bladder neck. In a second pass, the free edge of the urethropelvic fascia is included. The suture extends medially to incorporate a large segment of the periurethral fascia. With forceps in the retropubic space, medial retraction of the vaginal incision allows the exposure of the margin of the urethropelvic fascia (Fig. 2.14).

The sutures must incorporate the urethropelvic ligament (Fig. 2.15). Since a bladder neck suspension is not indicated on these patients.

Medial traction is applied to the vaginal wall, and the perivesical fascia at the bladder neck and the periurethral fascia at the proximal and midurethra are incorporated. The passage is extended medially in order to create a strong hammock of the anterior vaginal wall and the monofilament sutures, acting like a sling under the urethra. The same maneuver is done at least twice and the end traction is applied to the sutures to confirm a strong anchor (Fig. 2.16).

The perivesical and periurethral fascia are incorporated in a similar fashion on the contralateral side. The suture passage is extended medially in order to create a stronger suburethral hammock (Fig. 2.17).

Traction of the sutures confirms the strong anchor of the vaginal wall and urethropelvic fascia (Fig. 2.18).

A small puncture is performed in the suprapubic area. We perform only a midline puncture to avoid any lateral placement of sutures that can impact the inguinal innervation and cause suprapubic pain (Fig. 2.19).

Under finger control in the retropubic space, a double-pronged needle passer is used to transfer the sutures from the vagina to the suprapubic area. The distance between the tips of the double passer is 1 cm (Fig. 2.20).

The tips of the suture passer are exposed in the vaginal incision, and the sutures are transferred through the eyes of the needle for a distance of 10 cm to prevent dislodgement during the passage of the passer to the suprapubic area (Fig. 2.21).

The sutures have been transferred to the suprapubic puncture area (Fig. 2.22). The vaginal wall is closed with delayed absorbable sutures and all retraction is removed.

Cystoscopy is performed to rule out any bladder or urethral injury (Fig. 2.23). Keeping the sheet of the cystoscope in a 45° angulation, each of the sutures is tied individually without tension. Because there is a 1-cm space between the double needles, the tie of the sutures will be supported by the abdominal wall for this distance.

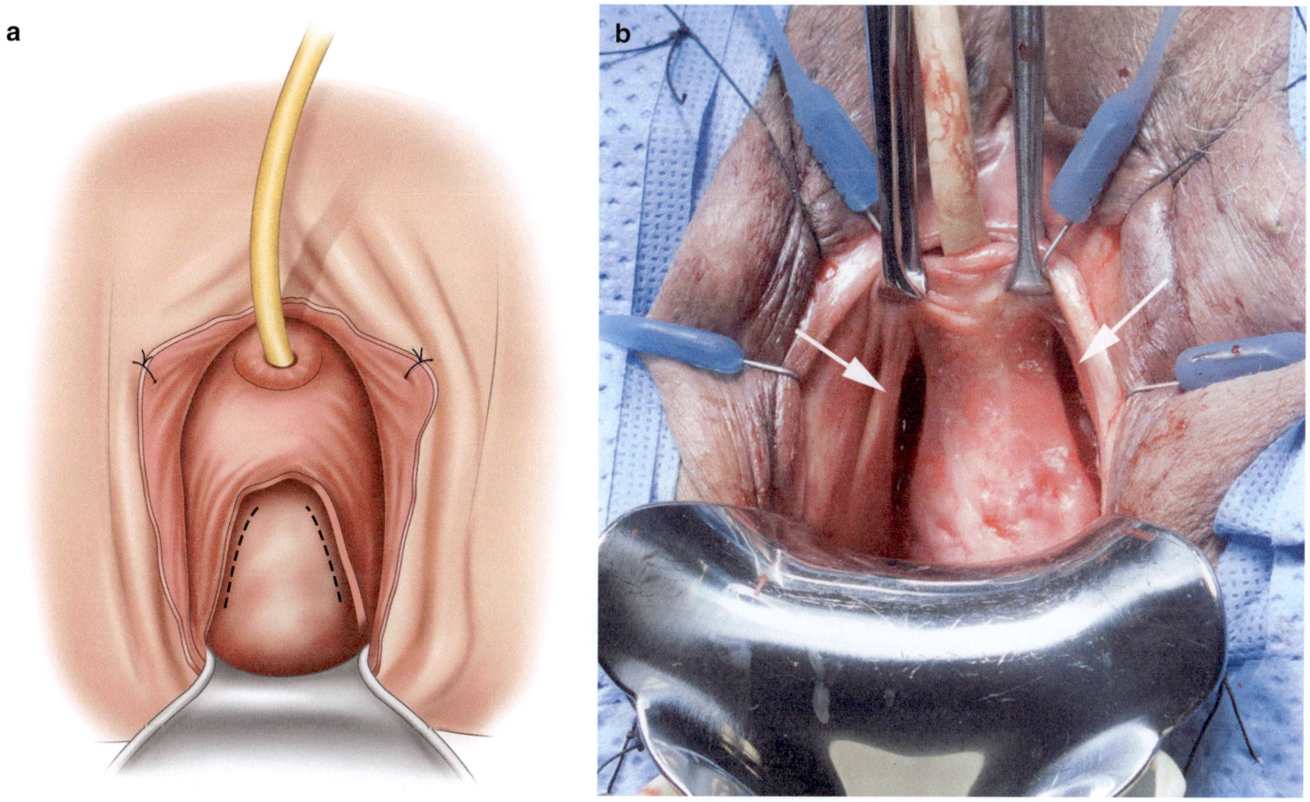

Fig. 2.10 (**a**) Two oblique incisions are made in the anterior vaginal wall, extending a few centimeters proximal to the bladder neck. The incision is made 1 cm from the lateral vaginal wall. (**b**) Two Allis clamps are placed on each side at the apex of the incisions (*arrows*) for traction and improved exposure

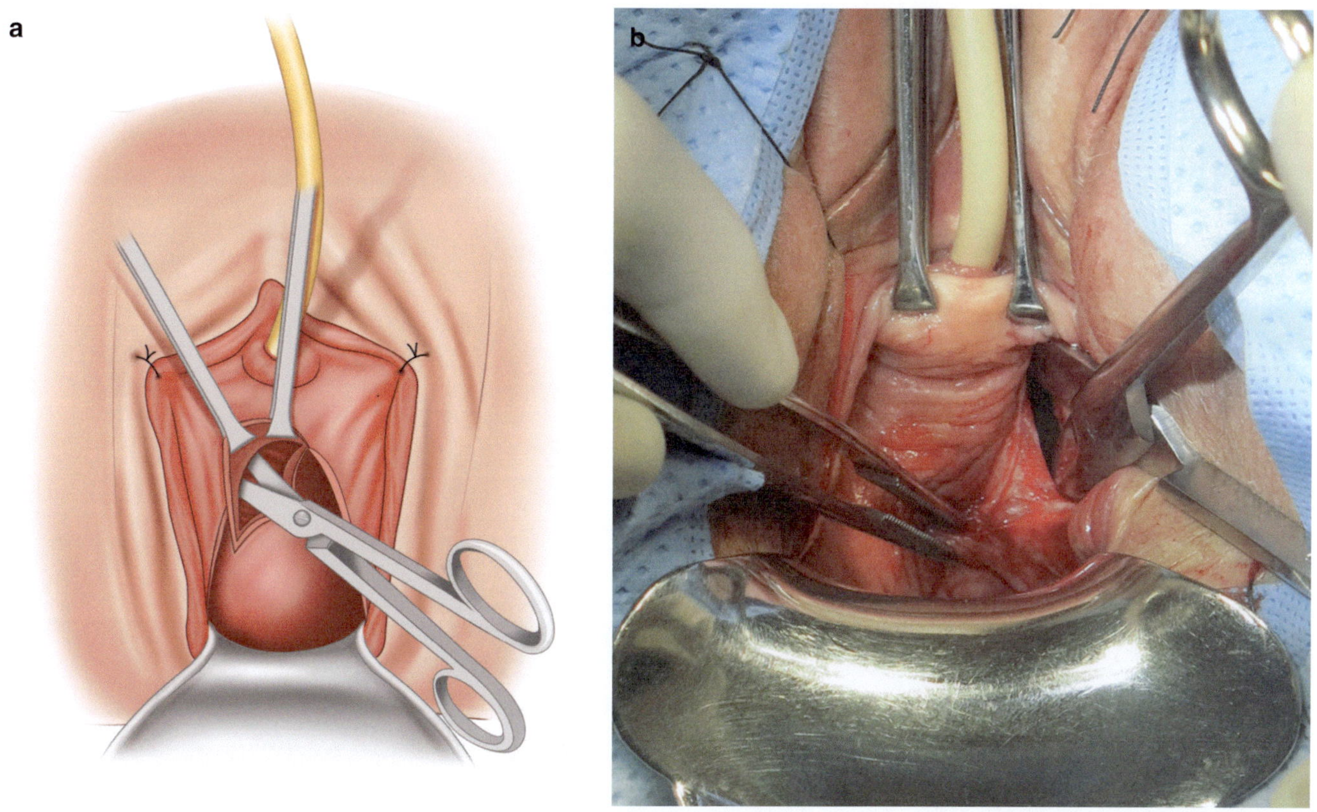

Fig. 2.11 (**a**, **b**) To enter the retropubic space, curved scissors are placed parallel to the urethra, under the pubic bone and in an upward direction, abutting the pubic bone at all times

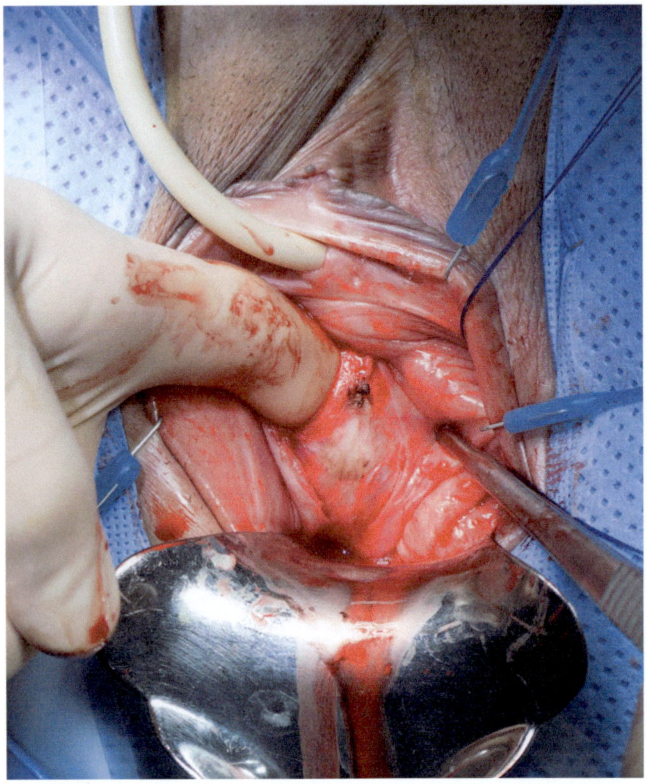

Fig. 2.12 A finger is placed in the retropubic space, exposing the lateral edge of the urethropelvic ligament

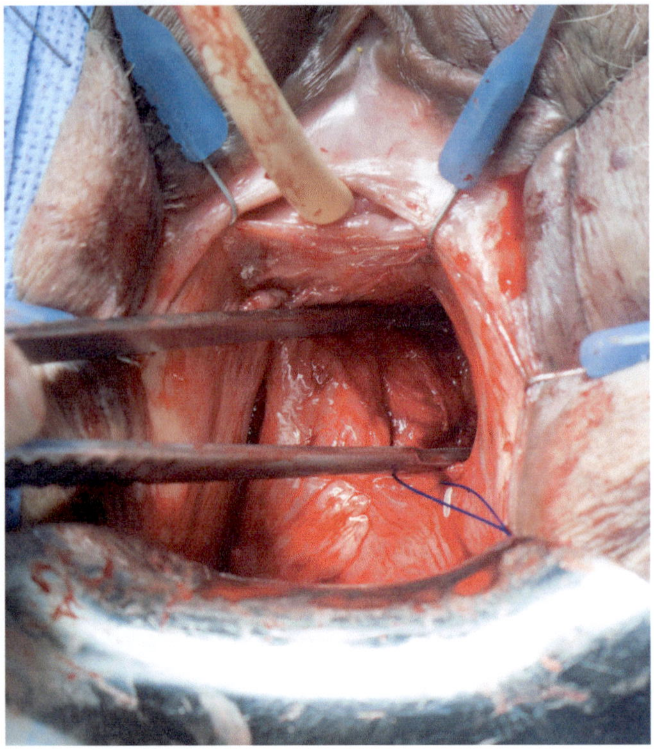

Fig. 2.14 The sutures are initially applied at the level of the bladder neck, incorporating the vaginal wall (excluding the epithelium)

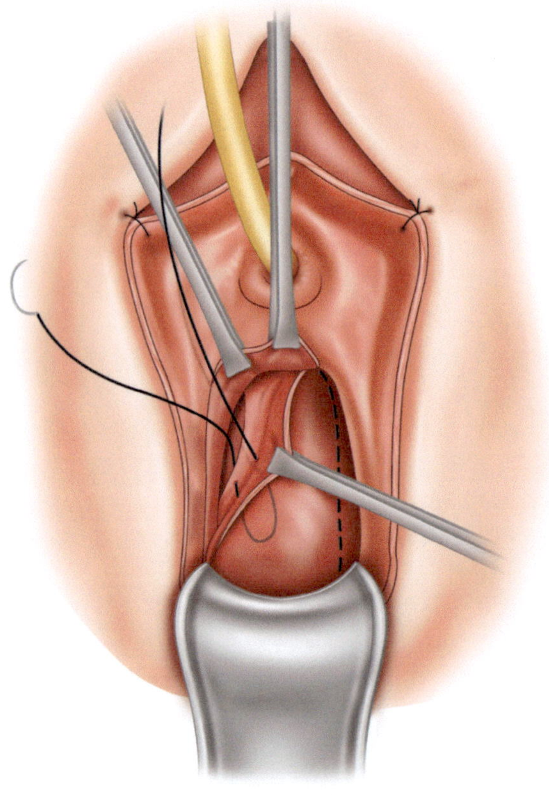

Fig. 2.13 Placement of the bladder neck suspension sutures used to create the suspension

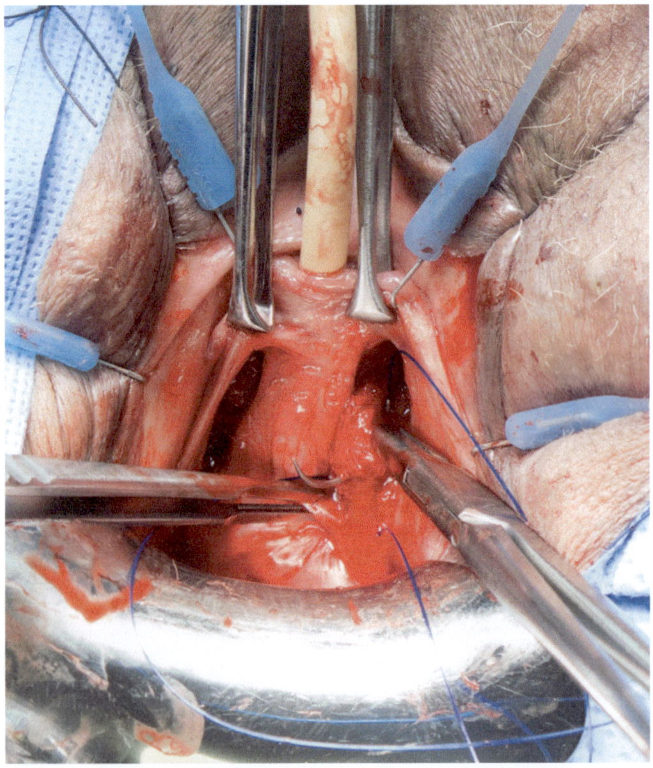

Fig. 2.15 A #0 monofilament nonabsorbable suture is used to incorporate the lateral margin of urethropelvic fascia. Care should be taken not to insert the needle deeply, to avoid penetrating the wall of the bladder or urethra

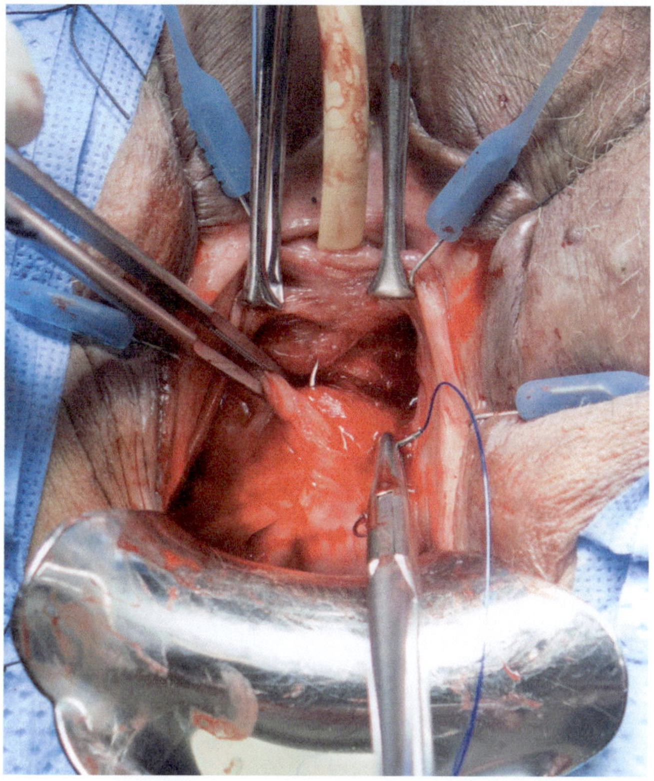

Fig. 2.16 The periurethral and perivesical fasciae are also included

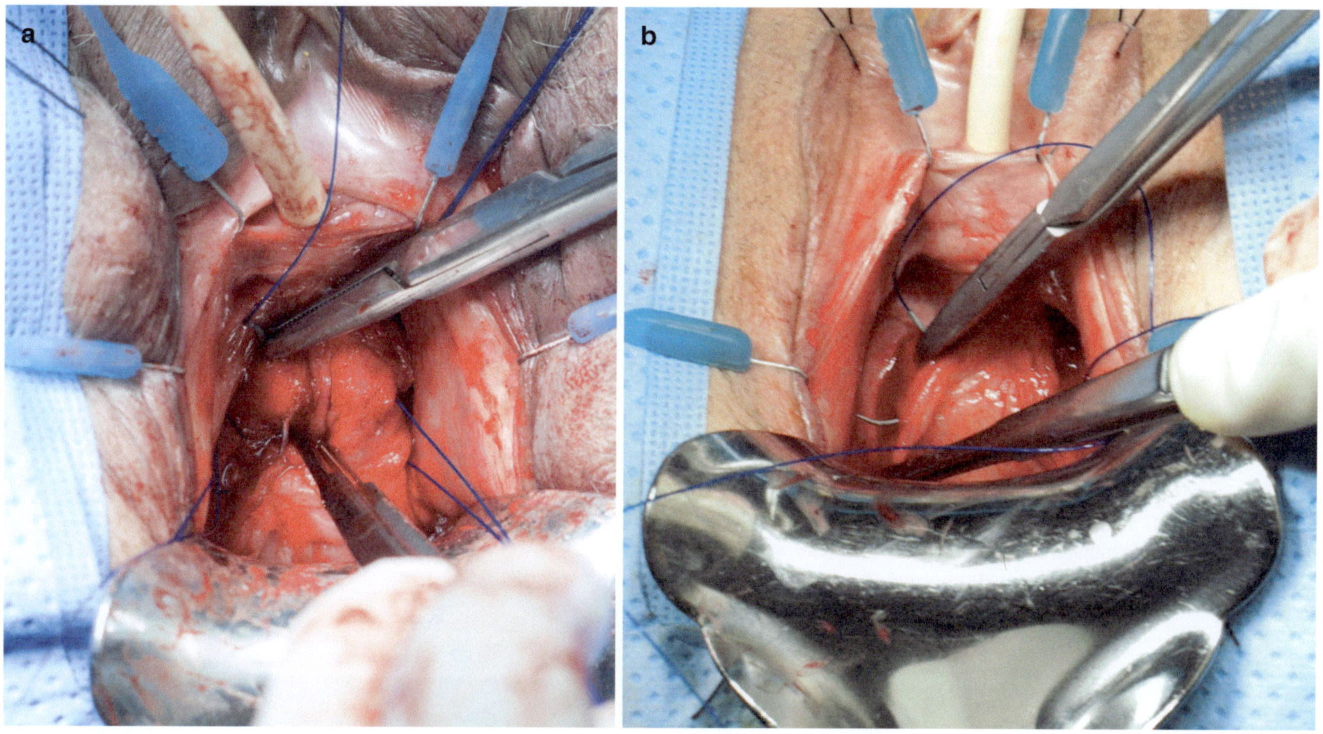

Fig. 2.17 (**a**, **b**) The same procedure is performed again on the contralateral side

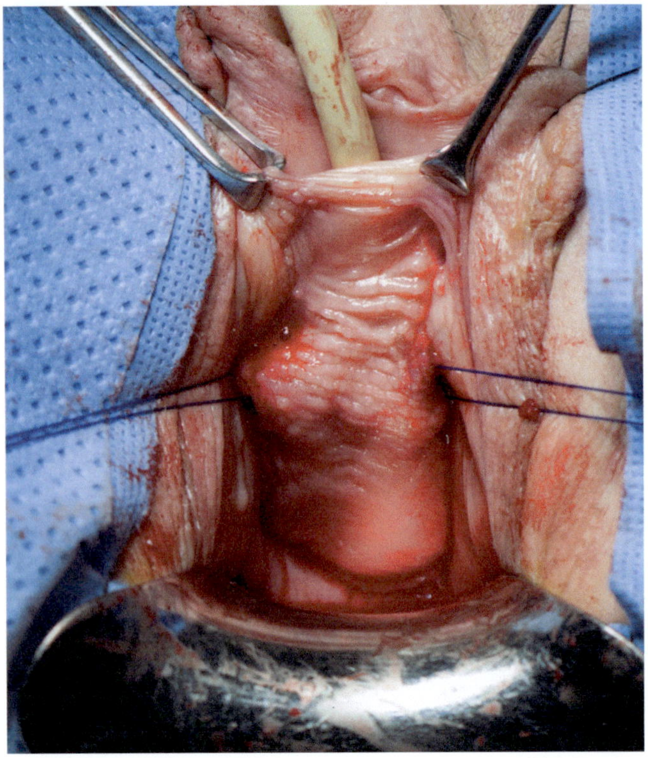

Fig. 2.18 By applying traction on the sutures, strong anchoring of the vaginal wall and periurethral tissues is confirmed

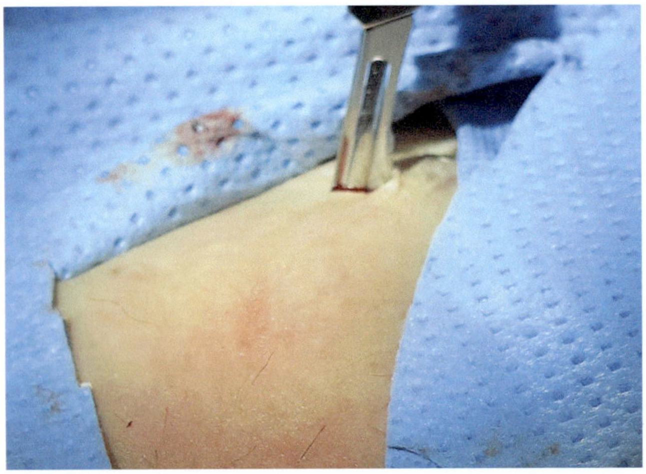

Fig. 2.19 A small puncture is performed just above the symphysis of the pubic bone. The puncture in the suprapubic abdominal wall is done as close as possible to the upper margin of the pubic bone to prevent suprapubic pain due to traction of the rectus musculature

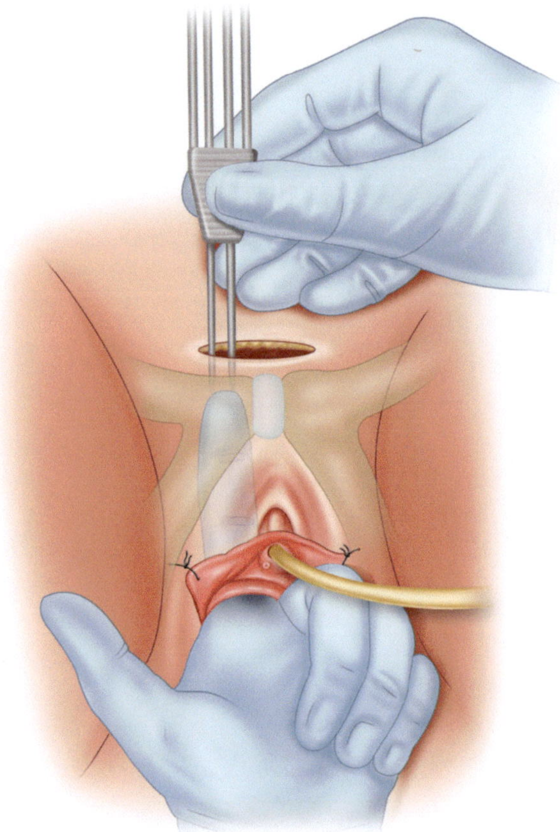

Fig. 2.20 A double-pronged ligature carrier (Raz needle passer) is used to transfer each of the Prolene® sutures from the vagina to the suprapubic region. Under finger control, the tips of the passer are transferred from the suprapubic incision to the vaginal incisions

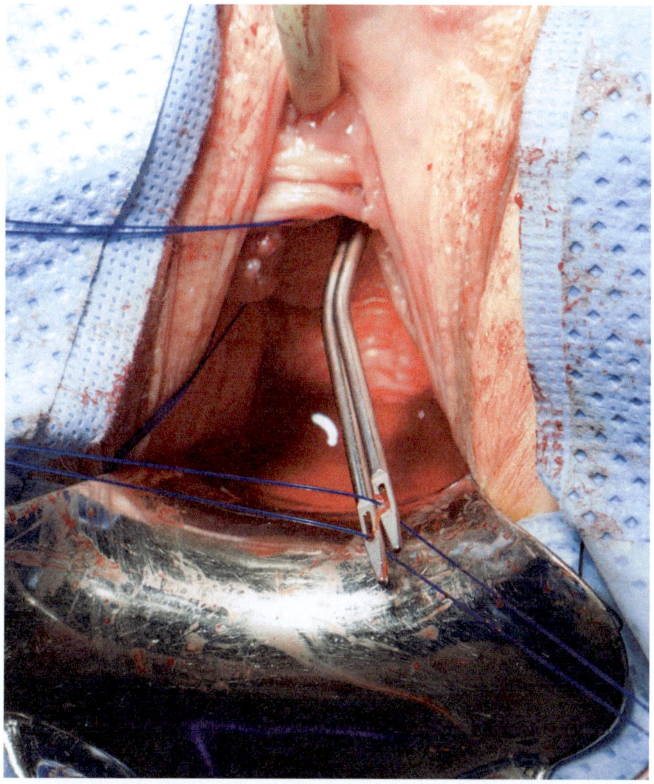

Fig. 2.21 The sutures are transferred through the eyes of the needle and retracted to the suprapubic area

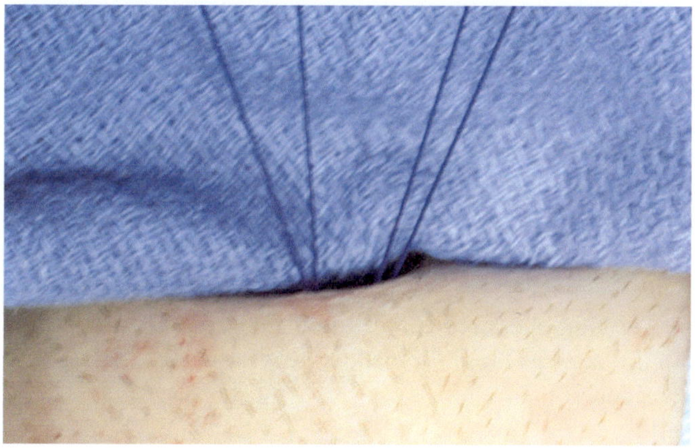

Fig. 2.22 The sutures are transferred to the suprapubic puncture area. The double-pronged carrier will permit the sutures to be tied over a 1-cm segment of the rectus fascia

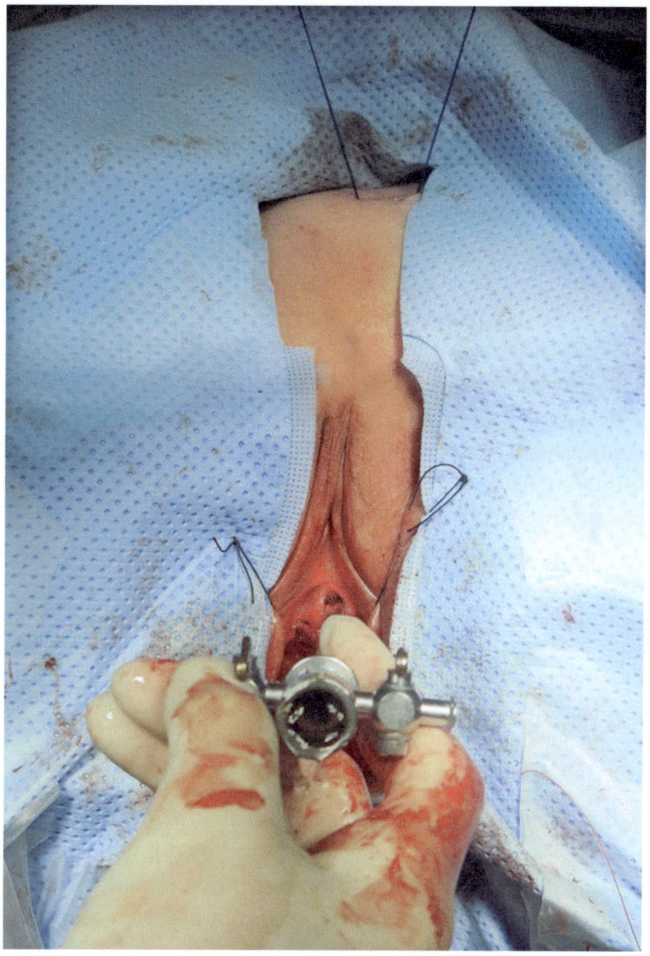

Fig. 2.23 In order to prevent undue tension on the sutures and urinary obstruction from the suspension, the cystoscope is inserted in the bladder and positioned at a 45° angle with the horizontal. The suprapubic sutures are tied individually over the rectus fascia, with the cystoscope sheath in place

2.5.4 Intraoperative Complications

Potential complications at the time of surgery are similar to those of other vaginal procedures and are discussed in another chapter. The most common potential complications are bleeding, urethral or bladder perforation during dissection, and urethral obstruction by the suspension sutures.

2.5.5 Postoperative Care

The procedure can be performed as an outpatient surgery. The vaginal packing is removed 2 h after surgery. The patient is discharged home with a Foley catheter that the patient will remove a few days later. The patient is discharged home after recovering from anesthesia, usually 2–3 h after surgery. Oral antibiotics when indicated, stool softeners, and pain medication are prescribed. There is minimal pain after surgery. Postoperatively, the patient is allowed to engage in normal activities like walking, driving, and performing simple chores. The patient is instructed to avoid high-impact exercise and sexual relations for 1 month.

2.5.6 Postoperative Complications

Risks of any sling procedure include delayed voiding, obstructive urinary symptoms, and even permanent urinary retention, but in our experience, no patient with non-neurogenic urethral incompetence has suffered from permanent retention. De novo overactive bladder without obstruction usually responds to anticholinergic medications. Vaginal shortening is another potential risk, although we have not yet found this to be a problem. Suprapubic wound infections are very rare and may require antibiotics, drainage, or both.

2.6 Distal Urethral Polypropylene Sling (DUPS)

2.6.1 Indications

The distal urethral polypropylene sling (DUPS) procedure for the treatment of stress incontinence is indicated in patients with mild to severe stress incontinence. After distal vaginal incisions are made bilaterally, a tunnel is made in the anterior vaginal wall between the two incisions, 2 cm from the external meatus. A segment of soft polypropylene mesh (10 × 1 cm) is prepared and a #0 delayed absorbable suture is applied at each end. The mesh is transferred through the vaginal tunnel. The sutures will be transferred under finger control in the retropubic space to a small suprapubic puncture. The mesh will be infiltrated by fibrous tissue, providing stability and support to the urethra and anterior vaginal wall during changes in abdominal pressure.

The diagnosis and preoperative considerations are the same as those for bladder neck suspension, discussed previously. We have encountered some patients who present with late complications due to the use of the mesh (erosions, exposure, and pelvic pain) even 7–10 years later. At this time, we will use this procedure very rarely.

2.6.2 Surgical Technique

The patient is placed in the dorsal lithotomy position. The lower abdomen and vagina are prepped and draped in a sterile fashion. If required, the labia are retracted laterally with stay sutures. A Foley catheter is inserted into the urethra, and the bladder is emptied. A weighted vaginal speculum is placed.

Figures 2.24, 2.25, 2.26, 2.27, 2.28, 2.29, 2.30, 2.31, 2.32, 2.33, 2.34, 2.35, 2.36, and 2.37 depict the sequence of steps in the placement of a Prolene® sling. At the end of the procedure, the vaginal wall is closed with multiple absorbable sutures, with extra care not to include the mesh during closure. Vaginal packing soaked in antibiotic cream is inserted in the vagina.

The intraoperative complications and postoperative care are the same as those for bladder neck suspension, discussed previously.

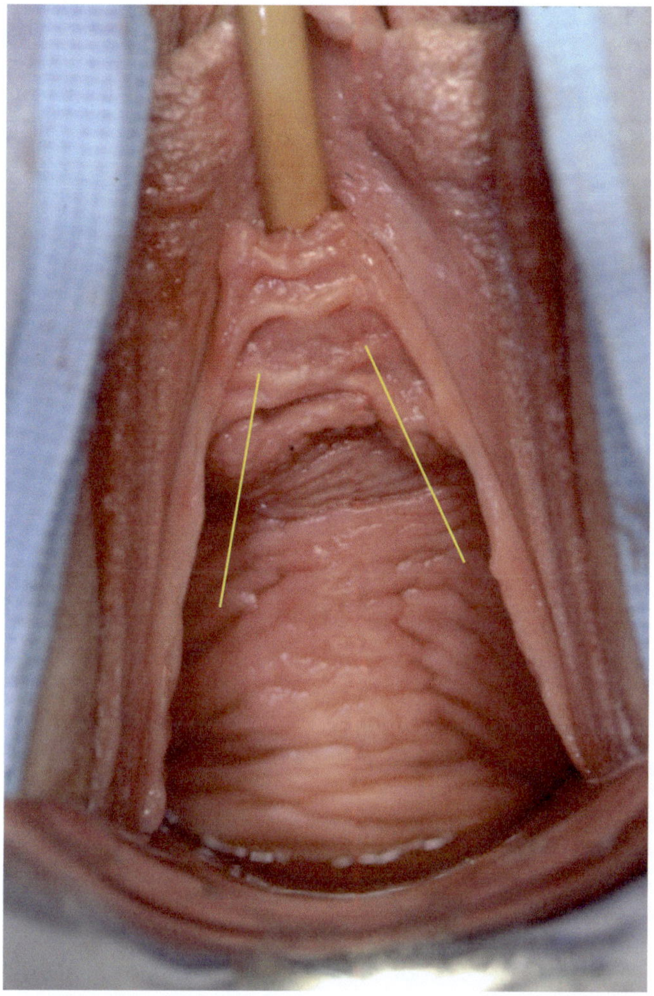

Fig. 2.24 Two oblique incisions are made in the anterior vaginal wall

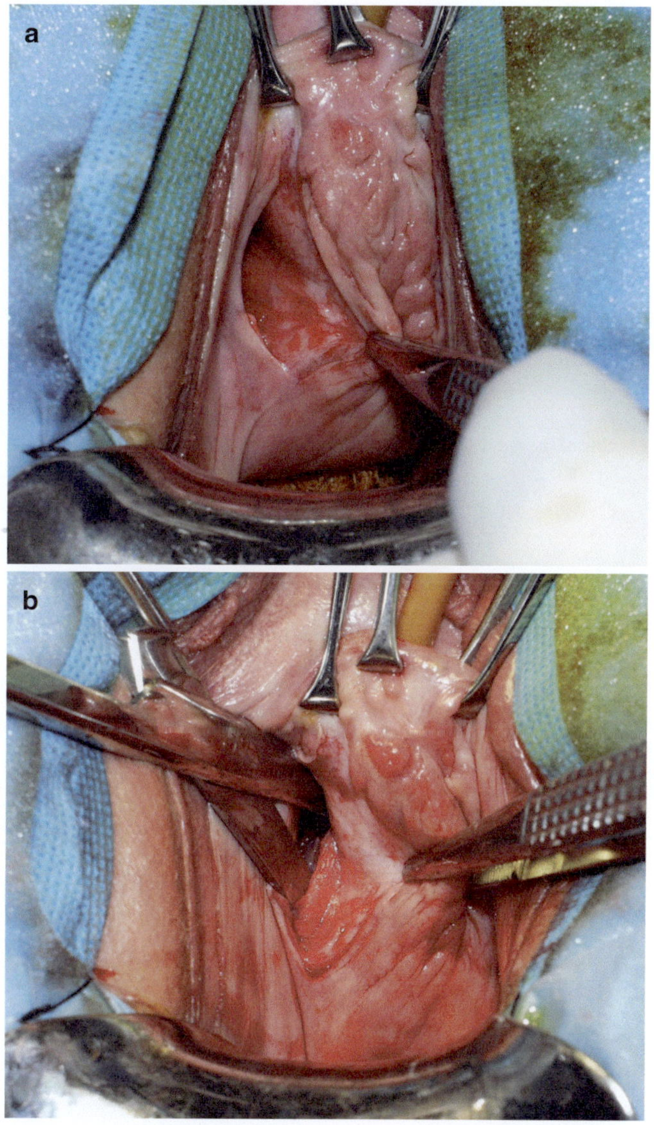

Fig. 2.25 (**a**) Allis clamps are used to grasp the anterior vaginal wall just proximal to the urethral meatus for traction. The oblique incision is dissected further to expose the periurethral fascia. (**b**) The vaginal wall is dissected laterally along the glistening white periurethral fascia toward the ipsilateral shoulder. With a curved scissors parallel to the urethra and pointing superiorly under the inferior pubic bone, the attachment of the urethropelvic fascia to the arcus tendineus fascia pelvis is entered. A small window is made in the retropubic space. The pubic bone can be palpated to confirm proper entrance into the retropubic space. All adhesions from prior surgeries are freed

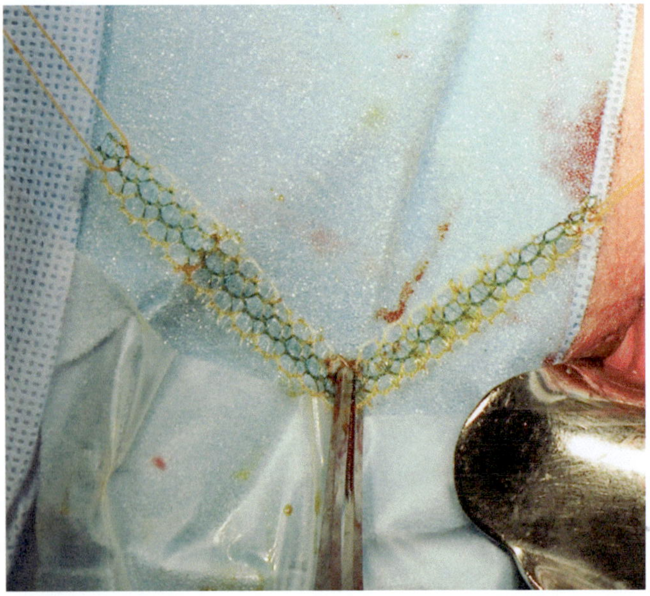

Fig. 2.26 A segment of soft polypropylene mesh measuring 10 × 1 cm is used. A #0 delayed absorbable suture is passed several times through the end of the sling to provide a strong anchor to the mesh. The mesh is kept soaked in antibiotic solution

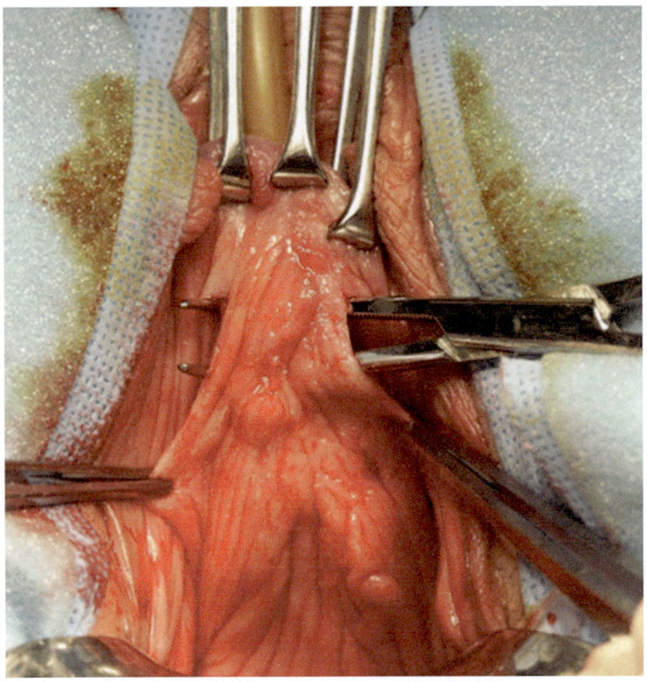

Fig. 2.27 Using a right-angle clamp, a tunnel connecting the two incisions is made under the vaginal wall, between the mid- and distal urethra

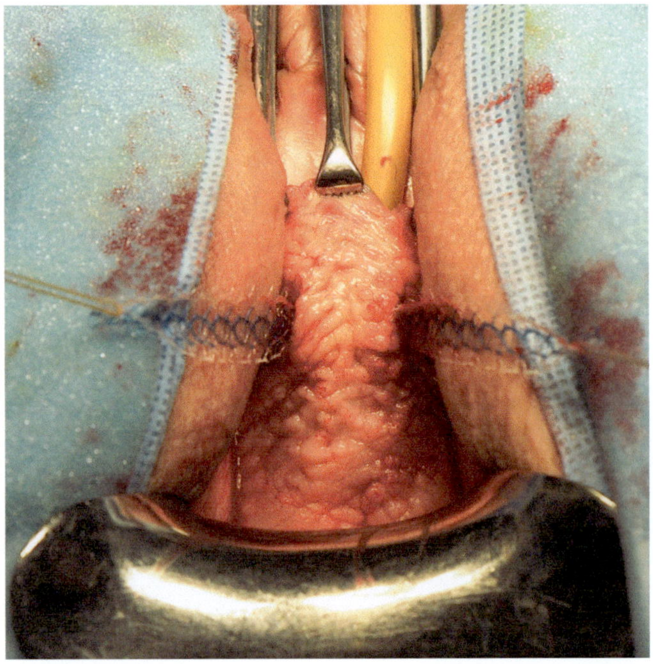

Fig. 2.28 Using a right-angle clamp, the mesh is transferred beneath the tunnel and positioned at the center of the incisions

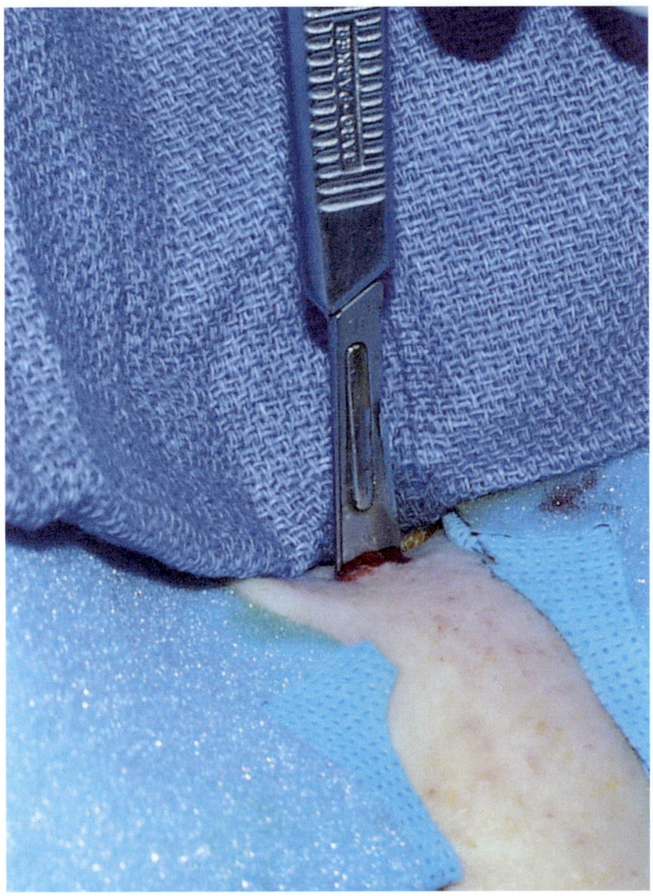

Fig. 2.29 A puncture is made in the suprapubic area just above the superior margin of the pubic bone

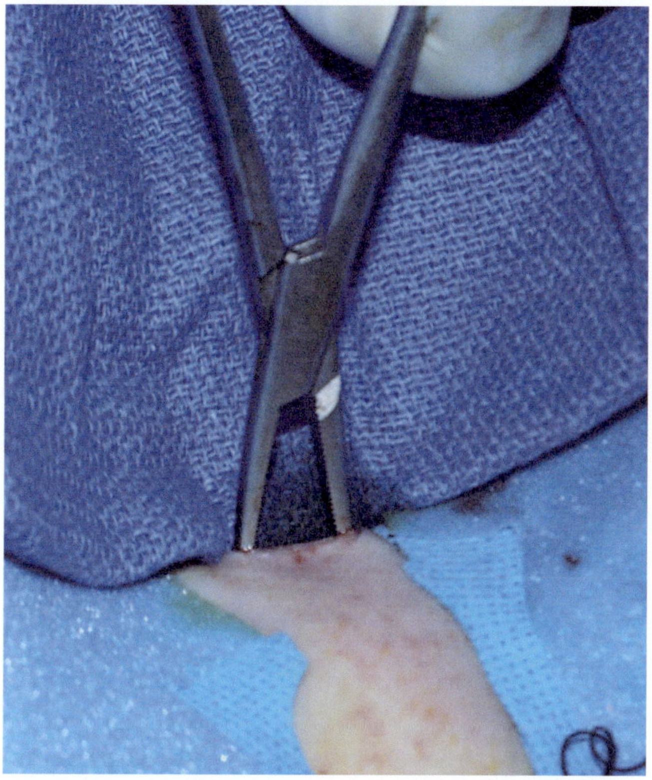

Fig. 2.30 A hemostatic clamp is used to create a pocket in the suprapubic area down to the rectus fascia, just superior to the symphysis of the pubic bone

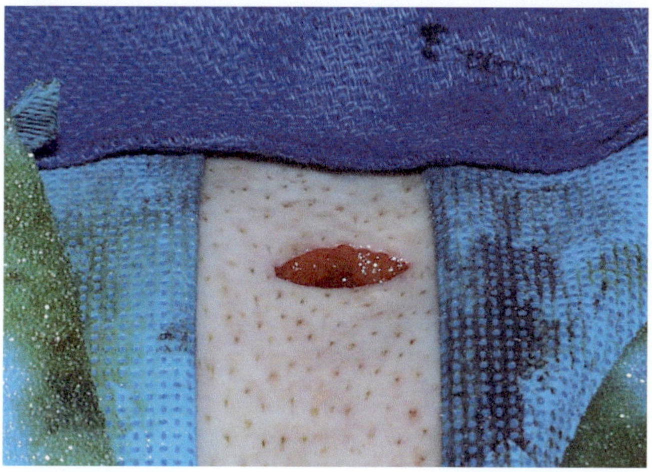

Fig. 2.31 The small incision over the suprapubic area is seen

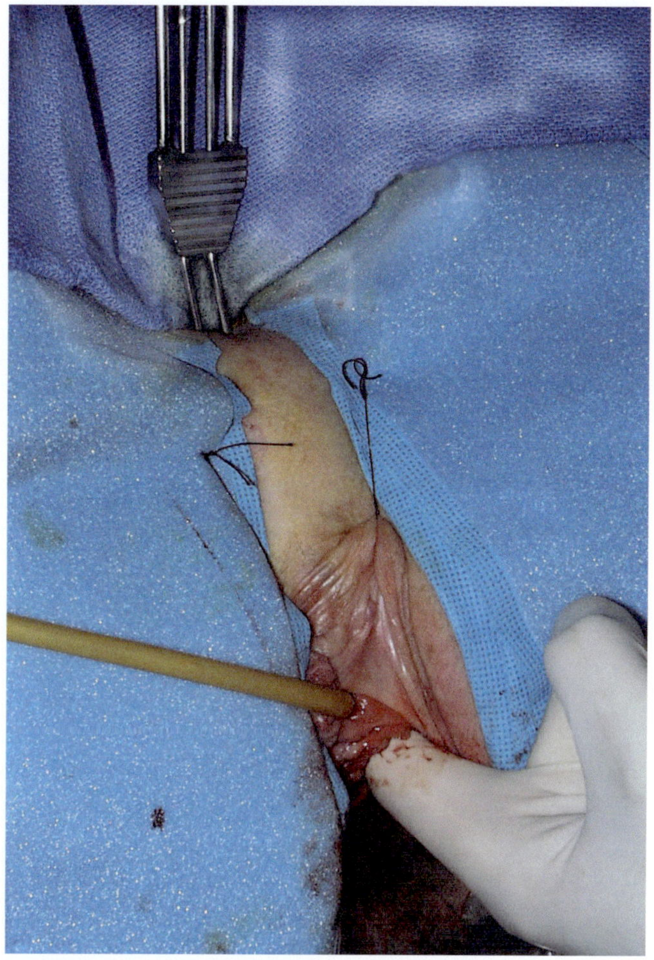

Fig. 2.32 A double-pronged ligature carrier is used to transfer the delayed absorbable sutures (DAS) from the vagina to the suprapubic region. Under finger control, the tips of the passer are transferred from the suprapubic to the vaginal area. Finger guidance in the retropubic space prevents inadvertent penetration of the bladder or urethra

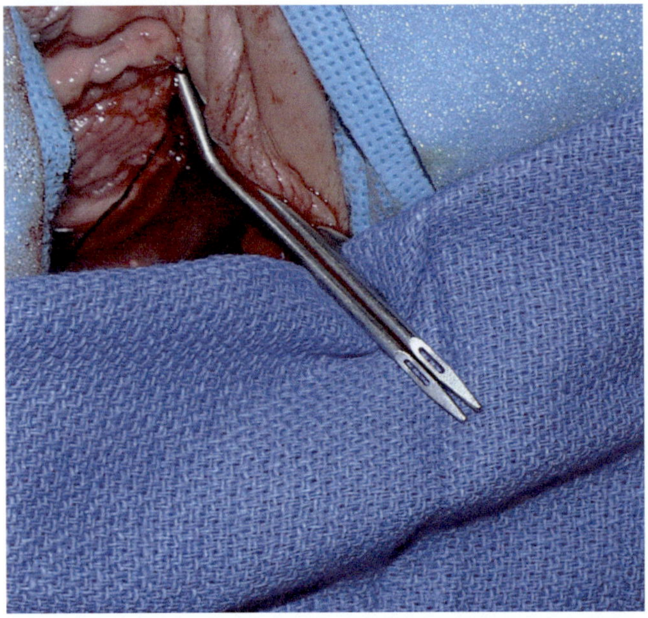

Fig. 2.33 The tips of the double-pronged passer are seen in the vaginal area after being transferred from the suprapubic area

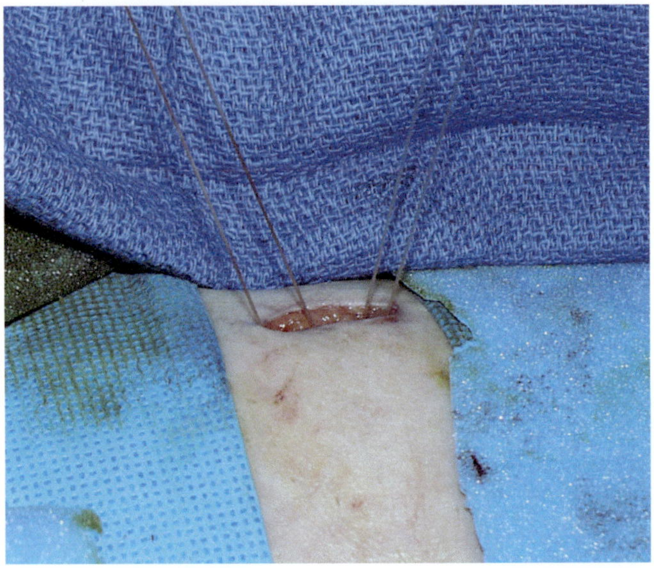

Fig. 2.35 The double-pronged passer is pulled up and retracted from the suprapubic area, allowing the retrieval of the sutures. The sutures are seen in the suprapubic wound

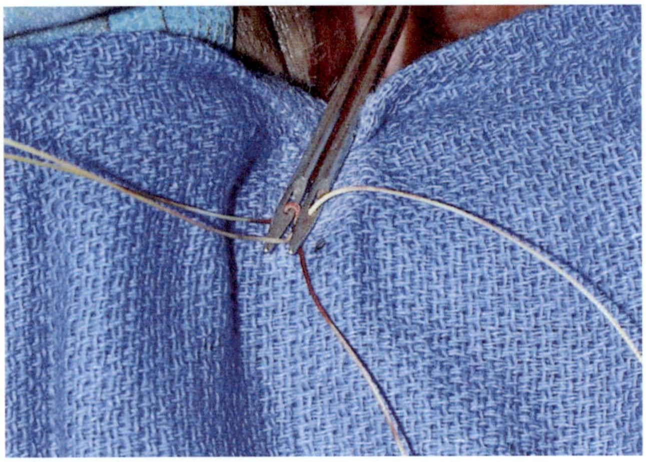

Fig. 2.34 The absorbable sutures are transferred through the eyes of the needle for a distance of 10 cm

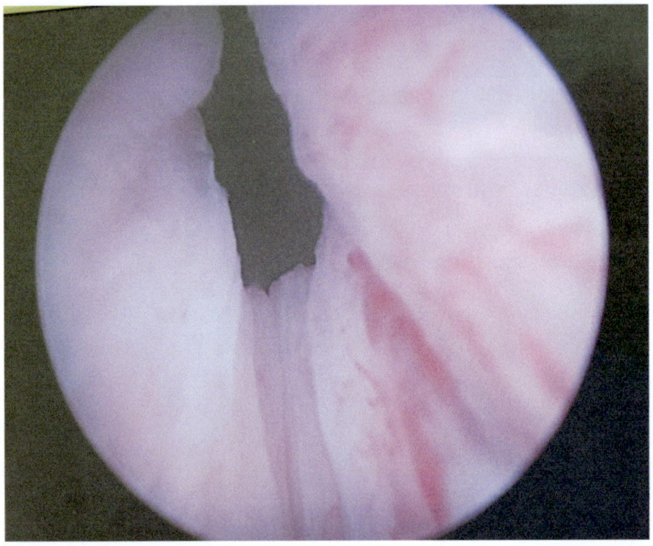

Fig. 2.36 Cystourethroscopy is performed to ensure that the bladder and urethra were not inadvertently injured

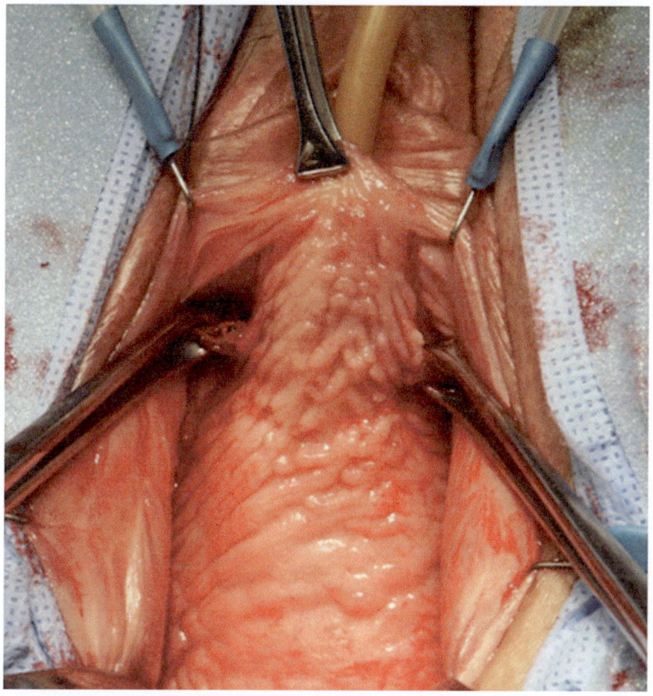

Fig. 2.37 Two Allis clamps are placed vaginally at each side of the mesh to prevent migration of the sling. The suprapubic delayed absorbable sutures (DAS) are tied individually, and the mesh is kept under slight traction to prevent excessive tensioning of the sling and urethral obstruction

2.6.3 Postoperative Complications

The complications of this procedure are similar to those of other anti-incontinence procedures. The potential for urethral obstruction with this technique may be higher because the mesh may shrink 20–30 % from its original size. The mesh should therefore lie loosely beneath the vaginal wall. Slight countertraction of the sling at the time of the tying of the suprapubic sutures will prevent excessive tensioning of the sling against the urethral wall. With the use of absorbable sutures, the potential for suprapubic infection is nearly eliminated. Infection of the sling or urethral perforation requires removal of the sling.

2.7 Abdominal Autologous Fascial Slings (Pubovaginal Sling)

Three types of autologous fascial sling procedures are described in this chapter: the classic U-shaped pubovaginal sling (Fig. 2.38), the omega shaped fascial sling (Fig. 2.39) and the spiral sling. While our original description of the spiral sling (Fig. 2.40) used mesh we currently have abandoned mesh and use exclusively autologous fascia lata.

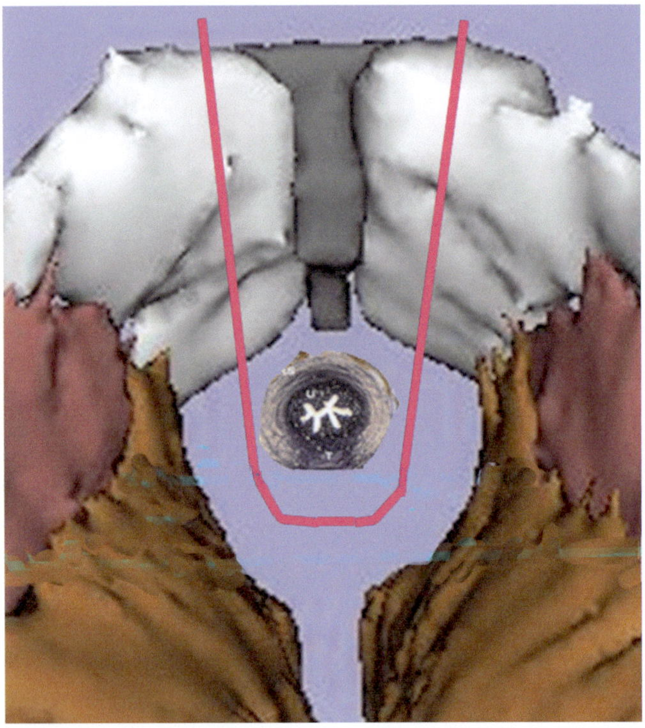

Fig. 2.38 Diagram of a U-shaped fascial sling: the fascial segment is placed in a U shape under the urethra. The sling is generally 10–12 cm long and is anchored to a small puncture in the suprapubic area

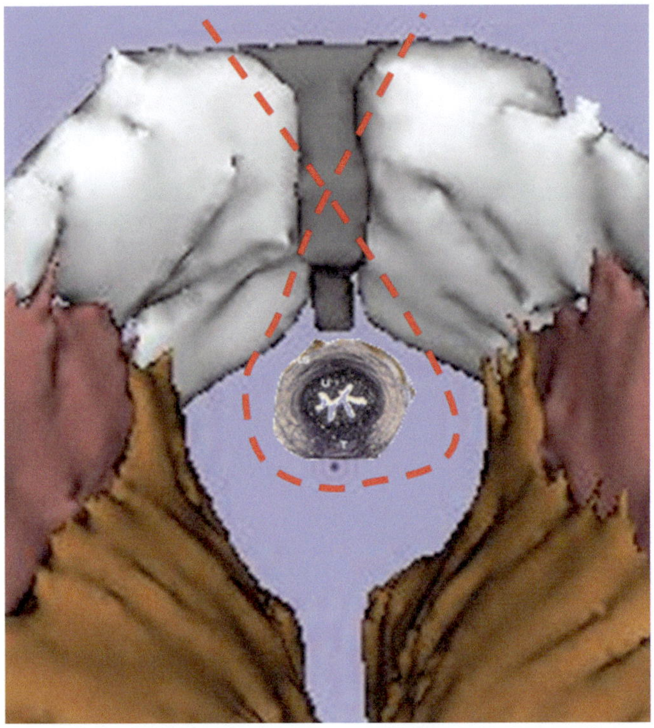

Fig. 2.39 Diagram of the omega-shaped fascial sling: the fascial strip is crossed in the retropubic space anterior to the urethra

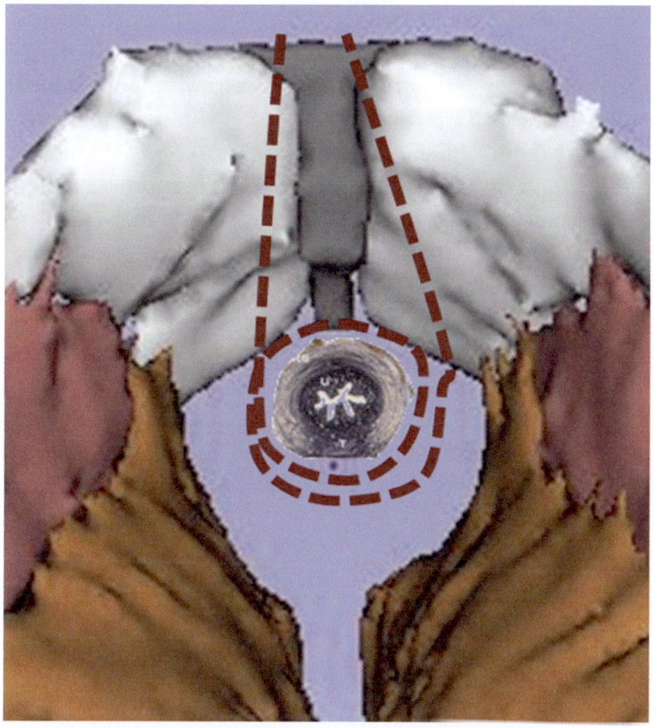

Fig. 2.40 Diagram of the spiral fascial sling: the sling surrounds the urethra in a circular fashion, providing the best possible urethral compression

2.7.1 Indications

The indications for this type of surgery include moderate to severe stress incontinence, failed prior surgeries, incontinence after mesh removal, or refusal of a mesh sling by a patient with stress incontinence. Most times, it is a secondary procedure.

2.7.2 Surgical Technique: Autologous Fascia Pubovaginal Sling

Figures 2.41, 2.42, 2.43, 2.44, 2.45, 2.46, 2.47, 2.48, 2.49, 2.50, 2.51, 2.52, 2.53, 2.54, 2.55, 2.56, and 2.57 illustrate the procedure for placement of a classic, U-shaped pubovaginal sling. For the classic fascial sling, a segment of autologous fascia is retrieved that is 2 cm wide and 10–12 cm in length. The segment of the fascia is usually obtained from the suprapubic area; rarely, it may come from other areas of the abdominal wall. It is not necessary to retrieve a long segment of the fascia, as the cure rate is the same with short segments, therefore diminishing the morbidity after surgery. At the end of the fascial strip, a #1 delayed absorbable suture is applied. The fascial strip is transferred under the tunnel and then passed toward a small suprapubic incision, using a double-pronged suture passer.

To prevent undue tension on the sutures and urinary obstruction from the suspension, two Allis clamps are used to keep the sling in an horizantal plane while the sutures are tied. We use two Allis clamps the sling can be maintained in an horizontal plane to prevent undo tensioning of the sutures. Once the cystoscope is removed, the urethral Foley catheter is replaced.

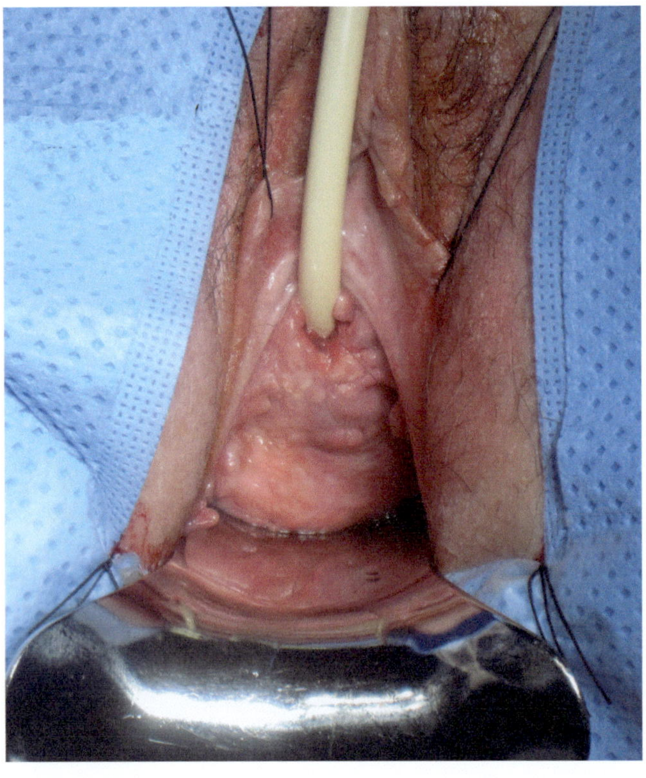

Fig. 2.41 The patient is placed in the dorsal lithotomy position. The lower abdomen and vagina are prepped and draped in a sterile fashion. A Foley catheter is inserted into the urethra, and the bladder is emptied. A weighted vaginal speculum is placed and a ring retractor with hooks is used to expose the anterior vaginal wall

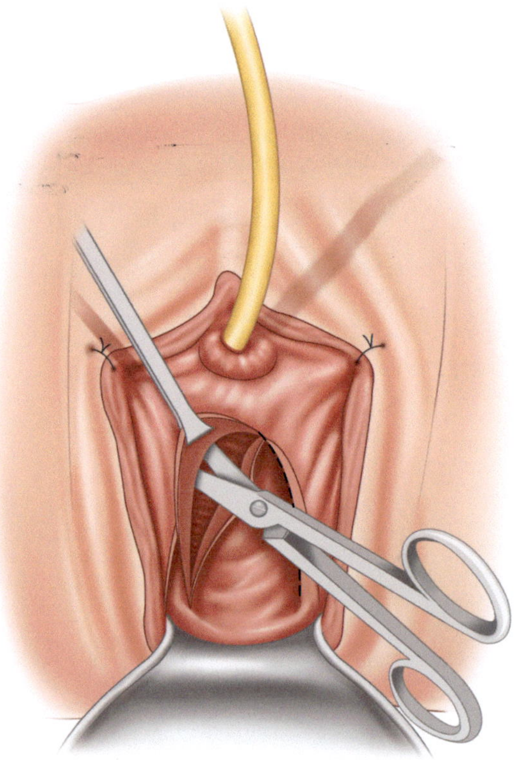

Fig. 2.42 Diagram depicting the oblique incisions that are made in the anterior vaginal wall. In a similar maneuver as described for bladder neck suspension surgery, dissection is carried out over the glistening surface of the periurethral fascia. A small window is made in the retropubic space to allow passage of a finger. All adhesions are freed

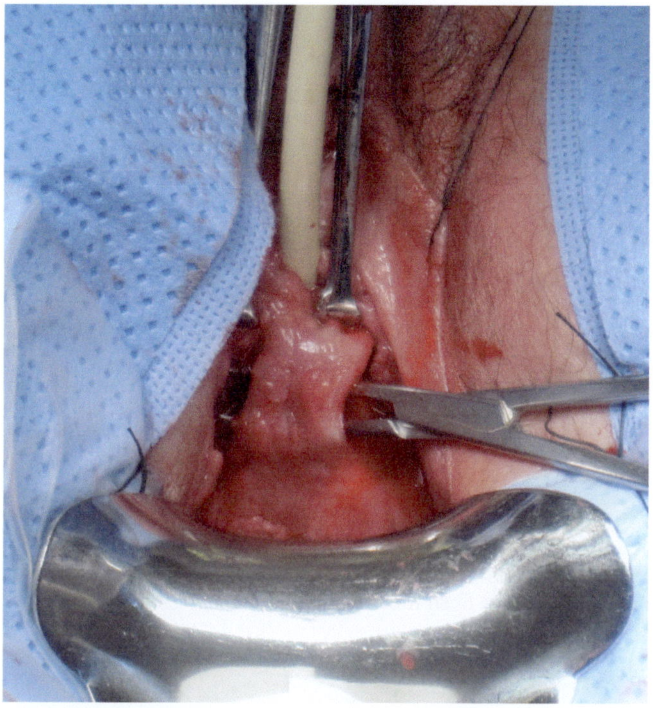

Fig. 2.43 Using a right-angle clamp, a tunnel is made under the vaginal wall, connecting the two incisions

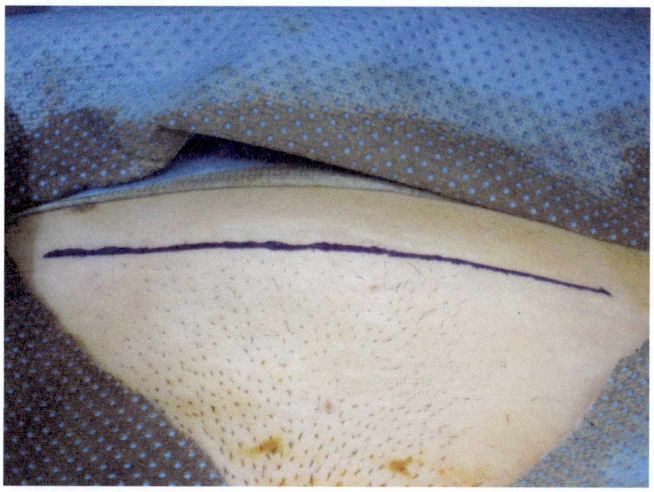

Fig. 2.44 Exposure of the lower abdomen is seen. The line of incision for fascial retrieval is marked

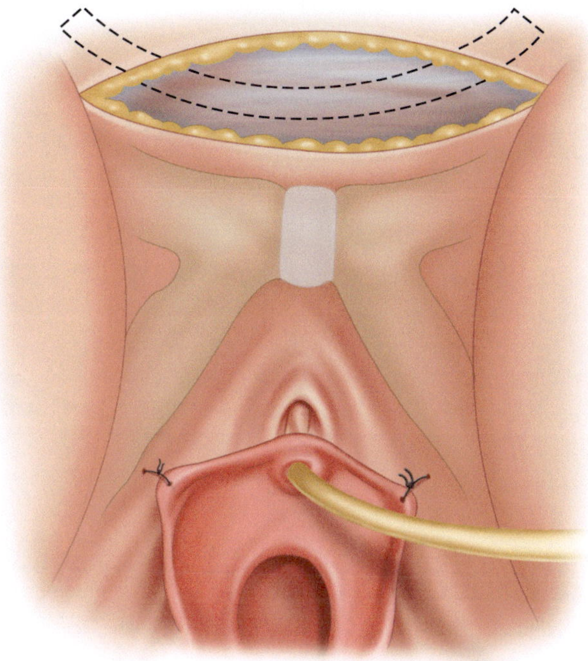

Fig. 2.45 Suprapubic exposure marking the area of fascial retrieval

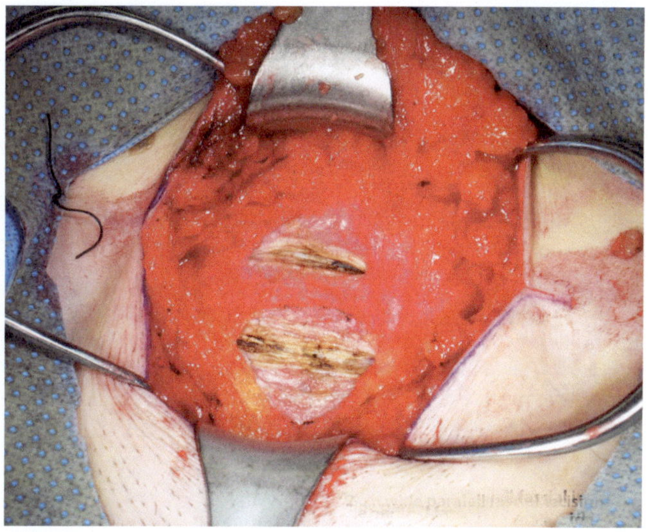

Fig. 2.46 The skin and subcutaneous are exposed. Two parallel incisions are made over the anterior abdominal wall fascia, 2 cm apart

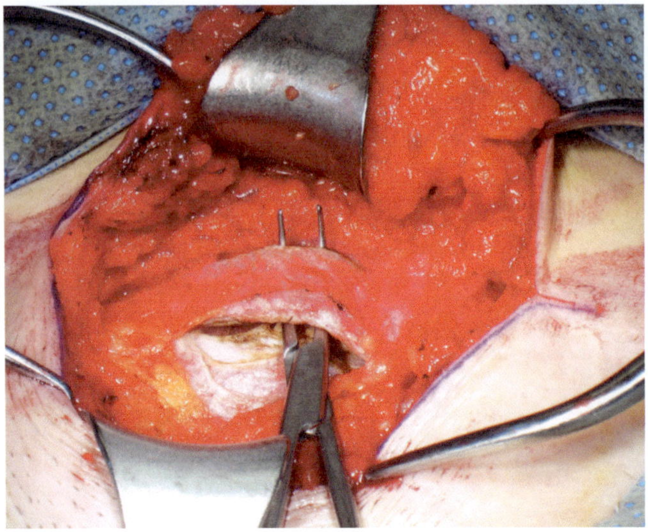

Fig. 2.47 A right-angle clamp is used to free underlying adhesions of the fascia to the anterior wall musculature

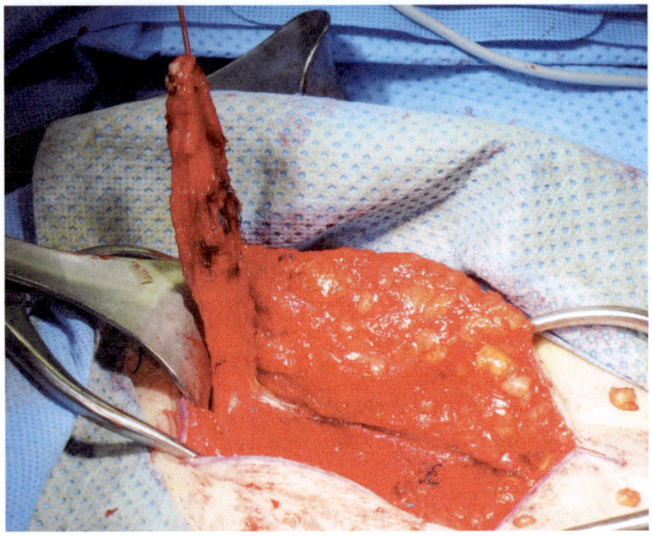

Fig. 2.49 The strip of abdominal wall is dissected toward the right side of the incision and freed from the abdominal musculature

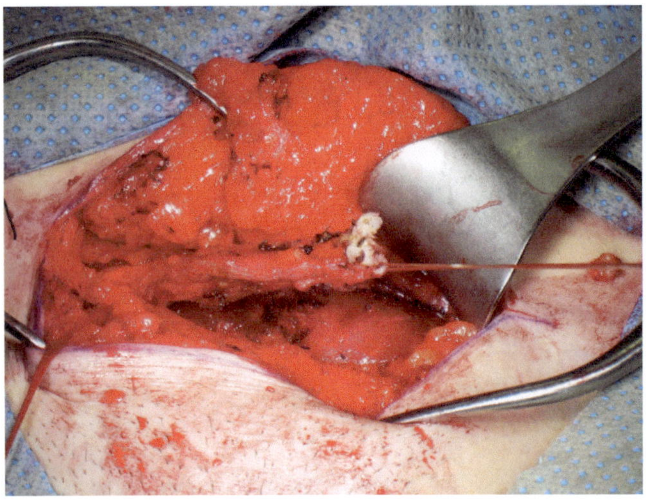

Fig. 2.48 The left side of the fascial strip has been detached from the lateral margin of the incision and multiple passes of a #1 delayed absorbable suture are applied to the end of the fascial strip

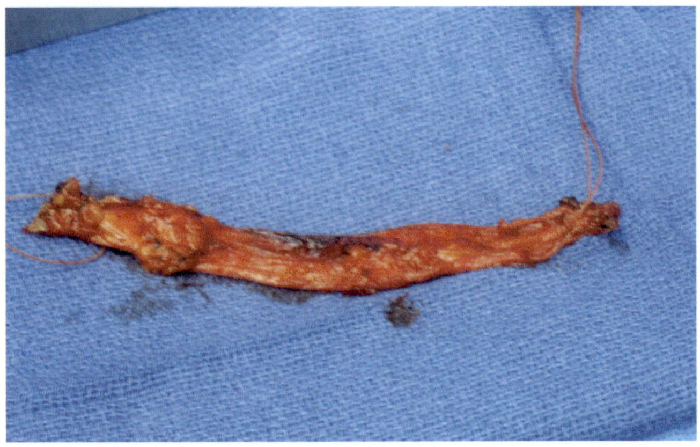

Fig. 2.50 The strip of abdominal wall fascia, measuring 2 × 12 cm, with multiple passes of #1 delayed absorbable at the end of the strip

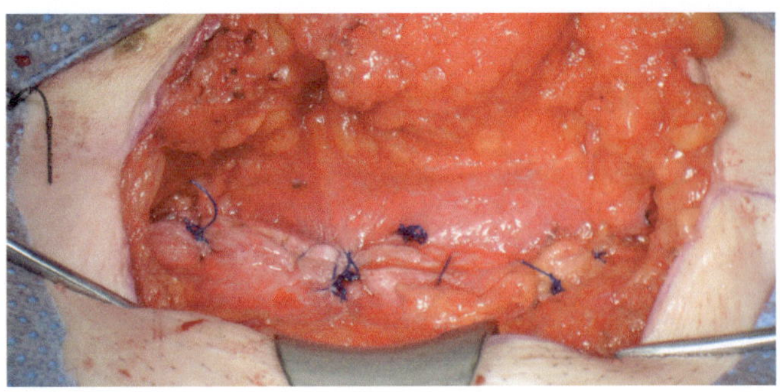

Fig. 2.51 The abdominal wall fascia is closed with multiple figure-of-eight sutures, using #1 delayed absorbable sutures

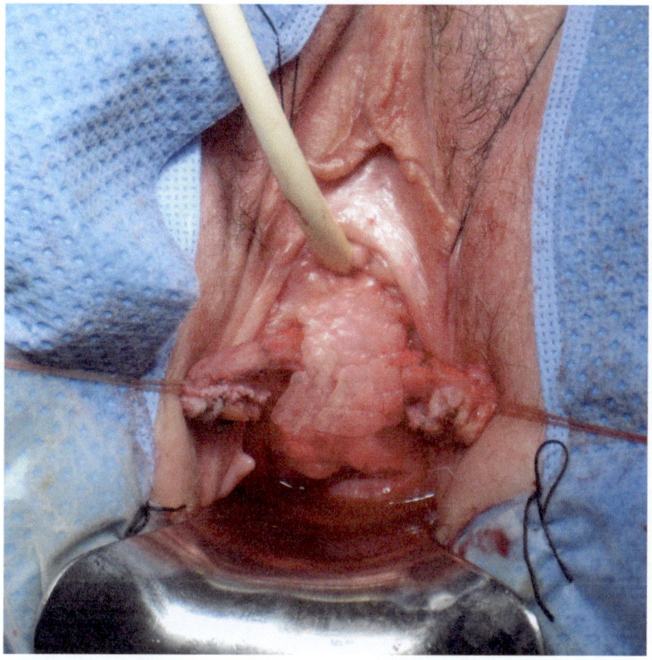

Fig. 2.52 The sling is transferred under the vaginal tunnel

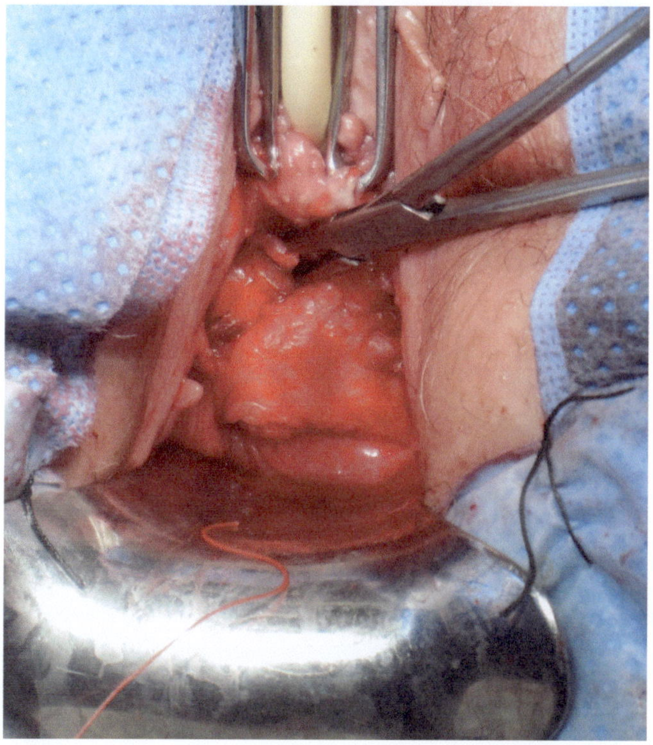

Fig. 2.53 The fascial strip is anchored to the periurethral fascia on the right side only, to prevent displacement during the tying of the sutures in the suprapubic area

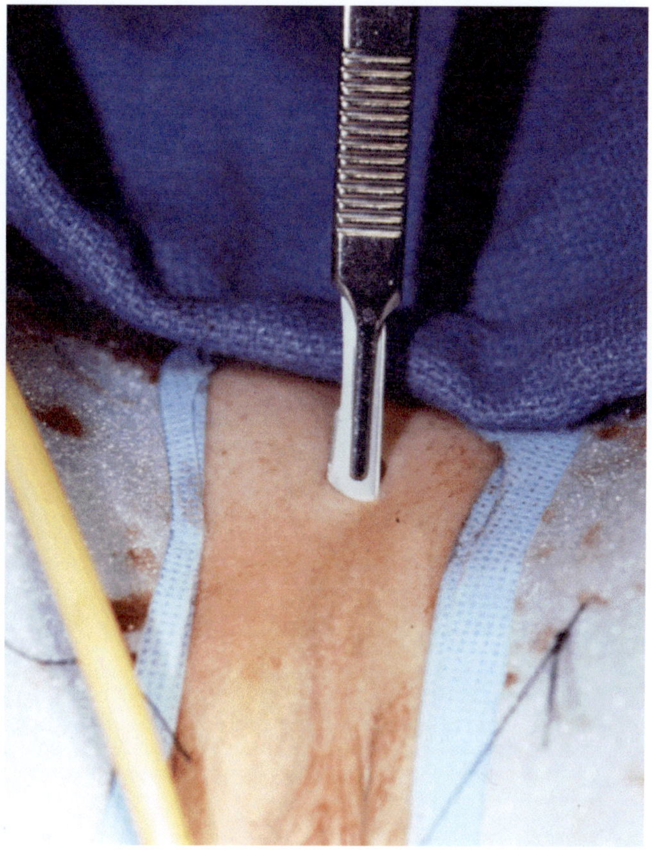

Fig. 2.54 A small suprapubic puncture is performed in the midline, just above the superior margin of the pubic bone. A clamp will be used to dissect a pocket down to the rectus muscle just above the pubic bone

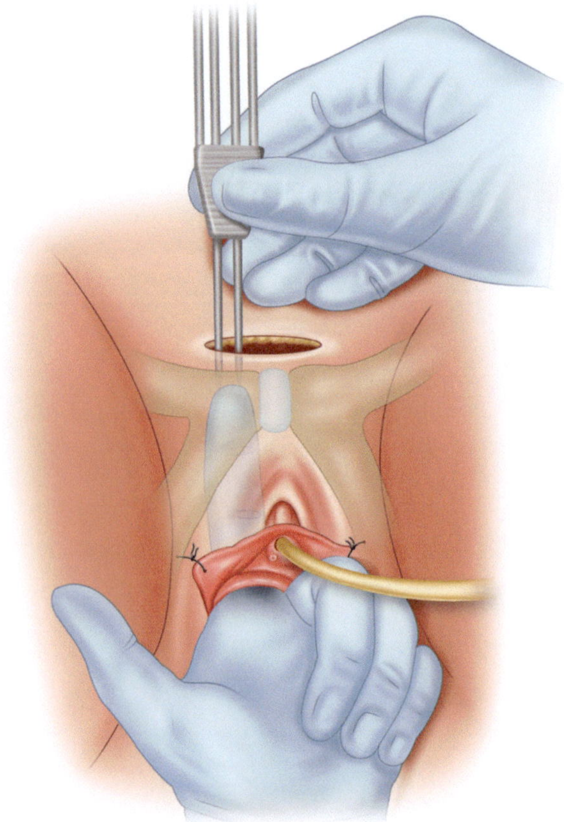

Fig. 2.55 Diagram of the passage of a double-pronged passer (ligature carrier) under finger control in the retropubic space

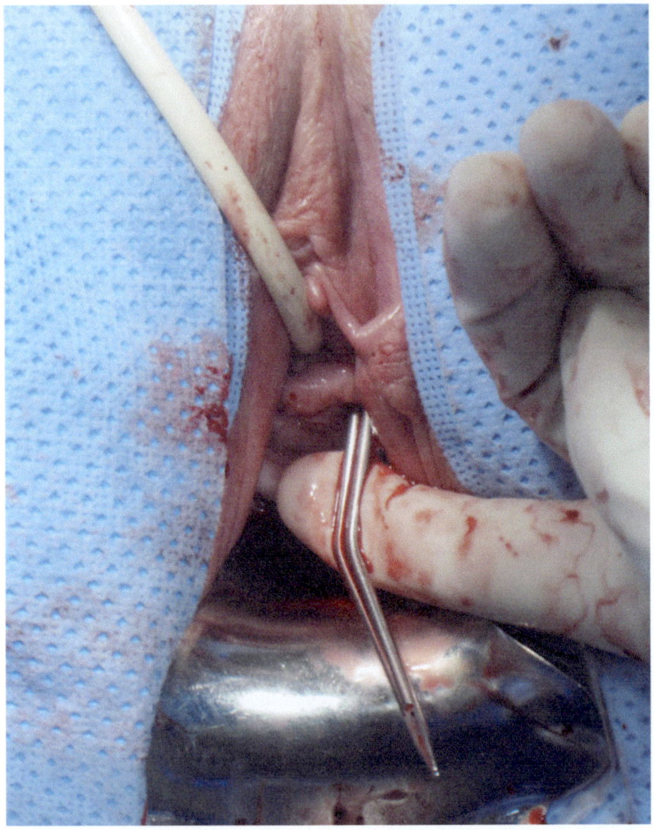

Fig. 2.56 The double-pronged passer is transferred to the vaginal area. The absorbable sutures at the end of the fascial strip are transferred through the eyes of the passer. The passer is retracted up and removed through the suprapubic incision, bringing with it the sutures attached to the sling. Proper positioning of the sling in the retropubic space must be confirmed, as outlined in the text

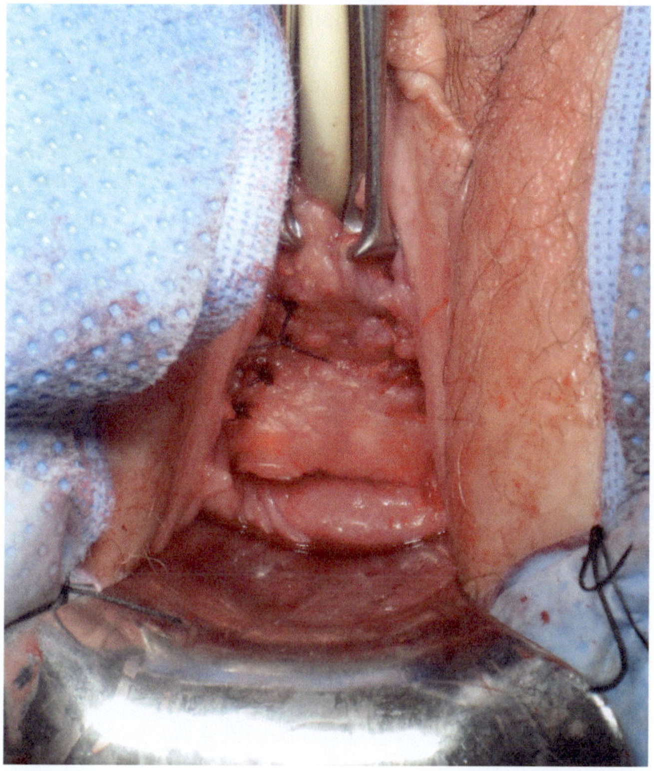

Fig. 2.57 After cystoscopy, the anterior vaginal wall is closed with multiple interrupted absorbable sutures

2.7.3 Surgical Technique: Omega-Shaped Autologous Fascial Sling

This fascial sling modification is used for patients with severe sphincteric damage with poor coaptation and severe incontinence. Instead of providing a U-shaped sling for urethral compression and support, the omega sling crosses anterior to the urethra (*see* Fig. 2.39), providing a more extended circular compression to the urethral wall. The technique is similar to the technique for placement of the classic fascial sling, but the difference is in the technique of passage of the fascial strip in the retropubic space (Figs. 2.58, 2.59, 2.60, 2.61, 2.62, 2.63, 2.64, and 2.65). After entering the retropubic space, all adhesions of the bladder and urethra to the posterior aspect of the pubic bone must be completely free in order to allow the crossover of the sling. Two punctures are performed in the suprapubic area. The double passer is transferred from the right suprapubic puncture to the left vaginal incision to capture the sutures attached to the sling. In the left suprapubic puncture, the passer is transferred through the retropubic space to the right vaginal incision, lateral to the urethra. The ends of the sling sutures are transferred to the suprapubic area. In the retropubic space, the sling is crossed anterior to the urethra, forming an omega-shaped compression.

In some patients with neurogenic incontinence, the sutures may be tied more tightly, to close an open urethra and create intentional urinary retention.

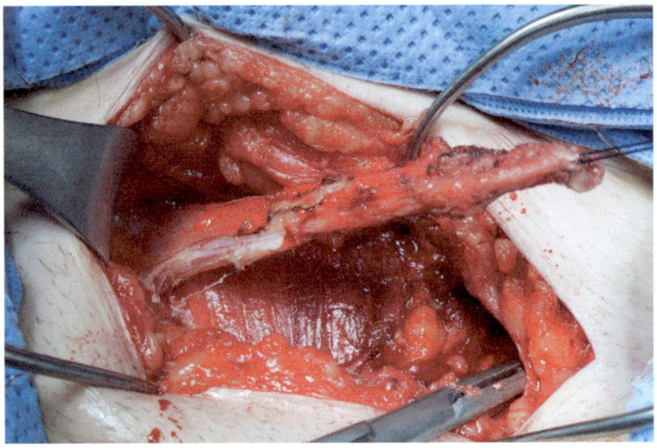

Fig. 2.58 A strip of anterior abdominal wall fascia (2 × 12 cm) is excised. At each end of the fascial strip, we apply #1 delayed absorbable sutures

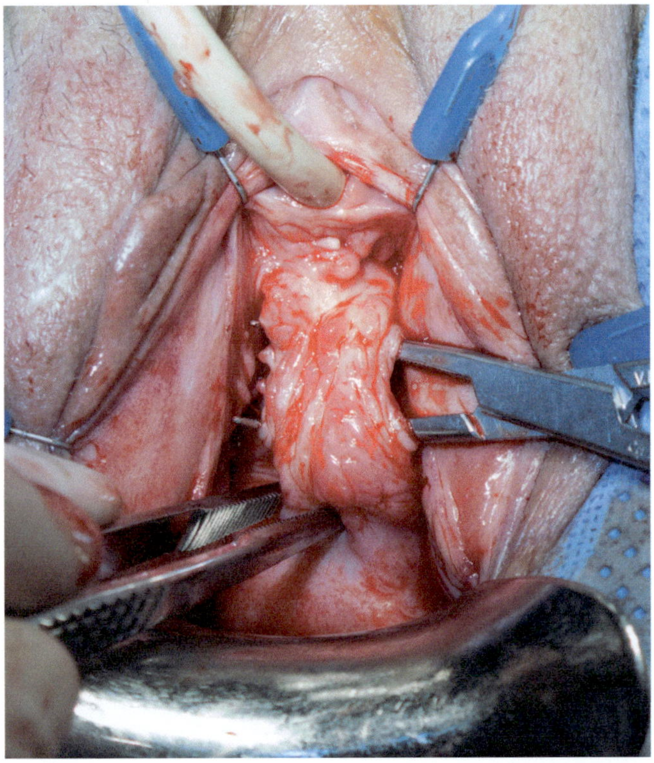

Fig. 2.59 A tunnel is made under the vaginal wall at the midurethral area

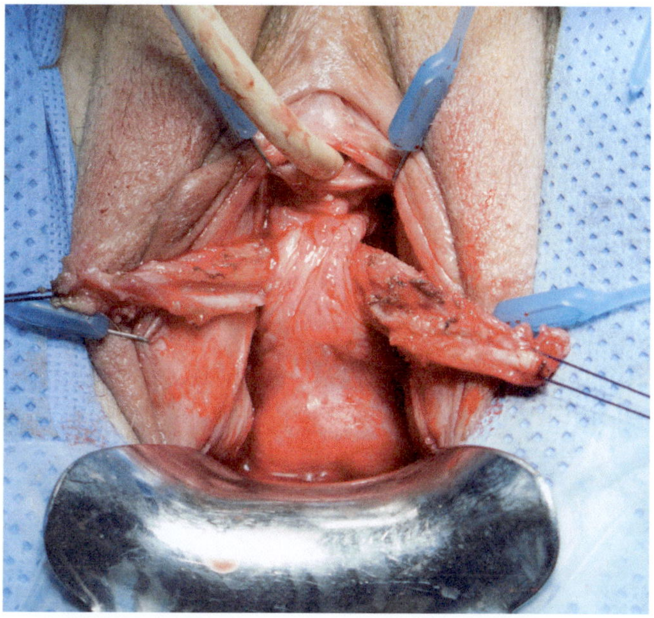

Fig. 2.60 The sling is transferred under the tunnel of the anterior vaginal wall at the midurethral level

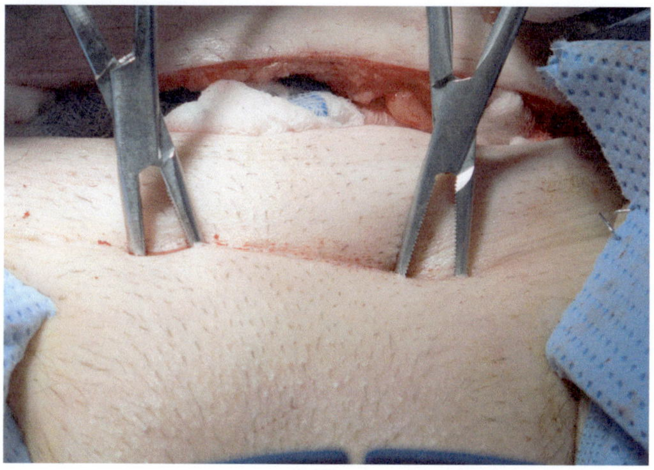

Fig. 2.61 Two punctures are performed in the suprapubic area, 10 cm apart. A clamp is used to create a subcutaneous pocket

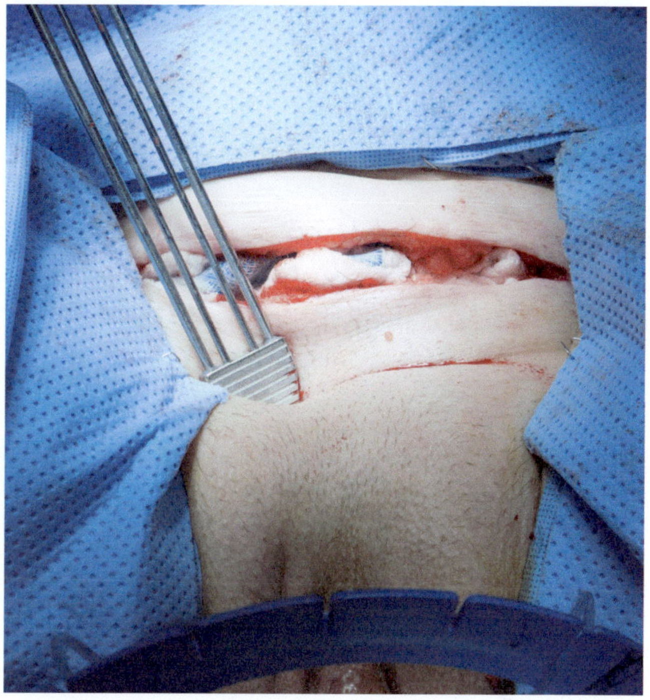

Fig. 2.62 A finger is inserted in the left vaginal incision and through the retropubic space. A double-pronged passer is inserted in the right suprapubic puncture, and the passer will be transferred under finger control to the left periurethral incision

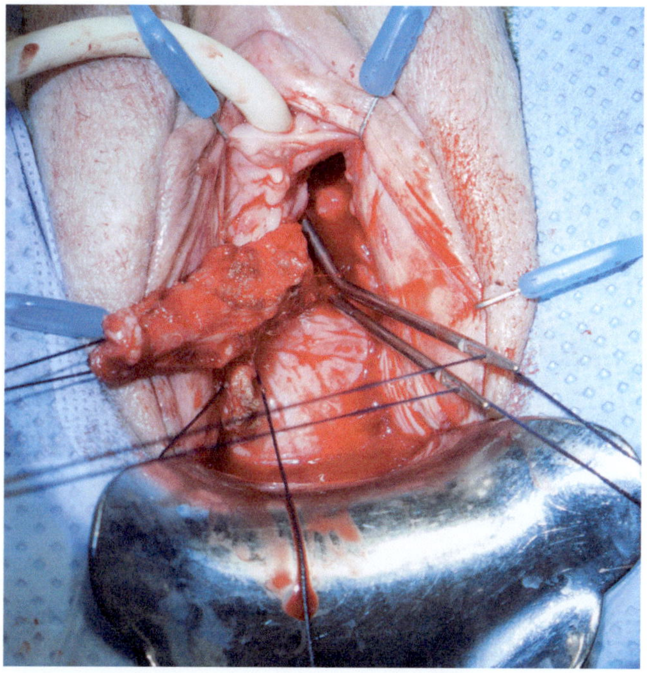

Fig. 2.63 The tips of the double passer are transferred to the left vaginal incision. The eyes of the needle are seen. The ends of the sling sutures are transferred through the eyes of the double passer for a distance of 10 cm. The same maneuver is performed on the contralateral side, transferring the passer from the left suprapubic puncture to the right vaginal incision. The sutures at the end of the right side of the sling are transferred to the left suprapubic area

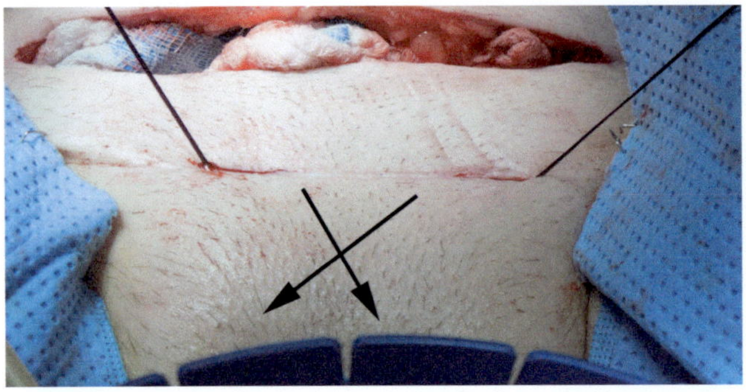

Fig. 2.64 The suprapubic area is seen after the sutures have been transferred. The suture in the right puncture anchors the left side of the sling, and the suture in the left puncture anchors the right side of the sling, creating the omega-shaped retropubic compression. The *arrows* indicate the direction of the double passer and the supporting sutures in the retropubic space

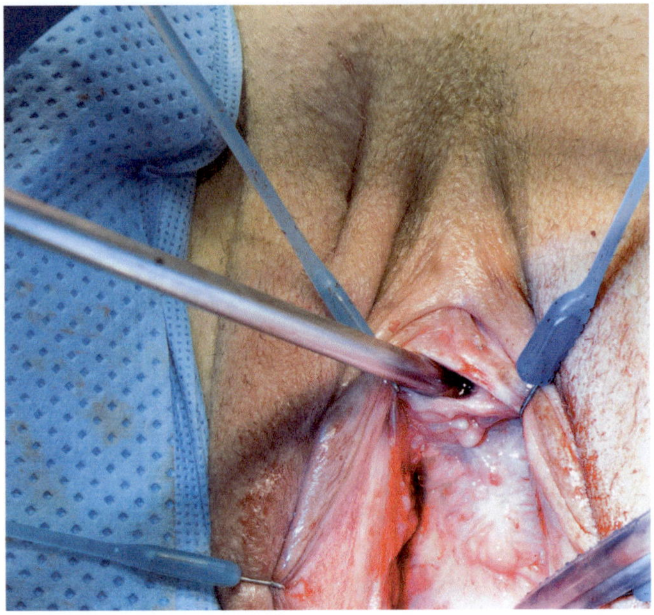

Fig. 2.65 Cystoscopy is performed to rule out any urethral or bladder injury. The suprapubic sutures are tied without tension

2.8 Fascia Lata Autologous Fascial Sling

2.8.1 Autologous Fascial Sling Using Fascia Lata

Although most surgeons used abdominal fascia for autologous fascial sling, we strongly prefer an old technique of fascial retrieval from the lateral thigh (iliotibial band of the tensor fascia lata) (Fig. 2.66). The technique is minimally invasive and is particularly useful in obese patients and patients with multiple abdominal surgeries. The tensor fascia lata and the gluteal muscle form a tendinous extension to the tibia called the iliotibial band. This strong tendon of the fascia lata extends lateral to the thigh inserting into the superior lateral tibial bone. A segment of 10–12 cm by 1–2 cm is retrieved, at the end of which we apply #0 or #1 delayed absorbable sutures. A tunnel is made under the vaginal wall and the sling material is transferred under the tunnel. Using a double-pronged passer, the sutures are transferred under finger control in the retropubic space from the vagina to the suprapubic area.

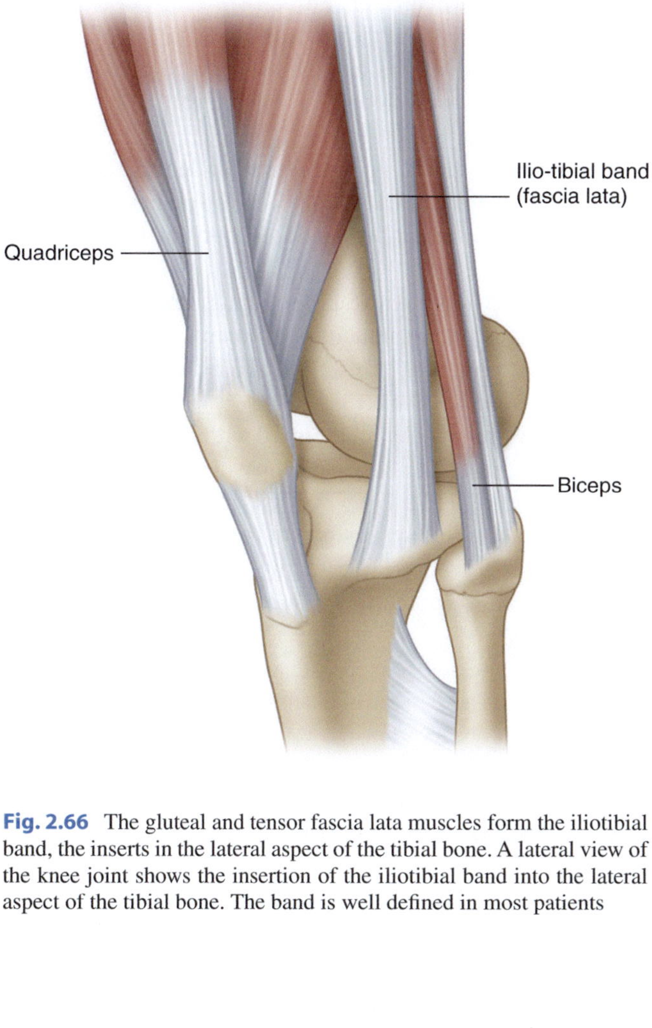

Fig. 2.66 The gluteal and tensor fascia lata muscles form the iliotibial band, the inserts in the lateral aspect of the tibial bone. A lateral view of the knee joint shows the insertion of the iliotibial band into the lateral aspect of the tibial bone. The band is well defined in most patients

2.8.2 Surgical Technique

The first part of the surgery is the retrieval of the fascial segment. The patient is placed in the tort position with elevation of the thigh and knee over a pillow. The inferior part of the lateral thigh and knee is prepared and draped (Fig. 2.67).

A horizontal incision is made on the lateral thigh 8–10 cm above the knee joint. Dissection is carried out of the subcutaneous tissues to expose the tendineus segment of the fascia lata (iliotibial band). The fascia is in general thick and different from the rest of the fascia covering the lateral musculature. The proper segment should be selected. Two parallel incisions are made 1–2 cm apart (Fig. 2.68).

A right-angle clamp is used to isolate the strip of the fascia from the underlying musculature (Fig. 2.69).

The fascia is transected inferiorly and #1 delayed absorbable sutures are applied to the free end of the fascial strip. Multiple passes of the needle are required to obtain a strong anchoring effect (Fig. 2.70).

Sharp and blunt dissection is used superior to the fascia to separate the fascia from the subcutaneous tissues for a distance of 10 cm. The fascia is also dissected sharply and bluntly from the underlying lateral musculature to facilitate the fascial incision (Fig. 2.71).

The Crawford fascial stripper is used. The device consists of two sliding elements with a rotational circular plate (*arrow*) that prevents the advancement of the cutting blade. The inner segment contains a cutting blade that transects the fascial strip when activated (Fig. 2.72).

The inner segment is retracted to show the cutting blade (*arrow*). Advancement of this segment will transect the sling at the desired point (Fig. 2.73).

The sutures applied at the end of the fascia are transferred through the tip of the fascial stripper, and the end of the fascia will also be transferred for a distance of 4–5 cm (Fig. 2.74).

A clamp is applied to the end of the fascial segment to provide countertraction at the time of the advancement of the stripper (Fig. 2.75).

The stripper is advanced in the subcutaneous tissues in the direction of the fascia lata fibers for the desired distance, in general 10–12 cm. The device is activated. The fascial strip is transected and retrieved from the incision (Fig. 2.76).

The fascial strip is removed and another #1 delayed absorbable suture is applied to the free end. The fascia lata segment is placed in antibiotic solution. The wound is closed in two layers of #2-0 delayed absorbable sutures in the subcutaneous and #4-0 in the skin (Fig. 2.77).

Pneumatic stocking is applied to the lower extremities, the patient is placed in lithotomy position, and the vaginal wall is prepared and draped.

Exposure of the anterior vaginal wall is obtained after insertion of a Foley catheter (Fig. 2.78).

Two oblique incisions are made in the distal lateral vagina. The retropubic is entered in each side and all adhesions are freed. A tunnel is made under the vaginal wall, 2 cm from the external meatus (Fig. 2.79).

The strip of fascia is transferred under the tunnel. A delayed absorbable suture is applied to the periurethral fascia and the fascial sling in one side, to prevent displacement (Fig. 2.80).

A small incision is made in the suprapubic area. Using a double-pronged passer, under finger control in the retropubic space, the sutures are transferred from the vagina to the suprapubic puncture area (Fig. 2.81).

The anterior vaginal wall is closed with interrupted figure-of-eight sutures after the cystoscopy and the tying of the siprapubic sutures (Fig. 2.82).

After the cystoscopy, cystocopy is performed to rule out intravesical lesions. Two Allis clamps are kept the horizontal plane and the suprapubic sutures tied without tension (Fig. 2.83).

A vaginal packing soaked with antibiotics will be inserted in the vagina. The patient is discharged home the same day or after a 24-h observation.

2.8.3 Postoperative Care

This is similar to other sling procedures.

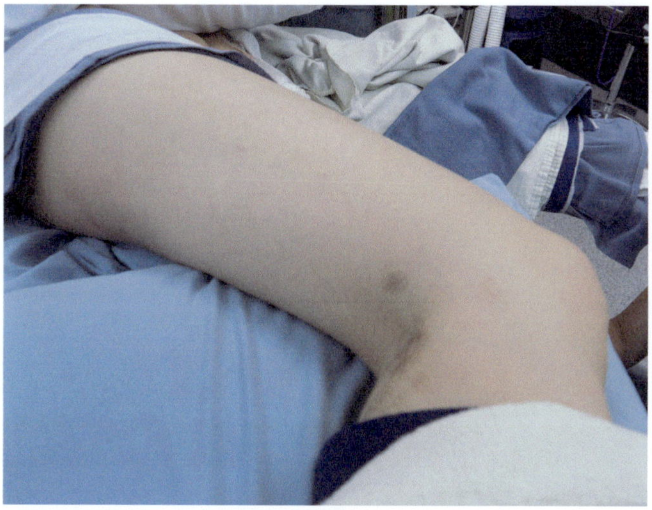

Fig. 2.67 The first part of the surgery is the retrieval of the fascial segment. The patient is placed in the tort position with elevation of the thigh and knee over a pillow. The inferior part of the lateral thigh and knee is prepared and draped

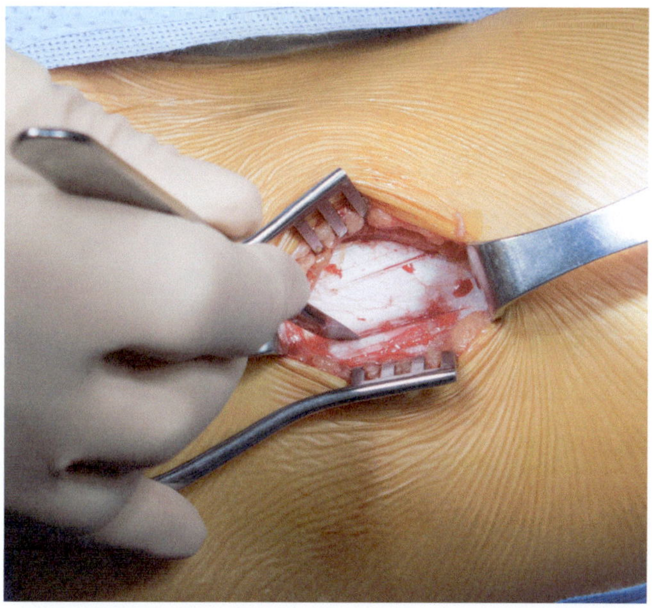

Fig. 2.68 A vertical is made on the lateral thigh 3–4 cm above the knee joint. Dissection is carried out of the subcutaneous tissues to expose the tendineus segment of the fascia lata muscle. The fascia is in general thick and different from the rest of the fascia covering the lateral musculature. The proper segment should be selected. Two parallel incisions are made 1–2 cm apart

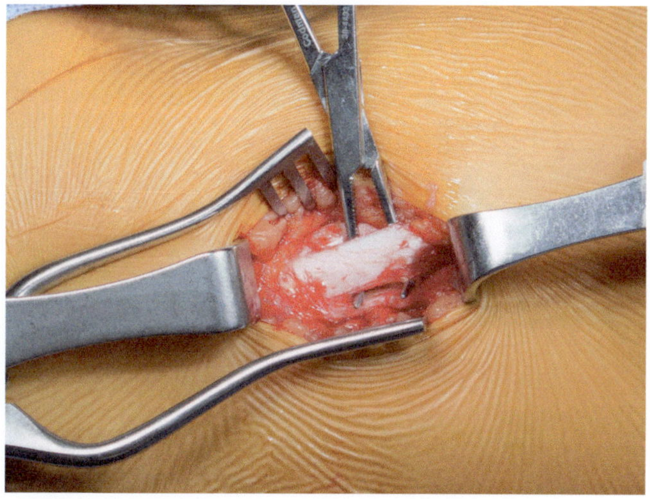

Fig. 2.69 A right-angle clamp is used to isolate the strip of fascia from the underlying musculature

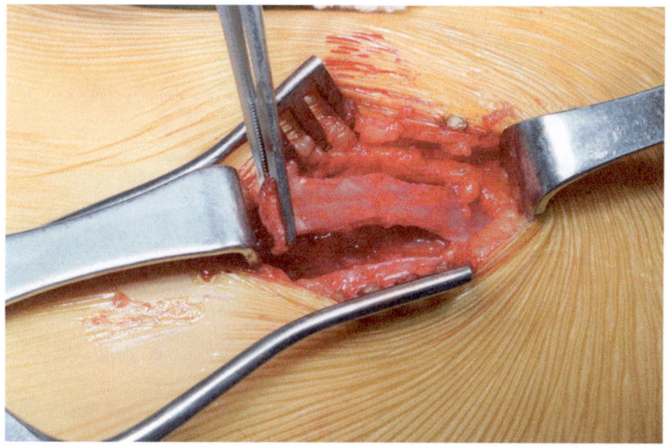

Fig. 2.70 The fascia is transected inferiorly and #1 delayed absorbable sutures are applied to the free end of the fascial strip. Multiple passes of the needle are required to obtain a strong anchoring effect

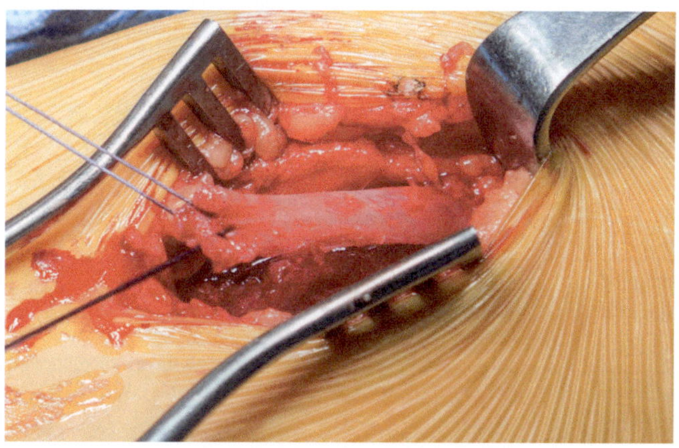

Fig. 2.71 Sharp and blunt dissection is used superior to the fascia to separate the fascia from the subcutaneous tissues for a distance of 10 cm. The fascia is also dissected sharply and bluntly from the underlying lateral musculature to facilitate the fascial incision

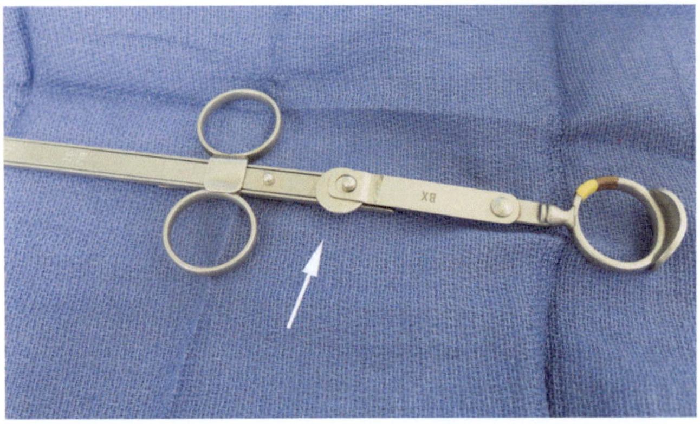

Fig. 2.72 The Crawford fascial stripper is used. The device consists of two sliding elements with a circular plate (*arrow*) that prevents the advancement of the cutting blade. The inner segment contains a cutting blade that will transect the fascial strip when activated

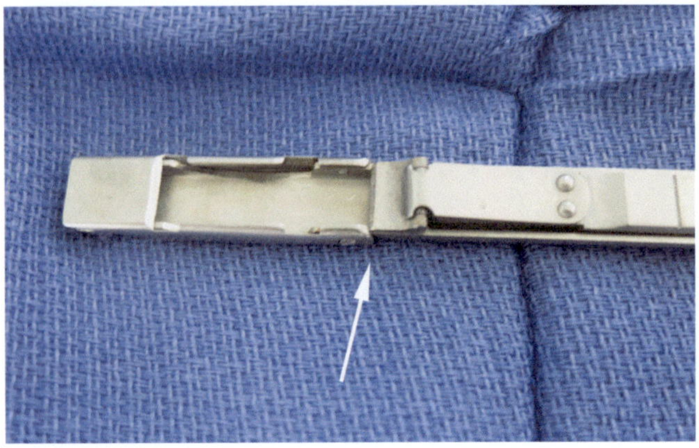

Fig. 2.73 Close view of the distal segment of the fascial stripper. The inner segment is retracted to show the cutting blade (*arrow*). Advancement of this segment will transect the sling at the desired point

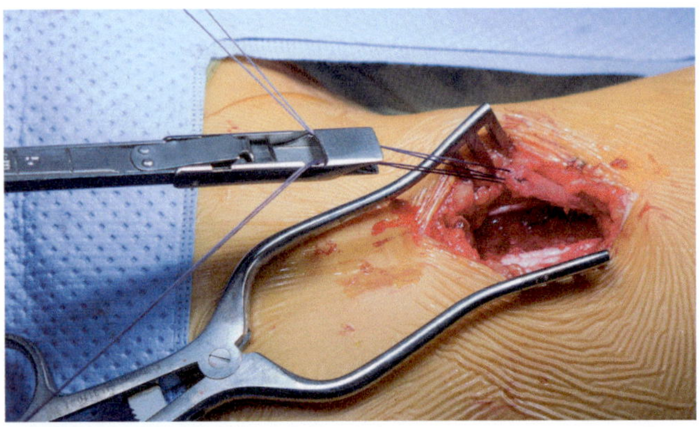

Fig. 2.74 The sutures applied at the end of fascia are transferred through the tip of the fascial stripper, and the end of the fascia will also be transferred for a distance of 4–5 cm

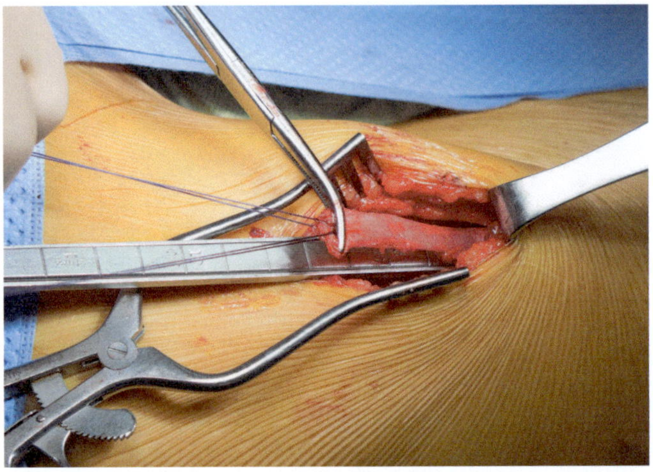

Fig. 2.75 A clamp is applied to the end of the fascial segment to provide countertraction at the time of the advancement of the stripper

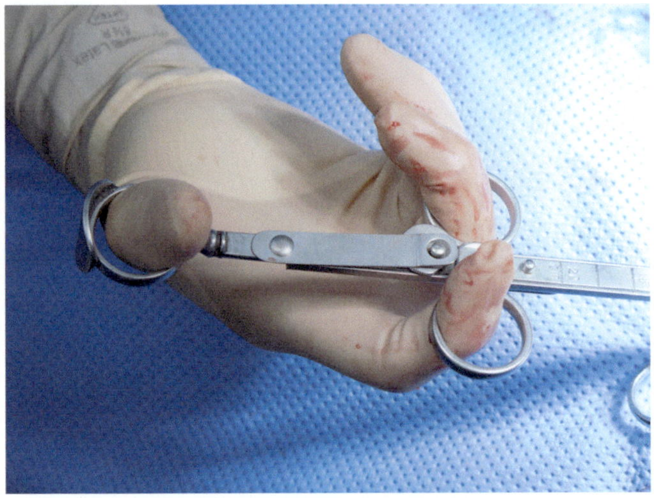

Fig. 2.76 The stripper is advanced in the subcutaneous tissues in the direction of the fascia lata fibers for the desired distance, in general 10–12 cm. The device is activated. The fascial strip is transected and retrieved from the incision

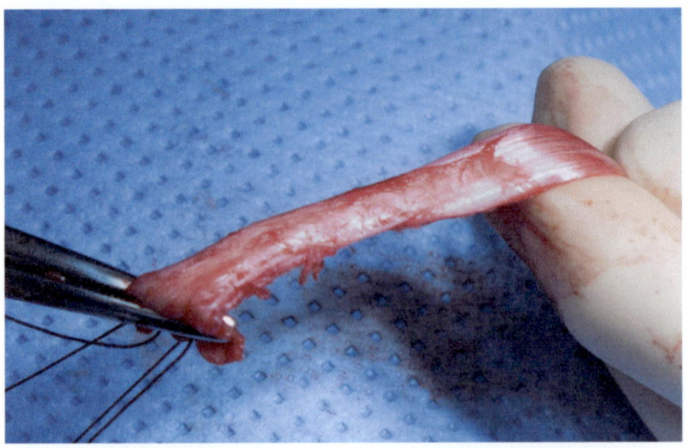

Fig. 2.77 The fascial strip is removed and another #1 delayed absorbable suture is applied to the free end. The fascia lata segment is placed in antibiotic solution. The wound is closed in two layers of #2-0 delayed absorbable sutures in the subcutaneous and #4-0 in the skin

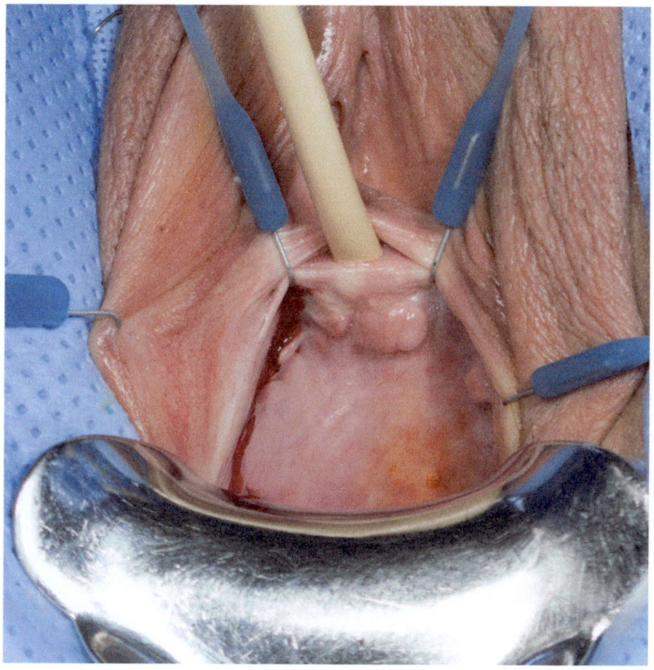

Fig. 2.78 Exposure of the anterior vaginal wall is obtained after insertion of a Foley catheter

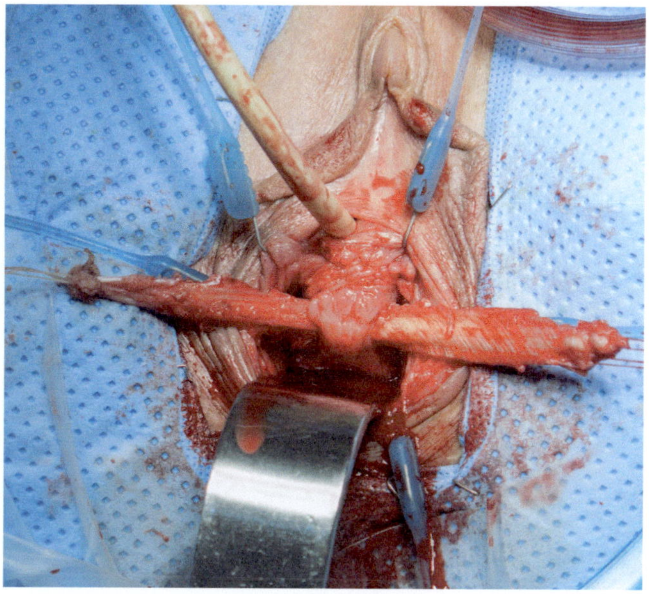

Fig. 2.80 A small incision is made in the suprapubic area. Using a double-pronged passer, under finger control in the retropubic space, the sutures are transferred from the vagina to the suprapubic puncture area

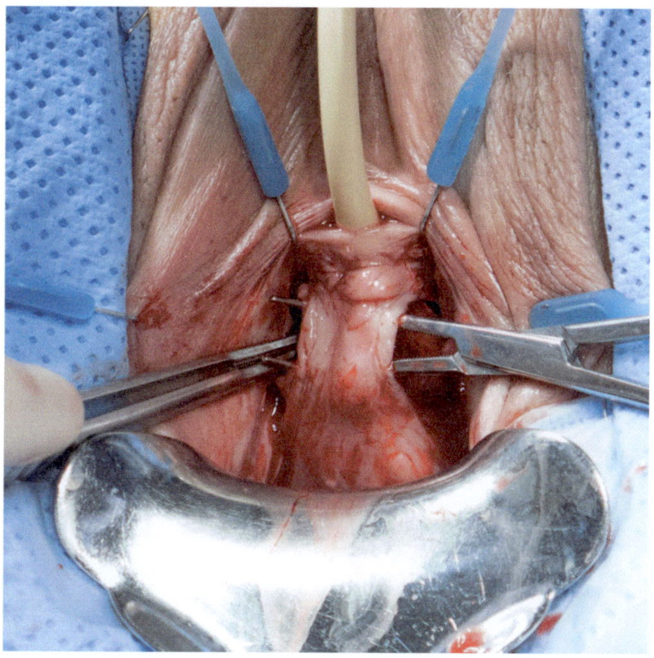

Fig. 2.79 Two oblique incisions are made in the distal lateral vagina. The retropubic is entered in each side and all adhesions are freed. A tunnel is made under the vaginal wall, 2 cm from the external meatus

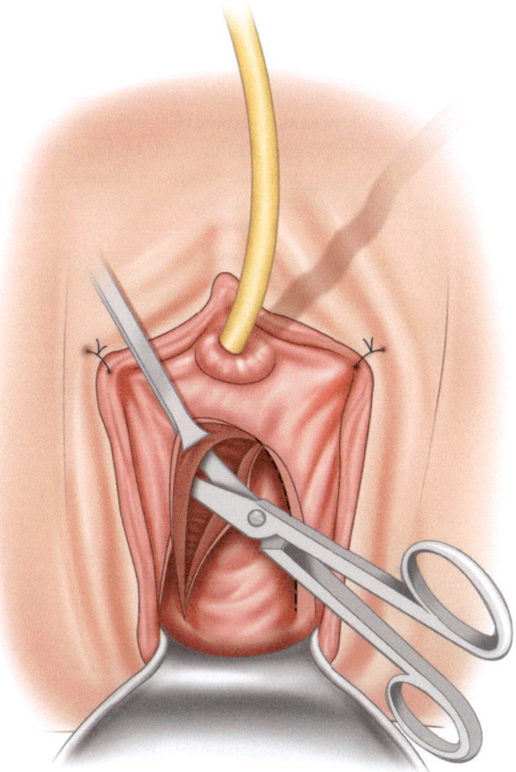

Fig. 2.81 The anterior vaginal wall is closed with interrupted figure-of-eight sutures

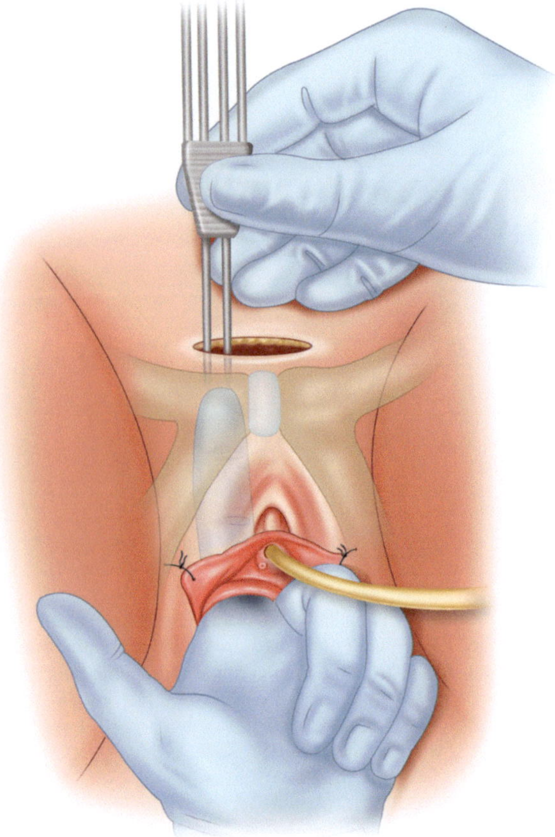

Fig. 2.82 After the cystoscopy, the sheet of the cystoscope is kept in a 45° angulation and the suprapubic sutures are tied without tension. A vaginal packing soaked with antibiotics will be inserted in the vagina. The patient is discharged home the same day or after 24-h observation

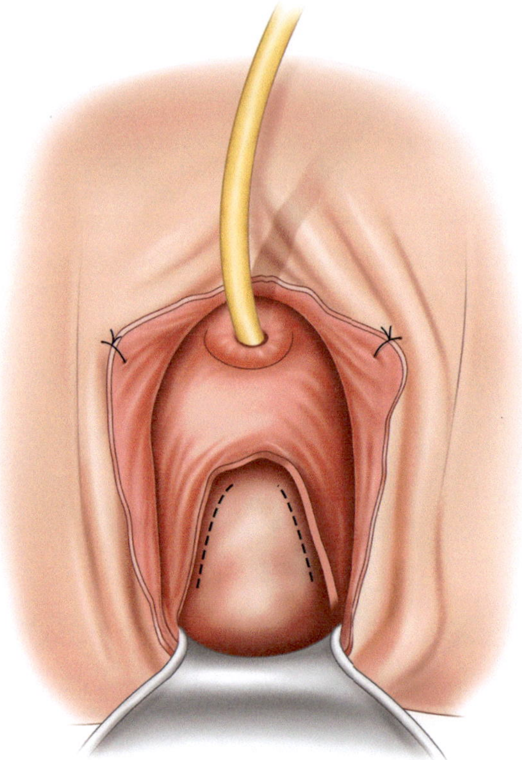

Fig. 2.83 Diagram of the exposure of the anterior vaginal wall, with two oblique incisions in the distal vagina

2.9 Spiral Slings

2.9.1 Indications-Surgical Technique

The spiral sling procedure is designed for the treatment of patients with severe stress incontinence. The patient is placed in the dorsal lithotomy position. The lower abdomen and vagina are prepped and draped in a sterile fashion. If required the labia are retracted laterally with stay sutures. A Foley catheter is inserted into the urethra and the bladder is emptied. A weighted vaginal speculum and a ring retractor with hooks are used (Figs. 2.84, 2.85, 2.86, 2.87, 2.88, 2.89, 2.90, 2.91, 2.92, 2.93, and 2.94). After distal vaginal incisions are made bilaterally, a tunnel is made in the anterior vaginal wall between the two incisions, 2 cm from the external meatus. A complete urethrolysis is performed, and all adhesions of the urethra and bladder to the posterior aspect of the pubic bone are freed. A segment of 15 × 1 cm of fascia lata segment is prepared and, at each end, a #1 delayed absorbable suture is applied. A Derra or other sharp angulated clamp is inserted into the retropubic space in one side of the vaginal incision and brought to the contralateral incision. The graft is transferred through the retropubic space. A right-angle clamp is passed under the vaginal tunnel from the left to the right side of the vaginal tunnel, and the end of the fascial strip is transferred to the left side of the vaginal incision. From the right side, the mesh is transferred from the left side of the vaginal incision to the right. On completion of the transfer, we have created a complete circle around the urethra. The sutures at the end of the fascial strip will be transferred to the suprapubic area and tied after a cystoscopy has been performed.

2.9.2 Surgical Technique

A vaginal packing soak with antibiotics will be inserted.

2.9.3 Postoperative Complications

The complications are similar to those of other anti-incontinence procedures. The use of this technique in patients with significant sphincteric damage increases the potential for temporary obstruction. Attention should be paid to tie the suprapubic sutures loosely. Light countertraction of the sling at the time of suprapubic suture tying will prevent excessive tensioning of the sling against the urethral wall. In case of urinary retention, the patient is instructed on self-catheterization. If retention continues after 6–8 weeks, a limited sling incision may be required.

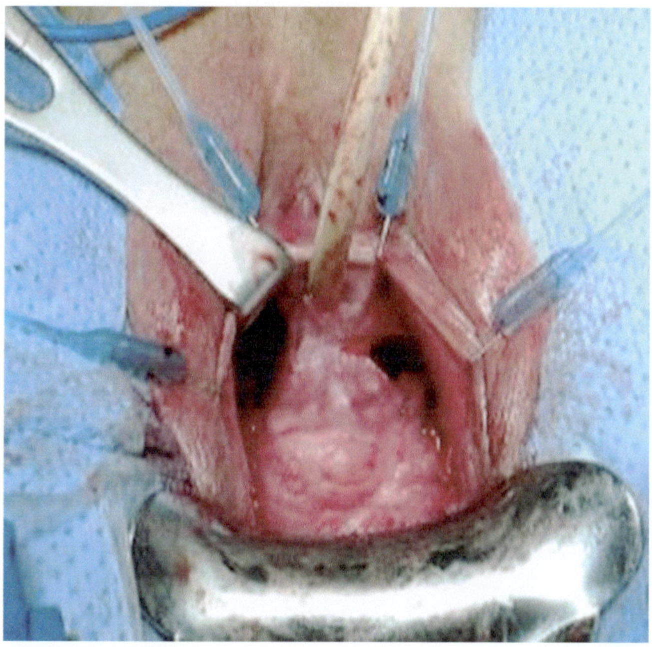

Fig. 2.84 Two oblique incisions are made in the anterior vaginal wall. The retropubic space is entered and all adhesions of the bladder and urethra are freed

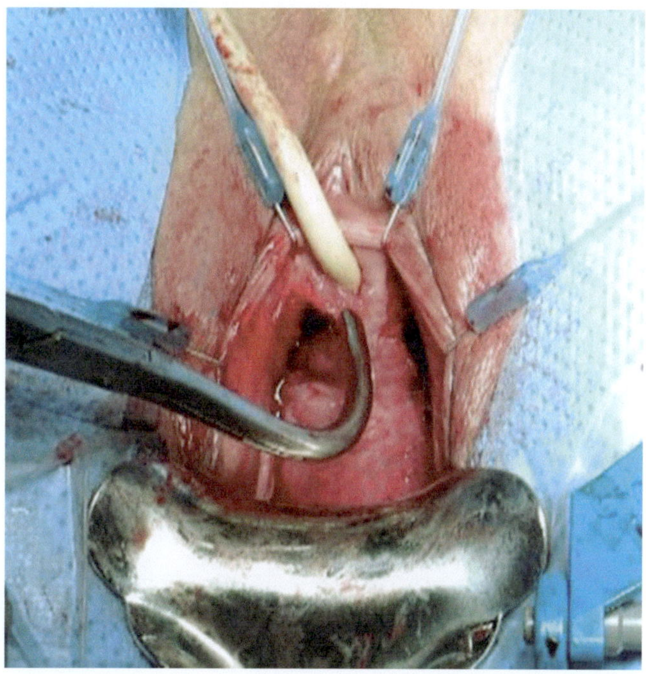

Fig. 2.85 A curved clamp is seen lateral to the vaginal incision

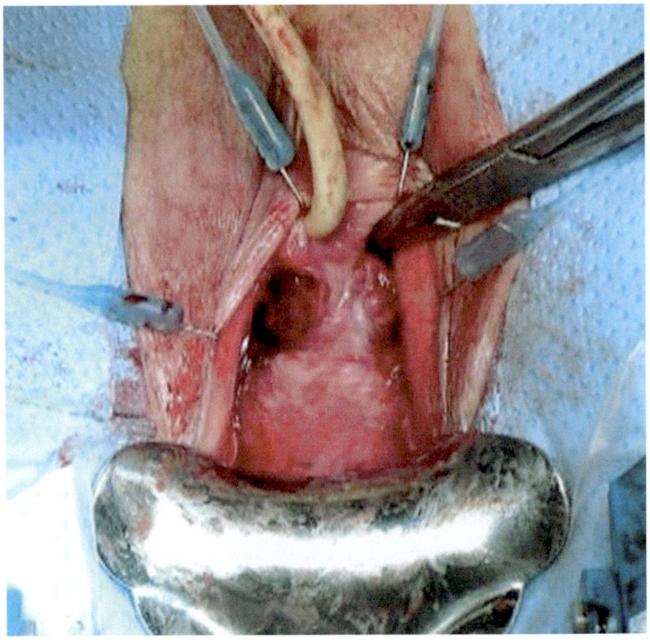

Fig. 2.86 Under finger control in the retropubic space just anterior and distal to the urethra, the clamp is transferred through the retropubic space from the left vaginal incision to the right side

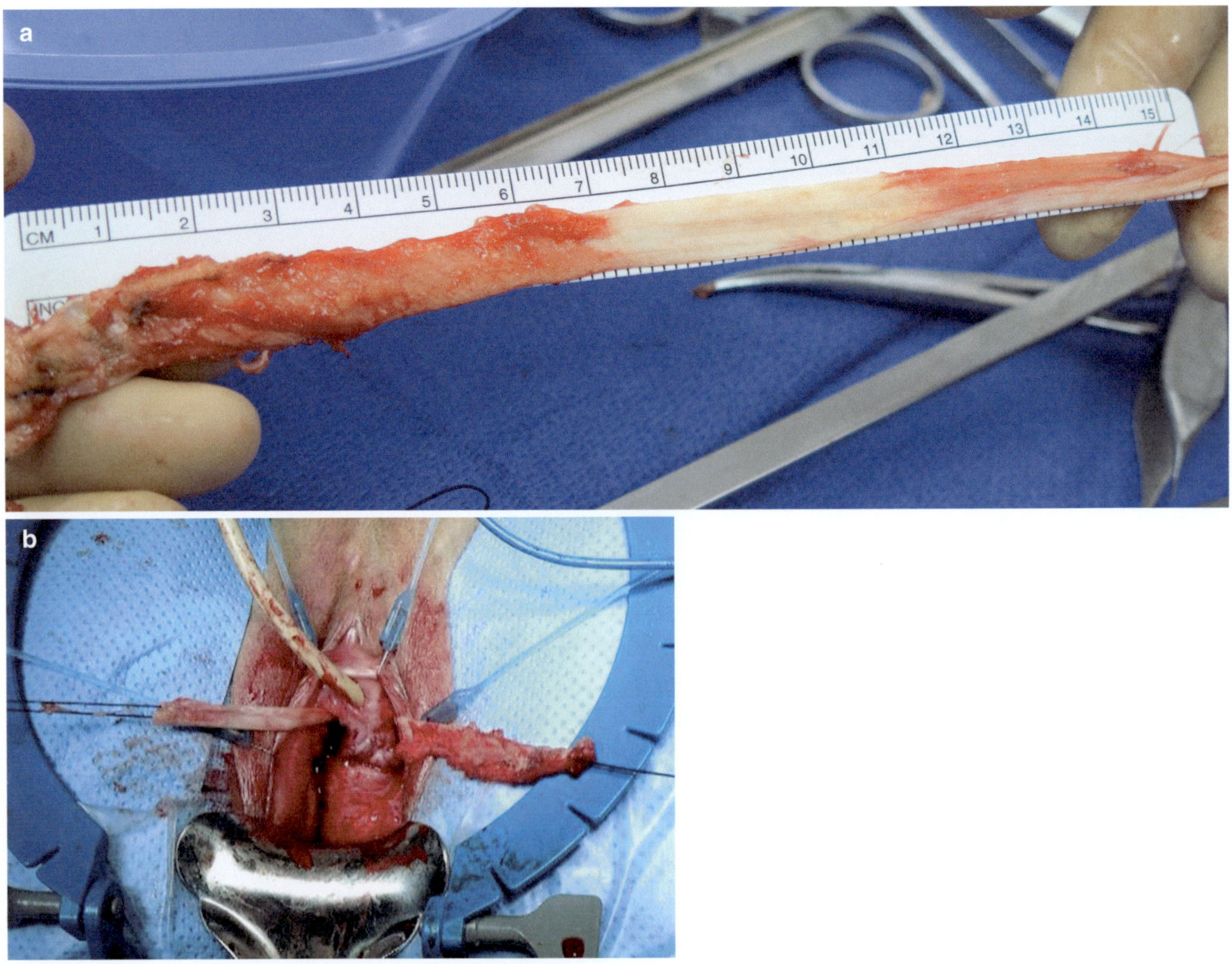

Fig. 2.87 (**a**) A 15 × 1 cm segment of fascia lata is prepared. At each end, a #1 delayed absorbable suture is applied. (**b**) The fascia is transferred through the retropubic space between the urethra and the pubic bone

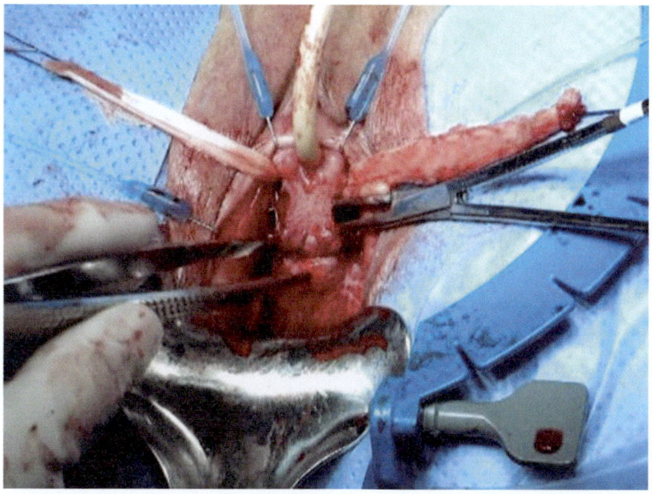

Fig. 2.88 A tunnel is made under the vaginal wall at the midurethral level

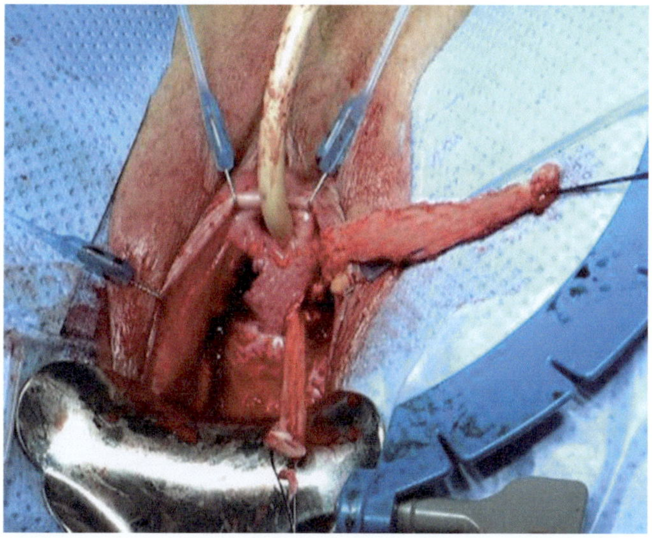

Fig. 2.89 The right side of the fascia is transferred under the vaginal tunnel to the left side

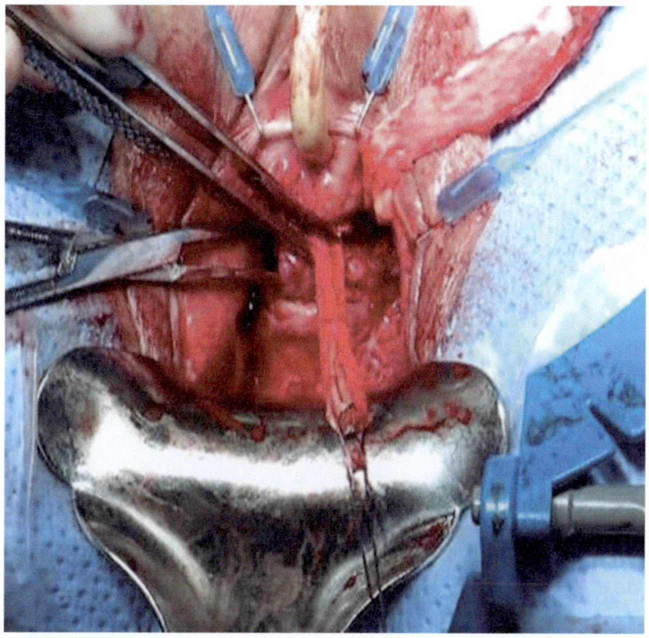

Fig. 2.90 The left side of the fascial segment will be transferred to the right side of the tunnel

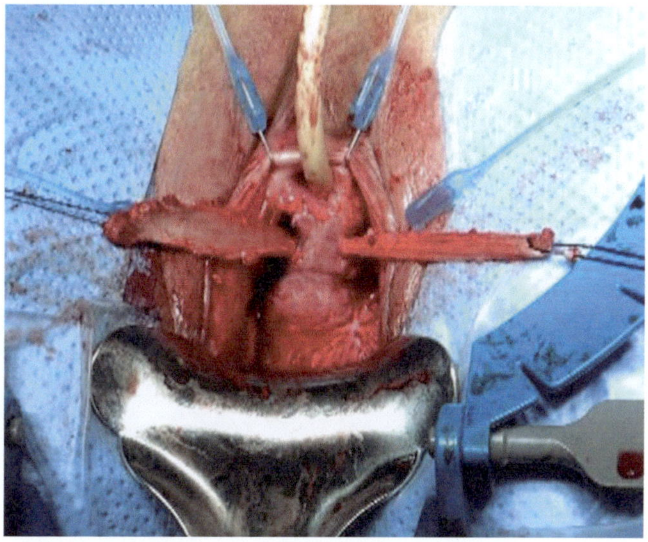

Fig. 2.91 Both ends of the fascial segment have been transferred, completing the circle around the urethra

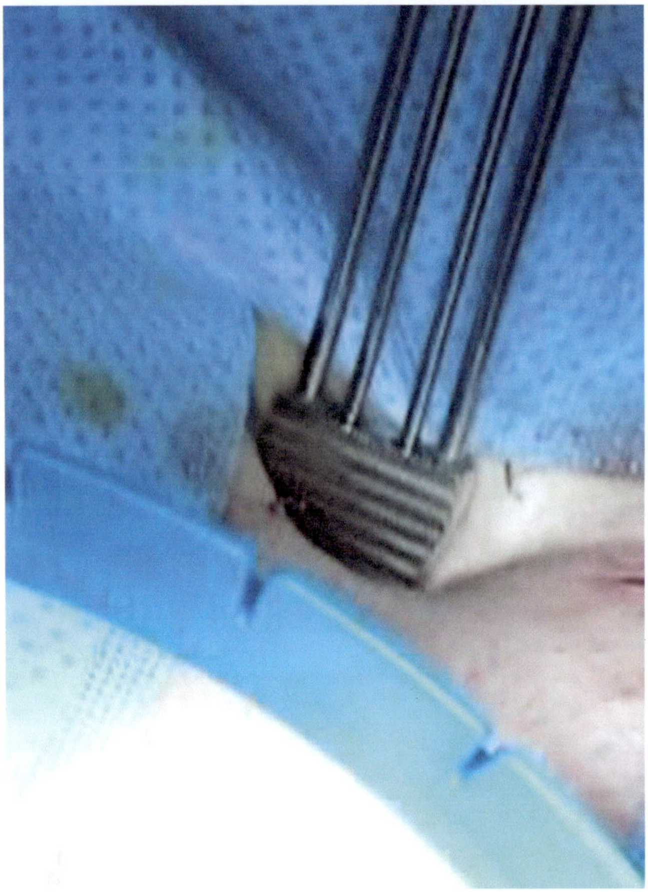

Fig. 2.92 A small suprapubic puncture is performed. A double-pronged passer is transferred, under finger control in the retropubic space, from the suprapubic to the vaginal area

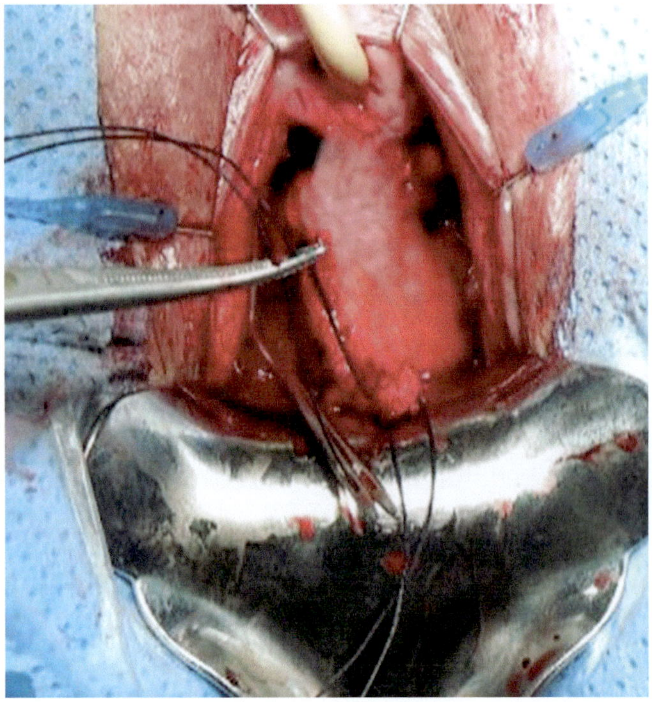

Fig. 2.93 The absorbable sutures are transferred through the needle holes of the passer for a distance of 10 cm. The passer is pulled to the suprapubic area, carrying the delayed absorbable sutures

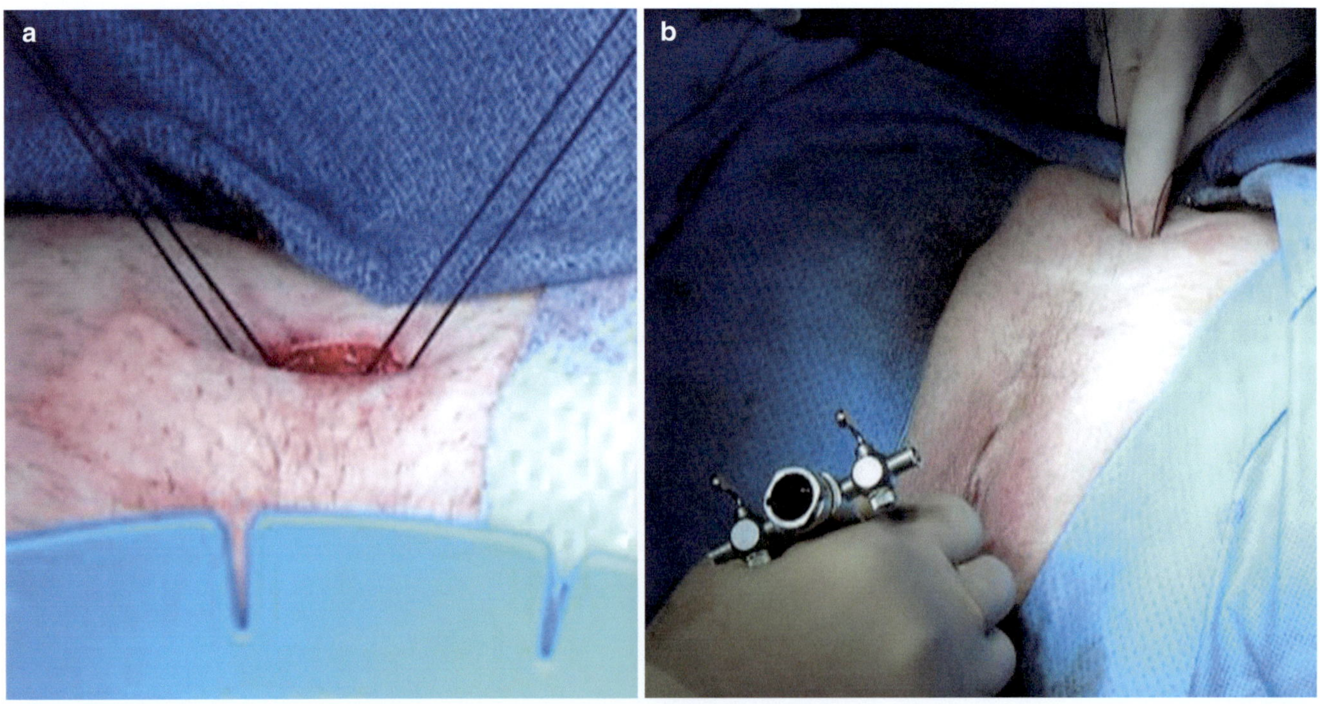

Fig. 2.94 (**a**) The suprapubic incision and sutures are seen. (**b**) Cystoscopy will be performed, the sutures will be tied using two Allis clamps to keep the sling in an horizontal plane and the anterior vaginal wall will be closed with several delayed absorbable sutures

Suggested Reading

Agur W, Riad M, Secco S, Litman H, Madhuvrata P, Novara G, et al. Surgical treatment of recurrent stress urinary incontinence in women: a systematic review and meta-analysis of randomized controlled trials. Eur Urol. 2013;64(2):323–36.

Albo ME, Richter HE, Brubaker L, Norton P, Kraus SR, Zimmern PE, Urinary Incontinence Treatment Network, et al. Burch colposuspension versus fascial sling to reduce urinary stress incontinence. N Engl J Med. 2007;356:2143–55.

Banakhar MA, Al-Shaiji TF, Hassouna MM. Pathophysiology of overactive bladder. Int Urogynecol J. 2012;23:975–82.

Brubaker L, Richter HE, Norton PA, Albo M, Zyczynski HM, Chai TC, Urinary Incontinence Treatment Network, et al. 5-year continence rates, satisfaction and adverse events of burch urethropexy and fascial sling surgery for urinary incontinence. J Urol. 2012;187(4):1324–30.

Chapple CR, Monassero F. Pathophysiology of stress incontinence. In: Raz S, Rodriguez L, editors. Female urology. 3rd ed. Philadelphia: Saunders-Elsevier; 2008. p. 301.

Committee Opinion No. 603: Evaluation of uncomplicated stress urinary incontinence in women before surgical treatment. Obstet Gynecol. 2014;123(6):1403–7.

Delancey J. What causes stress incontinence: fallacies, fascias and facts. Can Urol Assoc J. 2012;6(5 Suppl 2):S114–5.

deTayrac R, Deffieux X, Droupy S, Chauveaud-Lambling A, Calvanèse-Benamour L, Fernandez H. A prospective randomized trial comparing tension-free vaginal tape and transobturator suburethral tape for surgical treatment of stress urinary incontinence. Am J Obstet Gynecol. 2004;190:602–8.

Glazener CM, Cooper K. Bladder neck needle suspension for urinary incontinence in women. Cochrane Database Syst Rev. 2014;(12):CD003636. doi:10.1002/14651858.CD003636.pub3.

Leach GE, Dmochowski RR, Appell RA, Blaivas JG, Hadley HR, Luber KM, et al. Female Stress Urinary Incontinence Clinical Guidelines Panel summary report on surgical management of female stress urinary incontinence. The American Urological Association. J Urol. 1997;158:875–80.

Mansoor A, Vedrine N, Darcq C. Surgery of female urinary incontinence using trans-obturator tape (TOT): a prospective randomized comparative study with TVT. Neurourol Urodyn. 2003;22:488–9.

Nambiar A, Cody JD, Jeffery ST. Single-incision sling operations for urinary incontinence in women. Cochrane Database Syst Rev. 2014;(6):CD008709. doi:10.1002/14651858.CD008709.pub2.

Nilsson C, Falconer C, Rezapour M. Seven-year follow-up of the tension- free vaginal tape procedure for treatment of urinary incontinence. Obstet Gynecol. 2004;104:1259–62.

Petros P, Ulmsten U. An integral theory and its method for the diagnosis and management of female urinary incontinence. Scand J Urol Nephrol Suppl. 1993;153:1–93.

Porena M, Constantini E, Frea B, et al. Tension-free vaginal tape versus transobturator tape as surgery for stress urinary incontinence: results of a multicentre randomized trial. Eur Urol. 2007;52:1481–91.

Rehman H, Bezerra CC, Bruschini H, Cody JD. Traditional suburethral sling operations for urinary incontinence in women. Cochrane Database Syst Rev. 2011;(1):CD001754. doi:10.1002/14651858.CD001754.pub3.

Rodriguez LV, Raz S. Polypropylene sling for the treatment of stress urinary incontinence. Urology. 2001;58:783–5.

Tamussino KF, Hanzal E, Kölle D, Ralph G, Riss PA, Austrian Urogynecology Working Group. Tension-free vaginal tape operation: results of the Austrian registry. Obstet Gynecol. 2001;98:732–6.

Thor KB, de Groat WC. Neural control of the female urethral and anal rhabdosphincters and pelvic floor muscles. Am J Physiol Regul Integr Comp Physiol. 2010;299(2):R416–38.

Ward K, Hilton P. Tension-free vaginal tape versus colposuspension for primary urodynamic stress incontinence: 5-year follow-up. Br J Obstet Gynaecol. 2008;115:226–33.

3 Surgical Repair of Anterior Vaginal Wall Prolapse

3.1 Cystourethrocele

3.1.1 Indications

Anterior vaginal wall defects, or cystoceles, are very common. Approximately 50 % of women seeking routine gynecologic or urologic care have some degree of anterior prolapse. Most of these defects are asymptomatic, but as the leading edge of the prolapse extends beyond the hymen, the defect may become symptomatic. The cystocele may present itself as a vaginal bulge, or it may present with urinary symptoms of urgency, frequency, stress or urge incontinence, or even obstructive voiding symptoms. Risk factors for primary or secondary prolapse are age, menopausal status, parity, collagen defects, prior hysterectomy, increased body mass index, smoking, and chronic pulmonary disease.

3.1.2 Diagnosis

Many women with pelvic organ prolapse present with lower urinary tract symptoms that include stress incontinence with urethral hypermobility or incompetence, but some women are continent owing to a kinking or obstruction of the urethra. This symptom can be noted when a woman has to reduce her prolapse to void. This subset of women with an anatomic urethral obstruction may have symptoms of hesitancy, dribbling, poor stream, a sense of incomplete emptying, or urinary frequency with overflow incontinence. Additionally, a subset of patients with vaginal prolapse may experience urge incontinence that has developed de novo or from the obstruction of prolapse.

Evaluation should include a full medical and surgical history; a review of urinary, bowel, and sexual function symptoms; a voiding diary; urinalysis; and a post-void residual. On physical examination, the vaginal wall should be assessed for thickness, erosion, and friability. Each component of the vaginal vault—the anterior, posterior, apical, or superior areas—should be evaluated for the degree of prolapse, with evaluation for cervical-uterine prolapse, urethral hypermobility, and overt or occult incontinence. Transvaginal cystocele repair is rarely performed as a solitary surgery, as most patients require repair of other compartments or urethral supporting procedures (slings or suspensions).

The patient generally senses a bulging mass through the introitus, with or without stress urinary incontinence. On physical examination with a full bladder, the bladder base is seen bulging through the introitus at rest (Fig. 3.1). An increase in the protrusion can be detected when the patient coughs or strains. The degree of urethral hypermobility or any simultaneous rectocele, enterocele, or uterine prolapse should be properly diagnosed.

Cystoscopy may show hypermobility and funneling of the bladder neck and marked descent of the bladder base and trigone. The use of light during cystoscopic examination can be helpful in defining a cystocele defect, as sometimes they can be difficult to differentiate from an enterocele.

Radiological studies including a voiding cystourethrogram or video-urodynamics (VCUG) will show the bladder base to be descended well beyond the inferior rami of the symphysis. The bladder neck may be funneled, and stress-induced urinary incontinence may be present. During straining, the cystocele is further enlarged (Fig. 3.2). Commonly, patients void normally with low residuals, but some (particularly those with prior surgery) may show an obstructive pattern and an increase in post-void urinary residual. CT urogram or kidney ultrasound is indicated to rule out partial ureteral obstruction or hydronephrosis. MRI provides in a quick and noninvasive way to assess the degree of cystocele, diagnose rectocele or enterocele, and rule out hydronephrosis or any other pelvic pathology (Figs. 3.3, 3.4, and 3.5).

Electronic supplementary material The online version of this chapter (doi:10.1007/978-1-4939-2941-2_3) contains supplementary material, which is available to authorized users.

S. Raz, *Atlas of Vaginal Reconstructive Surgery*, DOI 10.1007/978-1-4939-2941-2_3

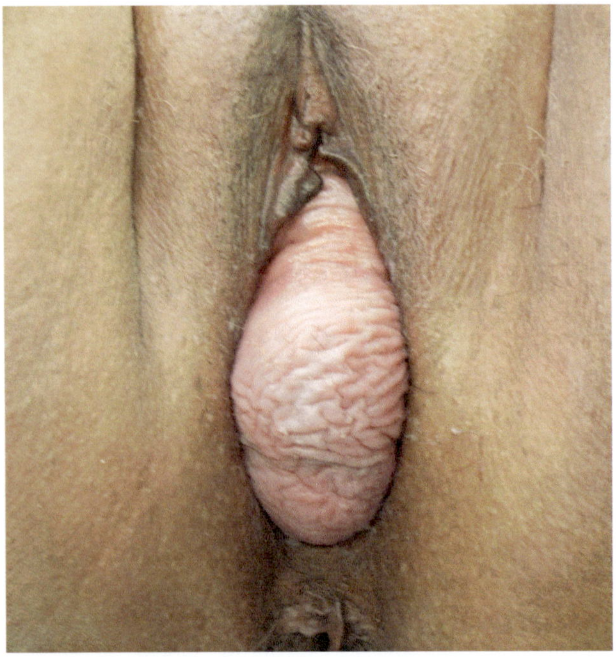

Fig. 3.1 Physical examination of a patient with significant cystocele coming outside the introitus. The patient has significant urethral mobility, enterocele, and rectocele that will be corrected at the time of the cystocele repair

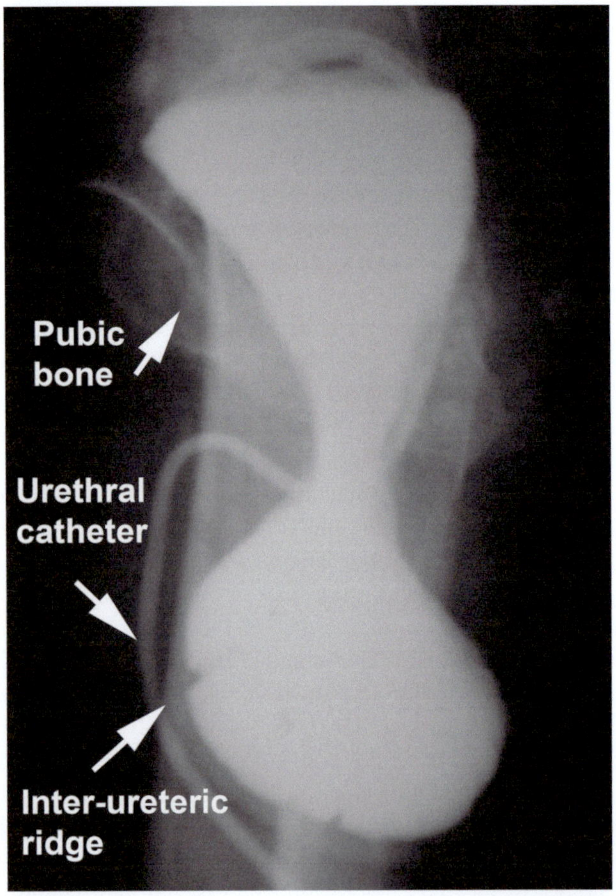

Fig. 3.2 Standing lateral cystogram of a patient with severe cystocele. The bladder base slides well below the inferior rami of the symphysis during straining. The inter-ureteric ridge is seen at the trigonal area

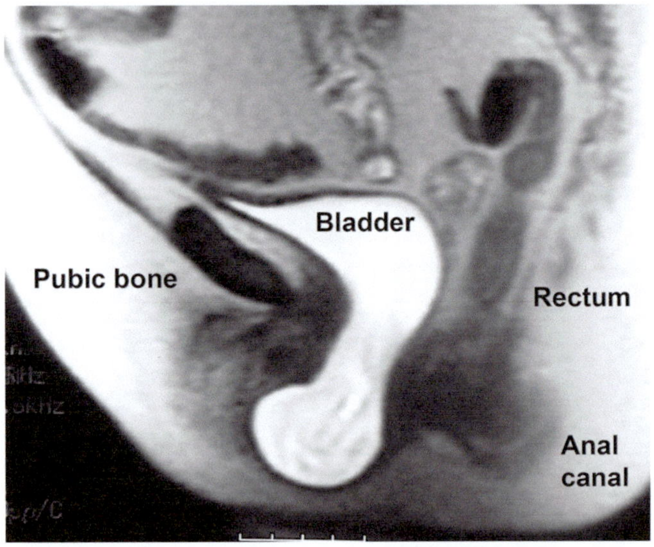

Fig. 3.3 Dynamic MRI showing the bladder descending below the inferior rami of the pubic bone. The urethra is also mobile and outside the vaginal canal

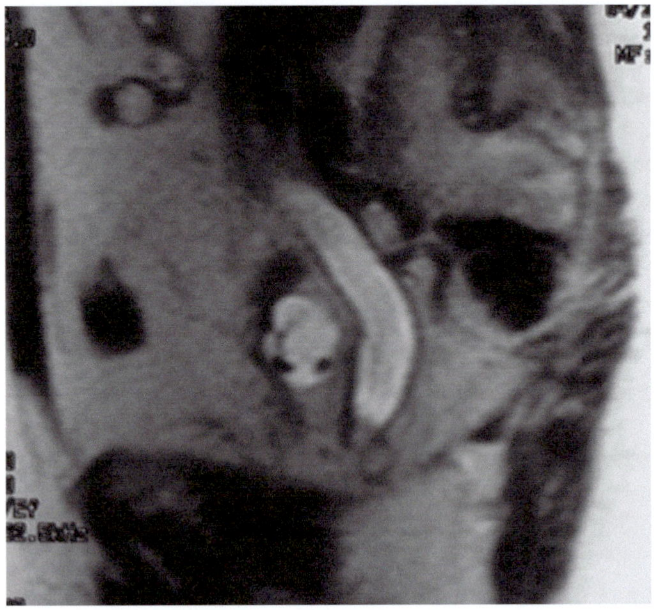

Fig. 3.4 Sagittal MRI showing significant dilatation of the ureter in a patient with severe cystocele and urinary retention

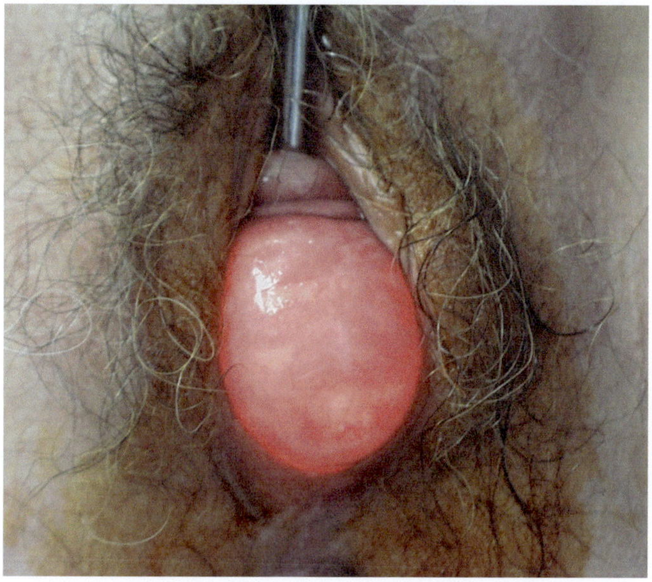

Fig. 3.5 During cystoscopy, transillumination of the bladder helps to outline the entire bladder wall in a patient with a severe vaginal bulge due to cystocele. This maneuver helps to define and diagnose an enterocele as a source of a large anterior and vault prolapse

3.1.3 Surgical Repair Techniques

This chapter describes five techniques of cystocele repair:

1. Repair of the central defect only. This technique is used very sporadically in selected patients with good lateral support. The repair can be reinforced with autologous fascia or a biological graft.
2. CRISP procedure (cystocele repair using interlocking sutures of polypropylene). In this technique, a central and lateral cystocele defect is repaired using interlocking polypropylene suture anchored to the lateral arcus tendineus fascia pelvis.
3. Four-corner bladder neck and bladder suspension for patients with lateral defects. In this technique, monofilament polypropylene sutures are used to support the bladder base, bladder neck, and urethra to the superior rami of the pubic bone.
4. A combination of central defect repair and four-corner bladder and bladder neck suspension for a lateral defect.
5. Lateral and central defect repair using autologus fascia lata.

The five techniques have many steps in common, and the differences are described in more detail.

We have abandoned the use of mesh for the repair of cystoceles or any other prolapse, relying instead on delayed absorbable sutures (polydioxanone [PDS]) and monofilament polypropylene sutures.

3.1.3.1 Repair of the Central Defect Only

Figures 3.6, 3.7, 3.8, 3.9, 3.10, 3.11, 3.12, 3.13, 3.14, 3.15, and 3.16 illustrate the surgical repair of a central defect alone.

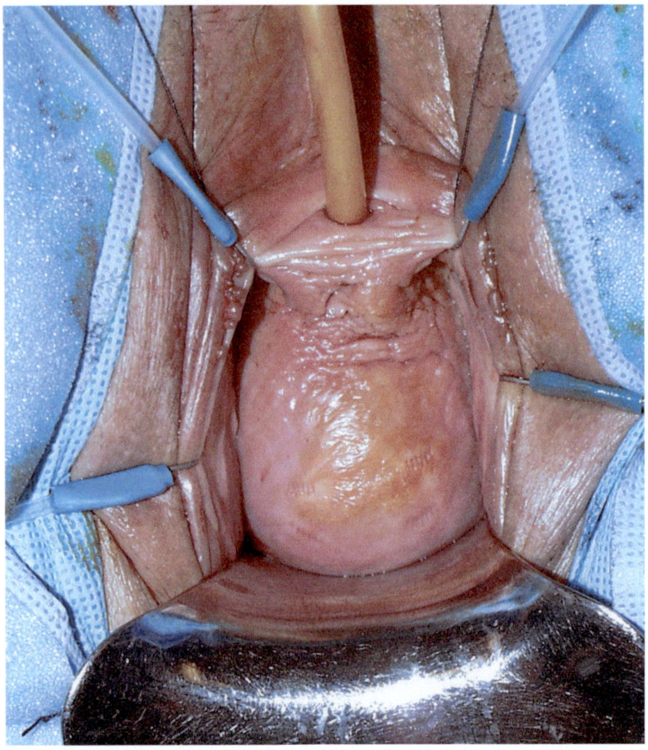

Fig. 3.6 Anterior vaginal wall exposure in a patient with significant central defect cystocele after prior lateral defect repairs

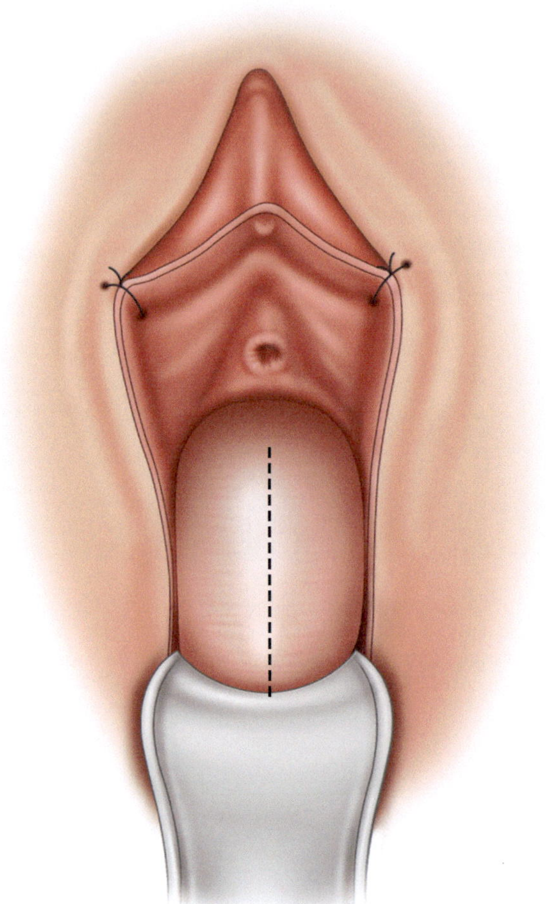

Fig. 3.7 Diagram showing the anterior vaginal wall and the extent of the incision that will be done from the bladder neck to the bladder base

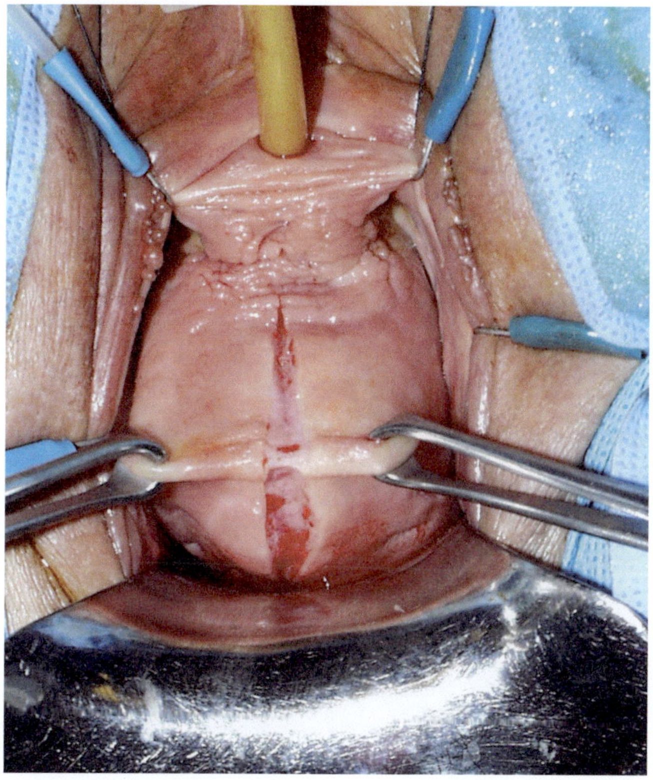

Fig. 3.8 Intraoperative photograph of the incision of the anterior vaginal wall. Usually a coagulation knife is used; we have not found it necessary to inject vasoconstrictors or do hydrodissection of the anterior vaginal wall

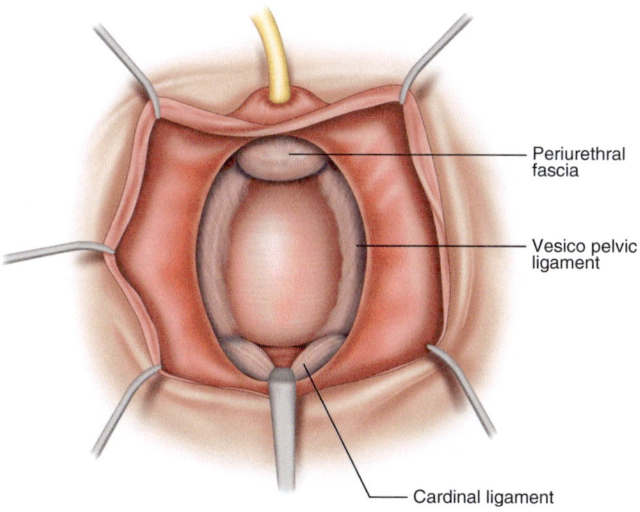

Fig. 3.9 Diagram of the anterior vaginal wall after dissection of the two lateral flaps. The periurethral fascia is seen superiorly and the cardinal–sacrouterine complex is seen inferiorly. The vesicopelvic fascia laterally support the bladder to the arcus tendineus fascia pelvis

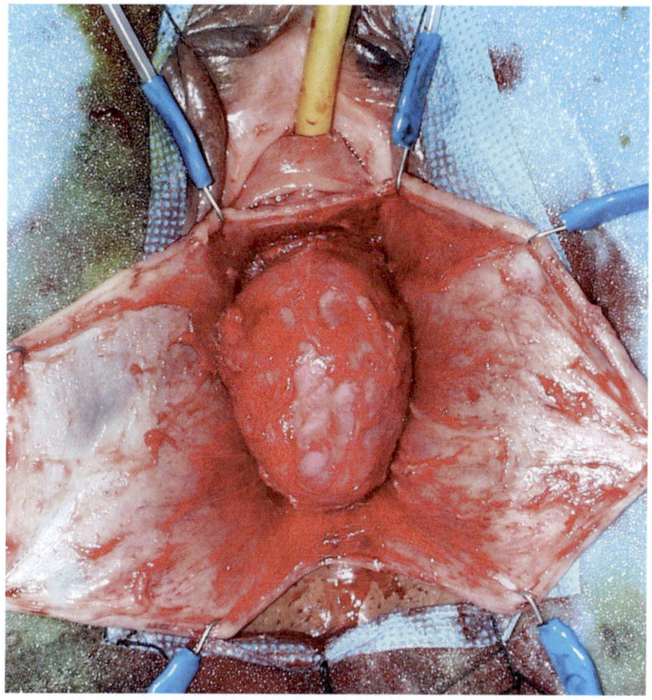

Fig. 3.10 Intraoperative photograph of the exposure of the anterior vaginal wall after the lateral dissection. Good hemostasis should be obtained. The dissection is carried out over the perivesical fascia, taking care to avoid bladder perforation

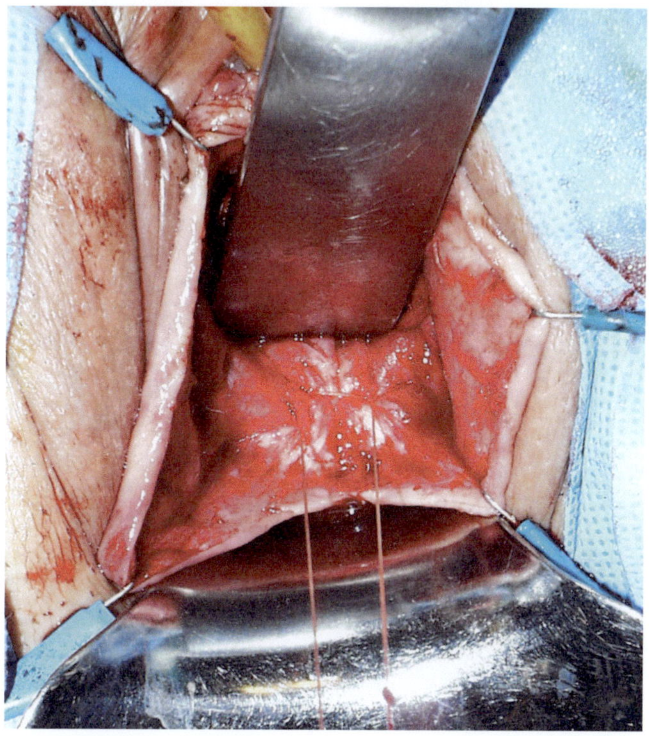

Fig. 3.11 The bladder is retracted to expose the vaginal cuff and the bladder base. The area of the cardinal–sacrouterine complex at the cuff is approximated to the midline using figure-of-eight delayed absorbable sutures

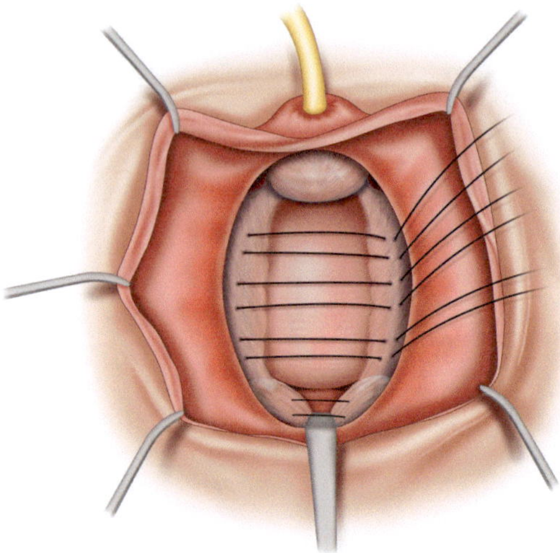

Fig. 3.12 Diagram showing the approximation of the perivesical fascia to the midline using horizontally placed figure-of-eight sutures

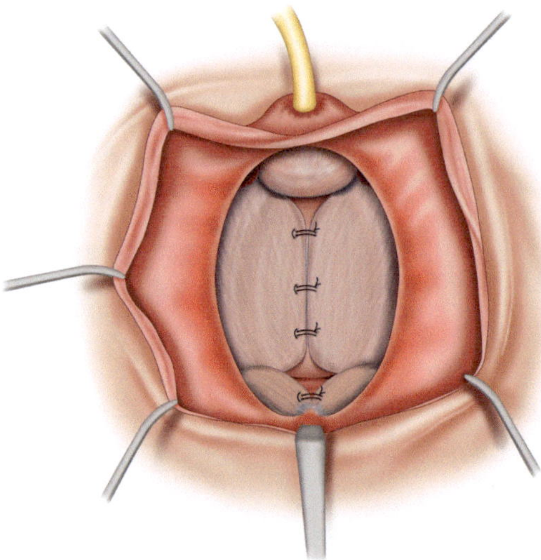

Fig. 3.13 Diagram showing the appearance of the anterior bladder wall after tying the central sutures

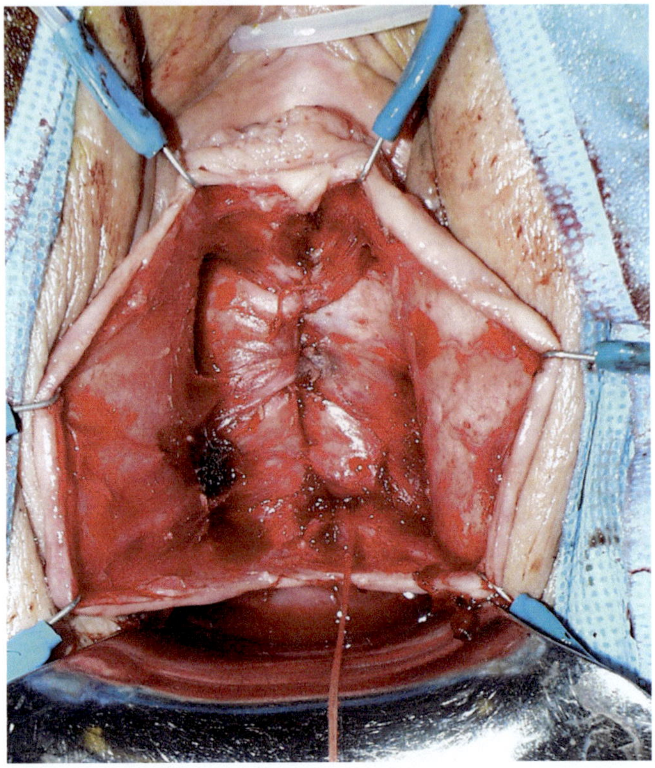

Fig. 3.14 Operative photograph showing the view of the anterior vaginal wall after the central sutures have been tied

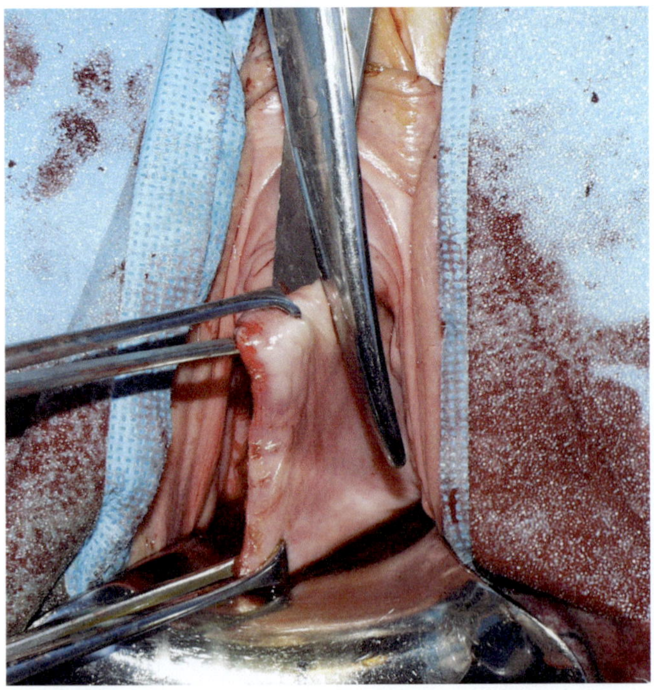

Fig. 3.15 The excess of the anterior vaginal wall is excised using scissors or a coagulation knife

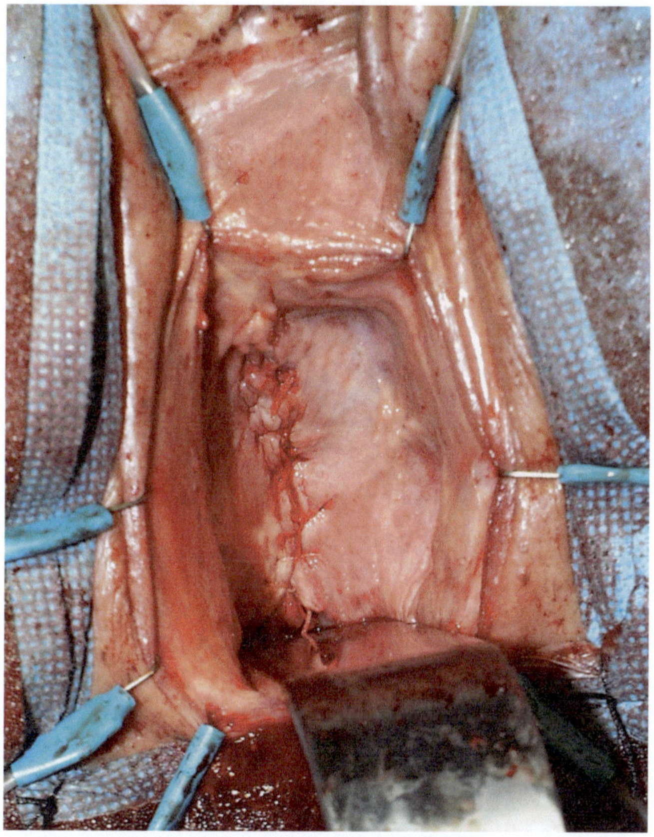

Fig. 3.16 The anterior vaginal wall is closed using delayed absorbable sutures. The sutures include the perivesical fascia in order to prevent any dead space or hematoma formation

3.1.3.2 CRISP Procedure: Cystocele Repair Using Interlocking Sutures of Polypropylene

In this technique (Figs. 3.17, 3.18, 3.19, 3.20, 3.21, 3.22, 3.23, 3.24, 3.25, 3.26, 3.27, 3.28, 3.29, and 3.30), the lateral defect is repaired by applying interrupted monofilament sutures to the lateral arcus tendineus fascia pelvis to incorporate the lateral margin of the bladder wall (vesicopelvic fascia). The central defect is repaired by using mattress monofilament sutures from the bladder neck to the bladder base. The central defect sutures are tied after interlocking each of them with the laterally placed sutures. The final result is a net of monofilament sutures supporting the lateral and central defects.

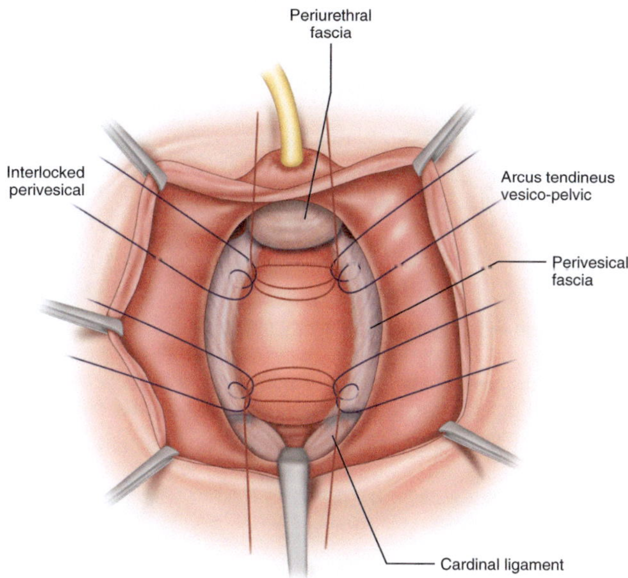

Fig. 3.17 Diagram showing the principles of the CRISP surgical procedure. The lateral sutures (*black–blue*) are applied to the vesicopelvic fascia and the arcus tendineus fascia pelvis and the central sutures (*red*) to the perivesical fascia

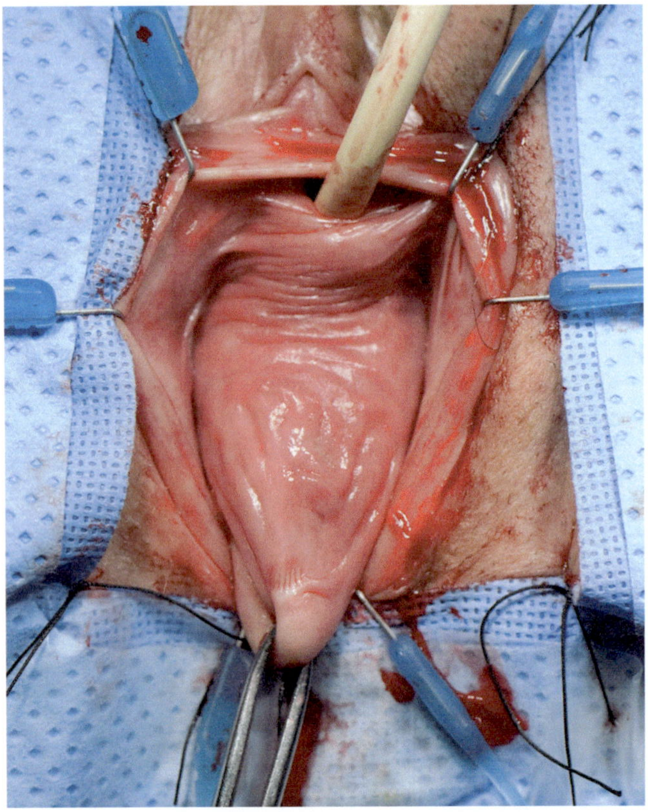

Fig. 3.18 Exposure of the anterior vaginal wall in a patient with lateral and central defect cystocele. The apex and the posterior vaginal wall also will be repaired

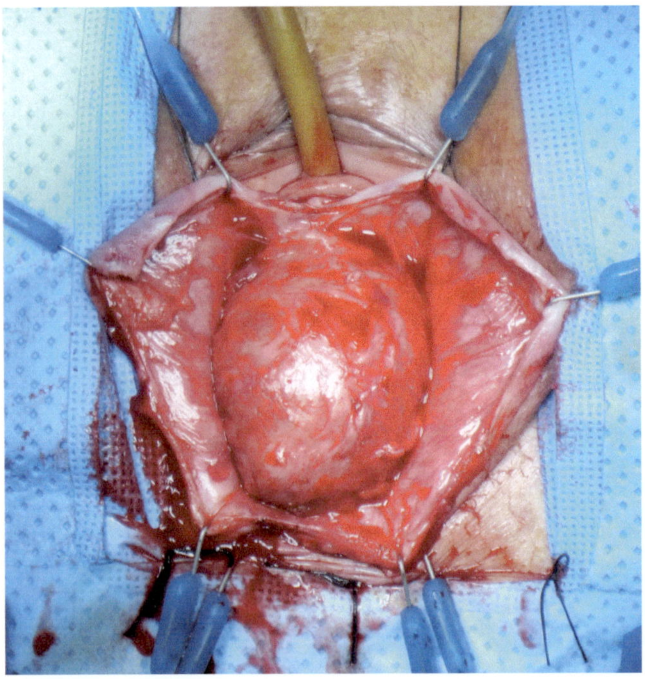

Fig. 3.19 A vertical incision is made in the anterior vaginal wall from the bladder neck to the bladder base

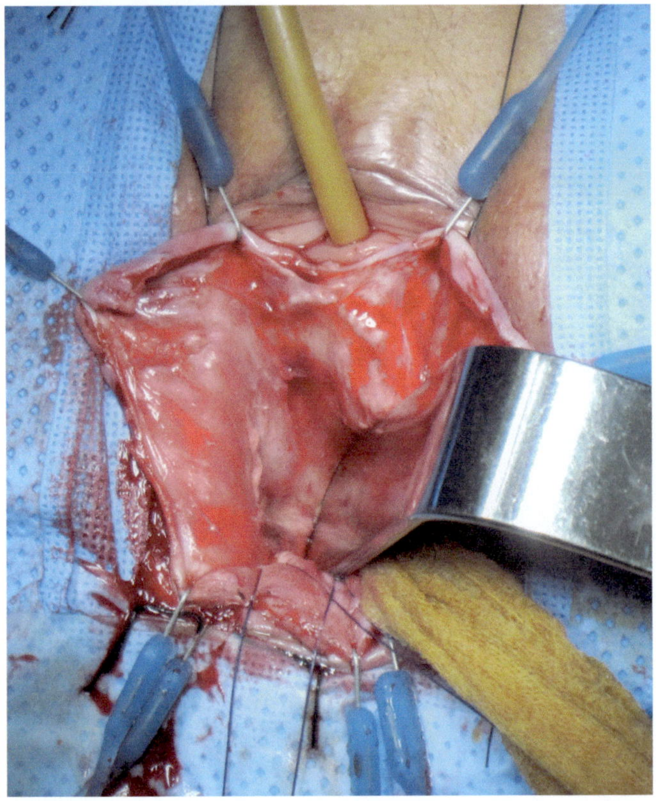

Fig. 3.20 The bladder is retracted, and exposure of the lateral anterior bladder wall exposes the attachment of the bladder to the arcus tendineus

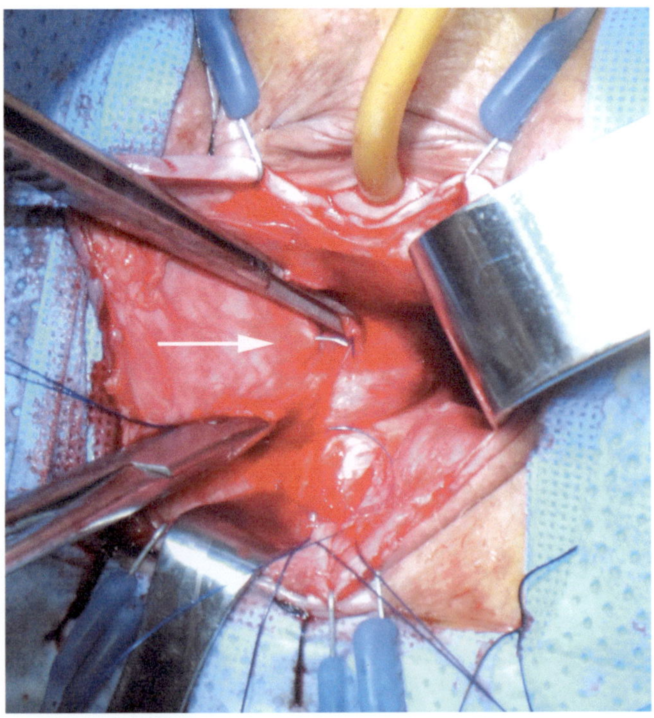

Fig. 3.21 A #3-0 figure-of-eight monofilament nonabsorbable suture incorporates the arcus tendineus, levator, and the vesicopelvic fascia laterally. Four sutures will be applied: two at the bladder base and two at the bladder neck. *White arrow* indicates the tip of the needle as the suture is applied

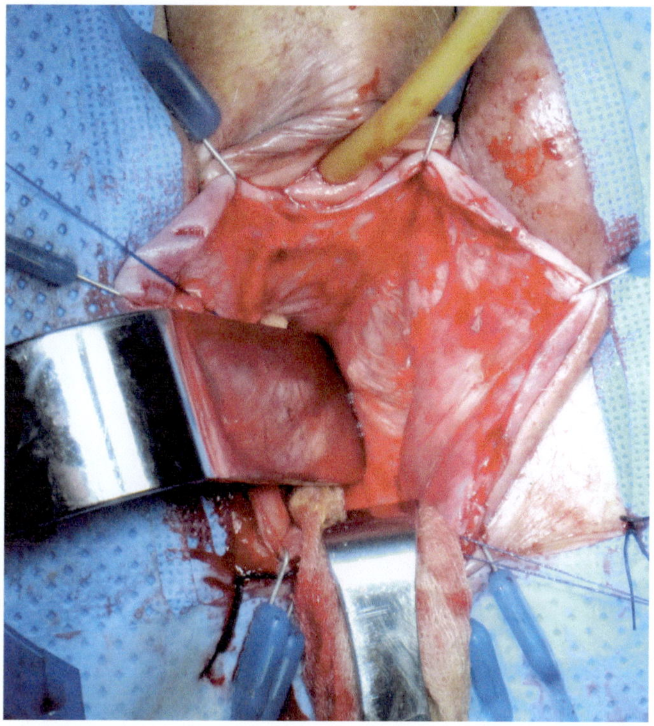

Fig. 3.22 Retracting the bladder exposes the left side insertion of the bladder to the lateral pelvic wall (arcus tendineus)

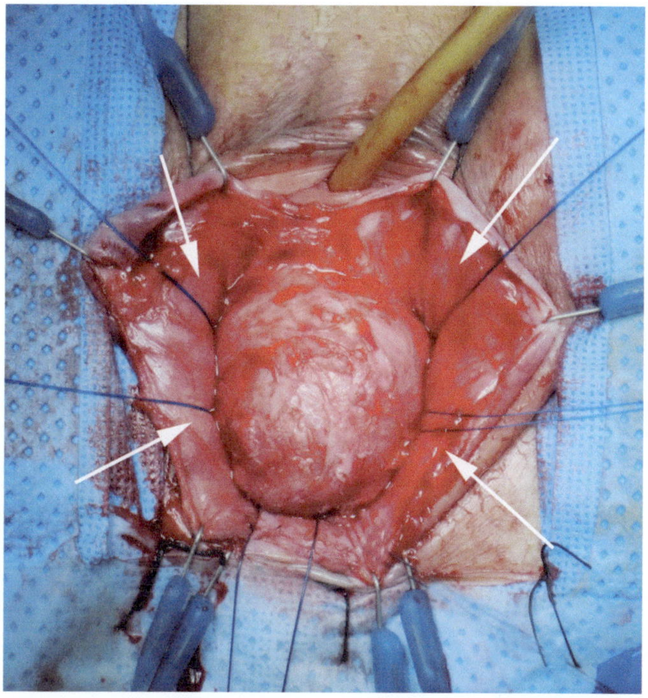

Fig. 3.24 The four lateral sutures and the central defect are seen. The *arrows* point to are of placement of the four lateral sutures

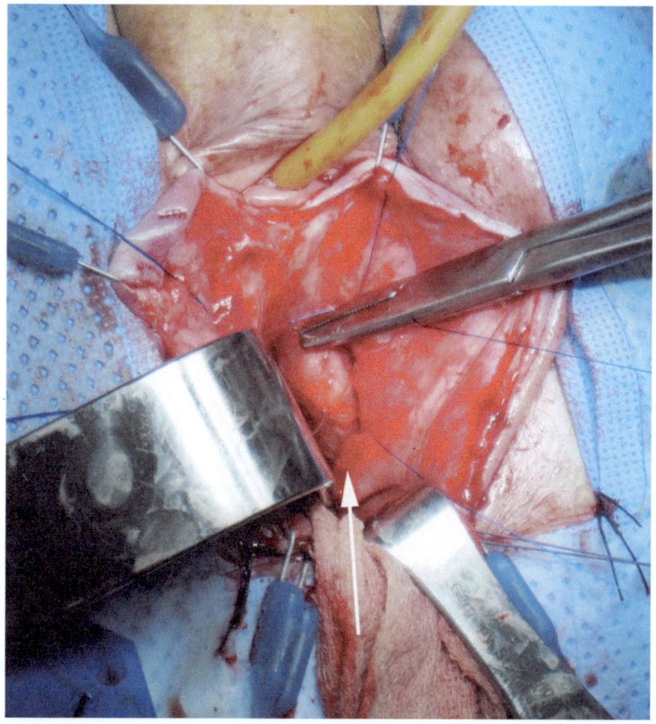

Fig. 3.23 Two figure-of-eight sutures are applied to the bladder base and bladder neck, incorporating the arcus tendineus area and levator musculatures. The *arrow* indicated the margin of the arcus tendinous fascia pelvis

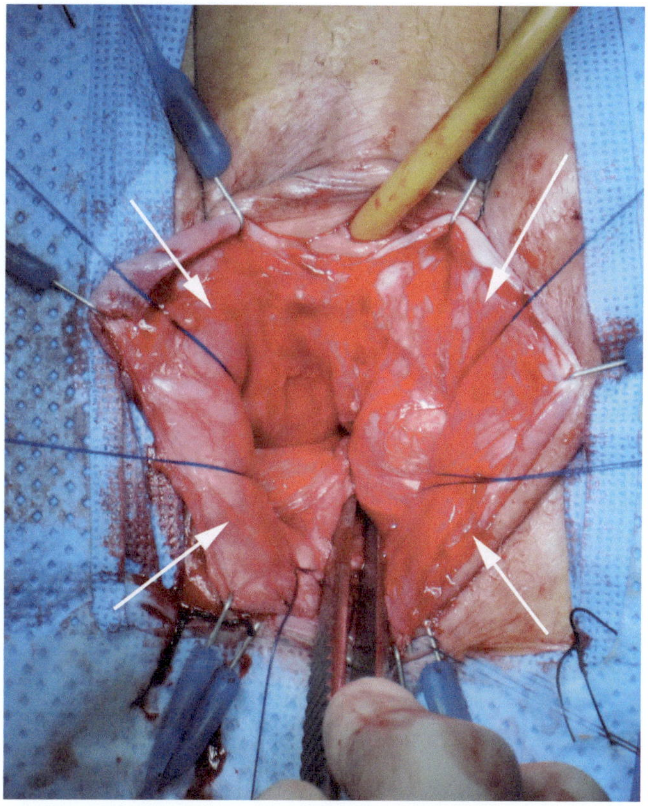

Fig. 3.25 The bladder is retracted posteriorly to expose the perivesical fascia, where the central defect sutures will be applied. The *arrows* point toward the dissected vaginal wall after the bladder is retracted

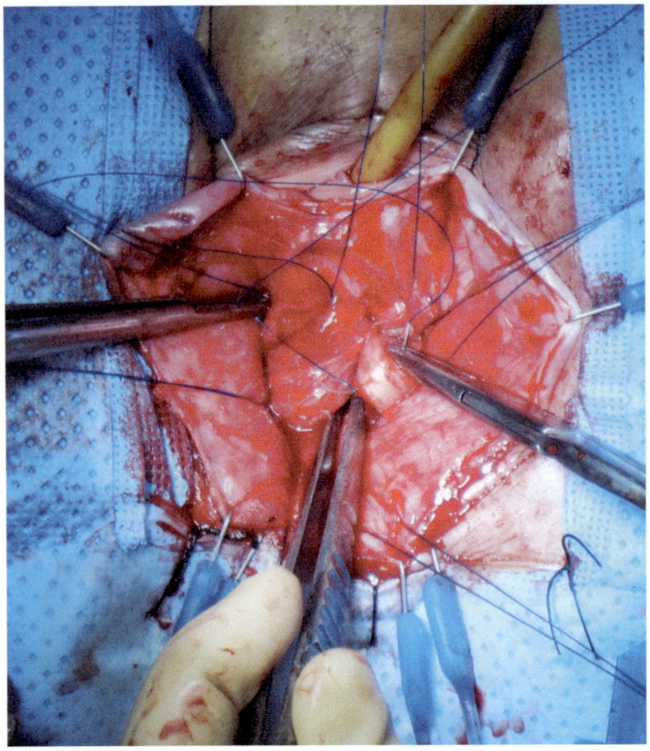

Fig. 3.26 Sequentially the perivesical fascia is approximated with horizontal mattress sutures from the bladder neck to the bladder base

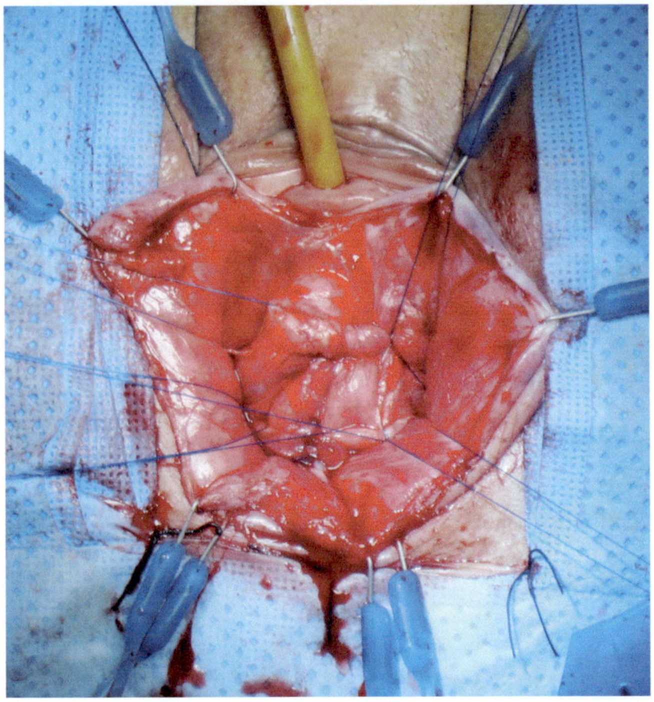

Fig. 3.28 The central sutures are tied. Prior to tying, each suture is transferred and interlocked with the lateral suture at the same level, providing a net of support to the anterior bladder wall

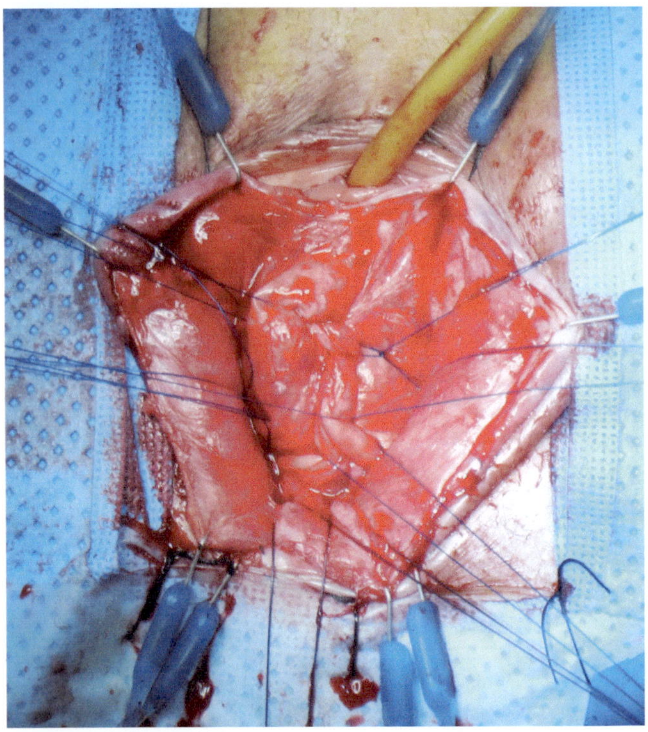

Fig. 3.27 Exposure of the central and lateral suture placement with reduction of the cystocele defect

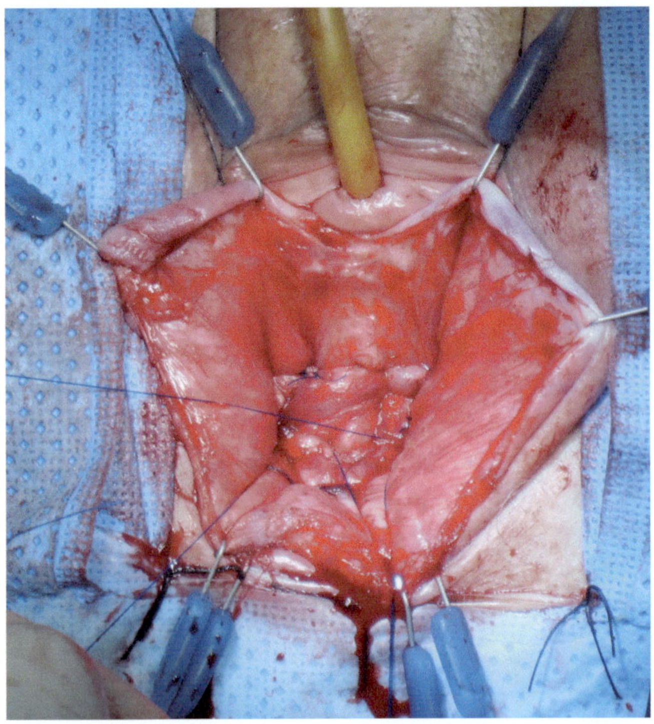

Fig. 3.29 The lateral sutures are tied after including one of the central sutures, completing the interlocked net of sutures

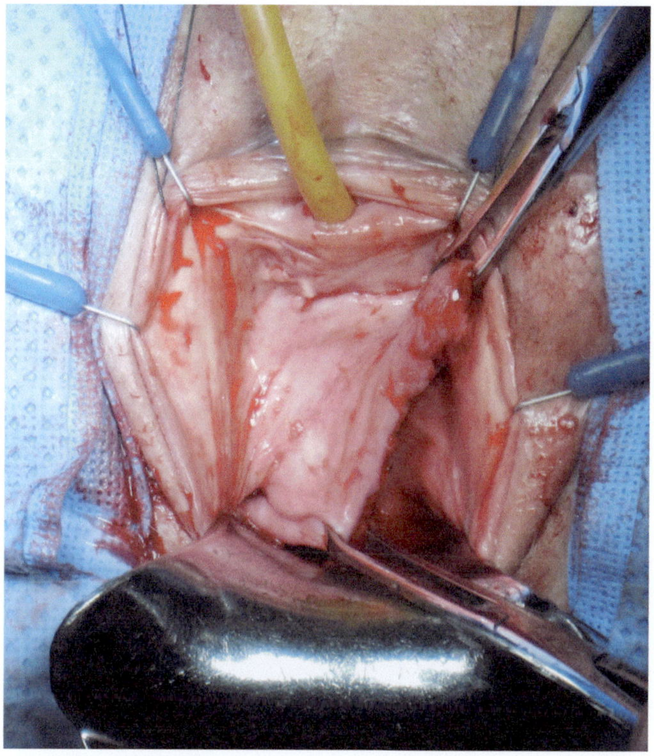

Fig. 3.30 The vaginal wall is excised in an asymmetric fashion. Most of the lateral vaginal flap is excised, and the right flap will cover the area of reconstruction, preventing protrusion of nonabsorbable sutures in the midline incision

3.1.3.3 Four-Corner Bladder and Bladder Neck Suspension for Lateral Defect Cystocele

This operation is indicated for patients with a moderate cystocele with a mainly lateral defect. The advantage of the operation is that the bladder and bladder neck are supported to the superior rami of the pubic bone, using nonabsorbable sutures. Four #0 monofilament polypropylene sutures are used to incorporate the urethropelvic and periurethral fascia at the bladder neck and the vesicopelvic and perivesical fascia at the bladder base. The sutures will provide lateral support to the anterior vaginal wall, including the urethra, bladder, and bladder base. The sutures are transferred and tied in the suprapubic area. Figures 3.31, 3.32, 3.33, 3.34, 3.35, 3.36, 3.37, 3.38, 3.39, 3.40, 3.41, 3.42, 3.43, 3.44, 3.45, and 3.46 illustrate this technique.

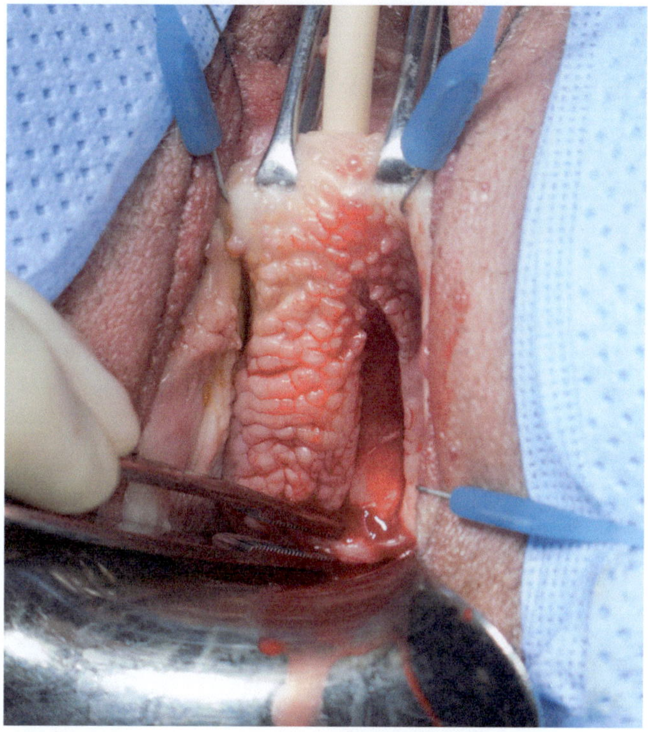

Fig. 3.31 Exposure of the anterior vaginal wall in a young patient with a lateral defect and mainly anterior vaginal wall prolapse. The uterus is mobile to the mid-vagina. Because of the young age of the patient, no hysterectomy is contemplated

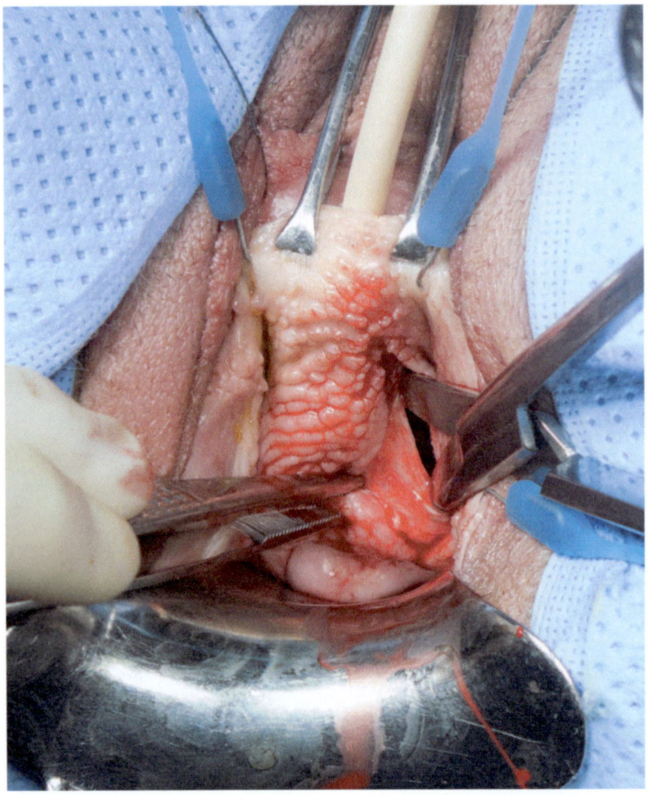

Fig. 3.32 Dissection is carried out around the periurethral fascia toward the inferior rami of the pubic bone. A pair of curved scissors is inserted as far lateral as possible, parallel to the urethra in a superior direction, just behind the posterior aspect of the pubic bone

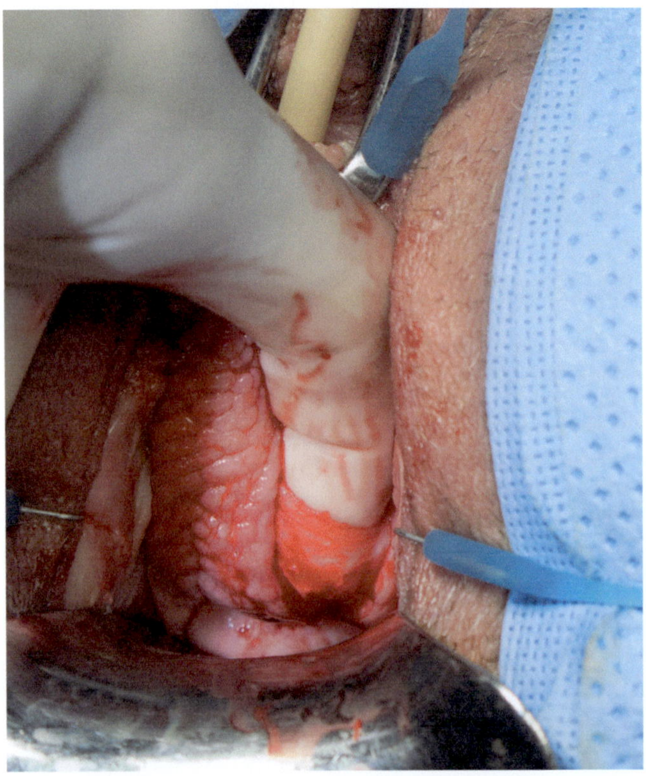

Fig. 3.33 A finger in the retropubic space allows the exposure of the detached urethropelvic and vesicopelvic fascia from the arcus tendineus fascia pelvis

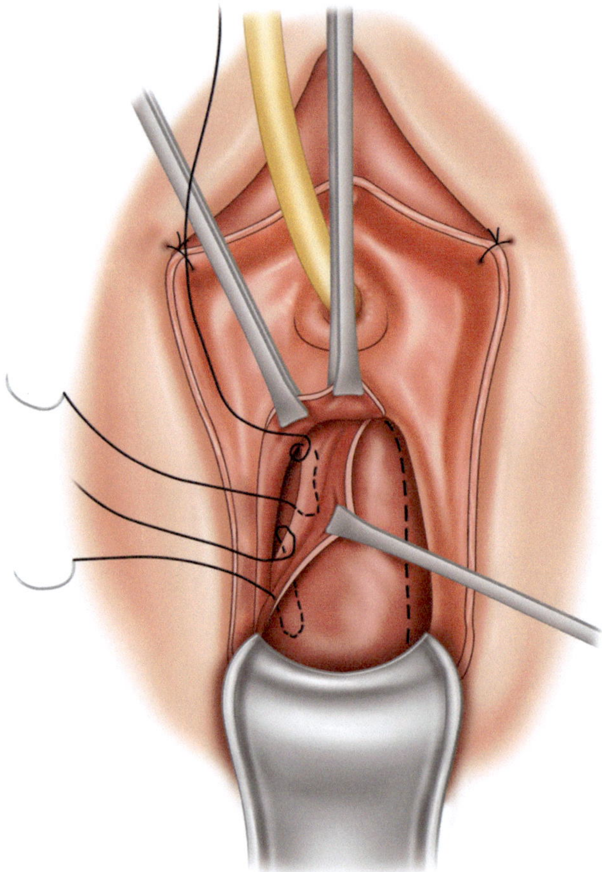

Fig. 3.34 Diagram showing the application of four #0 nonabsorbable monofilament sutures. At the bladder base, the sutures incorporate the vesicopelvic fascia in the retropubic space and with a wide passage of the needle under the vaginal wall to incorporate the perivesical fascia medial to the incision and at the bladder base. At the level of the bladder neck, the sutures incorporate the urethropelvic fascia in the retropubic space, the perivesical fascia at the level of the bladder neck, and the periurethral fascia at the level of the proximal and midurethra

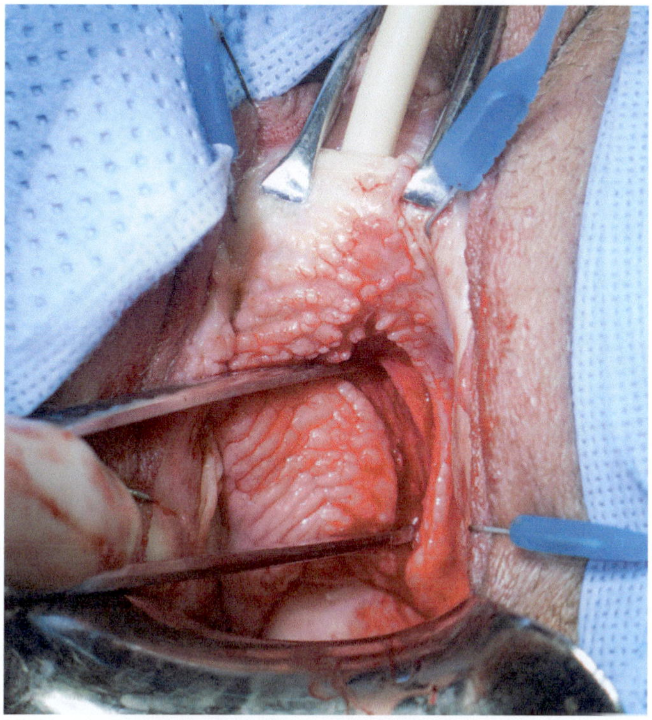

Fig. 3.35 A long forceps is used to retract medially the vaginal wall, exposing the vesicopelvic fascia detached from the arcus tendineus fascia pelvis

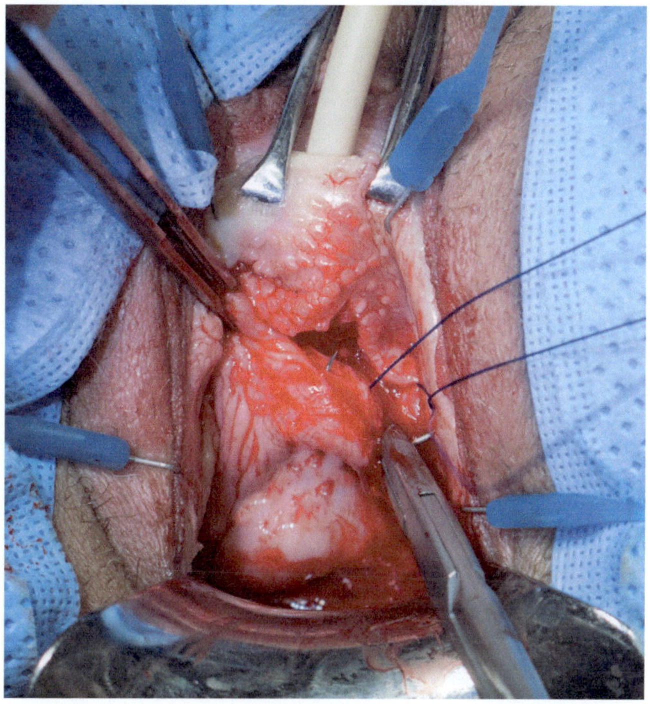

Fig. 3.37 A wide segment of the perivesical fascia is incorporated at the bladder base. Multiple passes of the needle incorporate again the vesicopelvic and perivesical fascia

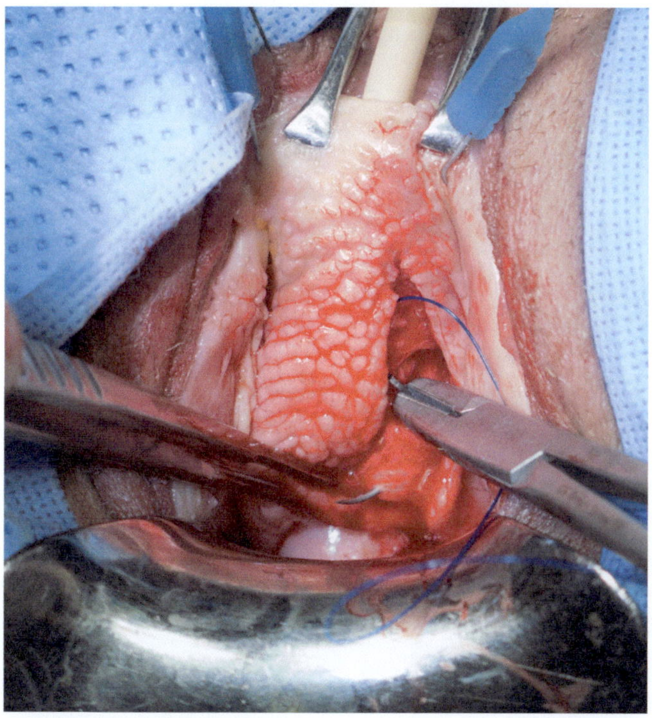

Fig. 3.36 At the bladder base, #0 monofilament nonabsorbable suture is used to incorporate the detached vesicopelvic fascia from the arcus tendineus

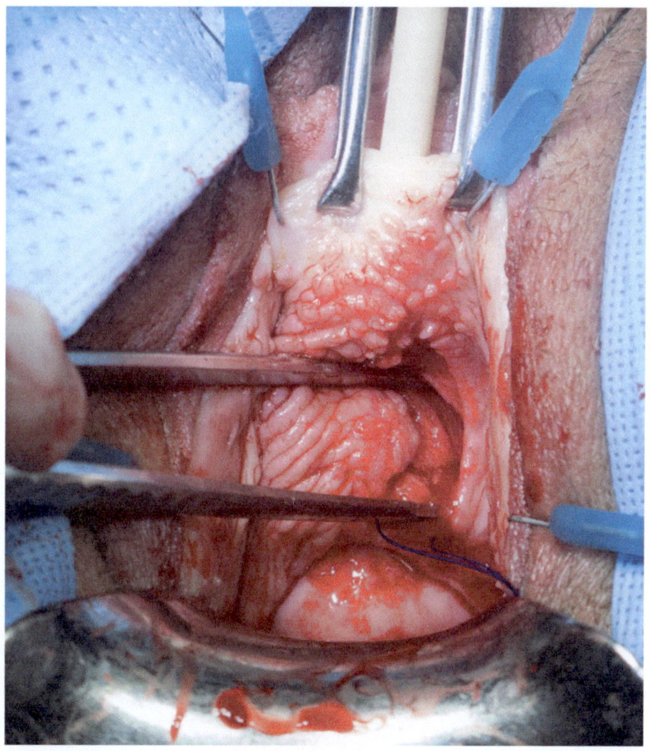

Fig. 3.38 A forceps in the retropubic space exposes the detached urethropelvic fascia at the level of the bladder neck

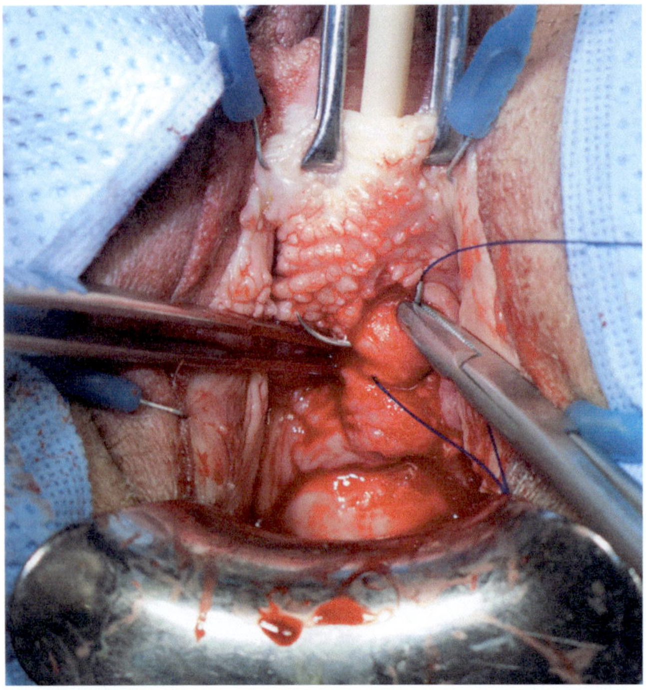

Fig. 3.39 At the level of the bladder neck, a #0 monofilament suture incorporates the urethropelvic fascia

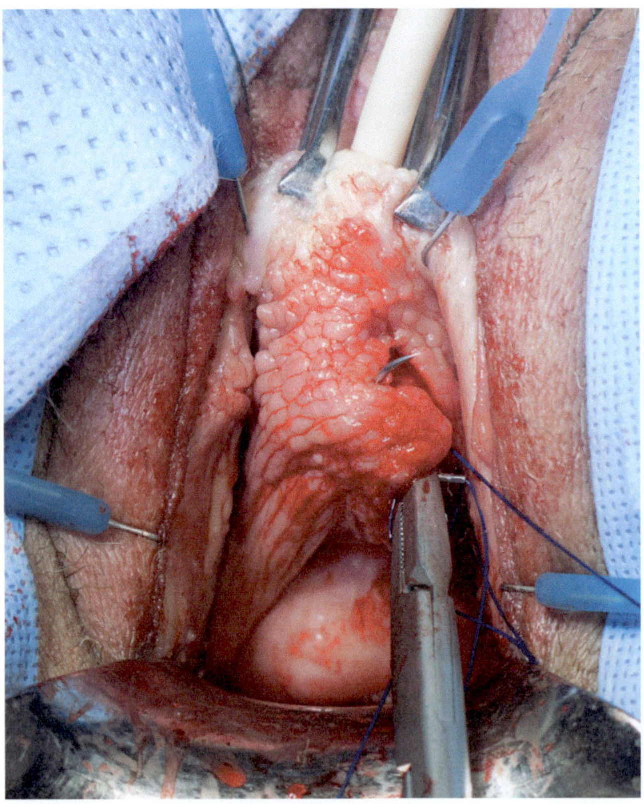

Fig. 3.40 The perivesical fascia at the bladder neck and the midurethral periurethral fascia are incorporated with the suture

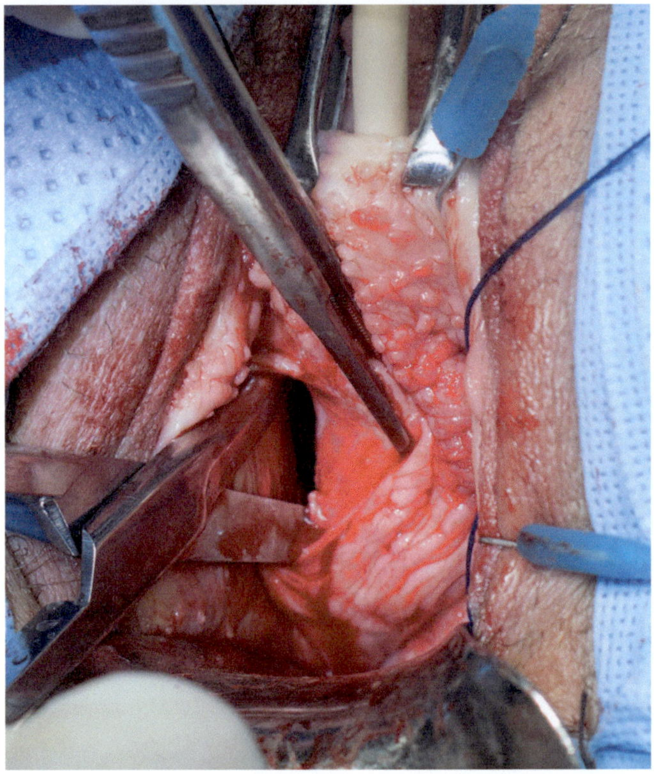

Fig. 3.41 The same maneuver is done in the contralateral side. An oblique incision is made in the left periurethral and perivesical area, and the retropubic space is entered with scissors, detaching the urethropelvic and vesicopelvic fascia from the arcus tendineus

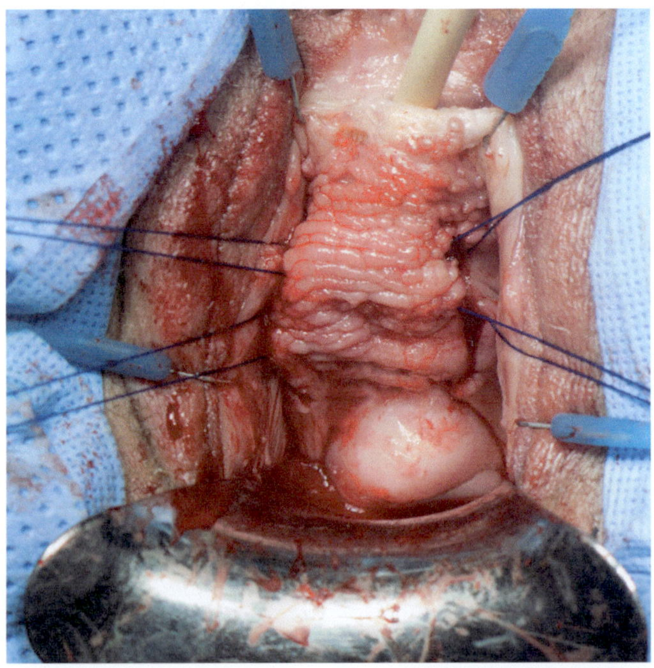

Fig. 3.42 The four sutures have been applied: two at the bladder base and two at the bladder neck and urethra. Pulling the sutures should confirm a strong anchor of tissue, to the point that the patient can be moved over the table

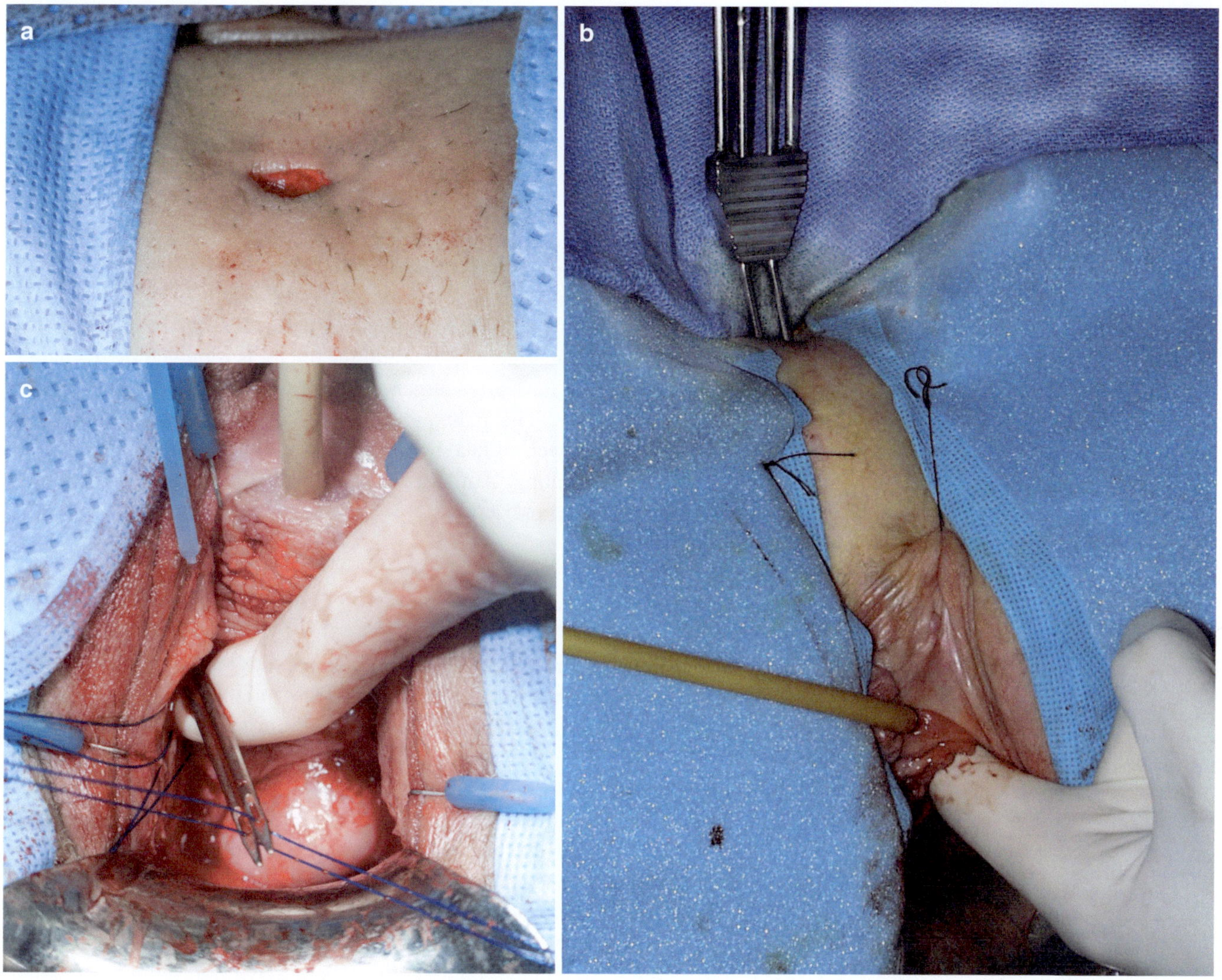

Fig. 3.43 (**a**) A small puncture is performed in the suprapubic area. (**b**) Under finger control in the retropubic space, a double-pronged passer is transferred from the suprapubic to the vaginal area. (**c**) The double passer is brought outside the vaginal incision, and the sutures will be transferred through the needle holes

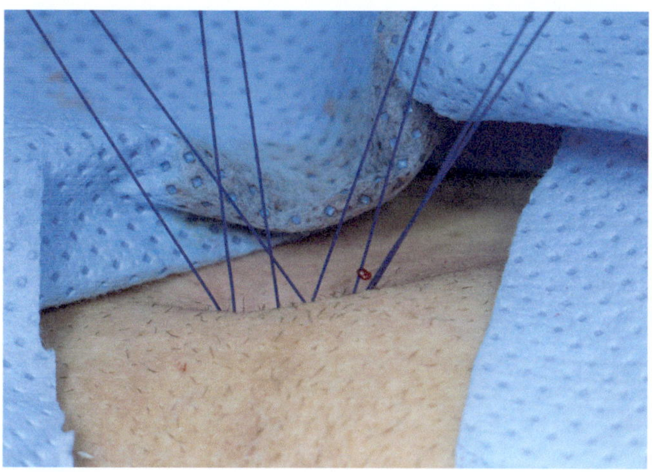

Fig. 3.44 The four sutures have been transferred to the suprapubic puncture area

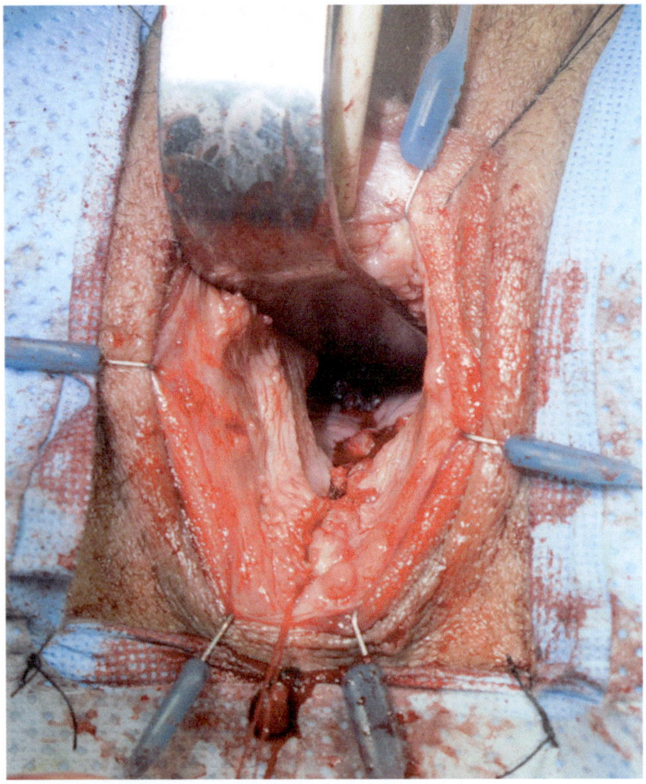

Fig. 3.45 After closure of the anterior vaginal wall with interrupted #2-0 delayed absorbable sutures, a posterior repair and uterine suspension procedure have been performed

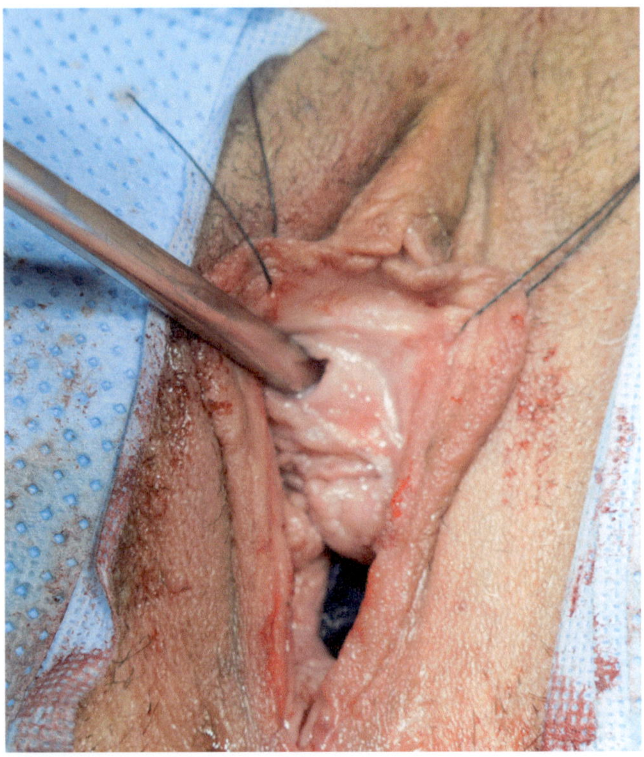

Fig. 3.46 Cystoscopy is performed after injection of indigo carmine. Keeping the cystoscope in a 45-degree angulation, the sutures in the suprapubic area are tied sequentially without tension. A vaginal packing soaked in antibiotics is inserted

3.1.3.4 Combination of Central and Lateral Defect Repair

Central and lateral defect cystocele correction using a combination of four-corner suspension and central defect repair is shown in Figs. 3.47, 3.48, 3.49, 3.50, 3.51, 3.52, 3.53, 3.54, 3.55, 3.56, and 3.57.

3.1.4 Postoperative Care

The vaginal packing and urethral catheter are removed 24 h after surgery. The urethral catheter is removed by the patient 2–7 days after surgery, depending on the extent of the procedure. The patient is allowed to walk, drive, climb stairs, shower, or take baths but is prohibited from heavy lifting or straining. Antibiotics, pain medication, and stool softeners are prescribed.

3.1.5 Intraoperative Complications

As in other vaginal procedures, the potential complications during surgery include bleeding, urethral or bladder perforation, and ureteral obstruction due to misplaced sutures. In these procedures, special attention should be given to the ureters because of their close proximity. The bladder and trigone should be retracted at the time of placement of midline sutures over the perivesical fascia. Cystoscopy should confirm the patency of both ureteric orifices; if in doubt, a stent should be inserted. If ureteric obstruction is found, the suspension or perivesical fascia sutures should be removed and replaced.

Bladder injury at the time of dissection should be repaired primarily using multiple layers of delayed absorbable sutures and prolonged bladder drainage. With an anterior bladder injury, a Penrose drain may be inserted in the retropubic space, using a percutaneous technique.

3.1.6 Postoperative Complications

Postoperative complications are similar to those with other vaginal reconstructive procedures. Prolonged urinary retention is rare and is managed by reinsertion of the indwelling catheter for a longer period. If the problem persists after 2 weeks, the patient is started on a program of self-intermittent catheterization until adequate bladder emptying resumes.

De novo or recurrent stress incontinence may develop as a result of inadequate support of the bladder neck and urethra. Stress incontinence also may result from an open, incompetent, nonfunctional proximal sphincteric area (intrinsic sphincter dysfunction). In this situation, the urethra is generally well supported. A fascial sling (with a donor site from the fascia lata or abdominal wall) should be used in this situations.

Recurrent prolapse of the bladder is rare and may result from inappropriate positioning of the sutures or from poor quality of tissues, especially when severe atrophic vaginitis is present. Another repair will be necessary using PDS sutures, biological graft, and very rarely abdominal wall fascia.

Concomitant surgical procedures such as hysterectomy or repair of an enterocele or rectocele are required in more than 75 % of patients with grade IV cystocele. Repair of the cystocele without repair of the other abnormalities may lead to their further aggravation, requiring another surgery. Secondary enterocele or rectocele (not present prior to surgery) may occur, as the transfer of the anterior vaginal wall to a high, supported position may facilitate the herniation of a weakened cul-de-sac and posterior vaginal wall.

Vaginal shortening may occur if excess vaginal wall is removed. If the concept of this surgery as a bladder suspension is kept in mind, very little vaginal tissue is excised, and this complication can be avoided.

Pain in the suprapubic area is rare and may result from nerve entrapment, tight knots, or a low-grade infection. Transfer of sutures in the midline will prevent damage to the ilioinguinal nerves.

Because these surgical procedures do not use mesh, complications with the use of synthetic materials such as chronic draining sinus, granulating tissue, infection of the mesh, urethral or bladder penetration by the synthetic material, and vaginal pain are obviated.

In spite of cystoscopic patency of ureters at the time of surgery, ureteric obstruction during surgery can result from kinking or obstruction of the ureters by the sutures. Undoing the surgical steps, suture removal, and release of any folds of the perivesical tissues should restore ureteric patency. If a complex surgical procedure has been performed and the cystoscopy shows ureteric obstruction with inability to pass a stent or guidewire, a ureteric reimplantation may be indicated. After complex reconstruction we prefer not to explore the area of ureteric obstruction transvaginally in order to avoid undue damage to an otherwise good anatomical repair. Discovery of ureteric obstruction after surgery requires full evaluation and possible percutaneous nephrostomy or later ureteric reimplantation.

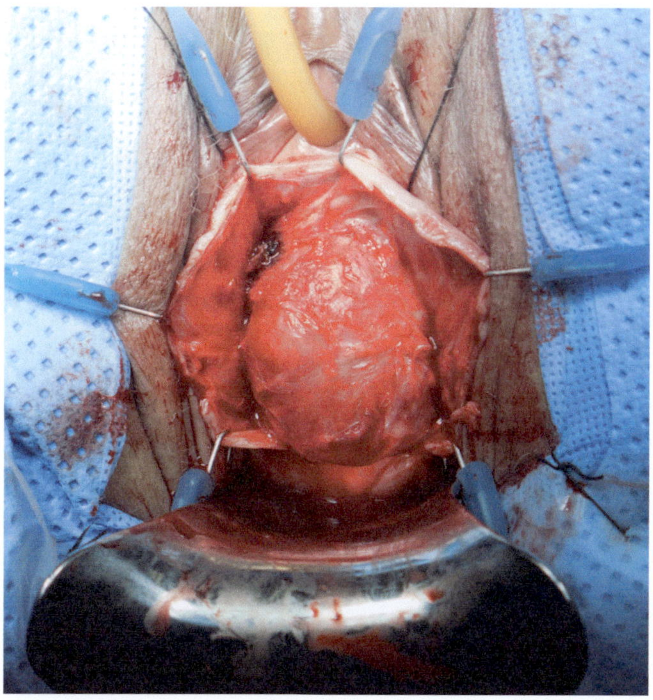

Fig. 3.47 In a patient with significant cystocele, a strip of the anterior vaginal wall has been excised to expose the perivesical fascia from the bladder neck to the bladder base

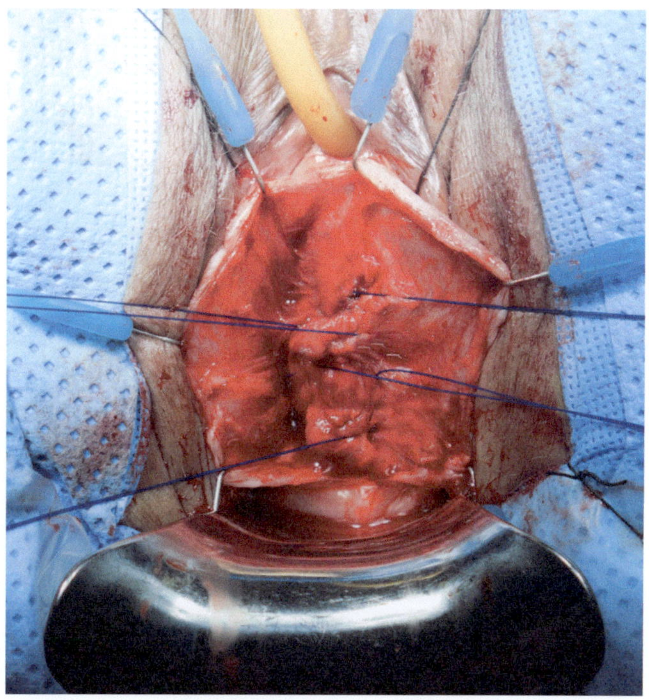

Fig. 3.48 The central defect is repaired by sequentially applying delayed absorbable sutures (PDS) to the perivesical fascia

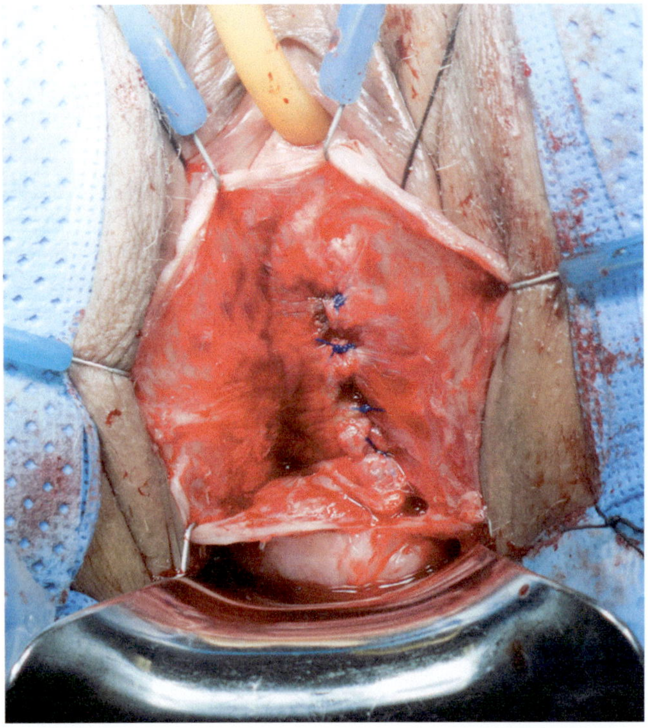

Fig. 3.49 The centrally placed sutures are tied to approximate the perivesical fascia to the midline

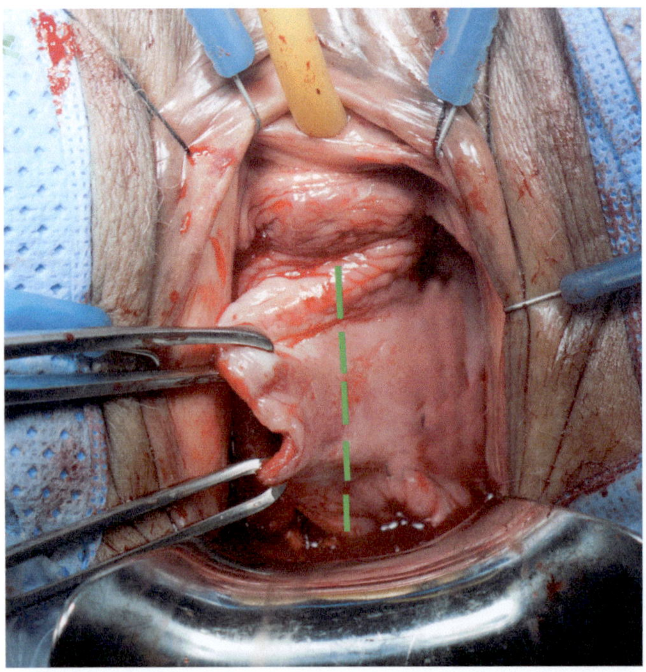

Fig. 3.50 The excess of the vaginal wall is excised and the anterior vaginal wall is closed with interrupted #2-0 delayed absorbable sutures. The *green dotted line* depicts the line of excision of the excess of vaginal wall

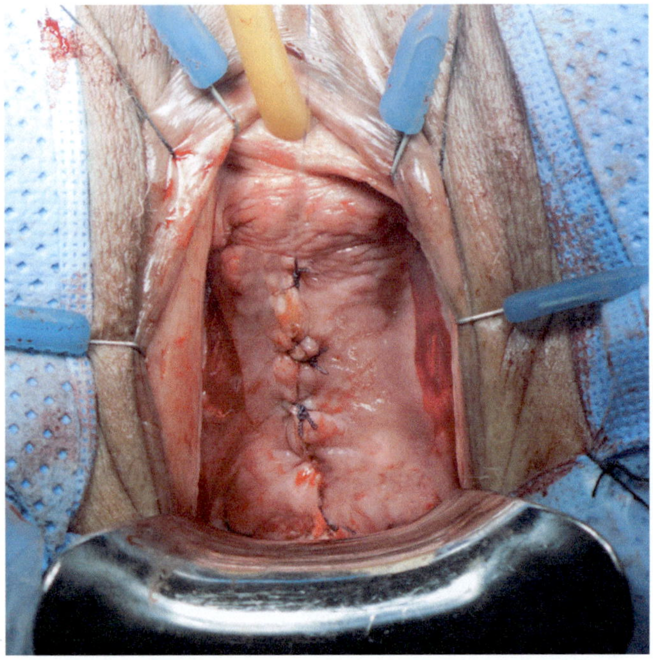

Fig. 3.51 The anterior vaginal wall is closed and two oblique incisions are made laterally from the midurethral area to the bladder base

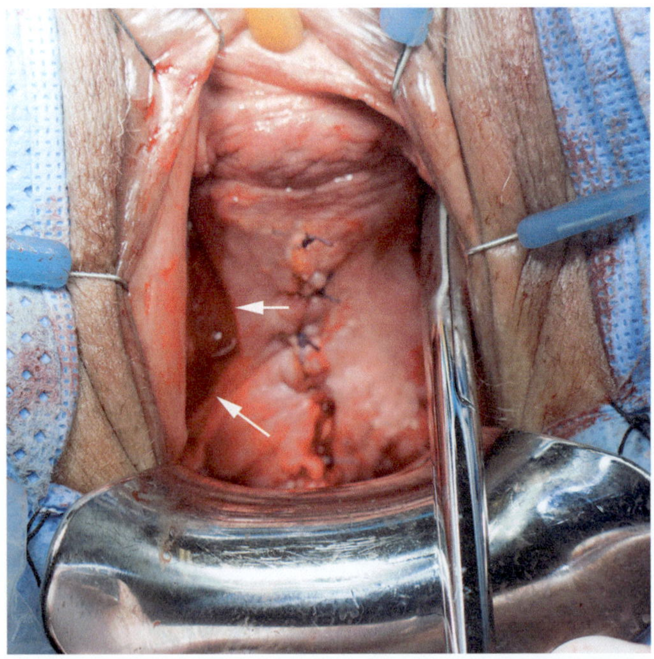

Fig. 3.52 Curved Mayo scissors are applied under the inferior pubic bone and parallel to the urethra, pointing the tip superiorly. *White arrows* indicate the lateral vaginal wall incision in the right side

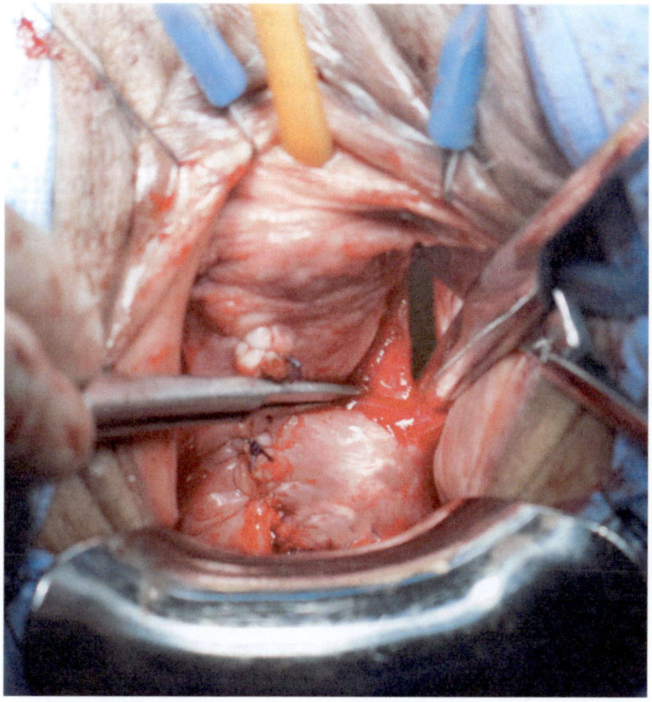

Fig. 3.53 The retropubic space is entered, detaching the urethra and vesicopelvic fascia from the arcus tendineus

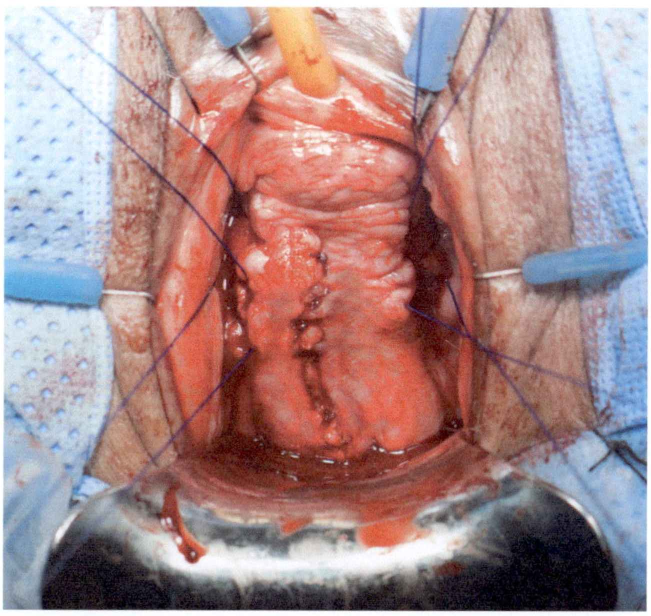

Fig. 3.54 In a similar fashion as described above, #0 monofilament nonabsorbable sutures are applied to the bladder base, the bladder neck, and periurethral area. Each pass includes the detached vesicopelvic and perivesical fascia at the bladder base and the urethropelvic fascia and periurethral fascia at the bladder neck and midurethral area. The placement of these sutures is similar to the four-corner bladder and bladder neck suspension (see Fig. 3.42)

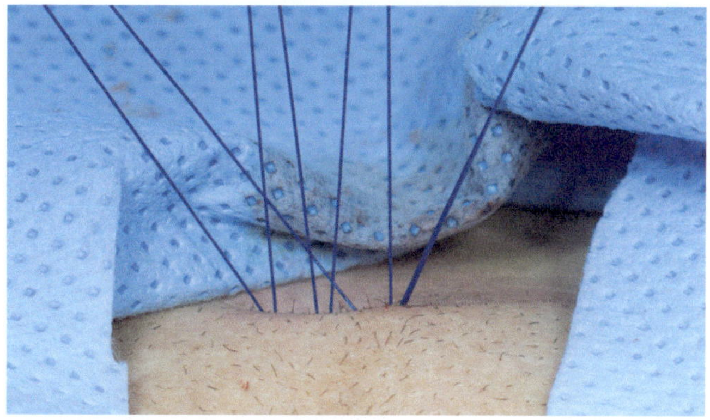

Fig. 3.55 The four sutures are transferred from the vagina to the suprapubic area using a double-pronged passer

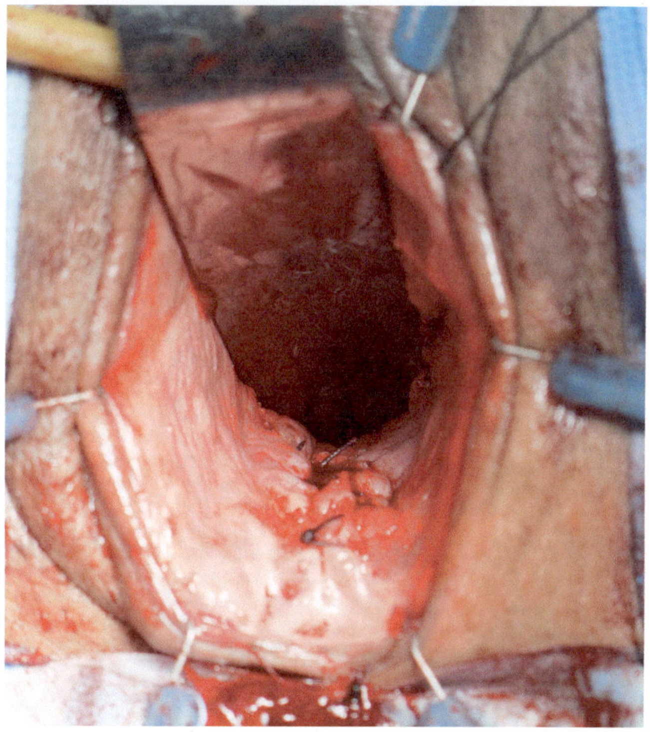

Fig. 3.56 The anterior vaginal wall is closed with interrupted #2-0 delayed absorbable sutures. A posterior repair has been performed

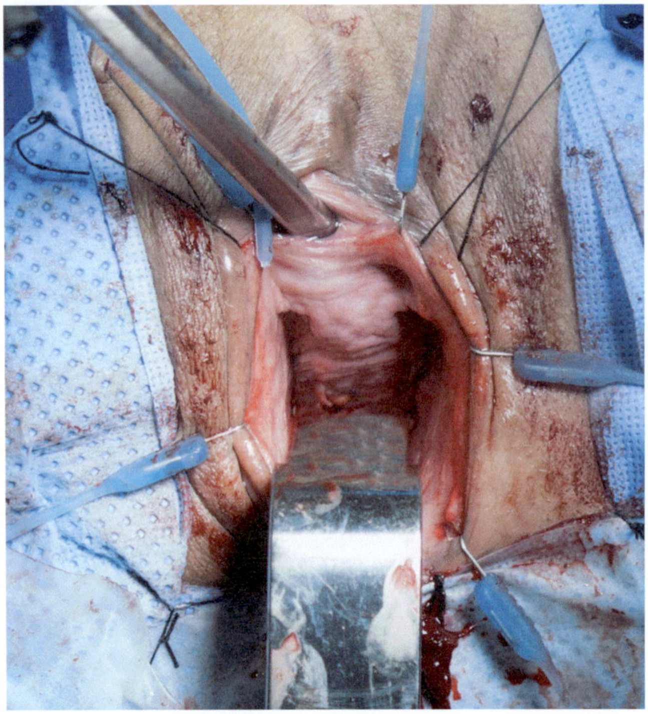

Fig. 3.57 Cystoscopy is performed after intravenous injection of indigo carmine. The suprapubic nonabsorbable sutures are tied sequentially, keeping the cystoscope in a 45-degree angulation in order to prevent unnecessary bladder and urethral overcorrection. A vaginal packing soaked with antibiotics will be inserted in the vagina. The suprapubic puncture is closed with a #4-0 delayed absorbable suture

3.1.7 Fascia Lata Lateral and Central Defect Repair in Patients with Recurrent Cystocele

After multiple failed cystocele repairs, it is not uncommon to find during the exploration of the anterior vaginal wall an absent periurethral fascia and a very thin bladder wall. Also commonly found is a lateral defect due to a detached and attenuated connective tissue that connects the bladder to the arcus tendineus fascia pelvis. Applying sutures for repair of the central defect or the lateral defect in the absence of perivesical tissue will end in another failed procedure.

We have designed a procedure using autologous fascia lata to repair the central and lateral defect in patients with multiple failed surgeries for cystocele (Figs. 3.58, 3.59, 3.60, 3.61, 3.62, 3.63, 3.64, 3.65, 3.66, 3.67, 3.68, and 3.69). We use two segments of autologous fascia lata that are approximated with interrupted sutures to form a large rectangular graft. At the end of both segments of fascia, a #1 delayed absorbable suture is applied. The paravesical space is entered in each side. A small suprapubic puncture is performed, and using a double-pronged passer, the sutures are transferred under finger control from the vagina to the suprapubic area. The graft is secured with interrupted sutures to the periurethral fascia and the base of the bladder to prevent displacement. Tying the suprapubic sutures will provide a central and lateral defect repair in patients with recurrent cystocele with absent tissue for a standard cystocele repair.

The procedure is minimally invasive, uses strong autologous tissue, and avoids the use of mesh. It provides an excellent lateral and central defect repair in patients with multiple failed cystocele repairs.

Postoperative care and complications of the procedure are similar to other anterior vaginal wall procedures.

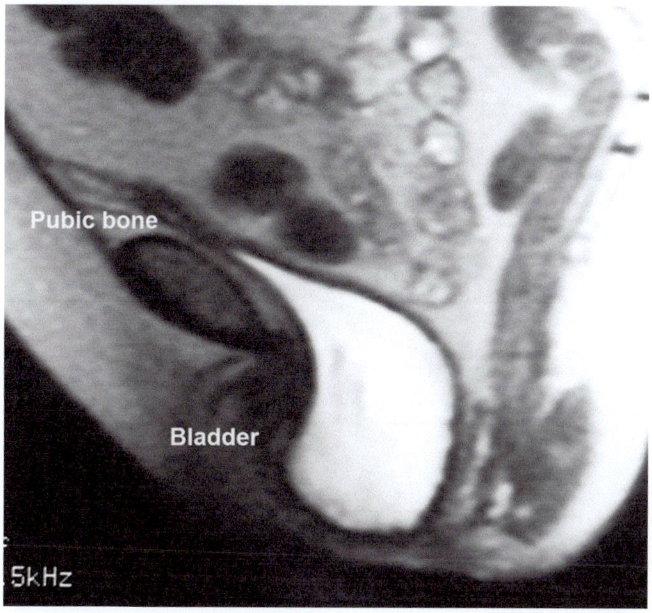

Fig. 3.58 Dynamic MRI of the patient with recurrent symptomatic cystocele. The patient had a cystocele repair with mesh resulting in erosion of the anterior vaginal wall and mesh removal. Subsequently she underwent two cystocele repairs that failed a few months later

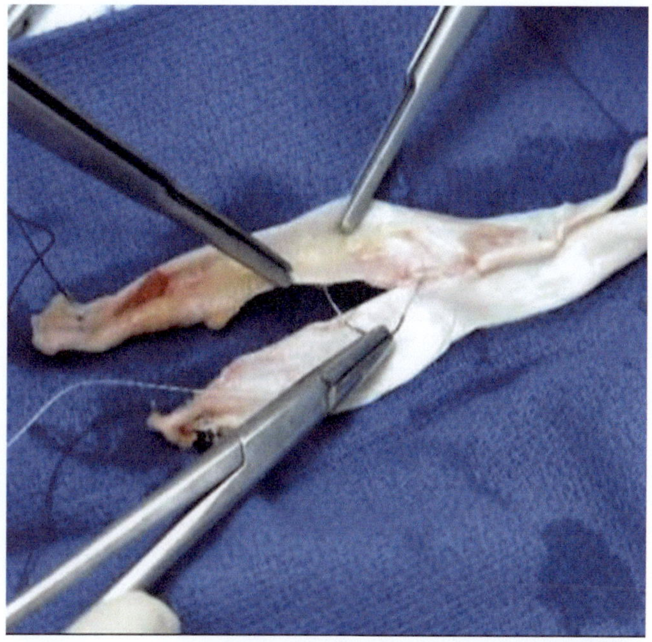

Fig. 3.60 The two segments of fascia are approximated using delayed absorbable sutures in order to create a wide rectangular fascial graft

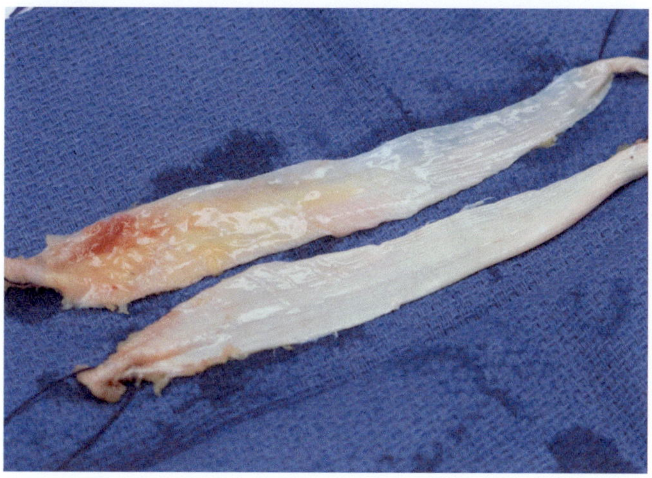

Fig. 3.59 Two segments of autologous fascia lata 10 cm long are obtained from the thigh through a 4–5-cm incision in the skin. The Crawford fascial stripper is used (see chapter on sling for incontinence using fascia lata)

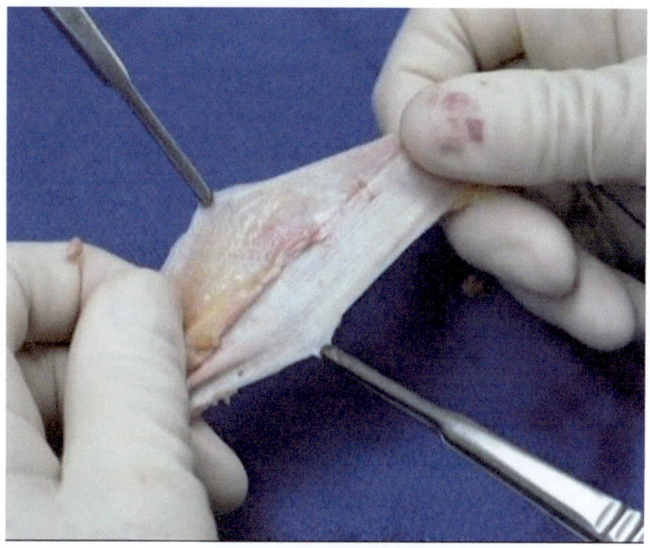

Fig. 3.61 The two joint segments of fascia are seen

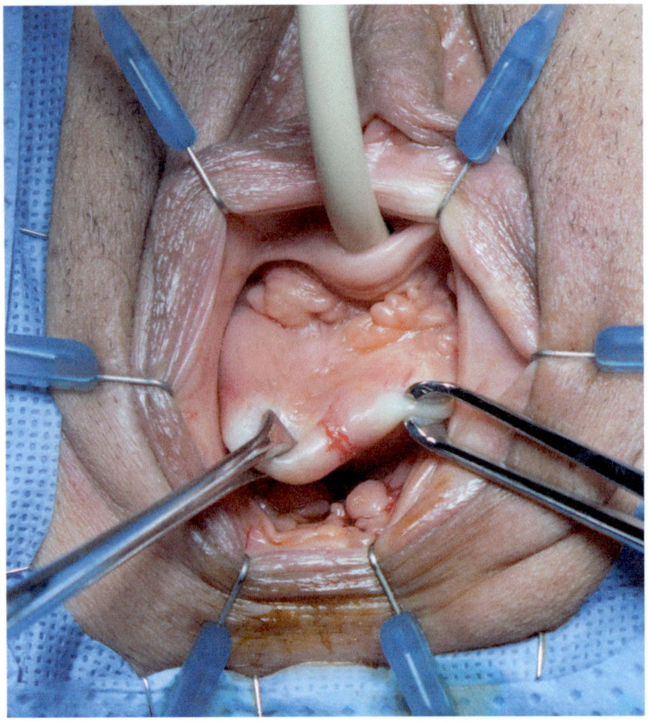

Fig. 3.62 A vertical incision is made in the anterior vaginal wall from the bladder neck to the bladder base

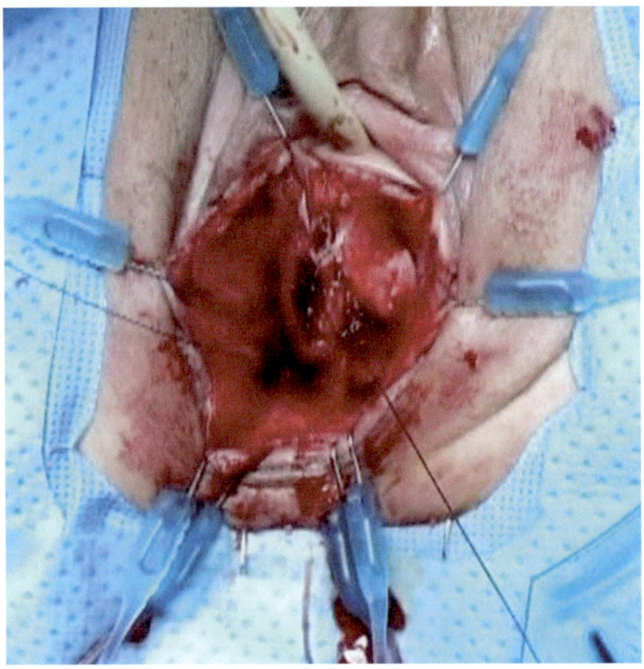

Fig. 3.63 The bladder wall is exposed and an absent periurethral fascia is found

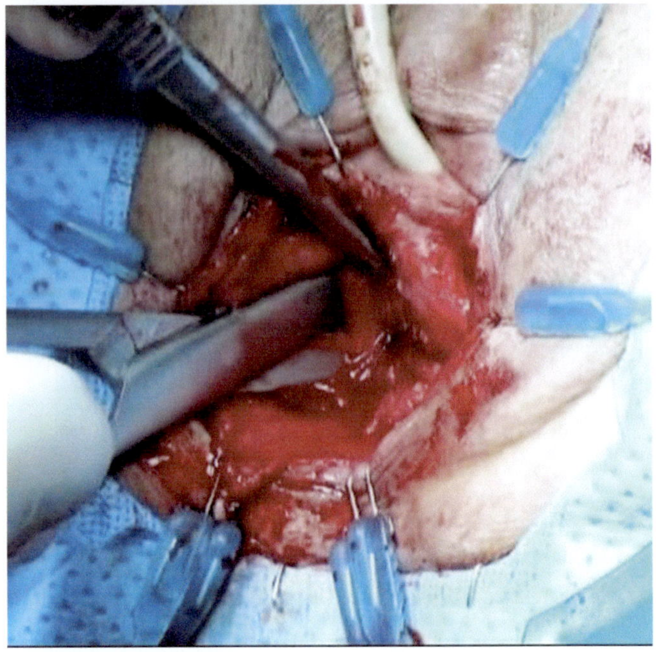

Fig. 3.64 Using scissors, the paravesical space is entered in each side and all adhesions are freed

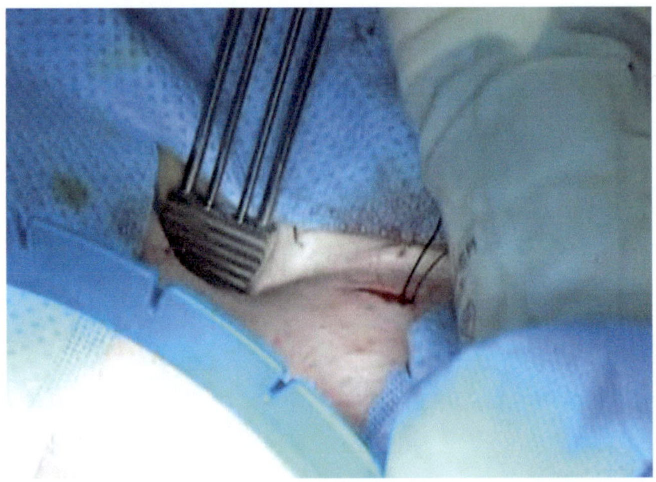

Fig. 3.65 Due to significant adhesions of the bladder in midline, two small punctures are performed in the suprapubic area. Under finger control in the retropubic space, a double-pronged passer is transferred from the suprapubic to the vaginal area

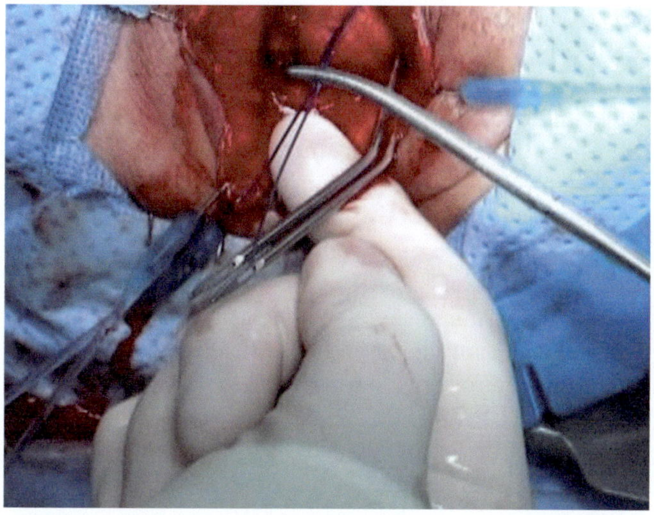

Fig. 3.66 The delayed absorbable sutures at the end of the fascial construct are transferred through the eyes of the needle passer. The passer is pulled back to the suprapubic area

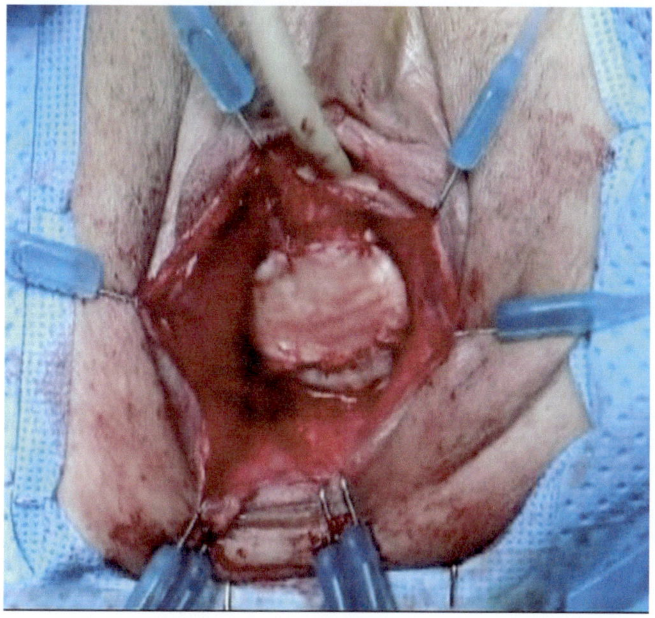

Fig. 3.67 Several #3-0 delayed absorbable sutures are used at the bladder base and bladder neck to secure the fascial segment to the perivesical tissues and prevent displacement

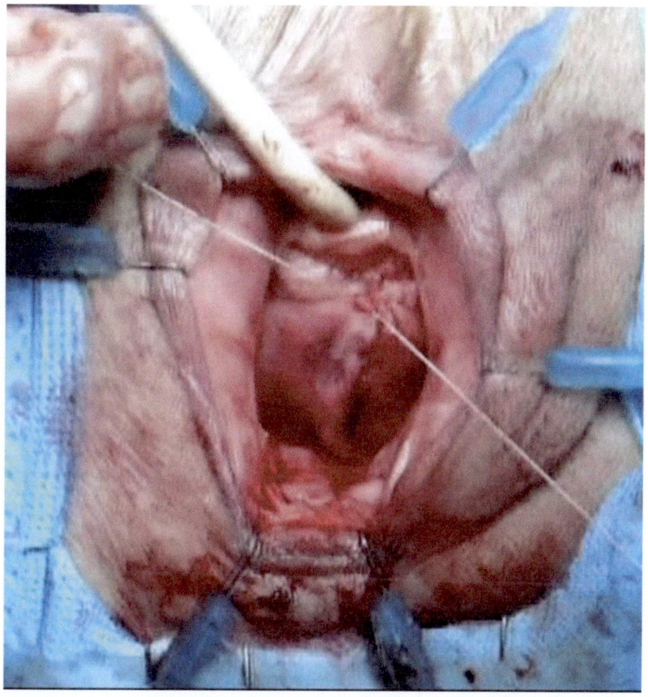

Fig. 3.68 The anterior vaginal wall is closed with delayed absorbable sutures

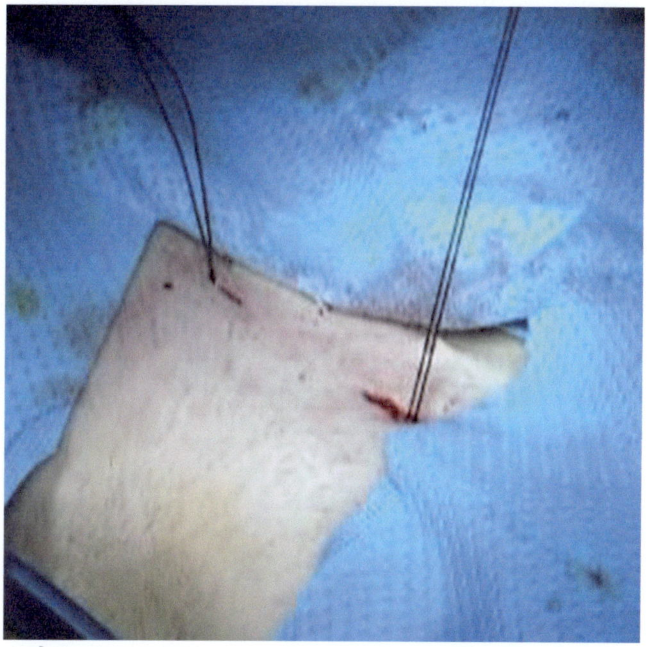

Fig. 3.69 View of the suprapubic punctures after the sutures are tied. The skin will be closed with a delayed absorbable suture

3.2 Vaginal Hysterectomy for Uterine Prolapse

3.2.1 Indications

Vaginal hysterectomy is in general indicated in cases of severe vaginal prolapse with concomitant uterine descent. Operations to provide support of the uterus are indicated in selected patients in particular patient that refuse to have hysterectomy or minimal uterine prolapse. In patients with uterine prolapse, the sacrouterine and cardinal ligaments, which normally are responsible for uterine support, are separated, detached, or stretched, allowing vault prolapse to occur. After completion of the hysterectomy, a defect is created between the perivesical and prerectal fascia, so it is important on completion of the vaginal hysterectomy to correct two defects, providing support of the vaginal cuff (vault suspension) and approximating the perivesical fascia to the prerectal fascia to close the posterior cul-de-sac. Uterine prolapse is rarely an isolated condition, and associated pelvic floor relaxation and prolapse of the bladder and rectum are very common.

Vaginal hysterectomy is not routinely indicated in patients with good uterine support who are suffering from stress incontinence. Relative contraindications include uterine size out of proportion to vaginal accessibility, adnexal tumor, acute or subacute pelvic inflammation, endometriosis, or malignancy of the ovaries or uterus.

3.2.2 Diagnosis

The diagnosis of uterine prolapse is easily made when physical examination reveals significant uterine descent. A clinical history of pelvic discomfort, vaginal mass, dyspareunia, or stress urinary incontinence associated with uterine prolapse is very common. Any history of vaginal bleeding must be fully evaluated to rule out uterine carcinoma. A bimanual pelvic examination will help to grade the degree of uterine prolapse from minimal (to mid-vaginal area) to moderate (mid-vagina to introitus) or severe (when the uterus is always outside the introitus). Any associated pelvic abnormality such as cystocele, rectocele, enterocele, stress incontinence, or pelvic floor relaxation should be clearly defined because they need to be repaired at the time of hysterectomy. If required, imaging by ultrasound or MRI may help to rule out other pelvic pathology (Fig. 3.70).

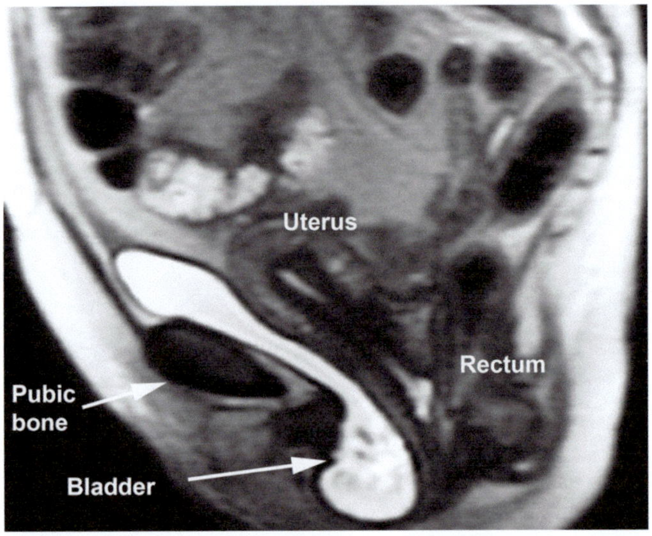

Fig. 3.70 Dynamic MRI of a patient with severe uterine prolapse without urethral or bladder prolapse. The uterus is seen coming out of the vaginal introitus

3.2.3 Surgical Technique

In patients with significant uterine prolapse, associated pathology such as cystocele or rectocele is very common and should be repaired simultaneously. If a cystocele is present, we perform the vaginal hysterectomy first, close the vaginal cuff, and then proceed with the cystocele repair. Figures 3.71, 3.72, 3.73, 3.74, 3.75, 3.76, 3.77, 3.78, 3.79, 3.80, 3.81, 3.82, 3.83, 3.84, 3.85, 3.86, 3.87, 3.88, 3.89, 3.90, 3.91, 3.92, 3.93, 3.94, 3.95, 3.96, 3.97, and 3.98 illustrate the technique of vaginal hysterectomy for severe uterine prolapse as an independent procedure.

3.2.4 Postoperative Care

Intravenous antibiotic prophylaxis is given before surgery. In selected patients further antibiotic therapy may be required. The vaginal packing is removed the morning after surgery. Patients are discharged after normal oral food intake is restored, usually on the second day after surgery. Pain medication and a stool softener are prescribed. The patient can immediately resume normal activities like walking, driving, or cooking. Strenuous activities and impact exercises are restricted for 1 month.

3.2.5 Intraoperative Complications

Potential complications at the time of surgery include bleeding (which may be severe if the uterine artery or vein is lacerated prior to completion of the lateral exposure of the cervix), ureteric injury, and bladder laceration.

3.2.6 Postoperative Complications

Complications after hysterectomy are not different from those of other vaginal surgery. A rare complication is postoperative ureteric obstruction, with the most commonly involved segment being the distal pelvic ureter immediately preceding its entrance into the bladder. Bladder fistulae are now seen less frequently and usually occur either cranially along the bladder base or at the trigone. Vaginal shortening may occur because of improper closure of the cuff, poor quality of the tissues, or excessive trimming of the vaginal wall during the closure of the cuff.

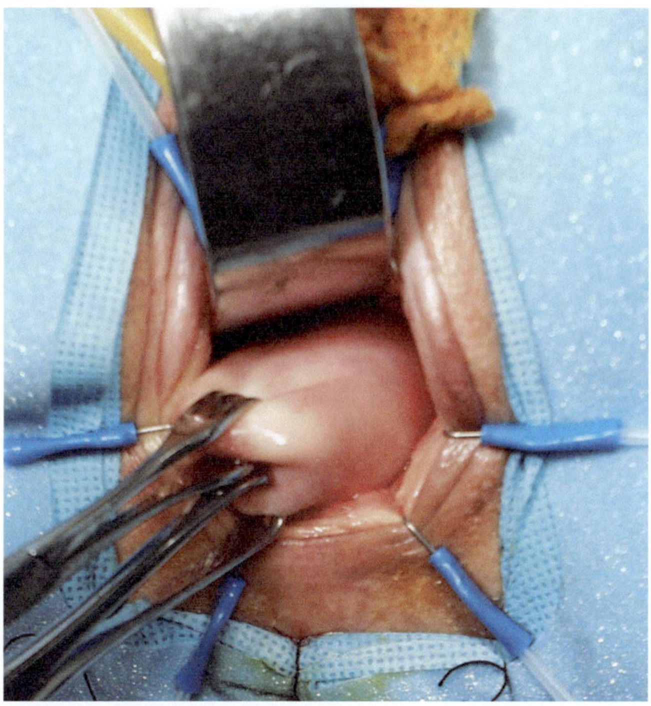

Fig. 3.71 A urethral catheter is used to empty the bladder. A ring retractor with multiple hooks is used to retract the vaginal margins. The cervix is grasped with two multiple-toothed tenacula (Lahey clamps), and the mobility of the uterus is once more assessed. One tenaculum is applied on the anterior margin of the cervix and one on the posterior margin. This maneuver will align the cervix and prevent accidental injury of the uterine pedicle during the initial dissection. The anterior and posterior cervical dissection can be performed in an avascular cleavage plane

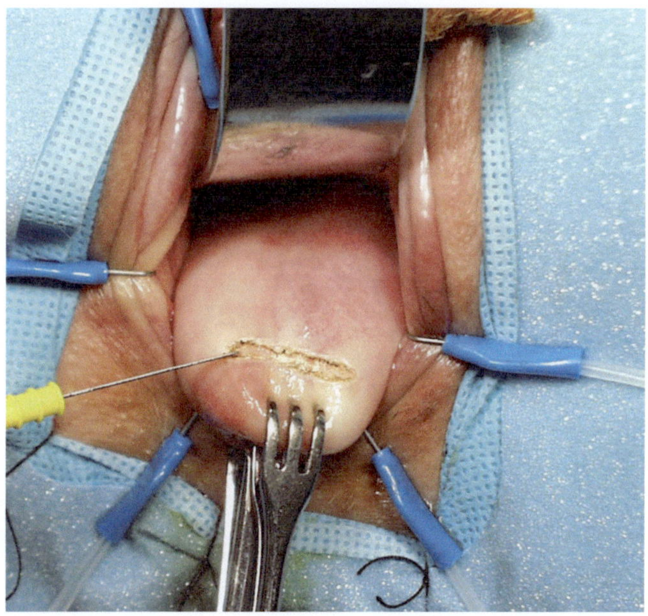

Fig. 3.72 Using a coagulation knife, a circumferential incision is made around the cervix, exposing the anterior cervical fascia

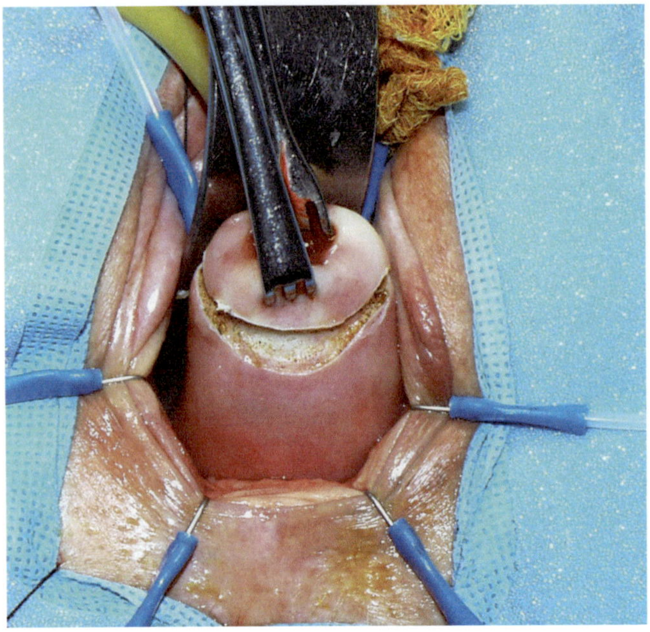

Fig. 3.73 The posterior vaginal wall is also incised using the coagulation knife to expose the posterior cervical fascia. The incision is extended laterally

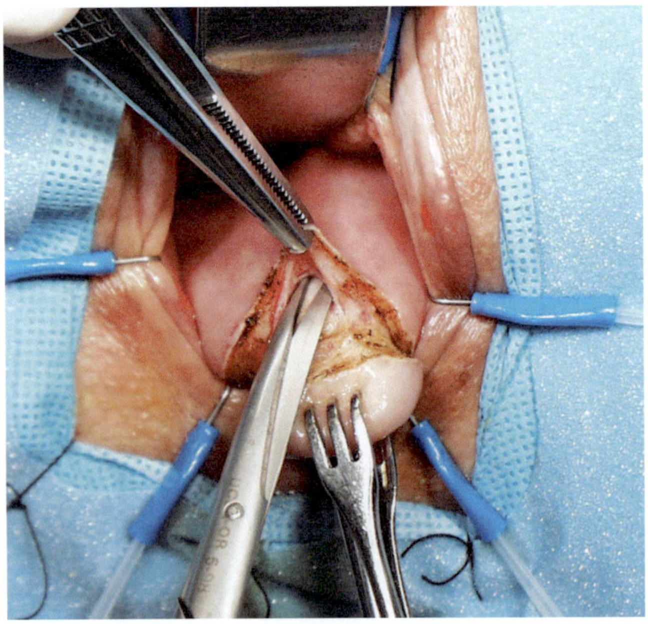

Fig. 3.74 The dissection is started over the glistening anterior surface of the cervix. Using Metzenbaum scissors, the plane between the anterior cervix and the posterior bladder wall and perivesical fascia is opened. Care is taken to stay close to the anterior cervical fascia to prevent accidental bladder injury

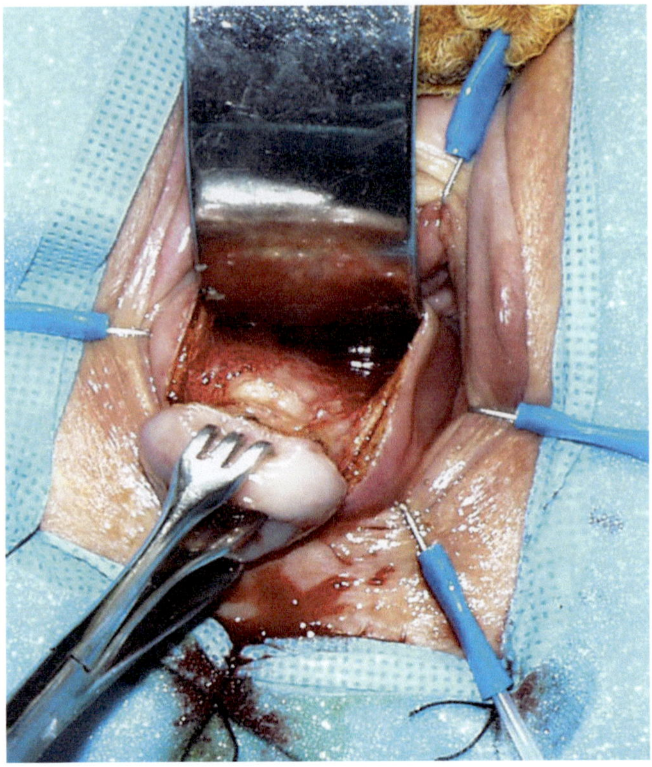

Fig. 3.75 The dissection is continued over the anterior surface of the cervix toward the anterior peritoneal fold, opening the vesicouterine space. A retractor is inserted in this space

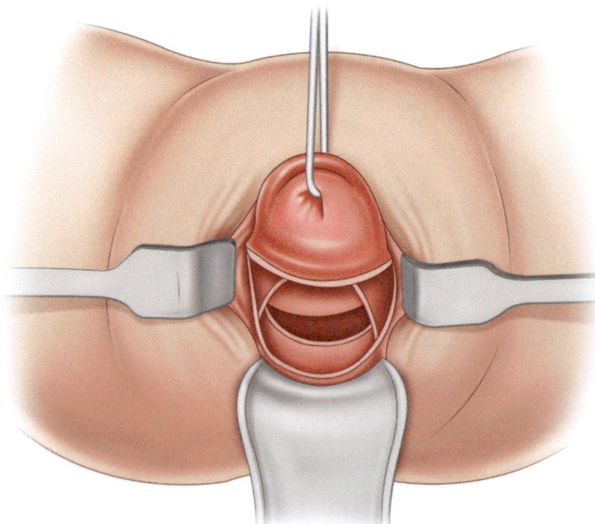

Fig. 3.76 Diagram showing the posterior dissection of the cervix before entering the cul-de-sac

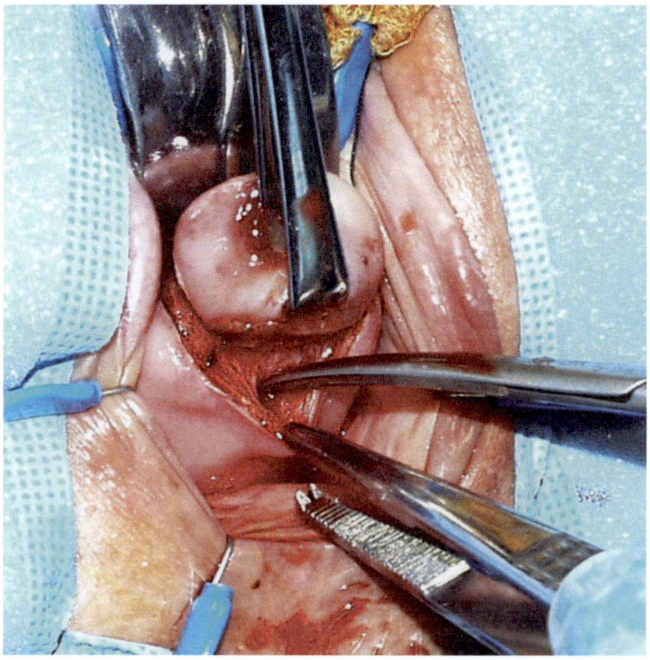

Fig. 3.77 With upward traction over the cervix, the dissection is carried out over the posterior cervical fascia until the peritoneal fold is reached. Care is taken to avoid lateral dissection in order to avoid damage to the uterine pedicle. The peritoneum is entered and a deep retractor is inserted in the cul-de-sac

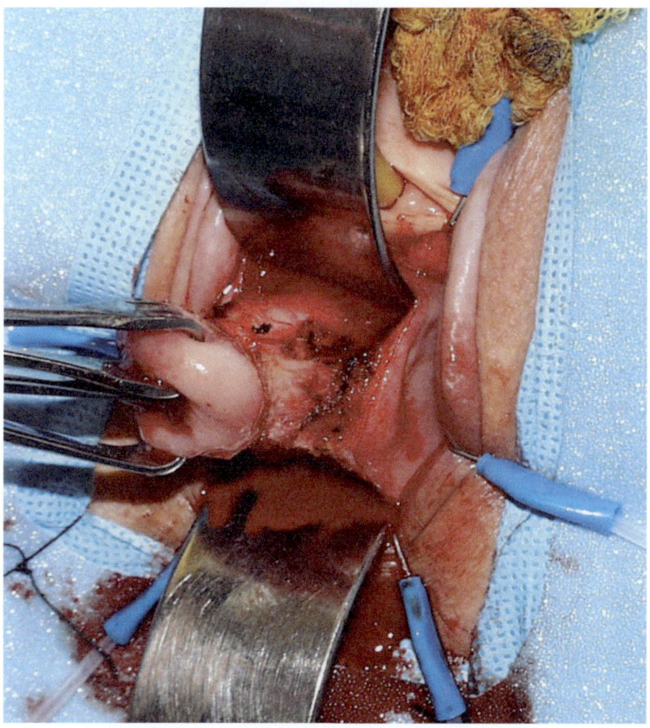

Fig. 3.78 With deep retractors in the anterior vesicouterine space and the posterior open cul-de-sac, lateral traction is applied to the cervix to expose the sacrouterine–cardinal complex

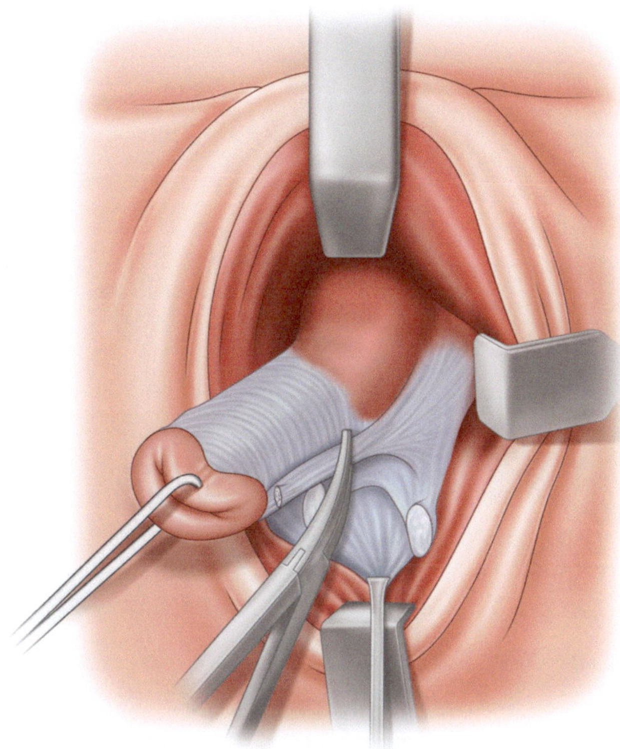

Fig. 3.79 Diagram showing the isolation of the cardinal and sacrouterine ligaments

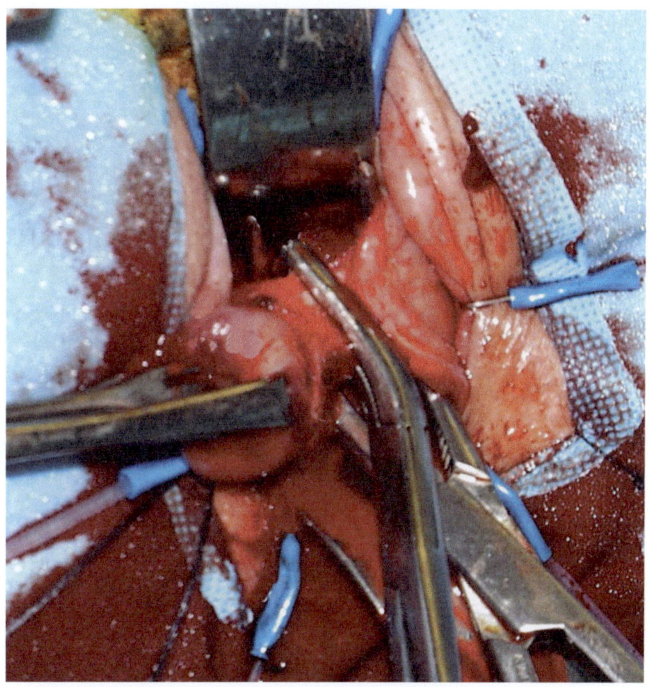

Fig. 3.80 The tip of a large right-angle clamp is introduced into the cul-de-sac to isolate the distal sacrouterine–cardinal complex. With the cervix under slight traction, using a curved Phaneuf clamp, the cardinal and sacrouterine ligaments are isolated and clamped 1–2 cm from the cervical junction. The ligaments are tied with figure-of-eight #0 delay absorbable sutures. The suture ends are left long, clamped, and secured lateral to one of the grooves of the ring retractor

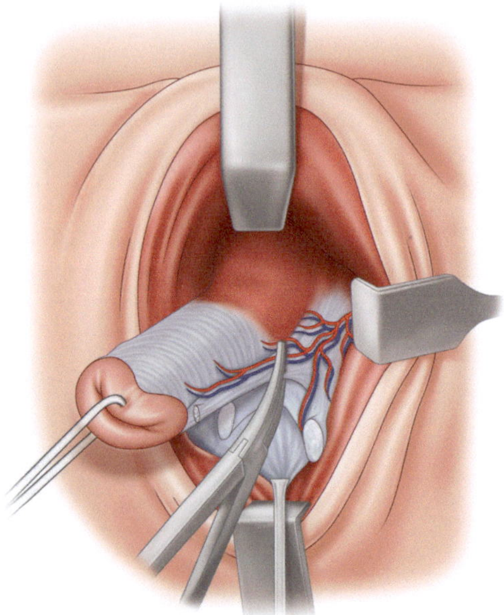

Fig. 3.81 Diagram showing the isolation of the uterine pedicle

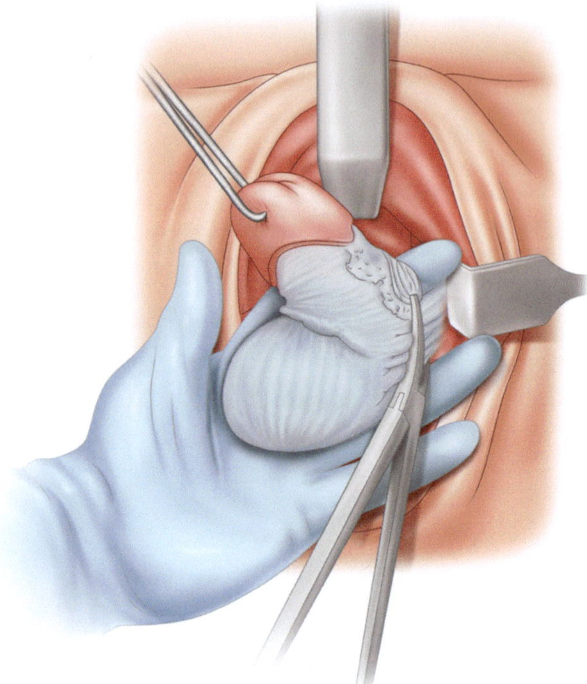

Fig. 3.83 Diagram of the eversion of the fundus of the cervix to expose the anterior peritoneum and broad ligaments

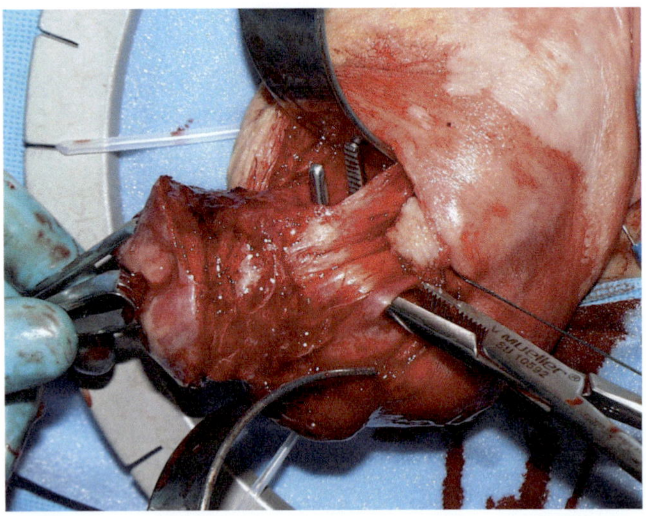

Fig. 3.82 With slight lateral traction on the cervix, the uterine artery and vein are identified and isolated using a right-angle clamp. Using a Phaneuf clamp, the pedicle is clamped and cut, and the pedicle is ligated as they run lateral to the cervix. The suture ends are left long, clamped, and secured to one of the grooves of the ring retractor

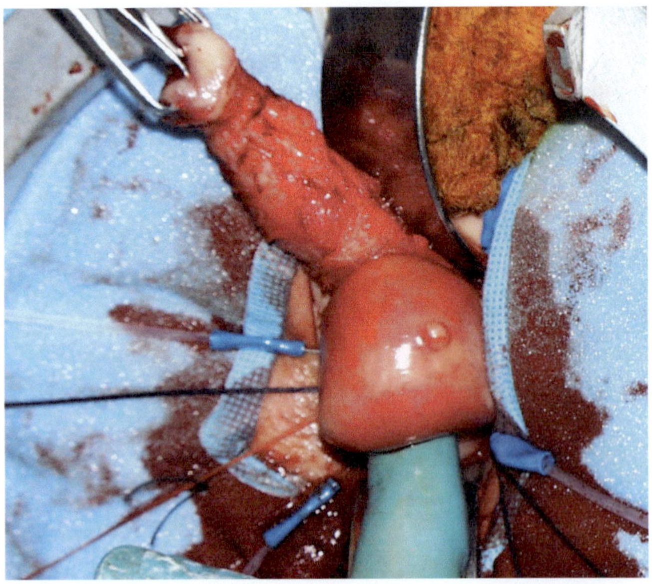

Fig. 3.84 The cervix is retracted upward and the fundus of the uterus is everted and brought outside the introitus. The thin, semilunar folds of the peritoneum can now be visualized attaching to the uterus. These folds are held with forceps, incised with scissors, and spread open. A retractor is inserted in the anterior peritoneum. The uterus is now attached only by the broad ligaments on each side

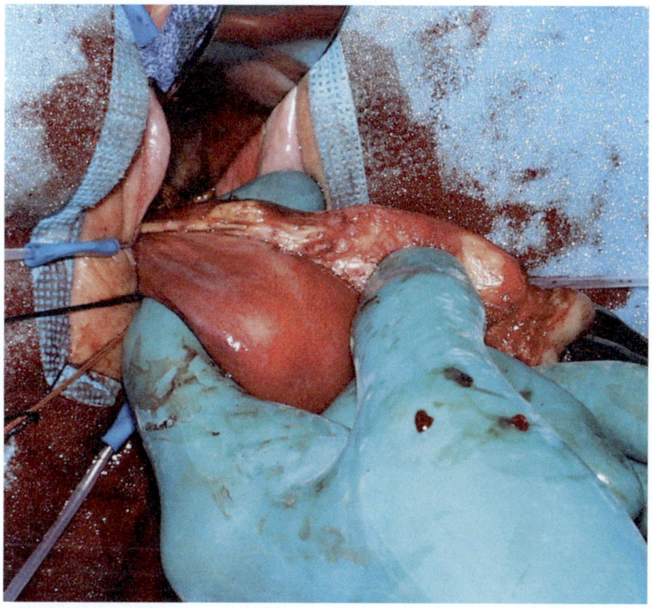

Fig. 3.85 The anterior retractor is now introduced in the anterior peritoneal space. The finger encircles the broad ligaments

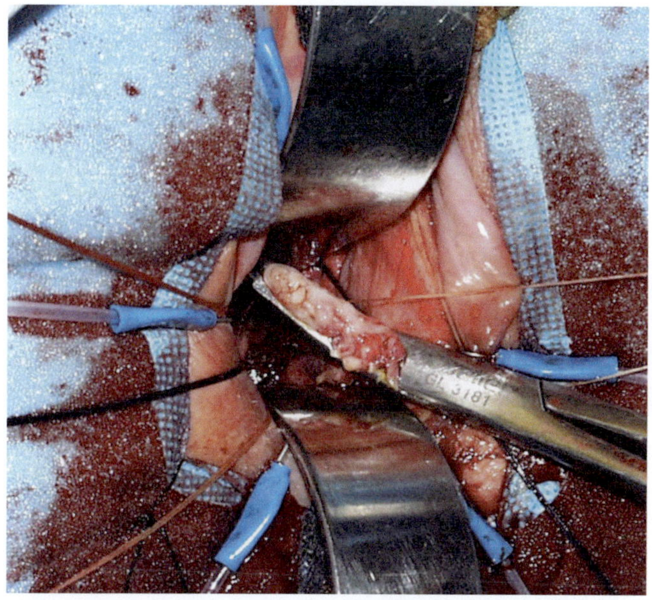

Fig. 3.87 The broad ligaments have been incised. The utero-ovarian ligament, the fallopian tube, and the round ligament are visible in succession from anterior to posterior and can be clamped, divided, and ligated with #0 delay absorbable sutures in one pedicle

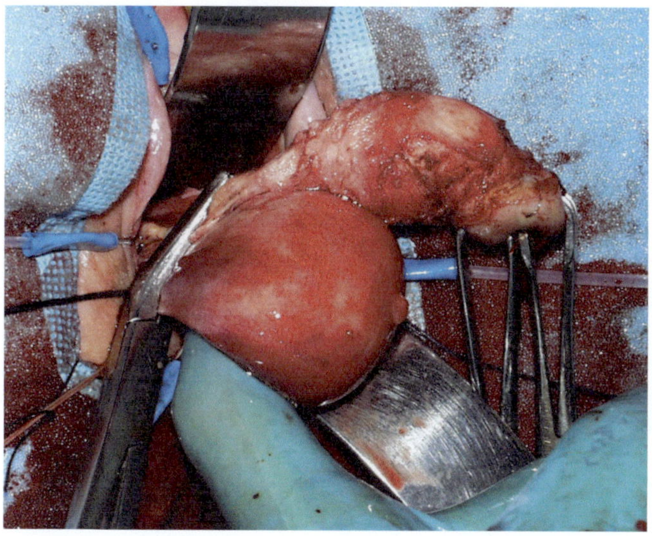

Fig. 3.86 If the adnexa are to be left behind, the broad ligaments are now clamped close to the uterine body

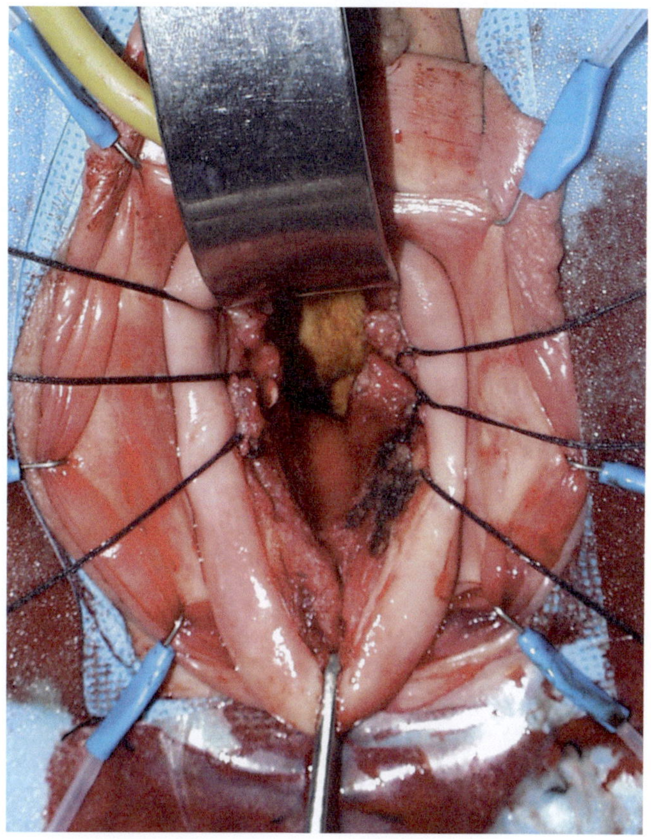

Fig. 3.88 After completion of the hysterectomy, three pedicles are observed on each side: the anterior includes the broad ligament, the middle includes the uterine artery, and the posterior includes the cardinal and sacrouterine ligaments. The closure of the cuff is performed with a pair of purse-string sutures to approximate the perivesical fascia to the prerectal fascia. The vault suspension will be done with a pair of culdosuspension sutures (to support the cuff) using #1 delay absorbable sutures, as described in the following section on enterocele repair

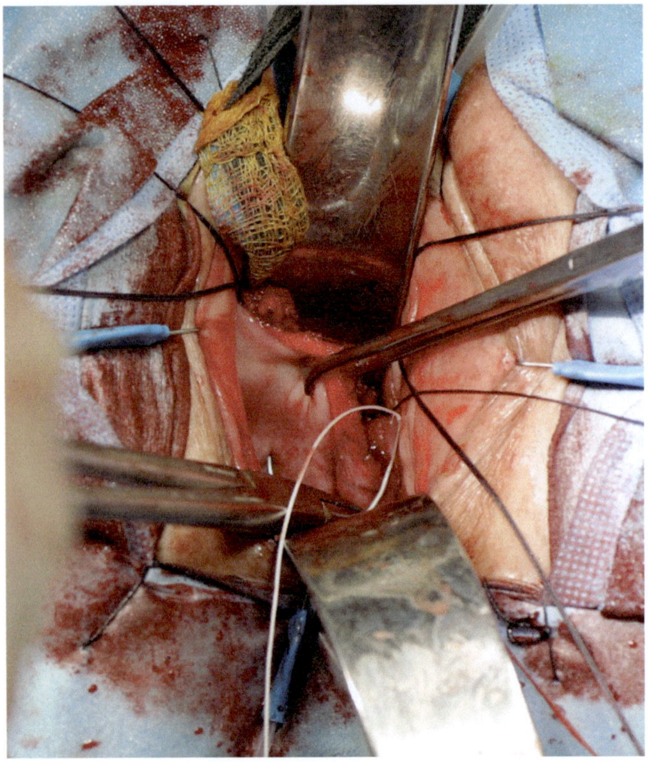

Fig. 3.89 A #1 slow absorbable suture (PDS) is placed through the posterolateral vaginal wall, high on the lateral fornix, and a few centimeters from the margin of the vaginal incision

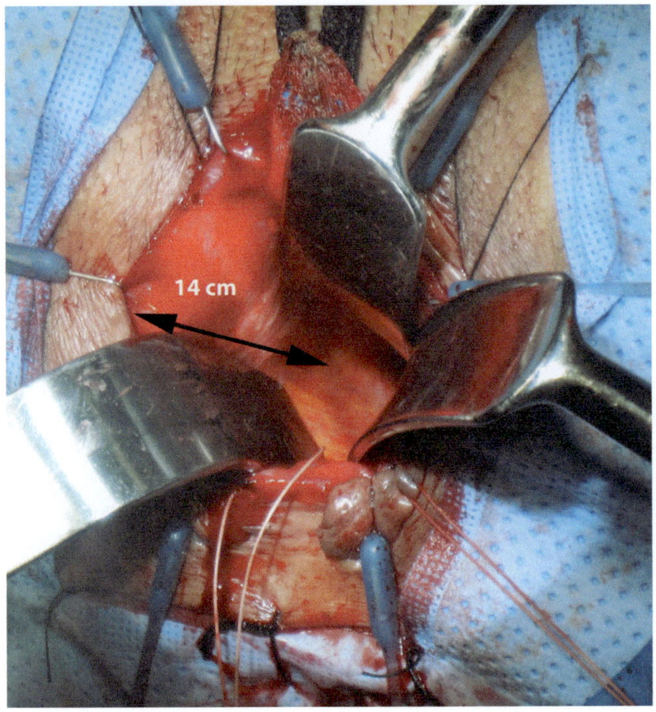

Fig. 3.90 With the suture in the peritoneum, the suture is successively passed through the prerectal fascia 4–5 cm from the cuff (to help correct a rectocele) and to the ipsilateral origin of the sacrouterine–cardinal complex. The sutures must incorporate a strong bite of tissue, and two passes of the needle are used. The suture is applied in pararectal fascia, medial to the levator musculature, lateral to the sacrum, and distal to the sacrospinous ligament and coccygeus muscle. The suture is brought outside the vaginal lumen 1 cm from the original site of entry. An identical suture is placed on the opposite side, starting from the contralateral vaginal fornix. These vault suspension sutures are left untied. The *arrow* indicates the distance of 14 cm between the introitus and the place of placement of the sutures in the groove lateral to the sacrum and distal to the sacrospinous ligaments

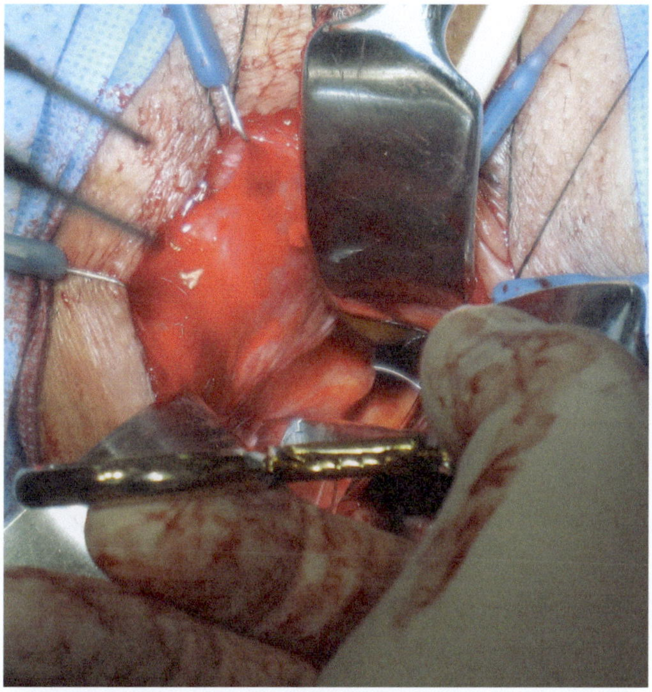

Fig. 3.91 Placement of the vault suspension suture at the origin of the sacrouterine ligaments in the pararectal area, lateral to the sacrum, medial to the levators, and distal to the sacrouterine ligaments

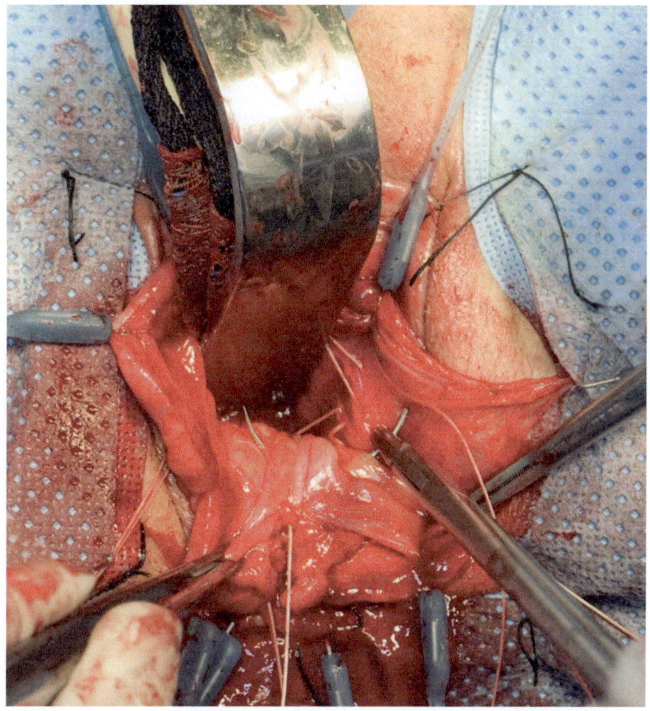

Fig. 3.93 Two purse-string sutures of #1 slow absorbable suture are applied distal to the vault suspension sutures. Posteriorly and distally, they incorporate the prerectal fascia

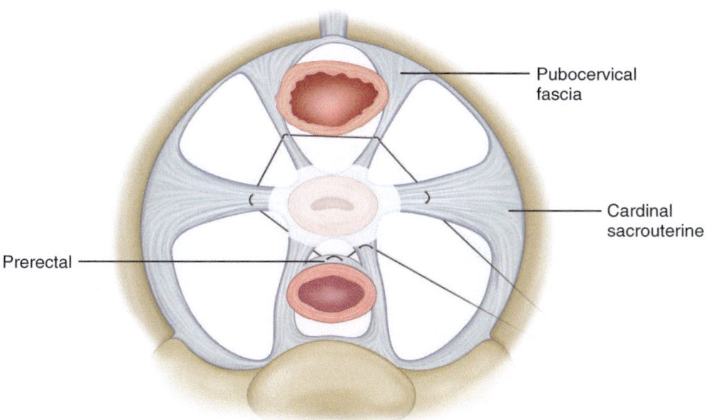

Fig. 3.92 Diagram of the placement of the purse-string sutures that will approximate the perivesical fascia to the prerectal fascia and close the peritoneal cavity

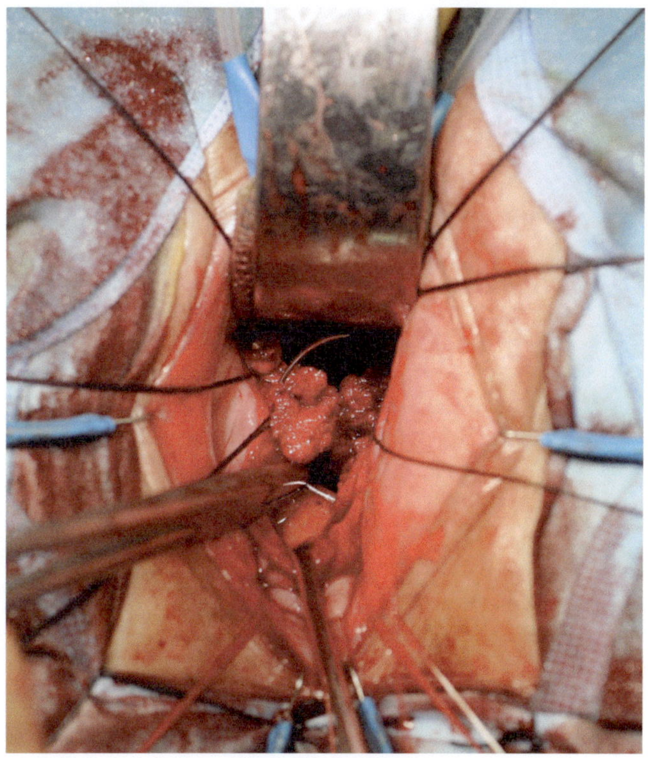

Fig. 3.94 The purse-string suture incorporates the sacrouterine–cardinal complex 1 cm inside the vaginal cuff and the prerectal fascia. The distal suture placement ensures adequate vaginal depth

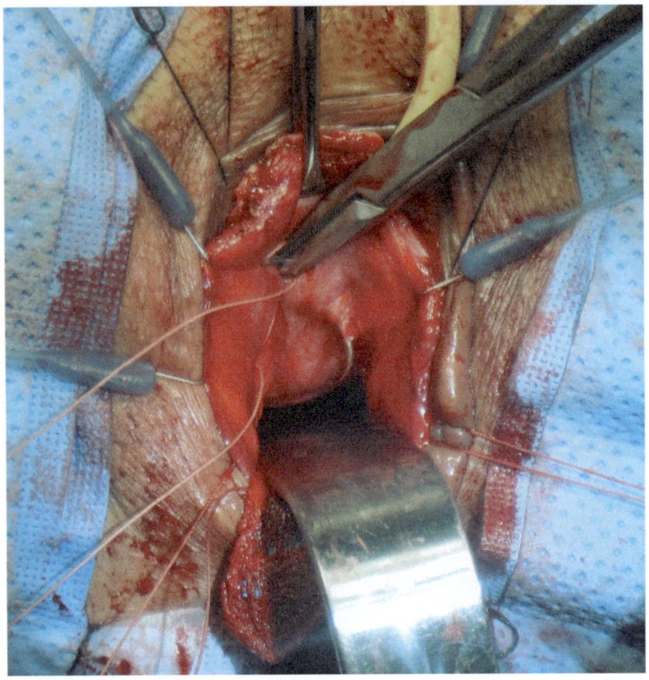

Fig. 3.95 The anterior segment of the purse-string suture includes the broad ligaments, the bladder base (the pubocervical fascia), and lateral peritoneum. Care should be taken not to apply the sutures high or lateral to the paravesical groove because of the close proximity to the ureter

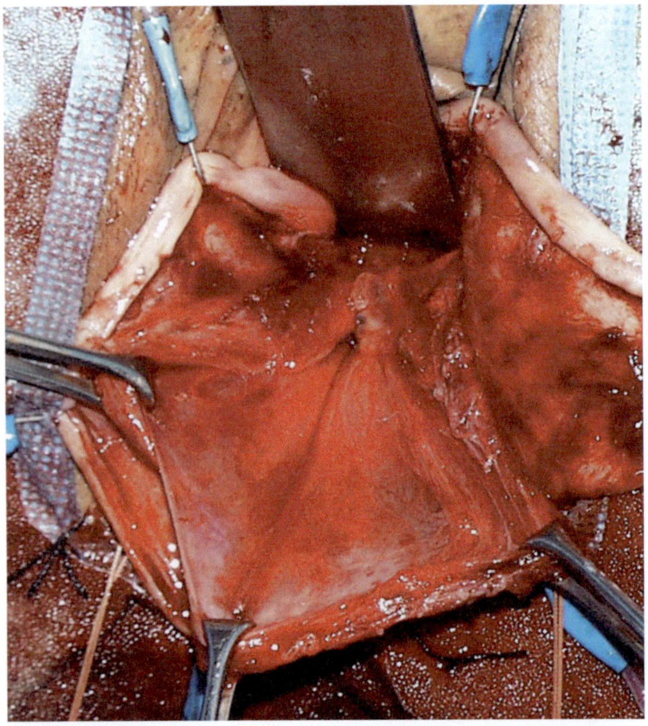

Fig. 3.96 A second purse-string suture is applied, the laparotomy pads are removed, and the purse-string sutures are tied. Prior to tying the sutures, the broad ligament sutures are approximated to the midline to keep the pedicles in an extraperitoneal location. In Figure 3.85 the vaginal cuff is closed with multiple running, locking, delay absorbable sutures after cutting the ends of the purse-string sutures. The vault suspension sutures are seen lateral to the closed cuff

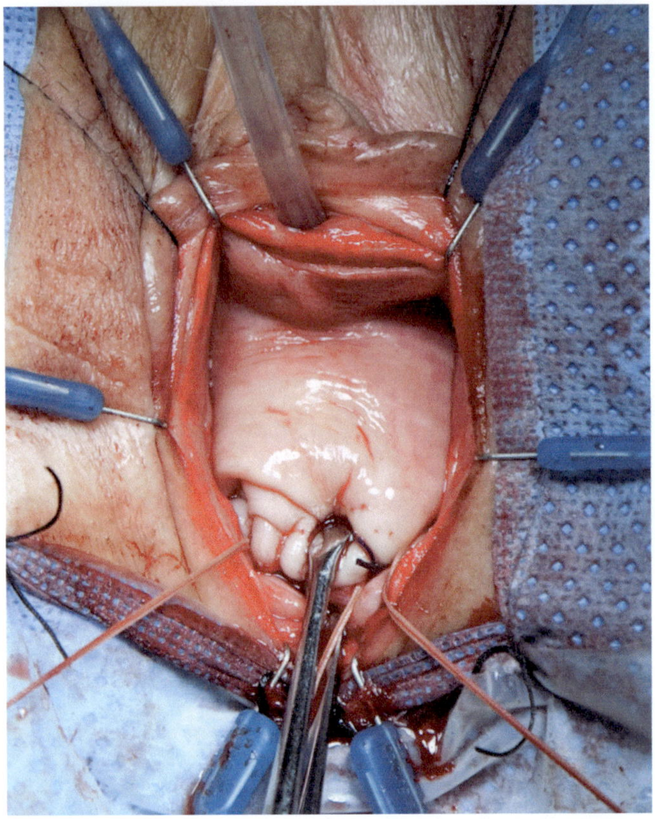

Fig. 3.97 After copious irrigation with antibiotic solution. the vaginal cuff is closed with multiple locking runs of delay absorbable sutures

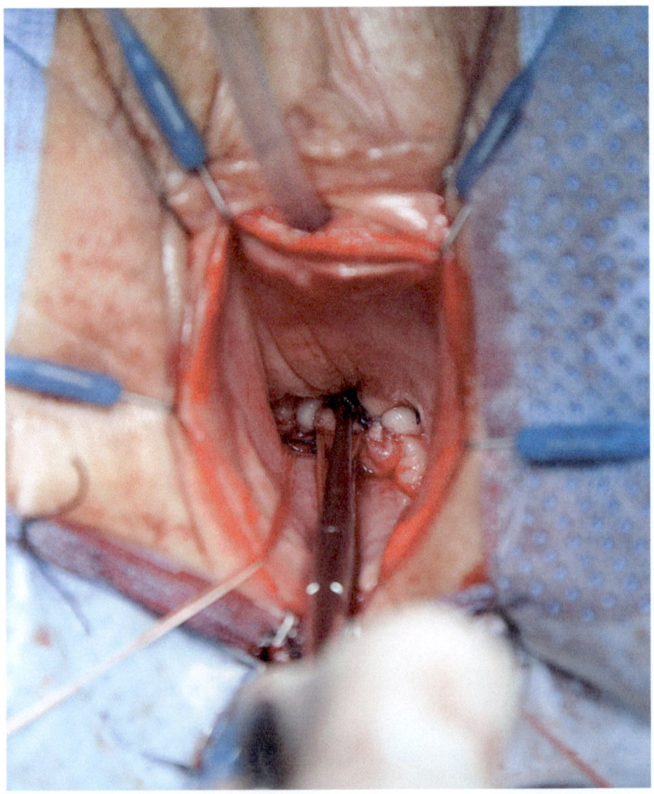

Fig. 3.98 If no other vaginal surgery is planned, the vault suspension sutures are cinched down and tied individually. Tying these suspension sutures pulls the vaginal cuff cephalad and posterior, restoring the normal axis of the vagina and providing vaginal depth. The vagina is packed with antibiotic-impregnated dressing

3.3 Transvaginal Repair of Enterocele and Vault Prolapse

An enterocele is a herniation of the peritoneum and its contents at the posterior vaginal wall or vaginal cuff. In unusual cases can be present with the uterus in place (Fig. 3.99a). Although a congenital enterocele may be present in a woman without previous vaginal surgery, most enteroceles are acquired as a result of a defect created at the vaginal apex by the separation or weakness of the sacrouterine ligaments after hysterectomy. A simple enterocele is an enterocele sac without vault prolapse; discontinuity between the perivesical and prerectal fasciae allows the peritoneum to herniate through the posterior cul-de-sac. Concomitant vault prolapse defines a complex enterocele (Fig. 3.99b). Most enteroceles are associated with vault prolapse of the vaginal cuff to the mid-vagina or outside the introitus. Often the enterocele defect may be more prominent in the distal posterior vagina and not at the cuff (Fig. 3.99c).

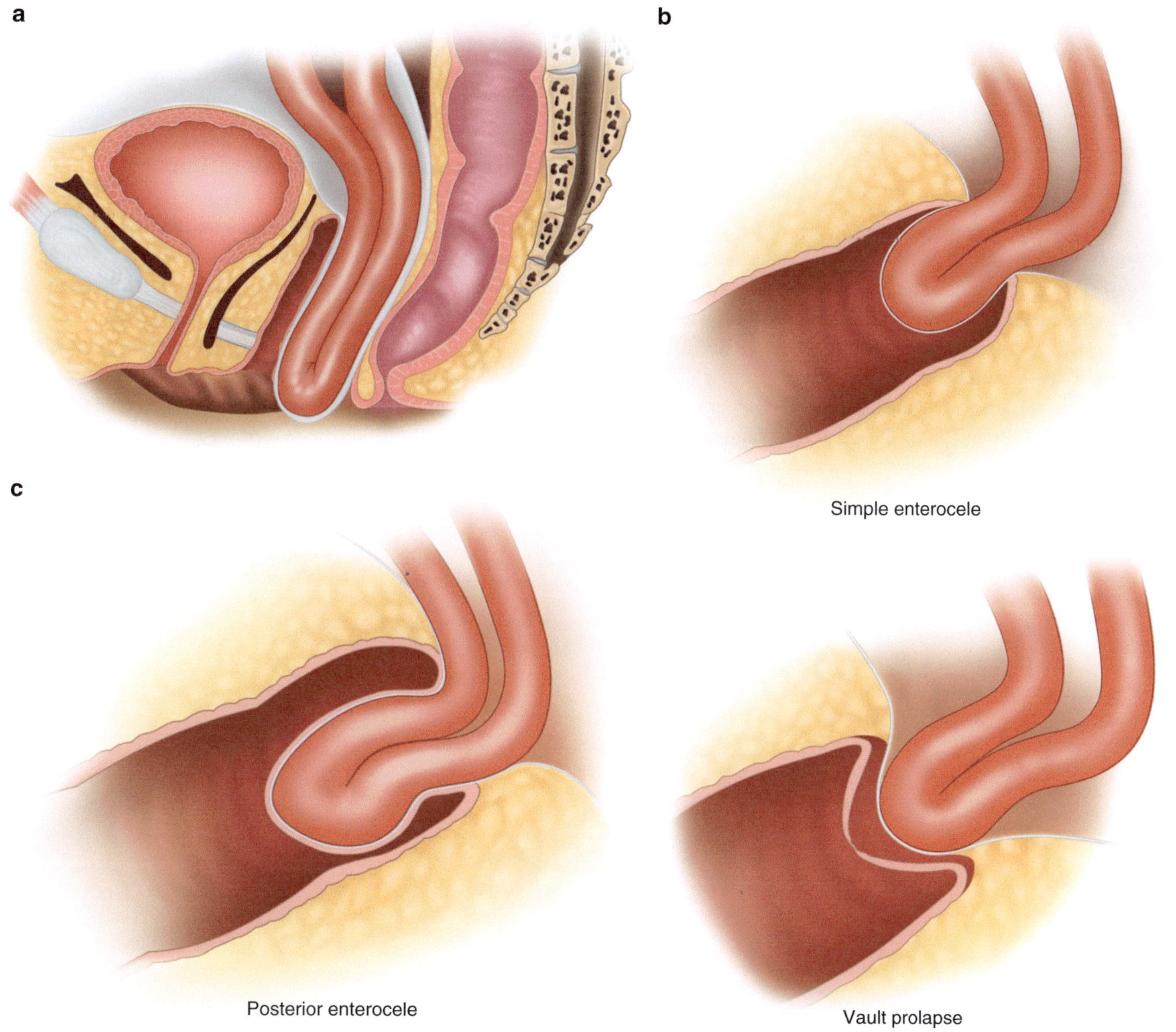

Fig. 3.99 (**a**) An enterocele is a herniation of the peritoneum and its contents at the level of the vaginal vault. (**b**) Concomitant vault prolapse defines a complex enterocele. Often the enterocele defect may be more prominent in the distal posterior vagina and not at the cuff. (**c**) Enterocele formation is most common after a hysterectomy but may occur after any surgery that displaces the vagina anteriorly (e.g., Burch colposuspension or sacrocolpopexy)

3.3.1 Indications

Enterocele formation is most common after a hysterectomy, but it may occur after any surgery that displaces the vagina anteriorly (e.g., Burch colposuspension or sacrocolpopexy). Anterior displacement of the proximal vagina, often in association with pelvic floor relaxation, exposes the cul-de-sac to increase the intra-abdominal pressure, thereby predisposing to enterocele formation. Patients with symptomatic enterocele typically note a vaginal bulge and often complain of vaginal discomfort or dyspareunia. In extreme cases, incarceration and bowel obstruction may occur.

The goal of surgery is to restore the herniated contents of the sac to the peritoneal cavity, to close the defect of the posterior cul-de-sac (by approximating the prerectal and perivesical fasciae), and to support the cuff to a normal anatomical and physiological location (S5) with restoration of the normal vaginal axis.

3.3.2 Diagnosis

Physical examination reveals a bulging mass at the vaginal apex or posterior vagina. The herniation most often lies posterior to the cervix or at the vaginal apex in post-hysterectomy patients. Based upon physical examination alone, it may be difficult to differentiate among cystocele, enterocele, and high rectocele. Very often the enterocele appears as a high continuation of the bulge in the posterior vaginal wall. The enterocele sac may contain bowel visible through the attenuated vaginal wall. With a finger in the rectum, the impulse of the enterocele hernia sac may be felt against the fingertip in the vagina during coughing (analogous to the impulse felt during examination for an inguinal hernia). Examination in the standing position may help to confirm the diagnosis in doubtful cases. Furthermore, placing a cystoscope and shining a light in the bladder can often help to differentiate between cystocele and enterocele (Fig. 3.100).

Sagittal cuts during dynamic MRI are not only useful in differentiating between the different types of vaginal prolapse (cystocele, rectocele, or enterocele) but also in differentiating the contents of a vault prolapse. A herniation of the small bowel is defined as enterocele (Fig. 3.101); herniation of the omentum is defined as an omentocele or fatocele (Fig. 3.102); herniation of the colon is defined as a sigmoidocele (Fig. 3.103).

3.3.3 Preoperative Considerations

Enterocele is commonly associated with other vaginal abnormalities (e.g., cystocele or rectocele) that should be repaired simultaneously. Proper bowel preparation is required in case of accidental injury to the rectum or small bowel. After general or spinal anesthesia is induced, the patient is placed in the dorsal lithotomy position. The lower abdomen and the vagina are prepped and draped in a sterile fashion. Perioperative antibiotics are given.

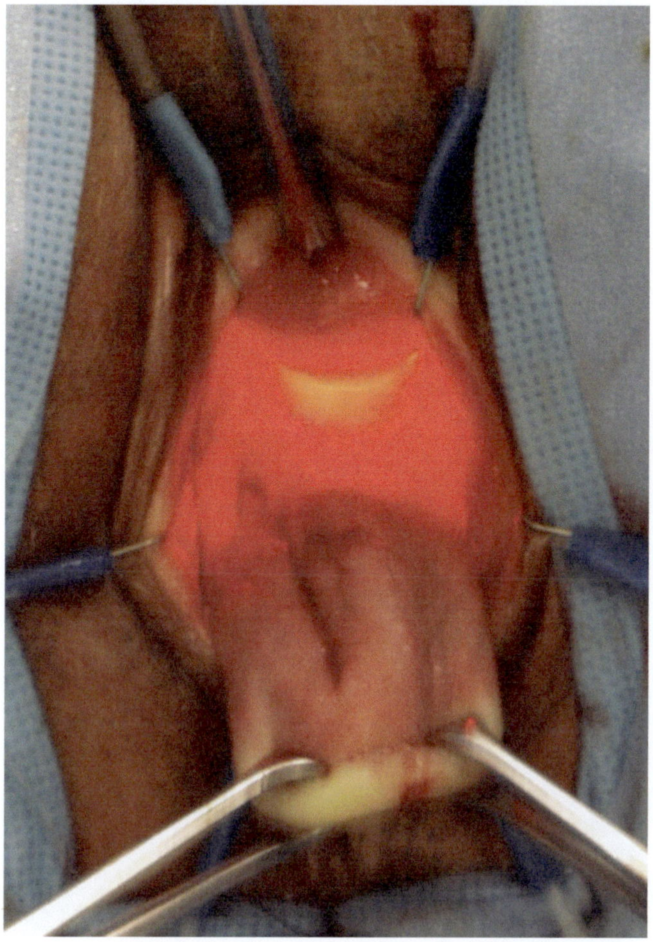

Fig. 3.100 Placing a cystoscope and shining a light in the bladder can often help to differentiate between cystocele and enterocele

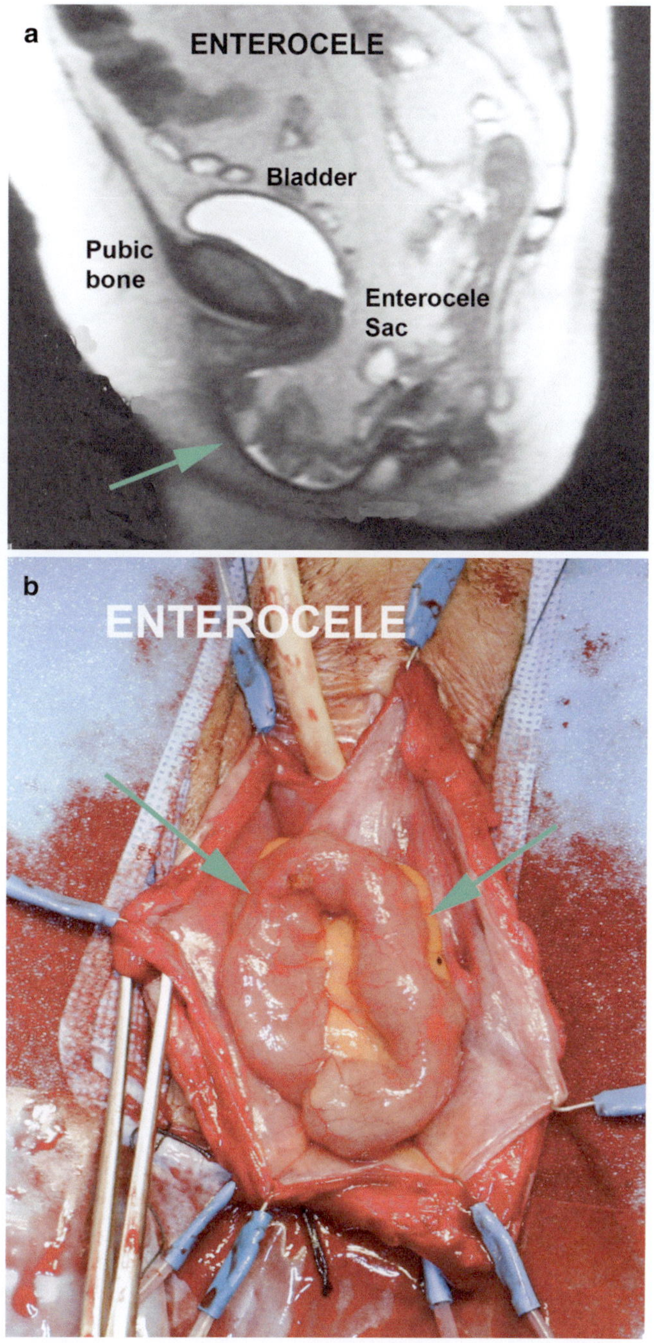

Fig. 3.101 A herniation of the small bowel is defined as an enterocele (*arrows*). (**a**) Sagittal T2 MRI of the pelvis showing a well-supported bladder and behind it a herniation of the cul-de-sac. The content of the hernia sac is small bowel (enterocele). (**b**) At the time of surgery, the hernia sac is open confirming the preoperative diagnosis of enterocele (the sac contains only small bowel)

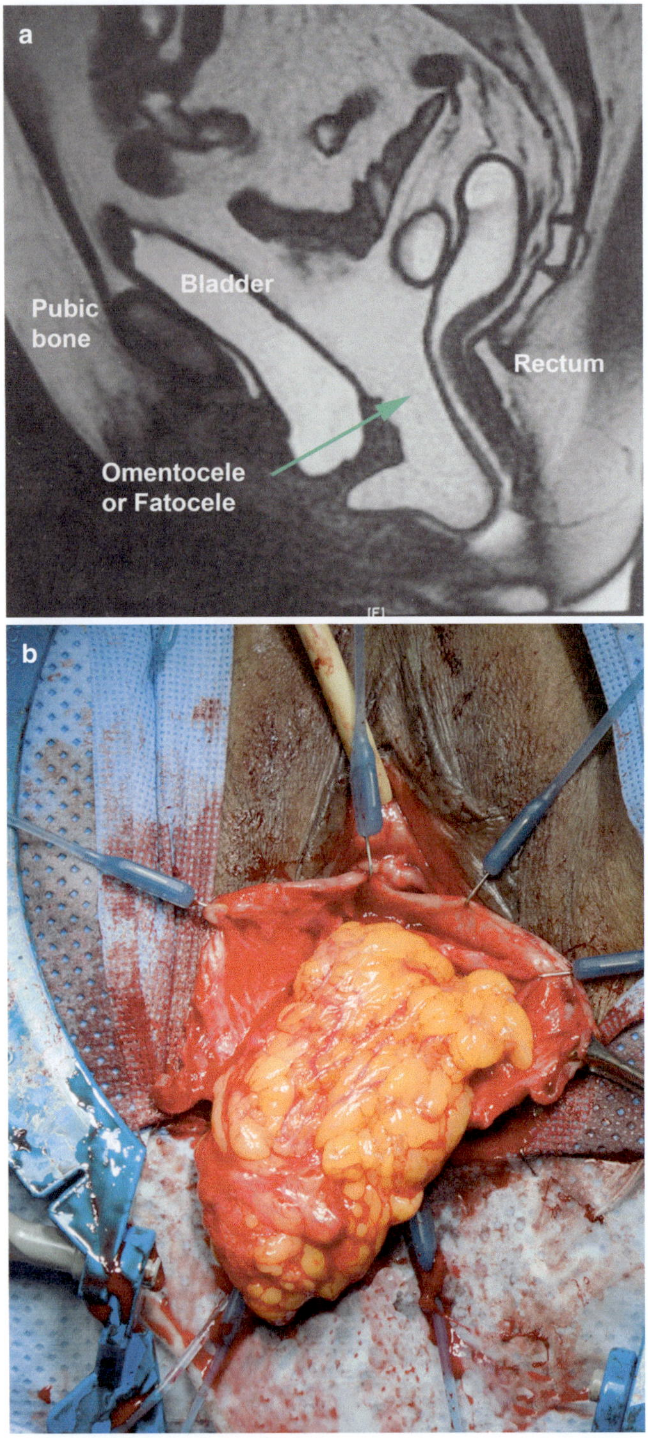

Fig. 3.102 Herniation of the cul-de-sac with omentum is defined as an omentocele or fatocele. (**a**) Sagittal MRI of a patient with a hernia of cul-de-sac containing only fatty tissue. The *arrow* indicates the large hernia sac filled with omentum (gray on MRI). (**b**) At the time of surgery opening the cul-de-sac, only omentum is found in the hernia sac

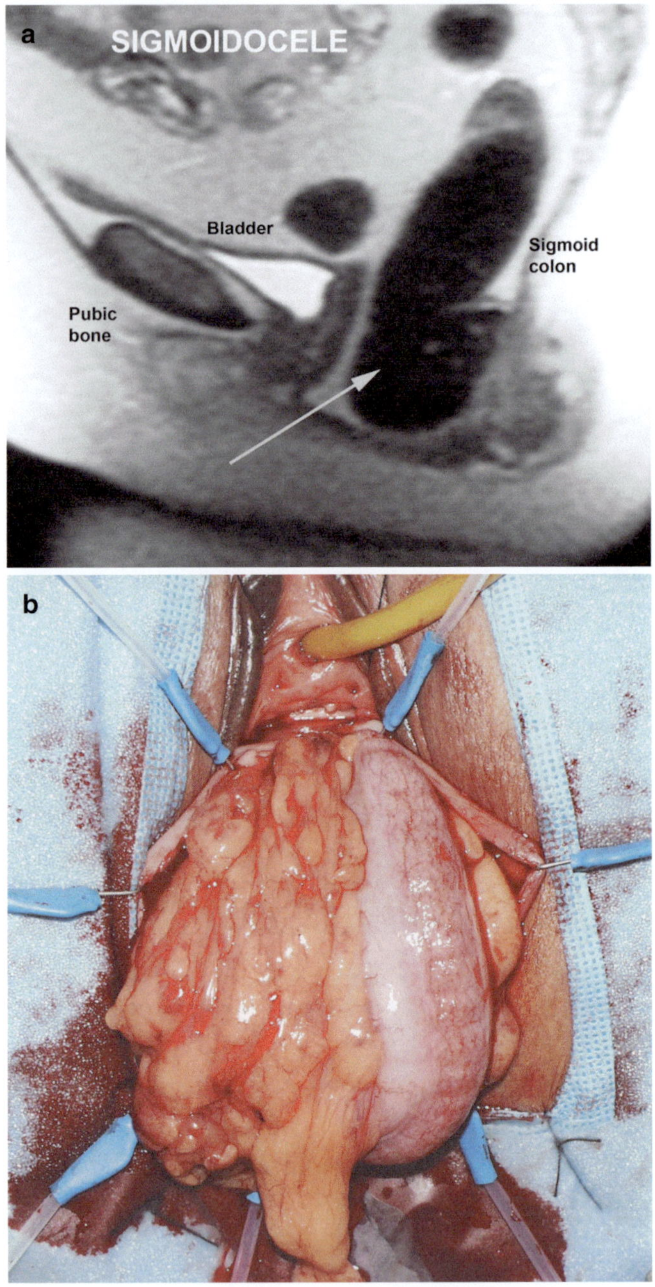

Fig. 3.103 Herniation of the cul-de-sac with the colon is defined as a sigmoidocele. (**a**) Sagittal MRI of a patient suffering from vault prolapse and herniation of the sigmoid colon in the cul-de-sac. The *arrow* indicated the segment of sigmoid colon contained into the hernia sac. (**b**) During surgical exploration the opening of the peritoneal sac reveals that most of the hernia sac is occupied by the sigmoid colon

3.3.4 Surgical Technique for Enterocele Repair

Repair of an enterocele must reduce the herniated contents of the sac, close the defect of the posterior cul-de-sac by restoring continuity between the prerectal and perivesical fasciae, restore the normal axis of the vagina, and support the vaginal vault (vault suspension) in order to prevent recurrent prolapse. Numerous surgical techniques have been described for enterocele repair, including transabdominal enterocele repair involving obliteration of the cul-de-sac followed by sacrocolpopexy, transvaginal sacrospinous fixation, laparoscopic or robotic enterocele repair using sutures or mesh, and simple colpocleisis. This chapter discusses our technique of transvaginal enterocele repair, illustrated in Figs. 3.104, 3.105, 3.106, 3.107, 3.108, 3.109, 3.110, 3.111, 3.112, 3.113, 3.114, 3.115, 3.116, 3.117, 3.118, 3.119, 3.120, 3.121, 3.122, 3.123, 3.124, 3.125, and 3.126. In this technique, two pairs of #1 delay absorbable sutures (PDS preferable) are placed. The first pair is vault suspension sutures that will provide support and depth to the vaginal vault to the area of S5, restoring the normal vaginal axis. The second pair is applied in a purse-string fashion to close the enterocele sac and approximate the prerectal fascia to the perivesical fascia.

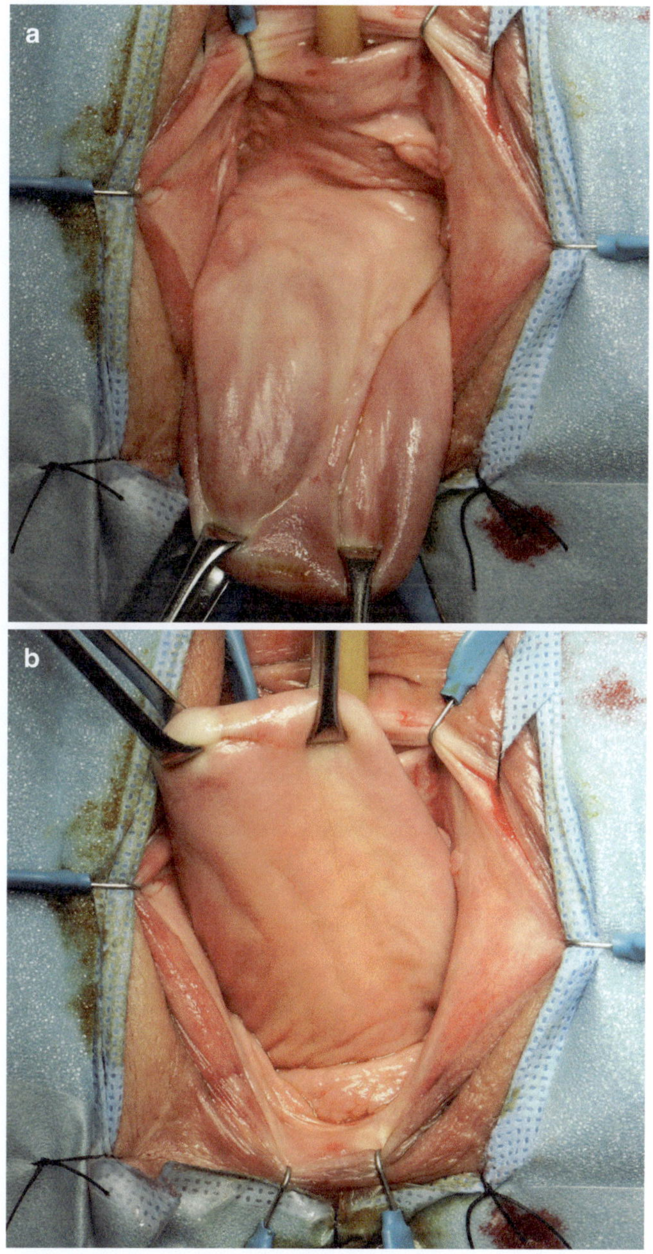

Fig. 3.104 (**a**) A ring retractor is positioned, the labia minora are retracted, and a urethral catheter is placed. The enterocele bulge is grasped with two Allis clamps. (**b**) #2-0 delay absorbable sutures are applied to the vaginal vault as marking sutures to further help in the placement of the vault suspension sutures

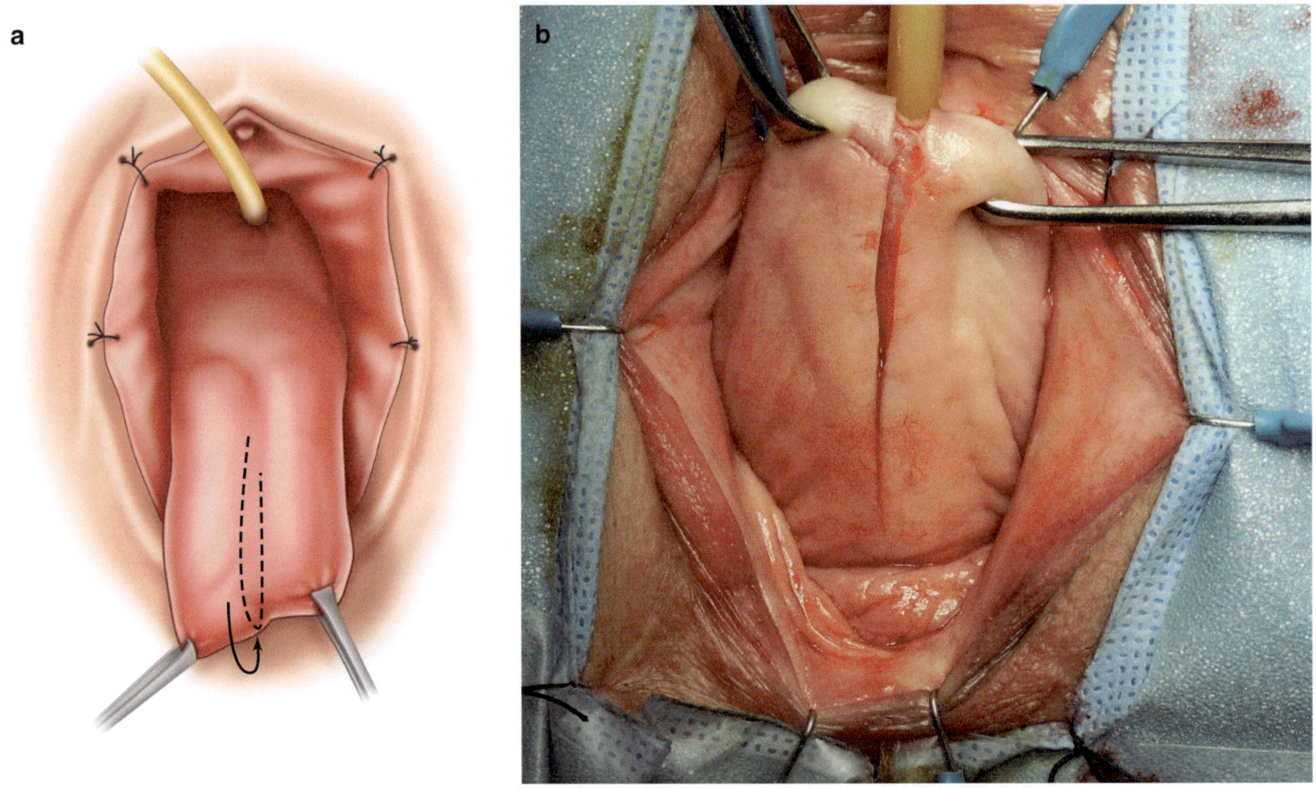

Fig. 3.105 (**a**, **b**) A vertical incision is made over the vaginal wall, extending anterior to the bladder base and posterior to the prerectal area

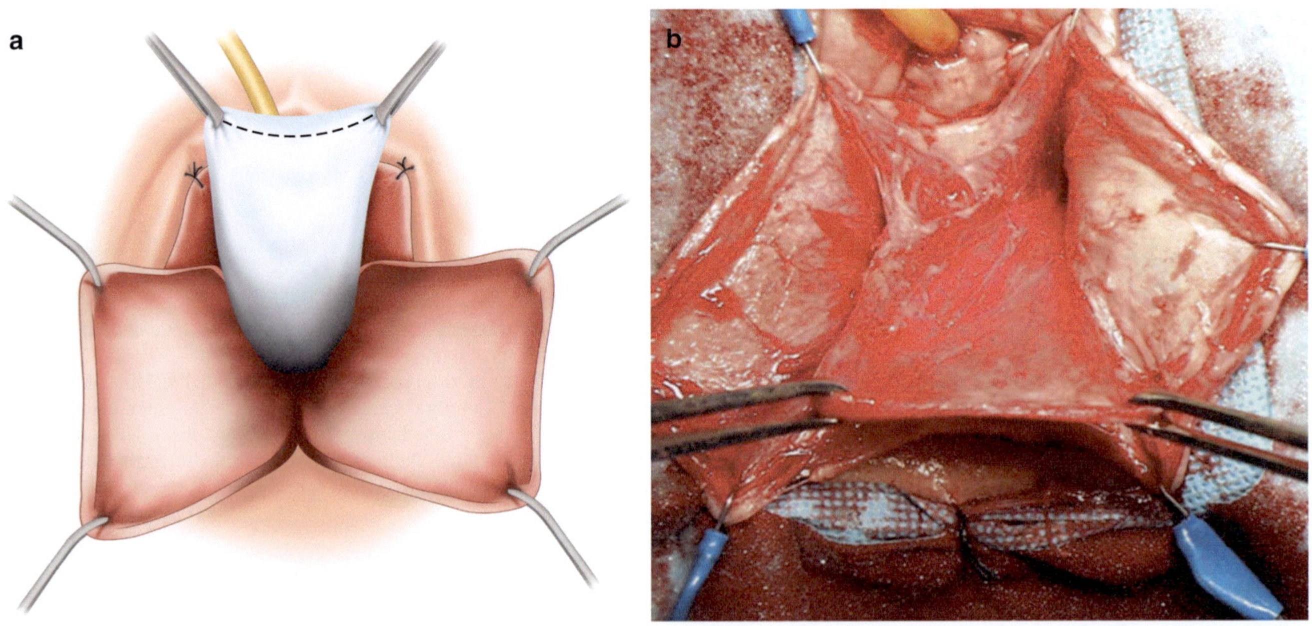

Fig. 3.106 (**a**, **b**) Using sharp dissection, the peritoneal sac is dissected free from the vaginal wall, posterior from the rectum and anterior toward the bladder base. The dissection is extended to isolate the base of the sac. Care should be taken to avoid bladder injury during the anterior dissection or rectal injury during the posterior dissection. A rectal finger can help during this phase of the surgery. Illumination of the bladder lumen with a cystoscopic light can help to define the bladder base. In case of doubt, the bladder should be irrigated in order to rule out perforation. Branches of the uterine artery are very often found at the base of the enterocele sac; they must be coagulated or suture ligated

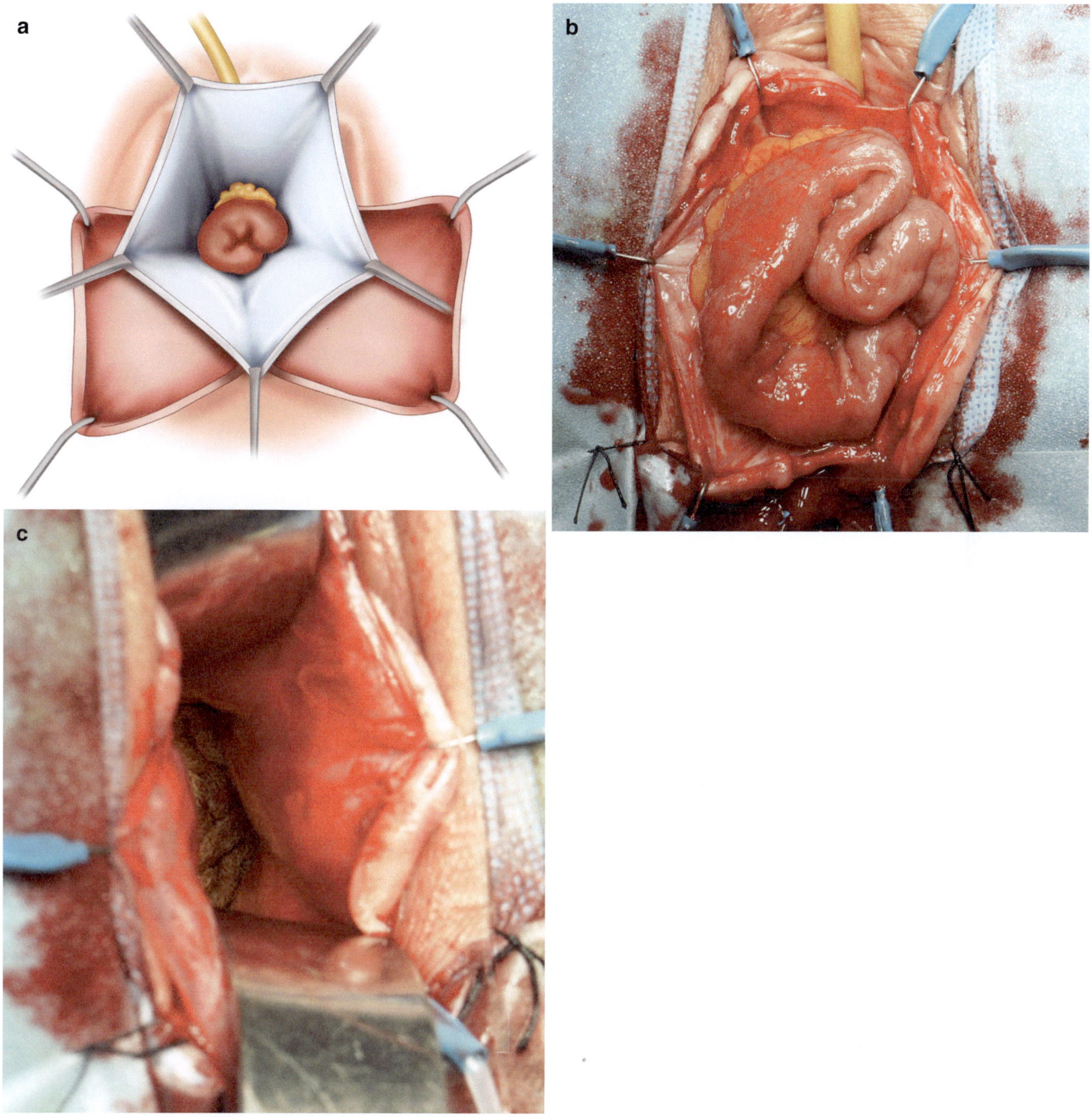

Fig. 3.107 (**a**, **b**) The peritoneal sac is opened, exposing the content. The bowel, omentum, or both are freed of any adhesions to the hernia sac. (**c**) Two laparotomy pads are inserted to reduce the peritoneal content, and the bladder is retracted anteriorly. A right-angle long retractor (Heaney) is placed over the iliococcygeus muscle (first laterally and then sliding inferiorly) to expose the groove between the rectum, the medial aspect of the sacrum, and the laterally located levator muscle. A third retractor is used to retract the rectum medially to facilitate the exposure. By forward and backward movement of the pararectal retractor, it is easy to identify the steplike feeling of the hard sacrospinous ligament transitioning to the soft iliococcygeus muscle

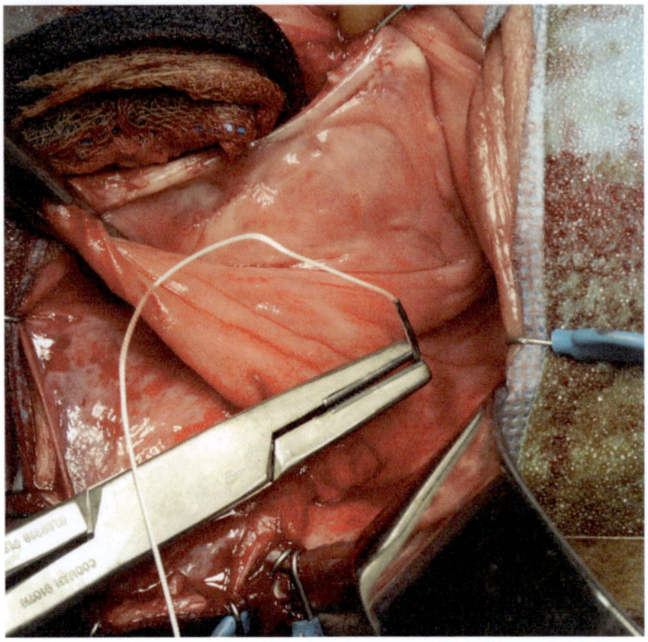

Fig. 3.108 Posterolateral to the cuff, from outside the vaginal wall at the level of the most dependent part of the cuff, a #1 delayed absorbable suture (polydioxanone [PDS]) is used to enter the peritoneal sac. With the needle in the peritoneum, the lateral prerectal fascia is incorporated 4–5 cm from the open cuff. Tying the vault suspension sutures will elevate and support the rectal wall, preventing secondary rectocele

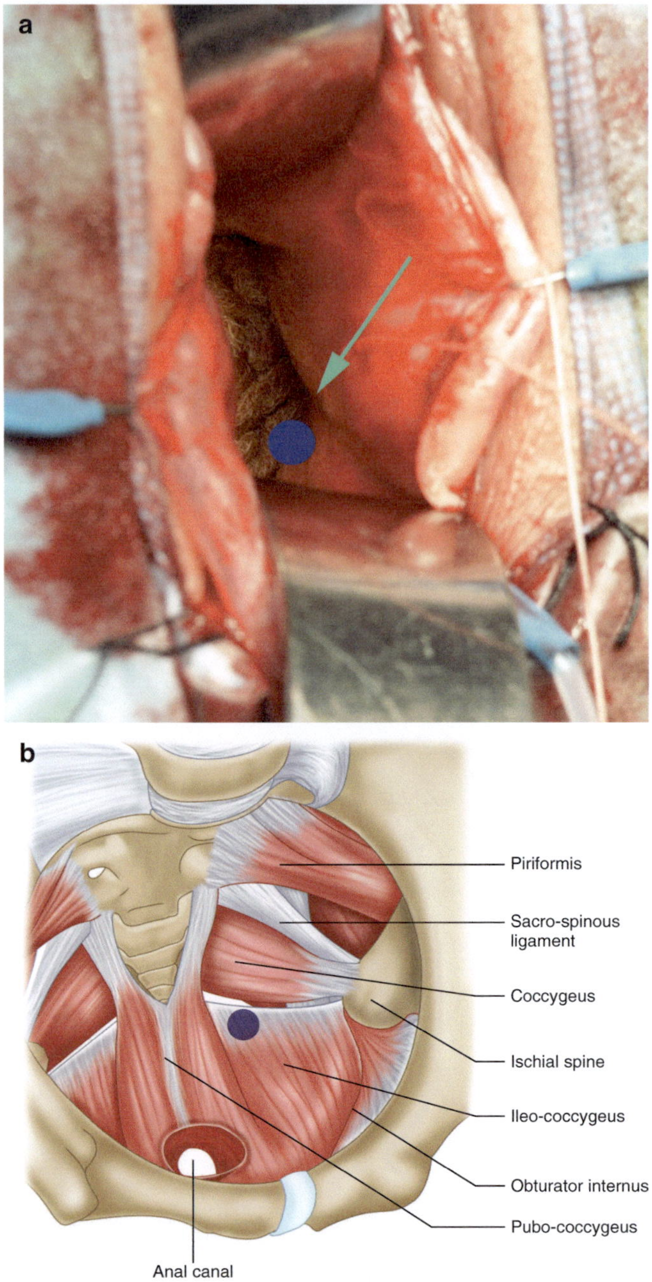

Fig. 3.109 (**a**) The point of anchoring sutures for the vault suspension (*blue dot*) will be 12–14 cm from the introitus in the groove lateral to the sacrum, medial to the iliococcygeus muscle, and distal to the sacrospinous ligament. The suture will incorporate the origin of the sacrouterine ligaments just distal to the coccygeus, providing a fibrous, strong anchoring tissue that will not cause postoperative pain; there are no vessels or nerves in the area. (**b**) Anatomical drawing showing the point of insertion of the vault suspension sutures, distal to the sacrospinous ligaments, lateral to the sacrum, and medial to the iliococcygeus muscle

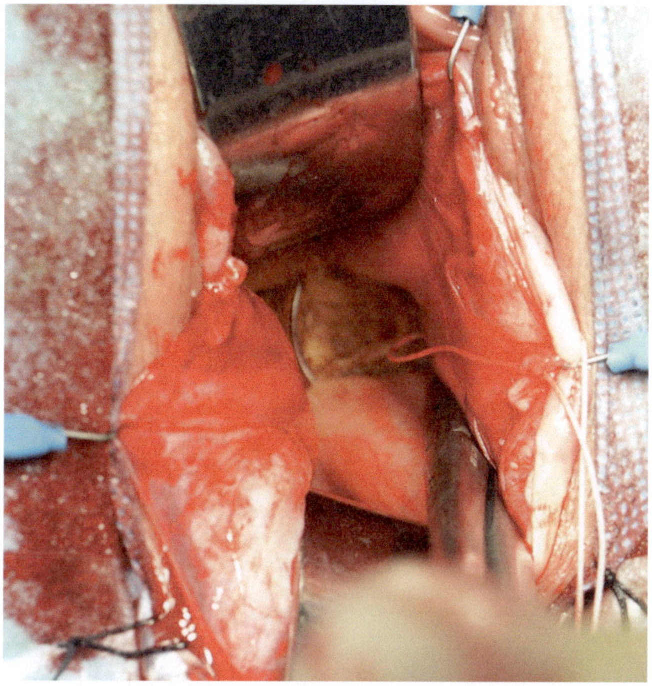

Fig. 3.110 The needle is transferred lateral to medial, distal to the sacrospinous ligament, lateral to the sacrum, lateral to the rectum, and medial to the iliococcygeus muscle. At least two passes of the needle are done to provide a strong anchoring point

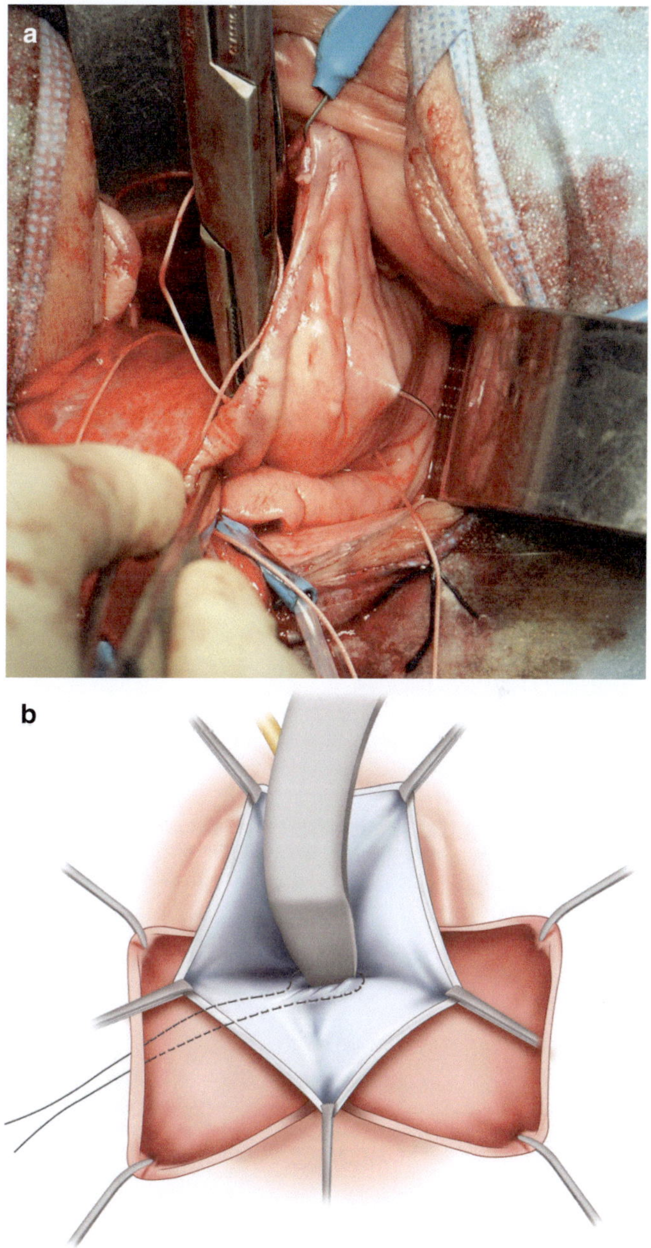

Fig. 3.111 (**a**) The needle is brought from inside the peritoneal cavity to outside the vaginal cuff, at least 1 cm from the original entrance. (**b**) Diagram of the final application of the vault suspension sutures with a point of insertion and exit in the posterolateral vaginal wall at the cuff

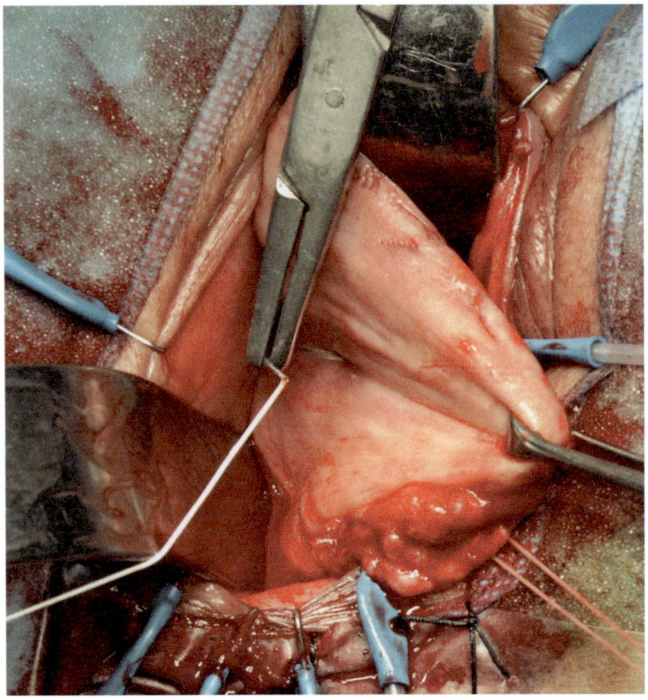

Fig. 3.112 A #1 PDS suture is inserted in the right posterior lateral aspect of the vaginal cuff

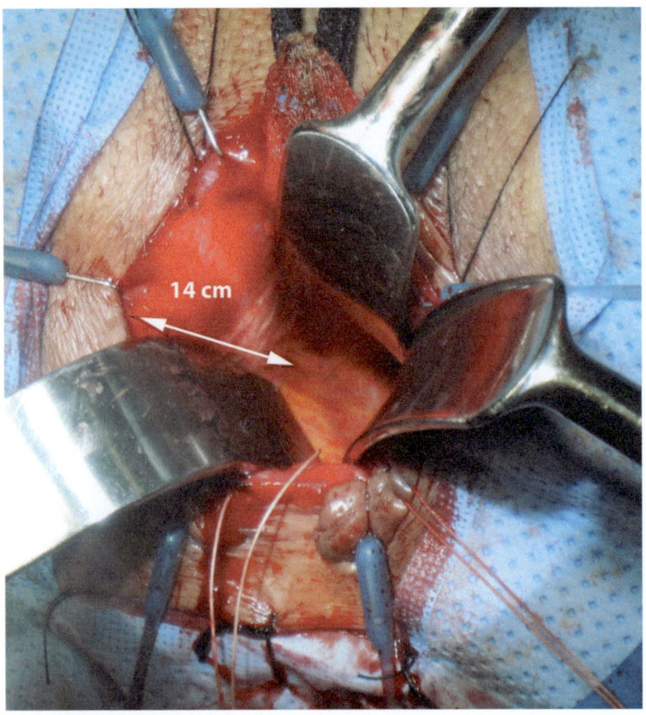

Fig. 3.113 The bladder has been retracted superiorly and the rectum medially. A Heaney posterior retractor exposes the right pararectal space. Palpation and forward and backward movement of the retractor help to localize the steplike feeling of the sacrospinous ligament. Just distal to the ligament and lateral to the sacrum, the strong avascular area where the sutures will be inserted is seen. The distance between the introitus and the selected point of insertion of the sutures is 12–14 cm

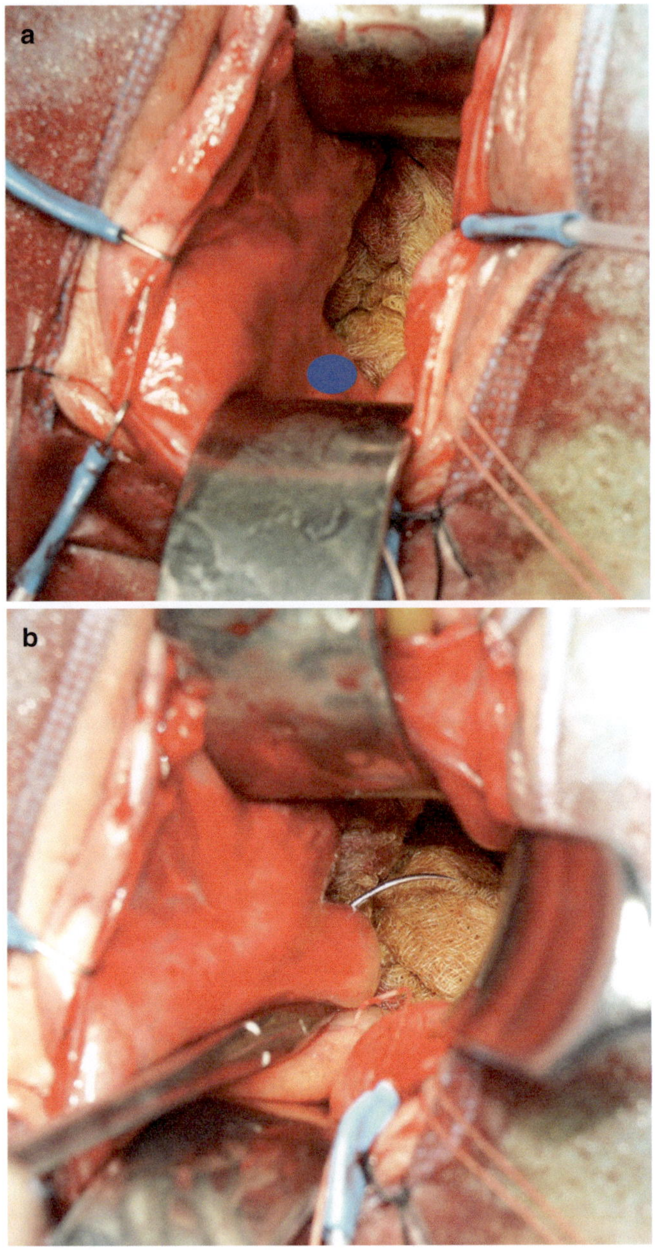

Fig. 3.114 (**a**) Exposure of the right pararectal space showing the point of insertion of the vault suspension sutures (*blue dot*). (**b**) The sutures incorporate the origin of the sacrouterine ligaments, lateral to the sacrum and distal to the sacrospinous ligament. A strong anchor of tissue is obtained

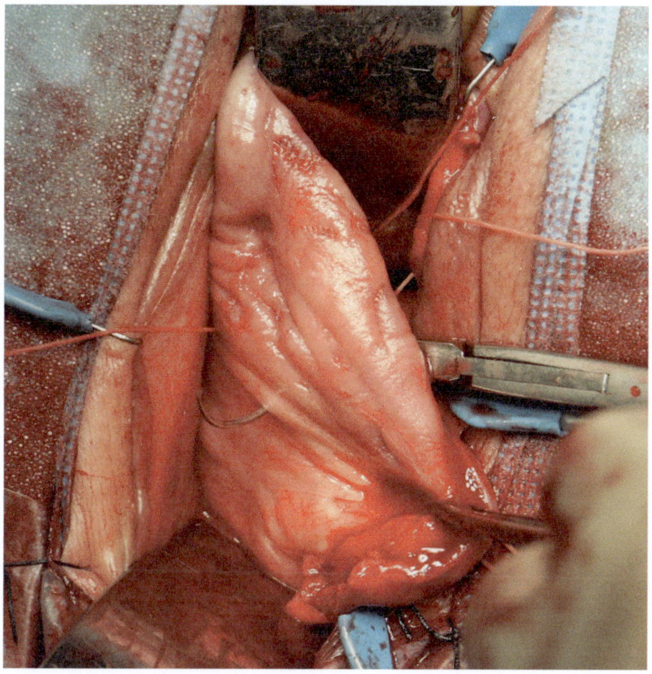

Fig. 3.115 The needle is transferred from the peritoneum to outside the vaginal wall, at least 1 cm from the original entrance

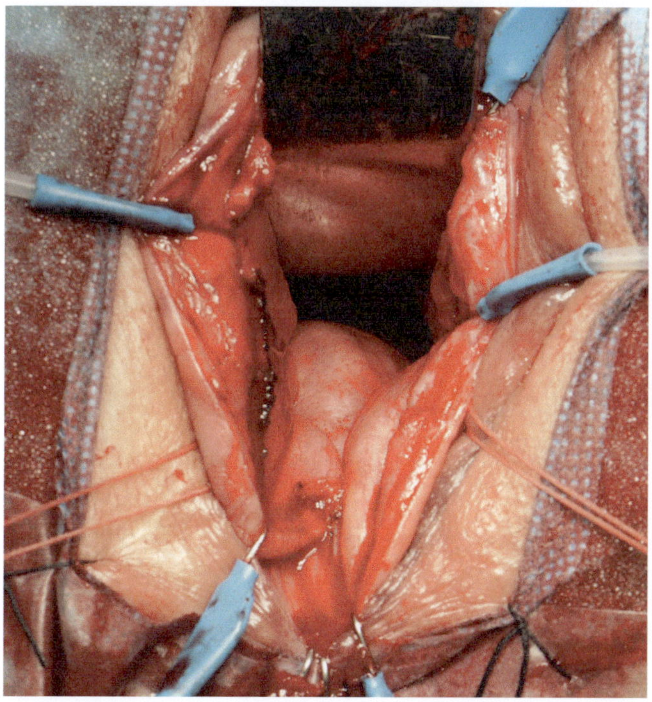

Fig. 3.116 The anterior vaginal wall is retracted and the rectum and posterior peritoneum are exposed. The two vault suspension sutures are seen in each side of the vaginal wall

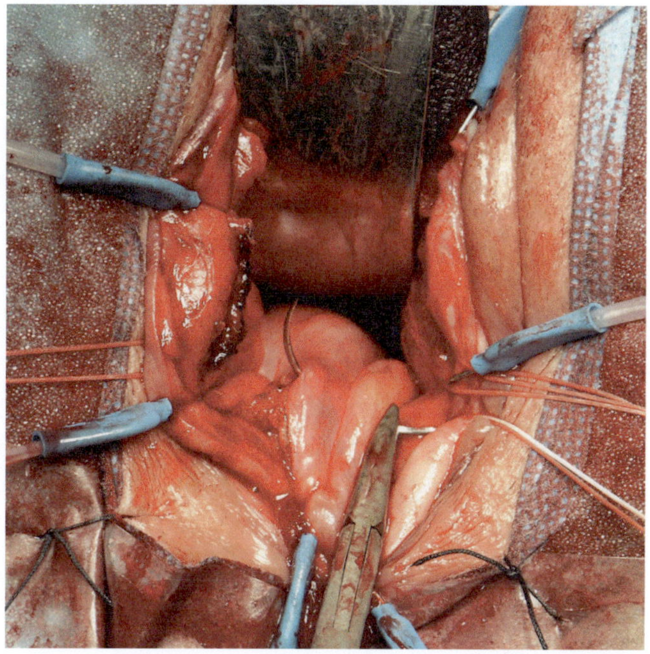

Fig. 3.117 Two #1 PDS sutures will be used to apply a purse-string suture to close the vaginal cuff. The first pass of the suture includes the prerectal fascia posterior to the distal segment of the cuff

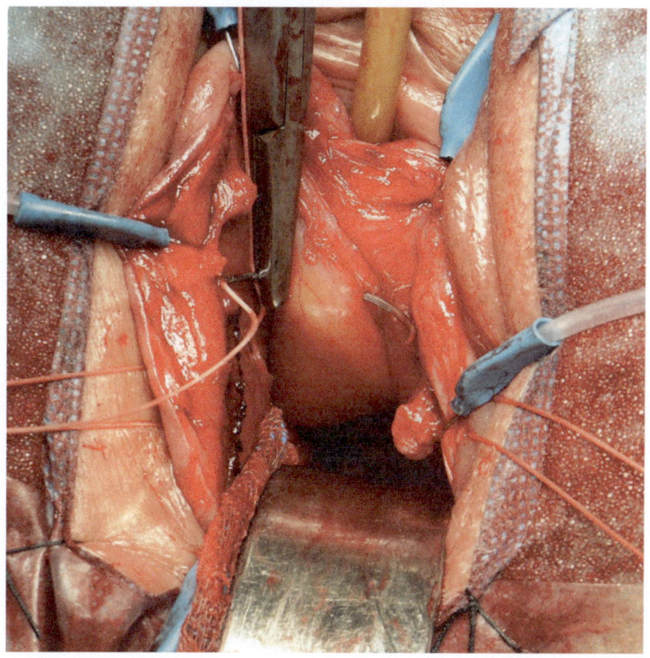

Fig. 3.118 After including the lateral peritoneum, the needle incorporates the bladder base to include the peritoneum and the pubocervical fascia. A large segment of tissue is incorporated

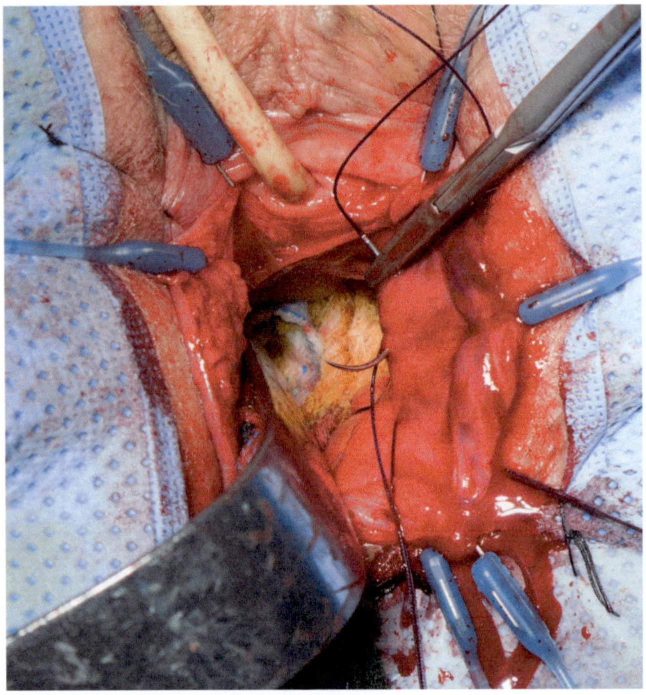

Fig. 3.119 Lateral peritoneal sutures are applied without incorporating the vaginal wall. The posterior peritoneum and prerectal fascia will be incorporated to complete the purse string. Two sutures will be applied

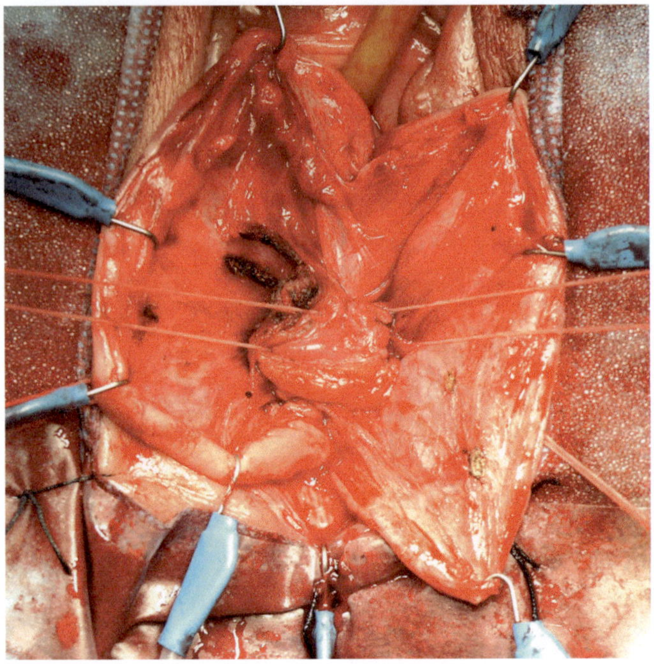

Fig. 3.121 After removal of the laparotomy pads from the peritoneum, traction is applied to the purse-string sutures, and they are tied individually. Optionally, the excess of peritoneum can be excised. Any posterior vaginal wall defect should be repaired at this time

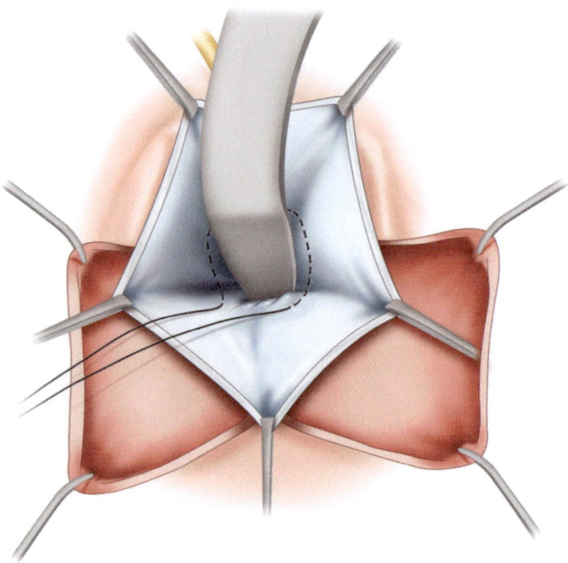

Fig. 3.120 Diagram showing the application of the purse-string sutures. The sutures will be tied individually to close the peritoneal sac and approximate the prerectal to the perivesical fascia

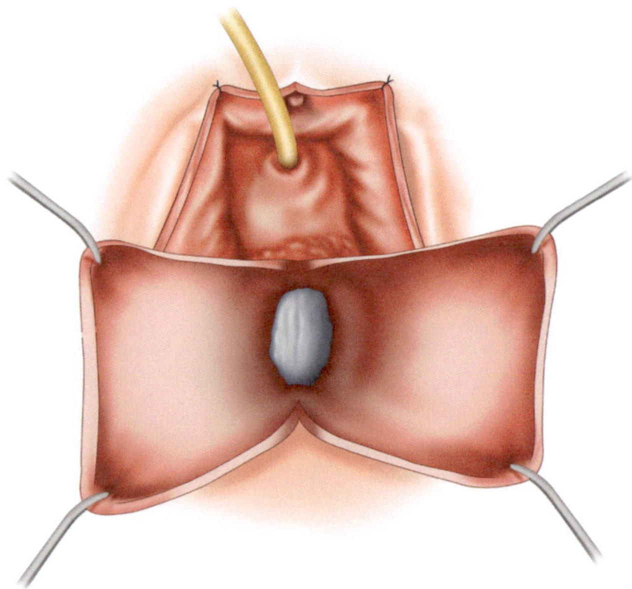

Fig. 3.122 Diagram of the closed peritoneal sac, showing the dissected excess vaginal wall on each side

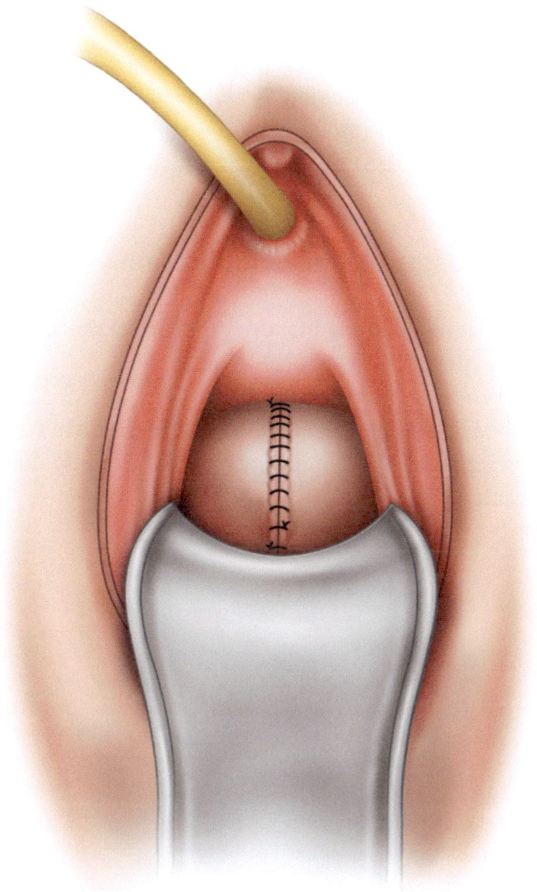

Fig. 3.123 Diagram showing the closed cuff after excision of the excess vaginal wall; #2-0 delayed absorbable sutures are used

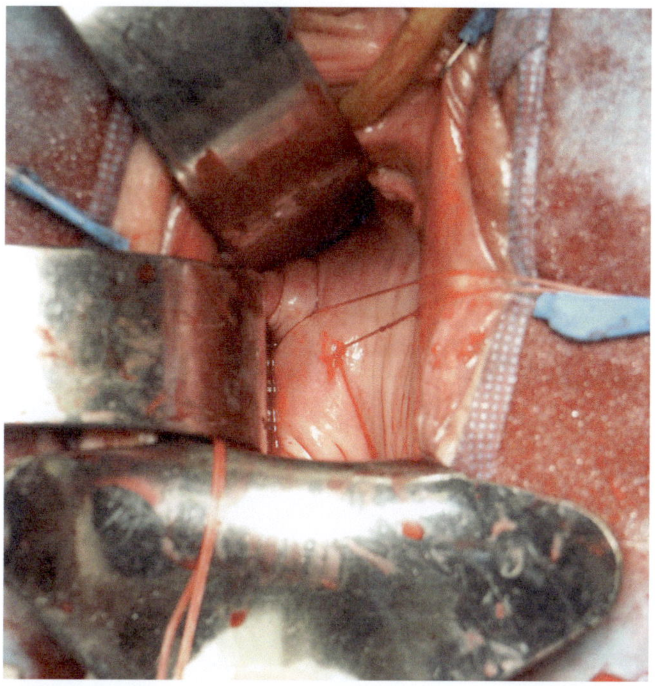

Fig. 3.124 The vault suspension sutures are tied individually. Traction is applied to eliminate any slack of the sutures

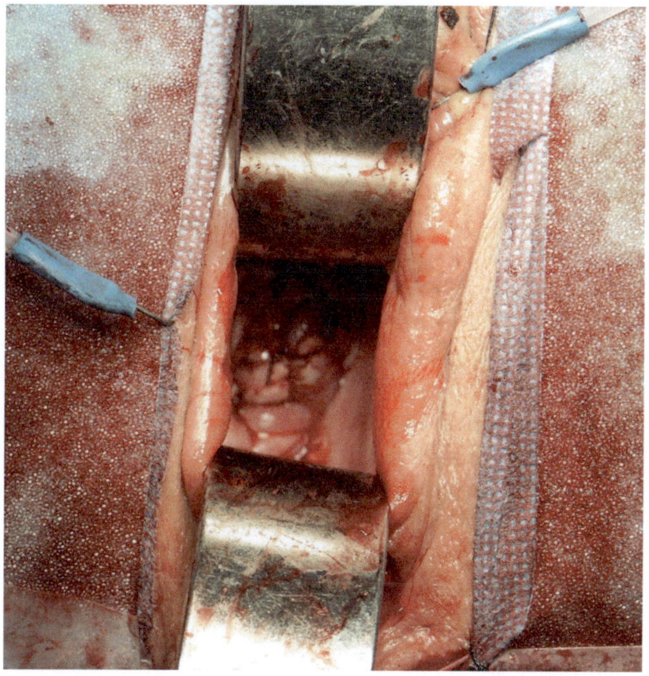

Fig. 3.125 The vaginal cuff is seen retracted high and posterior, restoring the normal vaginal axis toward S5

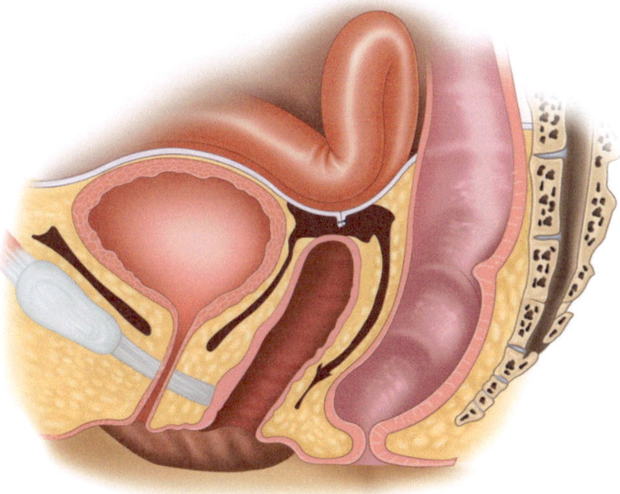

Fig. 3.126 Diagram of the final repair, showing an elevated vaginal cuff and closed peritoneal sac

3.3.5 Intraoperative Complications

Bleeding or injury to the ureters, bladder, or bowel can occur with any vaginal prolapse surgery. Ureteric injury is most likely during placement of the culdosuspension and the purse-string sutures, even though the anterior retraction of the bladder should protect the ureters. Placement of the vault suspension sutures should be done pointing the needle holder posteriorly toward the sacrum will also prevent ureteric obstruction. Intraoperative cystoscopy with intravenous injection of indigo carmine may be performed to assure the patency of the ureters. Urinary tract bleeding (blood in the Foley catheter) requires cystoscopy to rule out bladder injury. If the patient had adequate bowel preparation, any bowel injury can be repaired primarily. In case of stool contamination due to inadequate bowel preparation, a multiple-layer primary closure can be attempted with broad-spectrum antibiotic coverage, but colostomy may be required for extensive injury.

3.3.6 Postoperative Care

Most enterocele repairs can be performed as outpatient surgery. The vaginal packing is removed after 2 h. An oral cephalosporin or fluoroquinolone is administered for several days only if required. A voiding trial can be done after 24 h.

3.3.7 Postoperative Complications

Delayed complications include vaginal foreshortening, dyspareunia, ileus, or bowel obstruction.

Recurrent enterocele is unusual (less than 5 %). It may occur because of poor-quality tissues or technical failure and can be repaired in a similar fashion or using an abdominal approach.

3.4 Posterior Vaginal Wall Repair

3.4.1 Indications

In patients with good posterior vaginal support, herniation of the rectum into the vagina is prevented by the levator musculature and the strong prerectal and pararectal fasciae. When these fasciae and the levator sling are weakened, pelvic floor relaxation (PFR) develops. The distal half of the posterior vaginal wall is mainly supported by the levator sling. It pulls forward the distal vagina, creating an angulation of 45° with the vertical line. The proximal vagina is in a flat position of 100–110° with the horizontal line (Fig. 3.127). We like to compare the normal vaginal axis to the shape of a banana with the curvature pointing posteriorly toward the S4–S5 vertebra (Fig. 3.128). During surgery for PFR and rectocele, the final repair should restore the vaginal canal to the normal axis with preservation of vaginal depth and support with the prevention of stenosis.

The components of PFR include the development of a rectocele, widening and laxity of the levator hiatus, and perineal tearing and herniation. Several factors contribute to the weakening of posterior wall pelvic support. Childbirth and the passage of the child's head through the vagina causes stretching, damage, and tearing of the prerectal and pararectal fascia and weakening of the levator musculature, widening the levator hiatus and causing loss of the normal posterior angulation (banana shape) of the vaginal axis (Fig. 3.129). In this situation, the proximal vaginal axis, which is at a horizontal axis in the pelvis, may be changed to reside more vertically. Additionally, the pelvic organs slide downward along the vaginal axis as a result of loss of estrogen, aging, and chronic abdominal straining, facilitating further development of PFR.

Perineal body laxity caused by attenuation of the perineal musculature usually accompanies a rectocele, and therefore reconstruction of the posterior fourchette and perineum is carried out at the same time.

Surgery to the anterior vaginal wall or the vaginal cuff like in sacrocolpopexy can result in anterior displacement of the vagina, which can change the vaginal axis, thereby placing the posterior vaginal wall in the most dependent position, under the direct impact of intra-abdominal forces. Therefore, repair of PFR, when it is present, should be performed, as it will help to maintain the normal vaginal axis, prevent further prolapse, and improve the outcome of the anterior or vaginal vault surgery.

Many symptoms have been associated with PFR. Common presenting complaints are constipation, poor evacuation of stool secondary to stool pocketing in the rectocele, or the feeling of a vaginal bulge. Some patients require digital reduction of a rectocele in order to evacuate properly. Surgical correction may not cure these symptoms, but most patients who are symptomatic from PFR will be satisfactory candidates for repair. Repair of asymptomatic PFR at the time of surgery for incontinence surgery, anterior vaginal prolapse, or vaginal hysterectomy always should be considered, yet one must balance a risk of postoperative dyspareunia with worsening prolapse in unrepaired cases. It is our belief that simultaneously correcting posterior pelvic floor prolapse will result in restoration of the normal vaginal axis, will resist postoperative recurrence of prolapse, and may improve the results of anti-incontinence surgery as it creates a more solid pelvic floor.

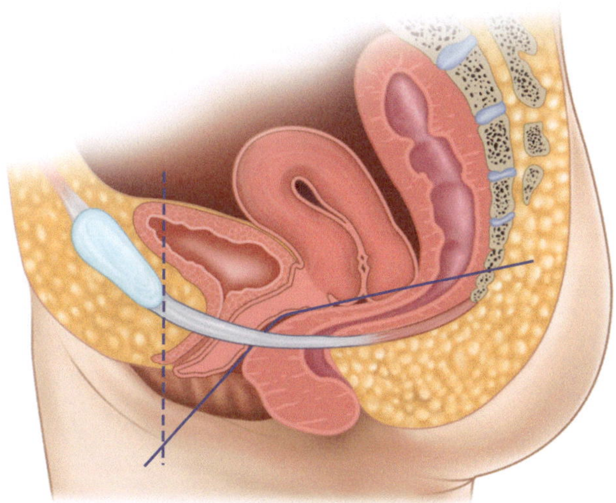

Fig. 3.127 Diagram of the posterior vaginal anatomy, with the distal third of the vagina in a 45-degree angulation and the proximal vagina in a more horizontal axis ending at the sacrococcygeal area

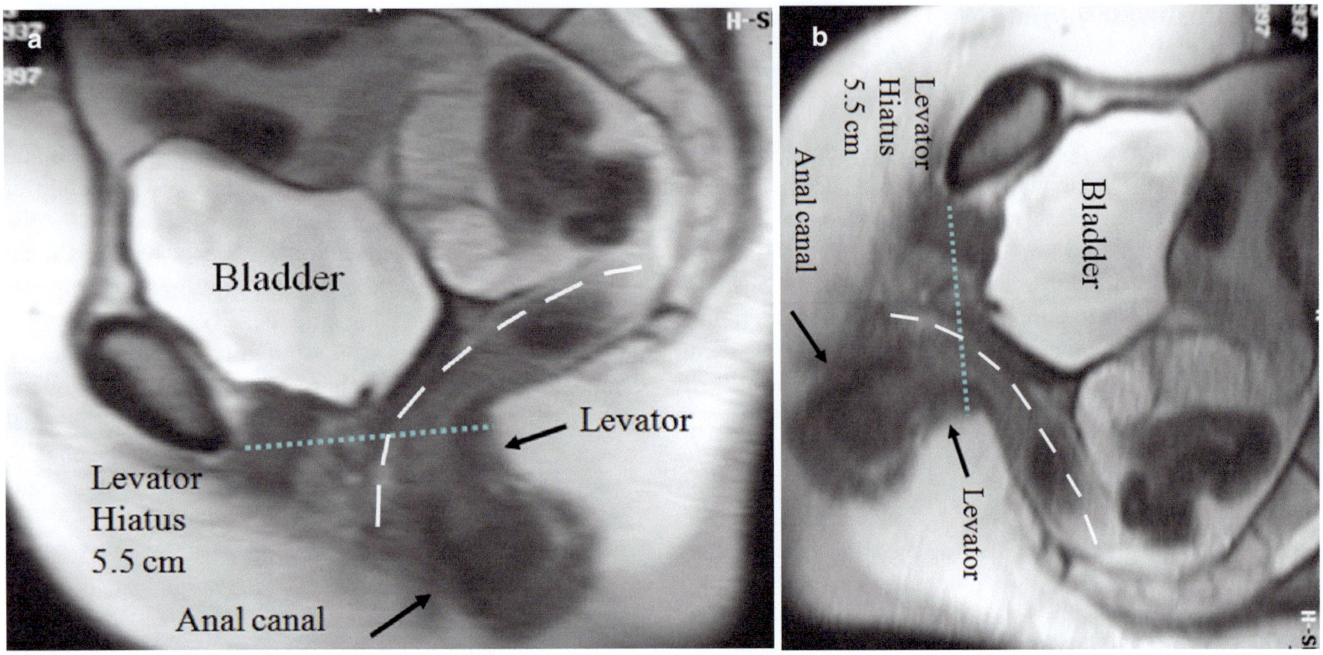

Fig. 3.128 (**a**) Sagittal dynamic MRI view of the pelvis in a young patient, showing the indentation of the levator (pubococcygeus and puborectalis) on the vagina, creating the elevation and angulation in its distal third. The size of the levator hiatus, the distance between the inferior rami of the pubic bone and the levator notch, is normally about 5.5 cm. The *white broken line* follows the axis of the vagina. (**b**) Rotating the same image 90° imitates the findings of the vaginal examination in the supine position; the vaginal canal has a banana shape with the distal vagina elevated and the proximal vagina reaching the sacrococcyx. The *dotted blue line* depicts the levator hiatus (the *arrow* points toward the beginning of the line)

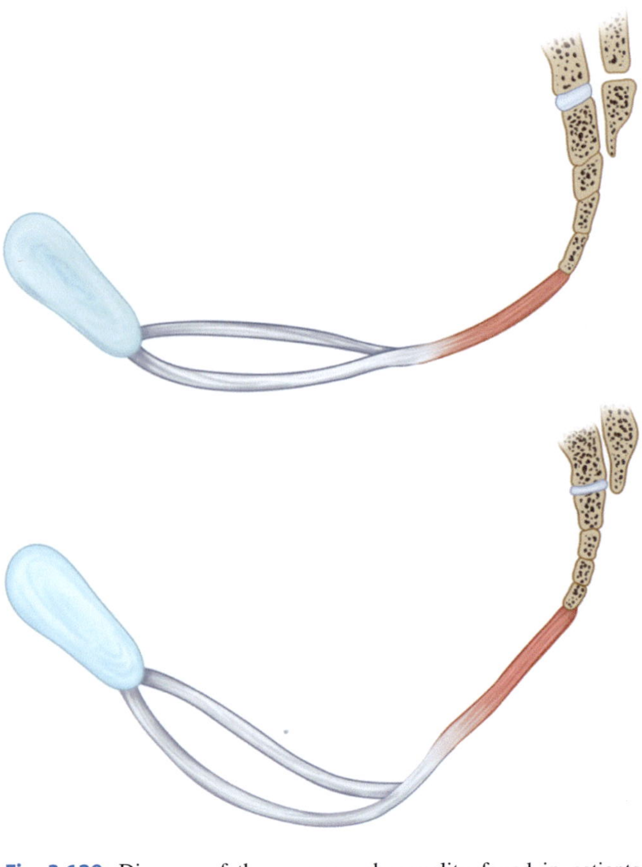

Fig. 3.129 Diagram of the common abnormality found in patients with pelvic floor relaxation. There is widening and descent of the levator hiatus and levator plate

3.4.2 Classification

Rectoceles (one of the components of PFR) may be classified as to their position in the vagina (low, medium, or high). The exact severity of the rectocele is graded according to the level of saccular protrusion. The Baden–Walker system and the pelvic organ prolapse–quantification classification can assess objectively the degree of posterior vaginal prolapse. Similarly, perineal tears are graded on a scale of I to IV:

- Grade I: a tear in the hymenal ring
- Grade II: a tear involving the perineal body but not the anal sphincter
- Grade III: a tear into the anal sphincter
- Grade IV: a tear into the anal mucosa

3.4.3 Preoperative Considerations

The patient begins a clear liquid diet 48 h prior to surgery and takes a laxative the night before surgery. Broad-spectrum antibiotics are administered intravenously immediately before surgery. The patient is anesthetized and placed in the lithotomy position. In selected patients with poor tissues or multiple surgeries, the rectum is copiously irrigated with an antibiotic solution prior to preparation and draping.

3.4.4 Diagnosis

The diagnosis of posterior relaxation starts with a good clinical history of traumatic deliveries, prior surgeries, defecatory changes such as constipation or stool incontinence, sensation of a posterior bulge, and the need for splinting the vagina or perineum to facilitate defecation. Clinical symptoms or findings do not always correlate to function; however, severe posterior vaginal prolapse may be asymptomatic, or mild prolapse can be very symptomatic. In complex cases with multiple surgical failures, unclear diagnosis, or disproportion of findings and symptoms, an objective evaluation in addition to the physical examination can be warranted. Figures 3.130, 3.131, 3.132, and 3.133 illustrate some of the objective diagnostic options.

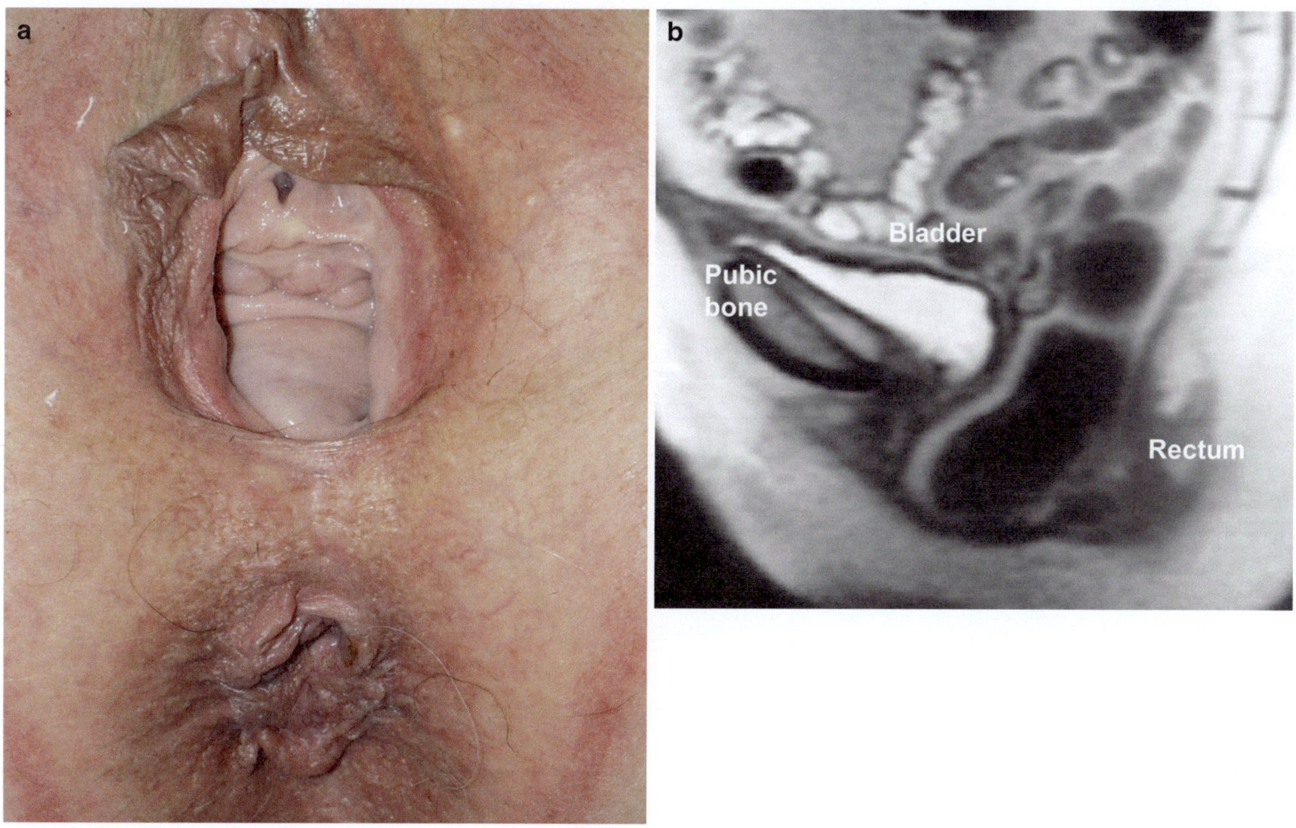

Fig. 3.130 (**a**) Physical examination of a patient with wide-open genital hiatus and a large posterior protrusion causing vaginal pressure, a bulge coming out of the vagina, and defecatory dysfunction with constipation and the need to splint the vagina in order to defecate. (**b**) Resting MRI using a T2 sequence showing the posterior vaginal wall (rectum) filled with gas. On straining, there is a displacement and a large herniation of the posterior vaginal wall emerging from the introitus (rectocele)

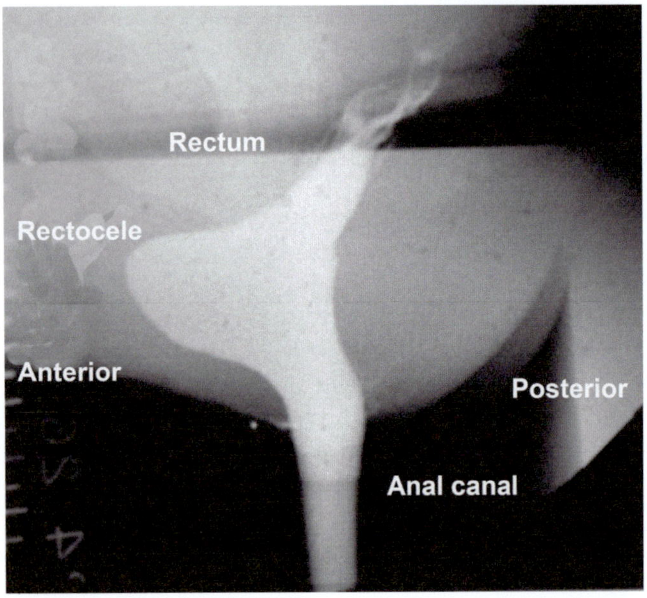

Fig. 3.131 Filling rectogram in the standing lateral position, showing the anterior bulge of a large rectocele

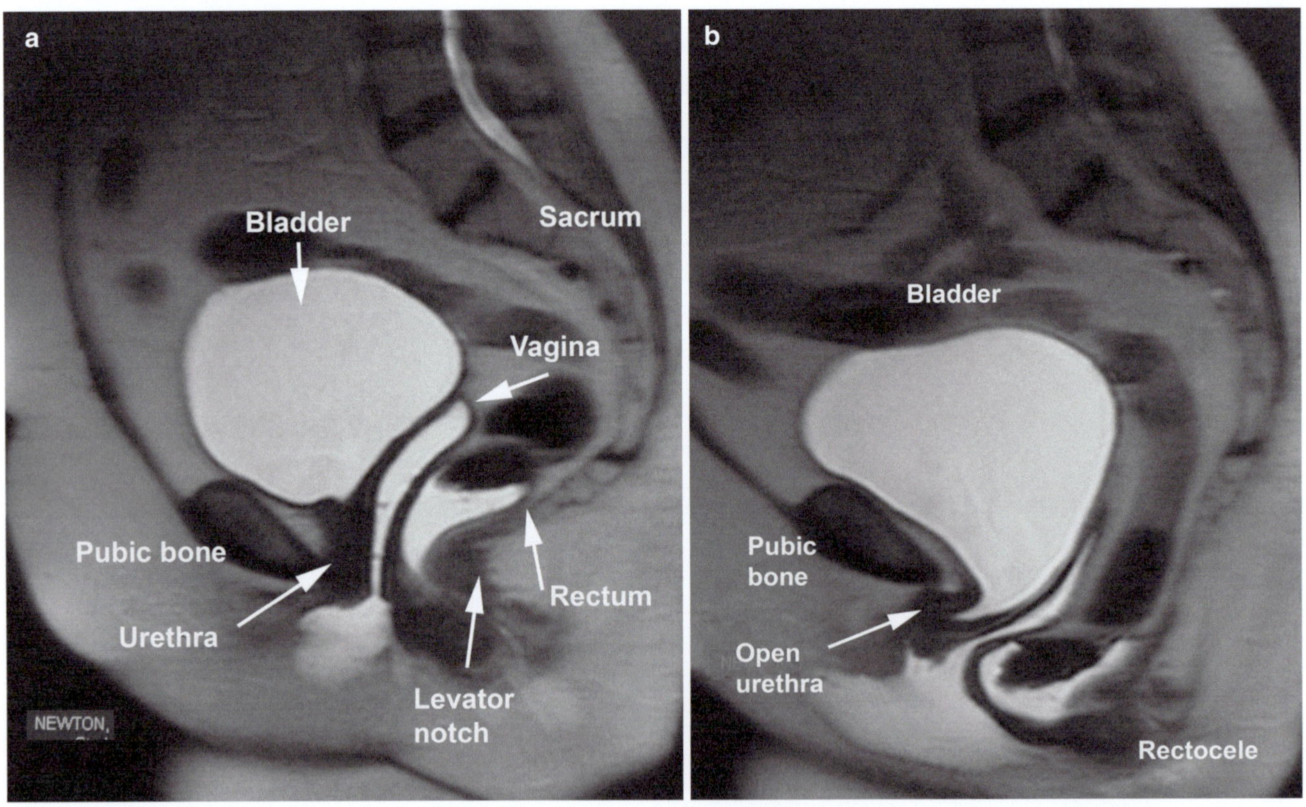

Fig. 3.132 (**a**) T2 sagittal view of the pelvis at the midline after the rectum and vagina were filled with a liquid gel. The bladder, urethra, vagina, and rectum are well defined. (**b**) On straining, a significant rectocele is visualized coming out of the introitus

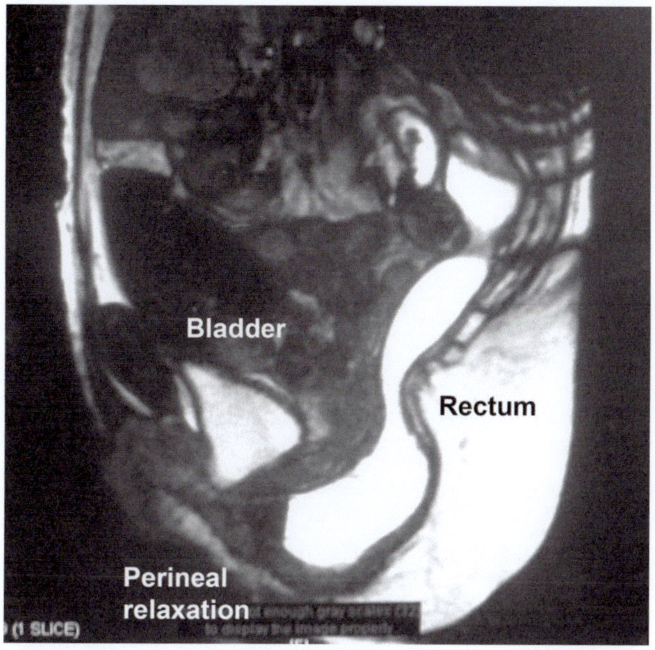

Fig. 3.133 In a patient with multiple failed surgeries and significant perineal laxity, an MRI defecogram shows the descent of the perineum and the increase convexity of the posterior levator due to the severe levator and fascial weakness

3.4.5 Surgical Technique

Figures 3.134, 3.135, 3.136, 3.137, 3.138, 3.139, 3.140, 3.141, 3.142, 3.143, 3.144, 3.145, 3.146, 3.147, 3.148, 3.149, 3.150, 3.151, 3.152, 3.153, and 3.154 show the surgical technique for posterior vaginal wall repair.

3.4.6 Postoperative Care

The surgery can be performed in the outpatient setting. The vaginal packing is removed 2 h after surgery. Stool softeners are continued for 1 month postoperatively. Oral antibiotics are administered if required for 2 weeks after surgery. Routine use of sitz baths is encouraged. Resumption of sexual relations is postponed for at least 1 month after surgery. Estrogen creams may facilitate wound healing and improve viscoelasticity.

3.4.7 Postoperative Complications

Recurrent rectocele is an uncommon complaint, but despite the best surgical efforts, it may occur in up to 10 % of patients. Dyspareunia and vaginal narrowing can be avoided by meticulous surgical technique, avoidance of over-resection of vaginal tissue, not leaving painful ridges, and not placing sutures directly into the levator musculature. Rectal injury should be repaired in layers, including the use of a Martius flap if required. Rectovaginal fistula is a very uncommon occurrence.

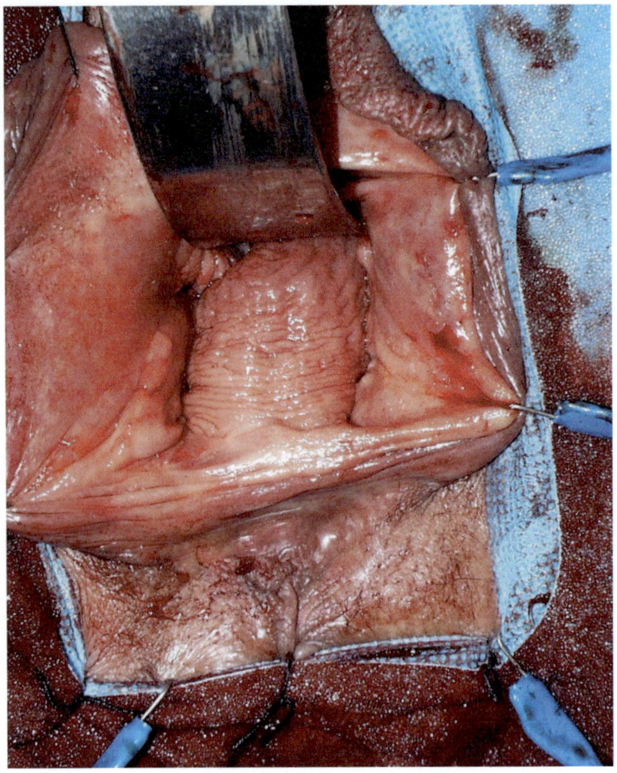

Fig. 3.134 A Foley catheter has been inserted, and a ring retractor with six hooks exposes the vaginal canal. A retractor is placed anteriorly to expose the length of the posterior vaginal wall. A large posterior defect is present

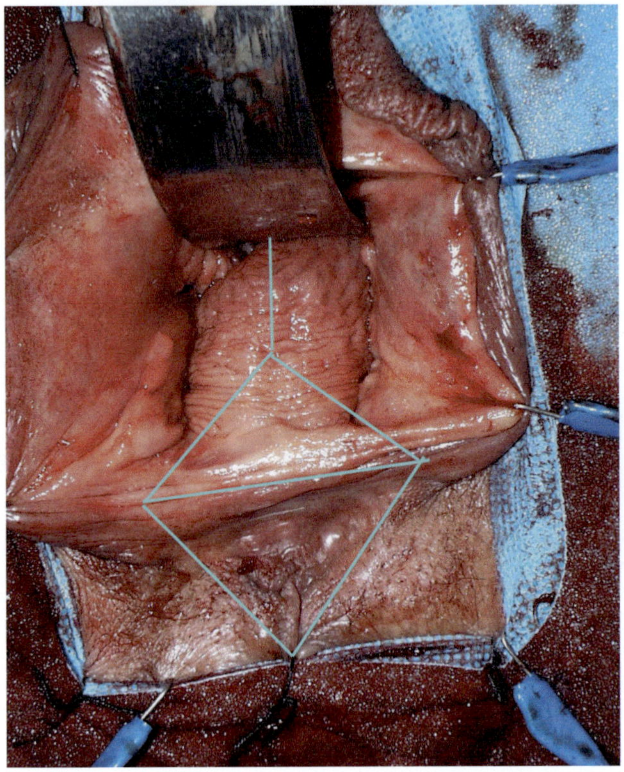

Fig. 3.135 Surgical picture outlining the surgical incisions: (1) a V-shaped incision in the perineum; (2) an inverted V-shaped incision in the vaginal wall, with the tip reaching 3 cm from the introitus (the level of the levator hiatus); (3) a straight incision extending to the vaginal cuff

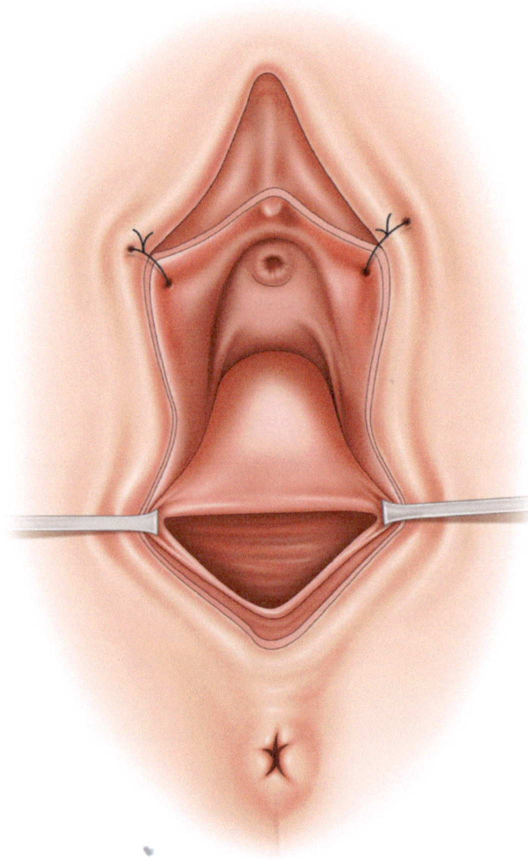

Fig. 3.136 Diagram depicting the triangular excision of the perineal skin and posterior fourchette

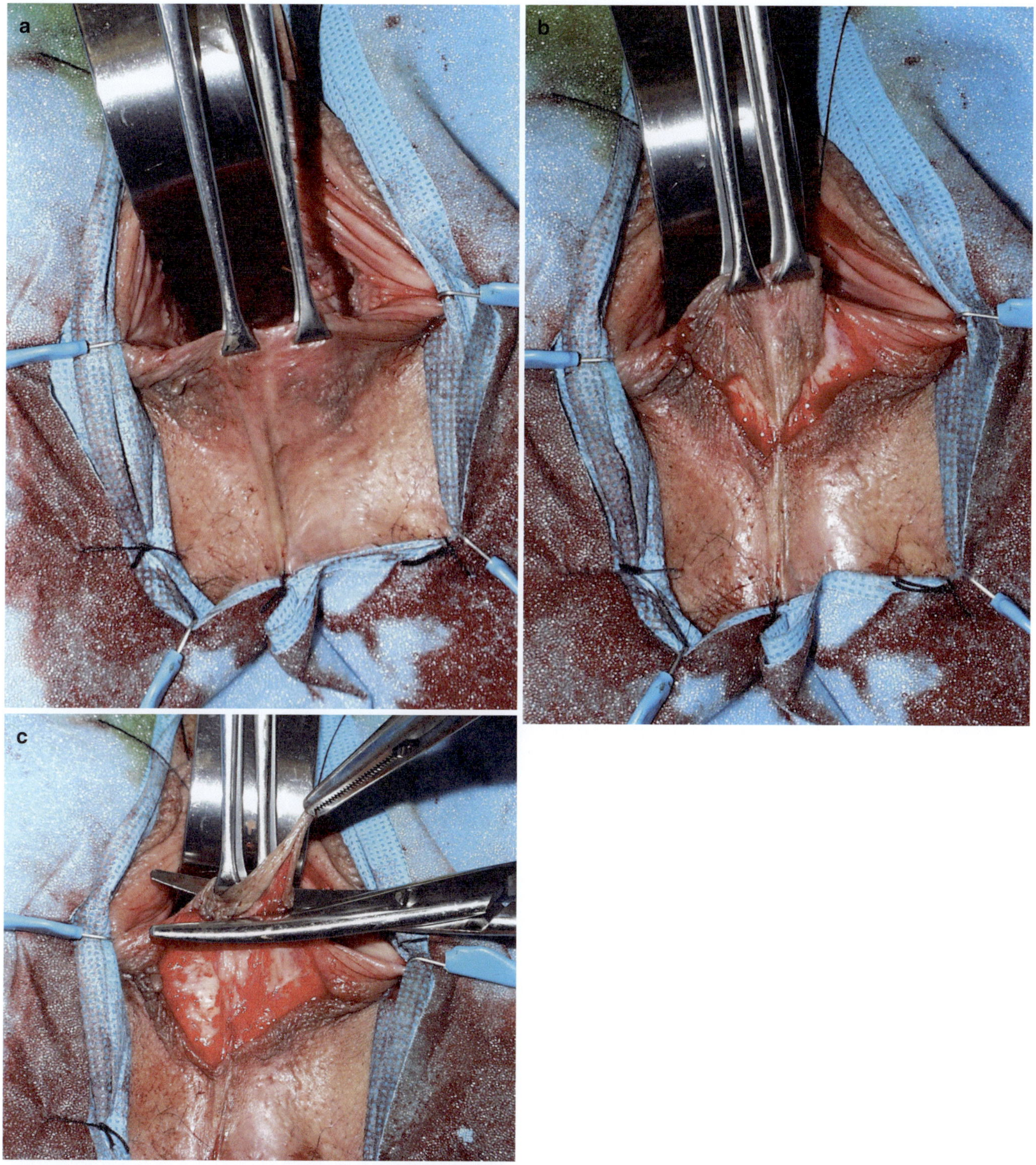

Fig. 3.137 (**a**) Two Allis clamps are placed at the margin of the introitus at the posterior fourchette, in the 5 o'clock and 7 o'clock positions. (**b**) A V-shaped incision is made from the posterior fourchette with the tip extending to the central tendon and external anal sphincter. The width of the V will depend on the degree of separation or widening of the posterior fourchette. (**c**) The skin is dissected free and the posterior fourchette is excised between the Allis clamps

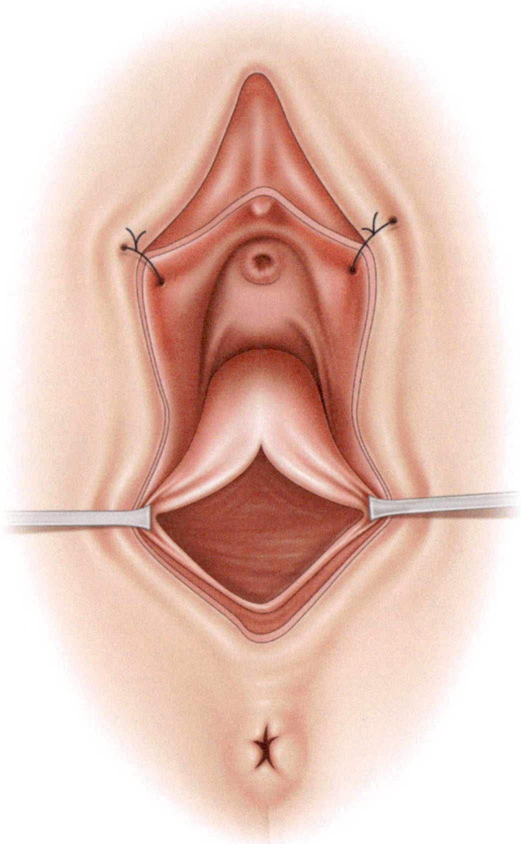

Fig. 3.138 Diagram showing the second step of the surgery: the excision of a triangular segment of the posterior vaginal wall extending 3 cm from the introitus

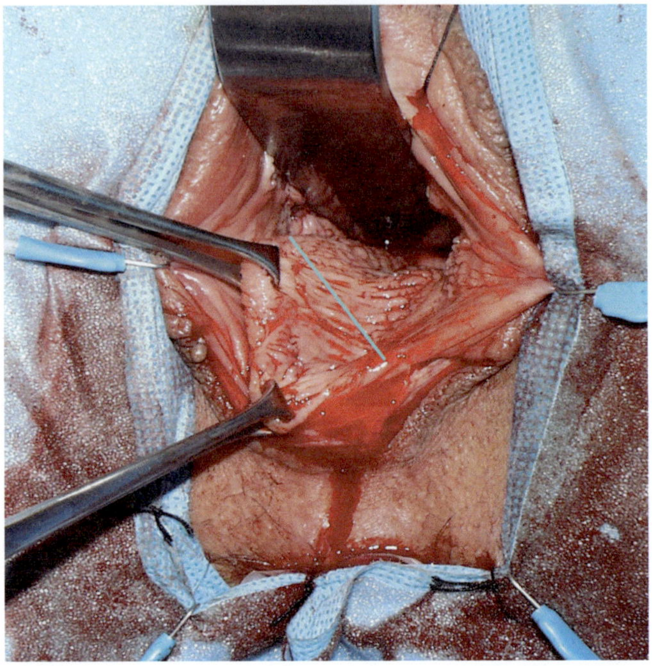

Fig. 3.139 Two Allis clamps are applied on the distal posterior vaginal wall. The upper Allis is usually applied 3–4 cm from the introitus, at the level of the levator hiatus. An oblique incision (*blue line*) is made from the levator hiatus distally toward the excised mucocutaneous junction at the posterior fourchette

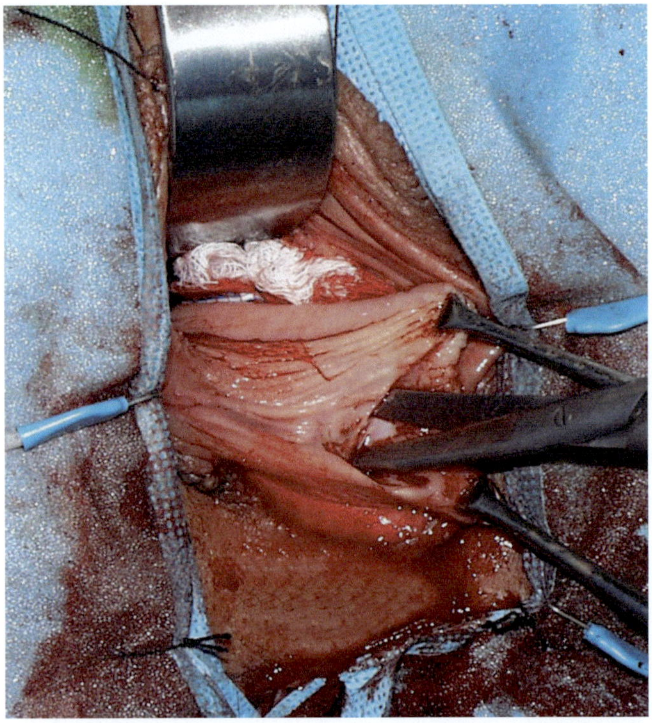

Fig. 3.140 Scissors are used to dissect the vaginal wall laterally, thereby exposing the attenuated prerectal fascia and the area of the perineal membrane that extends 3 cm into the vaginal canal

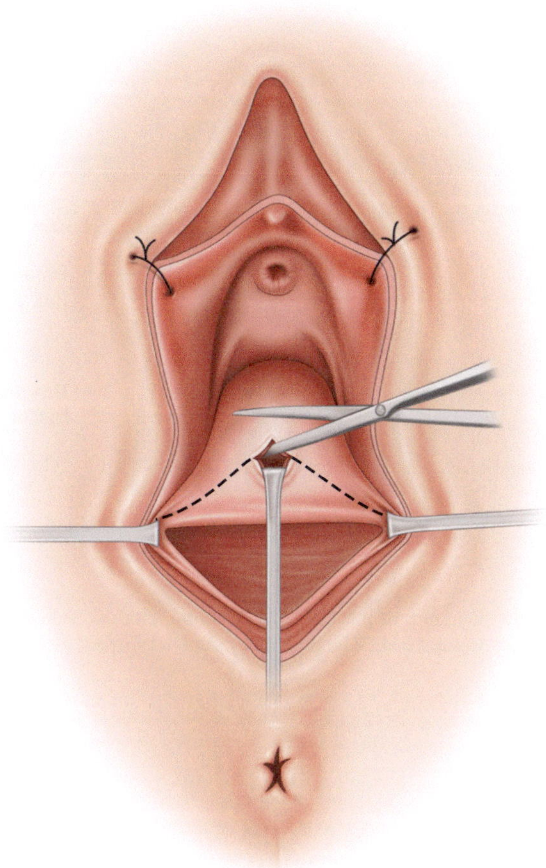

Fig. 3.141 Diagram of the triangular island of posterior vaginal wall (3–4 cm high) as it is excised

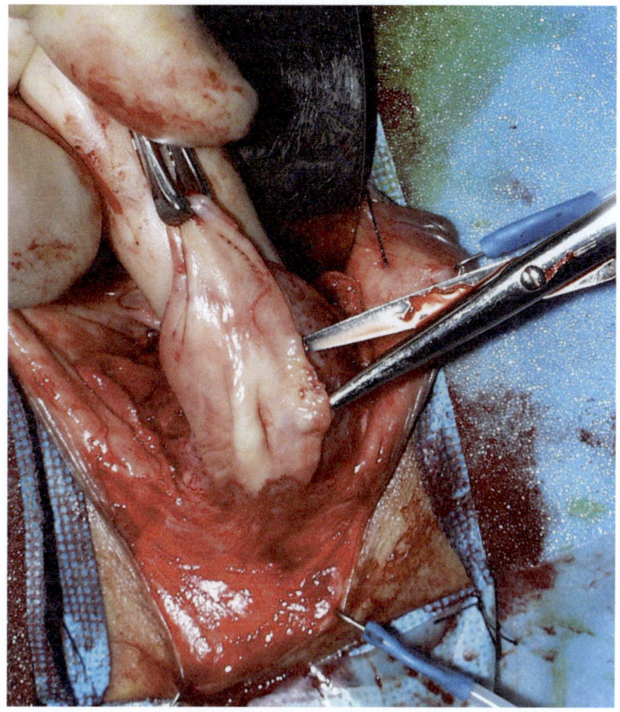

Fig. 3.142 The triangular island of vaginal wall will be sharply excised, revealing the prerectal fascia and the extension of the perineal membrane into the posterior distal vagina

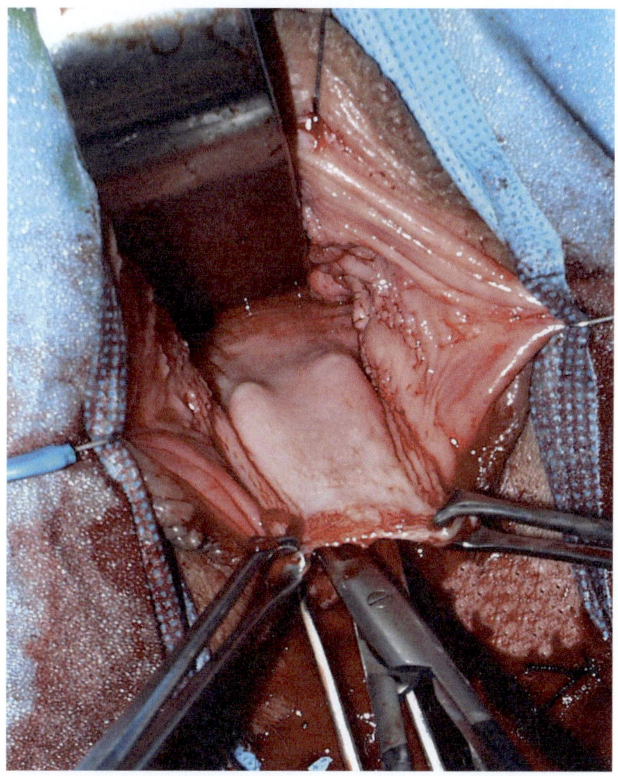

Fig. 3.143 Scissors are used to dissect under the vaginal wall toward the vaginal cuff to expose the prerectal fascia. With the anterior retractor under upward traction, a strip of the posterior vaginal wall is excised (with the width depending on the size of the posterior defect). The surgeon should be careful to refrain from excising an excessive amount of posterior vaginal wall, to avoid causing vaginal narrowing

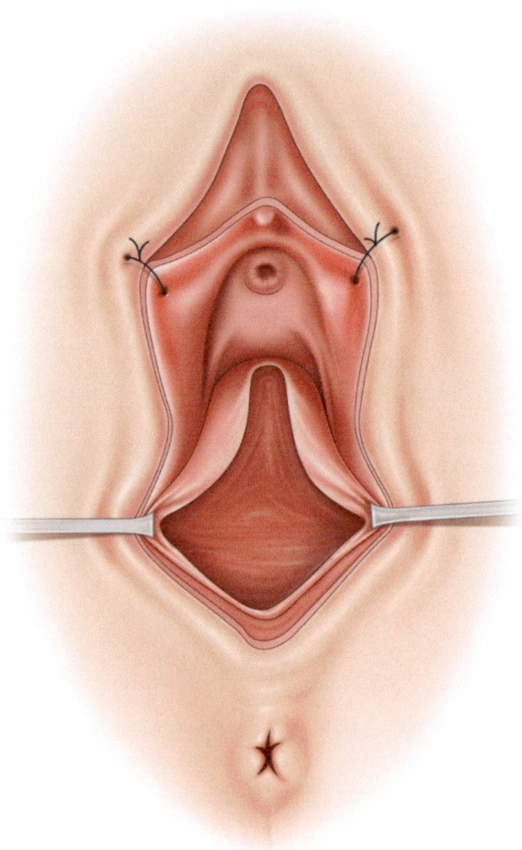

Fig. 3.144 Diagram of the posterior vaginal wall after excision of the strip

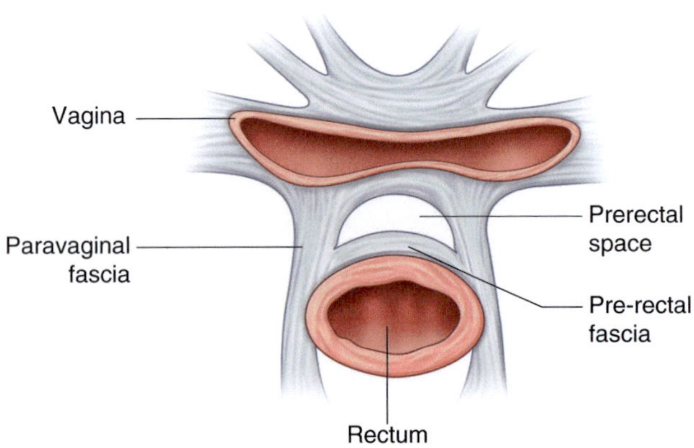

Fig. 3.145 Diagram of the vaginal canal and rectum with the laterally located paravaginal fascia or pillar of the rectum

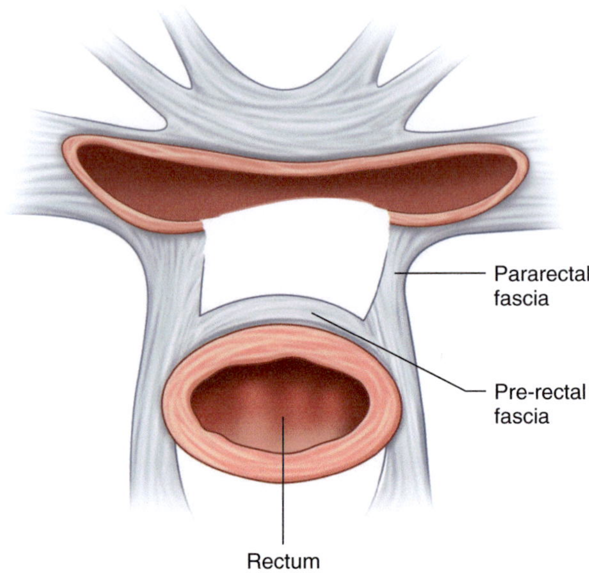

Fig. 3.146 Diagram of the vagina and rectum after excision of a strip of posterior vaginal wall. The prerectal fascia is exposed

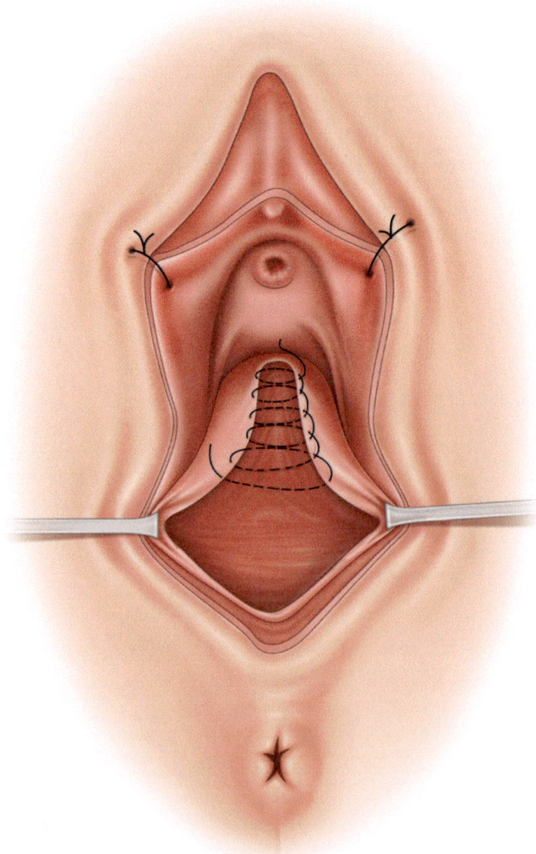

Fig. 3.147 Diagram of the closure of the rectocele defect using multiple running, locking #2-0 slow absorbable suture. We incorporate the edge of the vaginal incision; after insinuating the needle under the vaginal wall, strong segments of the pararectal and prerectal fasciae are incorporated

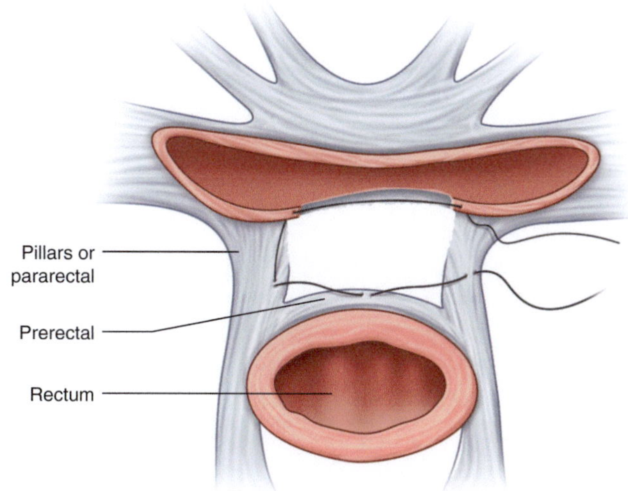

Fig. 3.148 Diagram of the closure of the rectocele defect. The suture includes the edge of the vaginal wall, the prerectal fascia, and the pillars of the rectum (pararectal fascia)

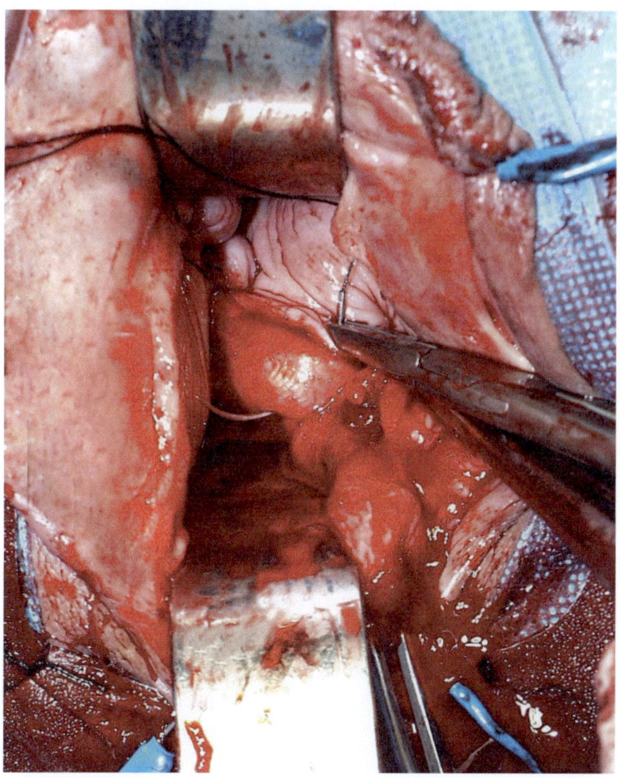

Fig. 3.149 Surgical photograph demonstrates the closure of the rectocele defect. The anterior vaginal wall is retracted upward, and the posterior rectal wall is retracted downward, both with the use of Haney or right-angle retractors. This maneuver facilitates the repair by protecting the rectum, reducing the rectocele, and allowing exposure of the prerectal and pararectal fasciae. The rectocele repair is undertaken by incorporating the prerectal and pararectal fasciae from the apex of the posterior vagina toward the levator hiatus, using a running, locking #2-0 slow absorbable suture. Each needle passage incorporates only the edge of the vaginal wall and generous amounts of the prerectal and pararectal fasciae bilaterally. The suture stops at the level of the triangular excision in the distal vagina, usually 3–4 cm from the introitus

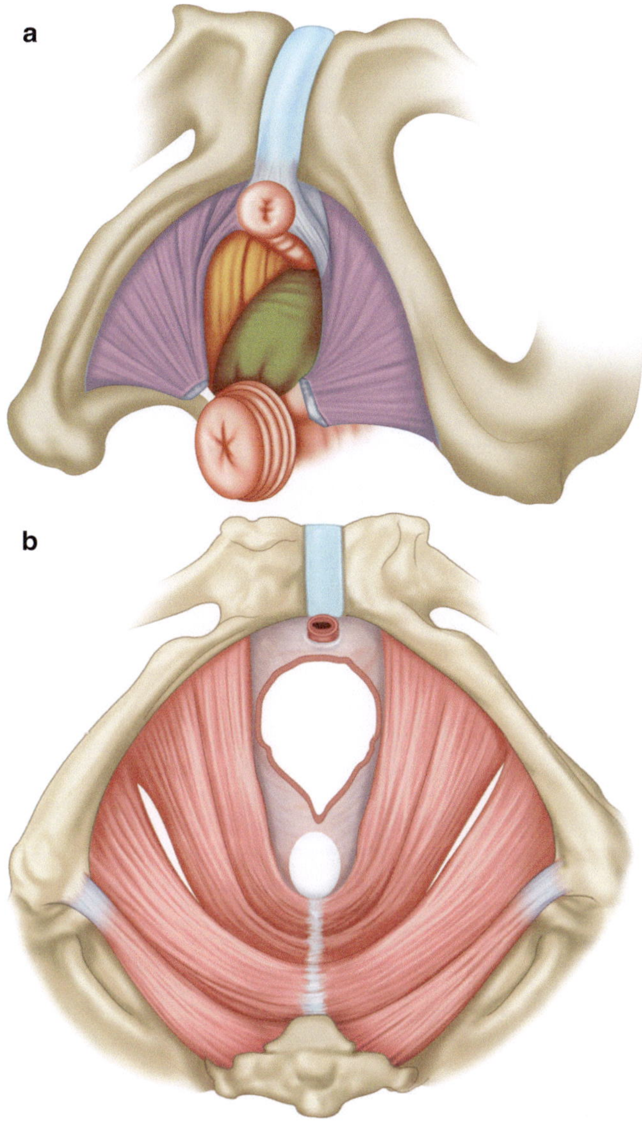

Fig. 3.150 (**a**) The perineal membrane inserts into the descending rami of the ischiopubis. Each half joins in the middle to form the perineal body, which extends 3–4 cm from the introitus inside the vagina. Perineal trauma such as vaginal delivery causes the loss of connection of each half, widens the levator hiatus, facilitates the formation of a rectocele, and decreases the size of the perineal body. The diagram depicts the separation of the perineal membrane and shortening of the perineal body. (**b**) Diagram of the pelvic floor showing a wide levator hiatus

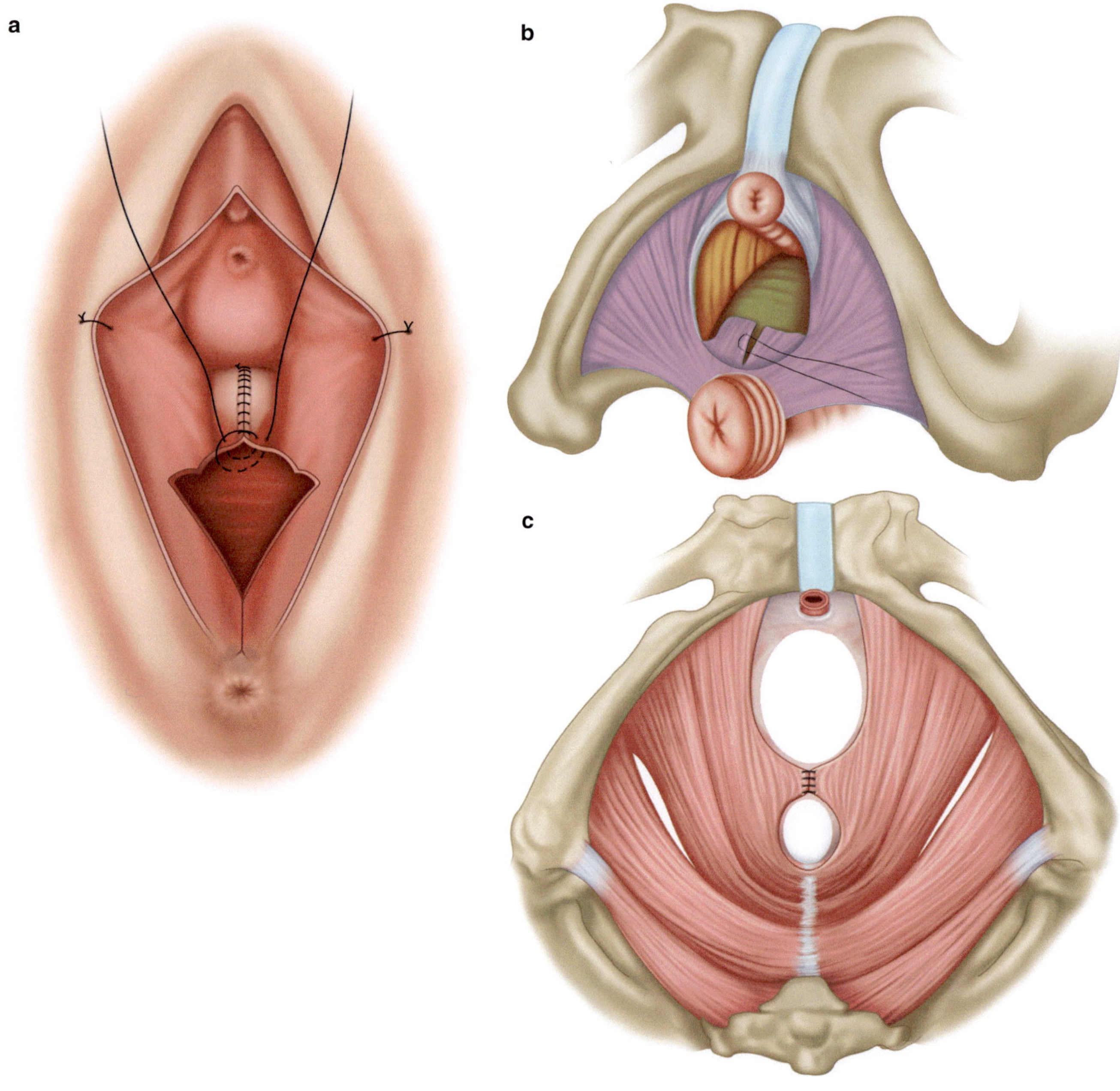

Fig. 3.151 (**a**) Diagram of the application of interrupted figure-of-eight sutures over the distal vagina, incorporating the perineal membrane and resulting in a narrower levator hiatus. Usually two or three sutures are required. They will elevate the distal vagina and rebuild the perineum. (**b**) Diagram depicting the repair of the distal vagina with figure-of-eight sutures approximating the perineal membrane and narrowing the levator hiatus. (**c**) Diagram of the reconstructed and narrowed levator hiatus. The levator muscles are not directly incorporated in the sutures

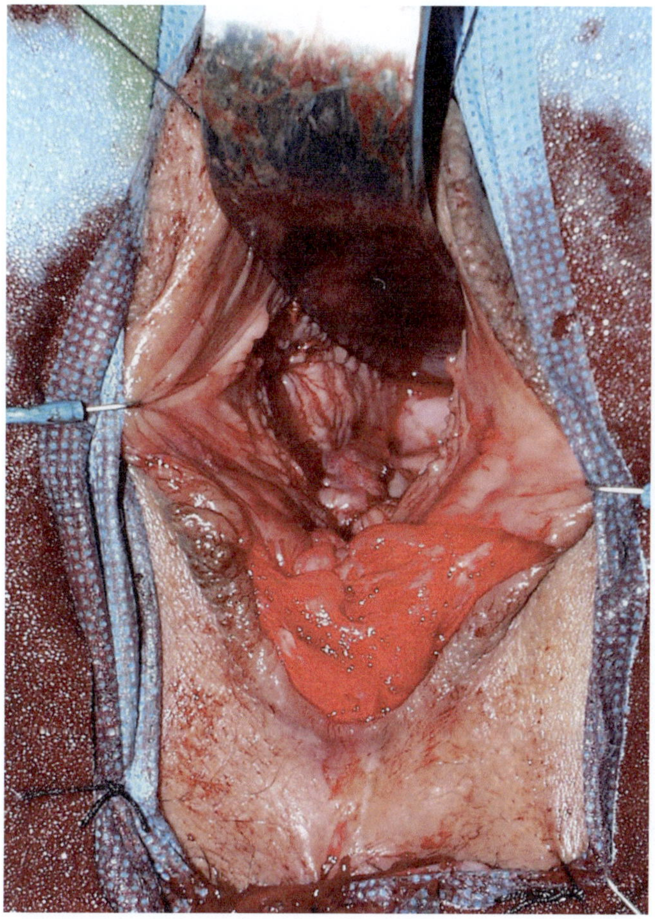

Fig. 3.152 The distal sutures have been applied, creating the narrowing of the wide levator hiatus and elevation of the distal vagina

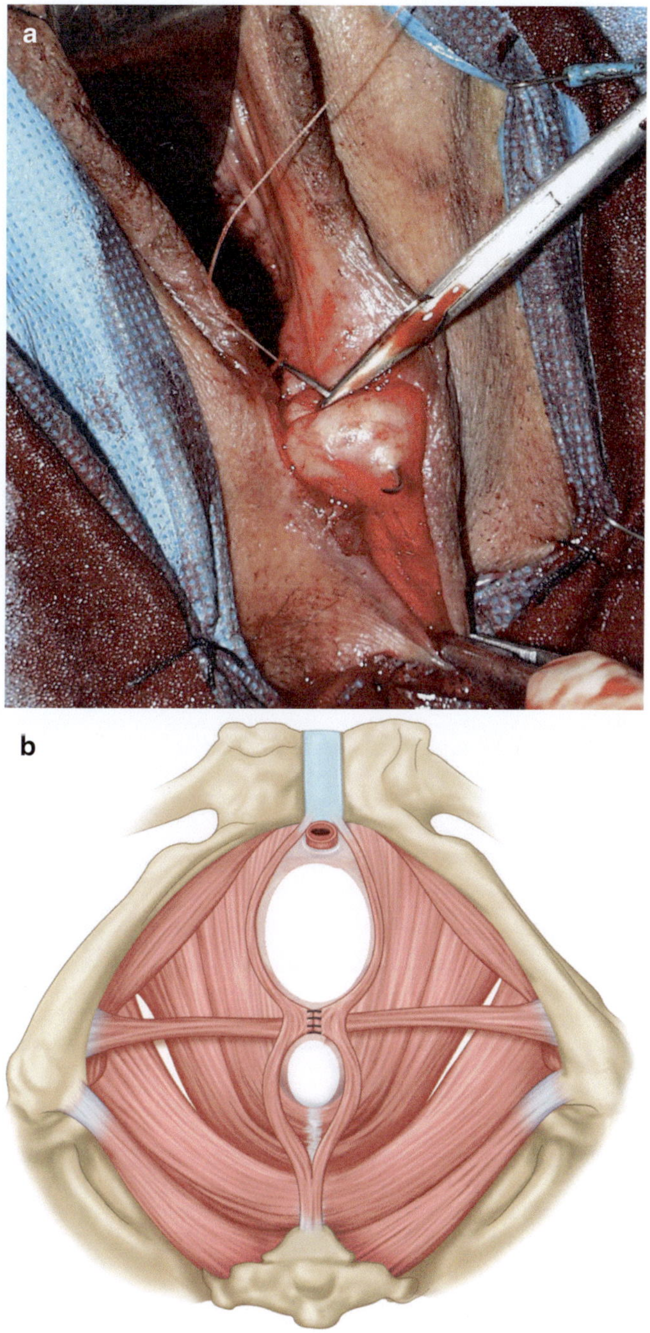

Fig. 3.153 (**a**) Vertical mattress sutures of #2-0 slow absorbable suture are used to approximate the bulbocavernosus, superficial transverse perinei muscles, and external anal sphincter muscles, allowing reconstruction of the urogenital diaphragm and support of the central tendon. (**b**) Diagram showing the reconstructed perineum after the repair

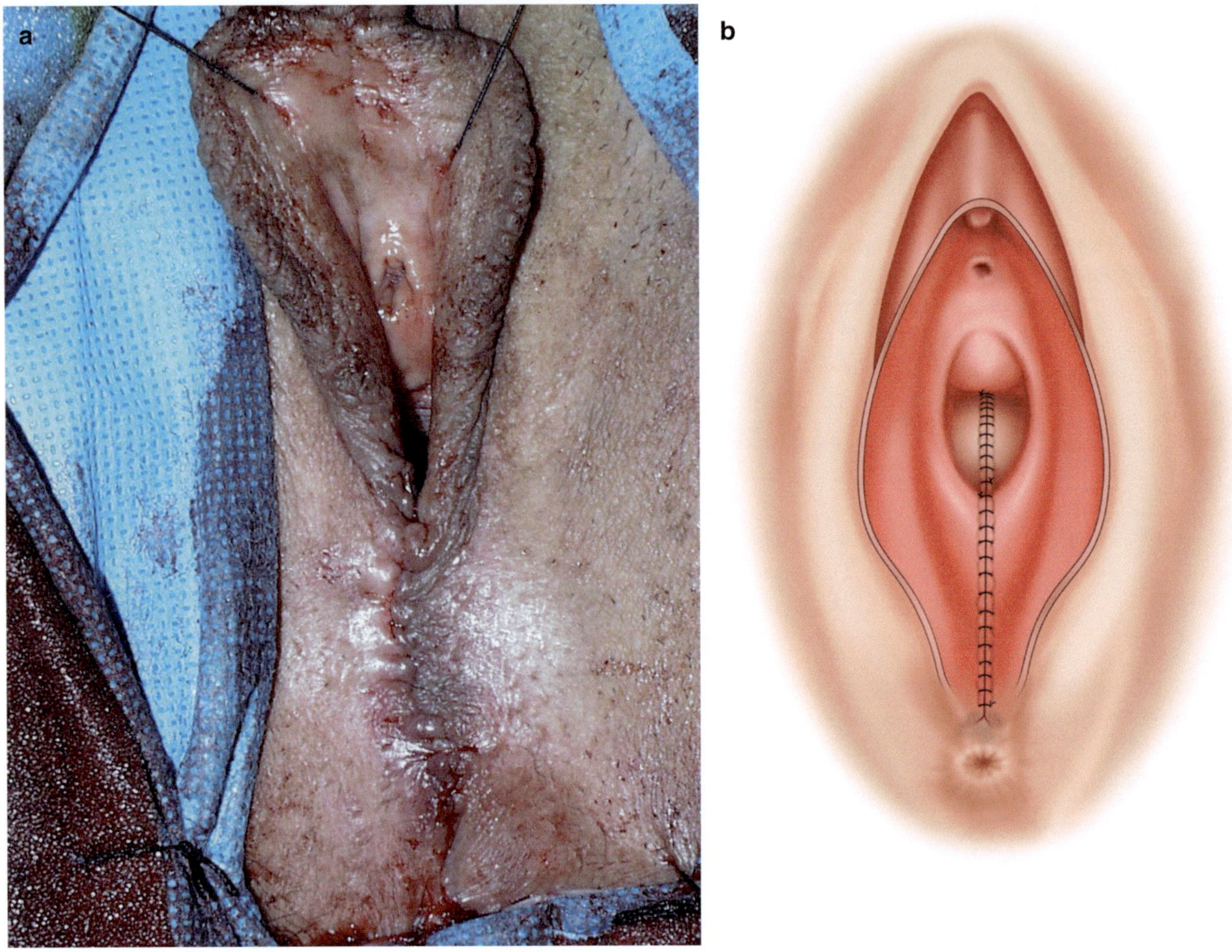

Fig. 3.154 (**a**) The skin of the perineum is approximated with a vertical line of delay absorbable sutures. Local anesthesia is injected to improve postoperative pain. (**b**) Diagram of the complete posterior vaginal wall and perineal reconstruction

3.5 Repair of Perineal Hernia

3.5.1 Indications

Perineal herniation is an often-overlooked condition in which the perineal musculature loses its supporting properties because of trauma, atrophy, weakness, or neuropathy. The vaginal examination may be normal or may have concomitant abnormalities. The main diagnostic feature is the presence of a bulge of the perineal musculature when the patient is straining. The normally flat perineum (Fig. 3.155) bulges on straining, appearing as a convex deformity. The herniation combines weakness and separation of the levator musculature in the perineum and loss of the fascial and muscle support (Fig. 3.156). The distal colon and the small bowel are often included in the hernia sac. Neuropathic pelvic floor damage such as sacral arc injury or pudendal neuropathy can cause significant perineal herniation through paralysis of the pelvic musculature.

Presenting symptoms include perineal pressure, constipation, and the need to use pressure to reduce the perineal herniation. The physical examination reveals the finding of the perineum bulging on straining. The vaginal examination reveals no prolapse or often other organ prolapse (Fig. 3.157). The distance between the posterior fourchette and the anal sphincter is increased and further increases with strain. Dynamic MRI has helped to better define the condition by objectively demonstrating the type and degree of the perineal defect (Figs. 3.158 and 3.159).

3.5.2 Preoperative Considerations

The bowel should be properly prepared before surgery. Mechanical preparation of the distal colon is advisable. Broad-spectrum antibiotics are used in the perioperative period.

The patient is in the lithotomy position.

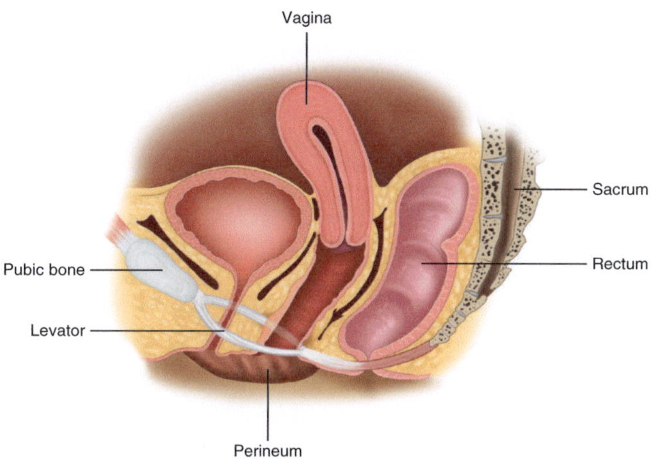

Fig. 3.155 Diagram of the normal anatomy of the perineum showing the flat space between the posterior fourchette and the rectum

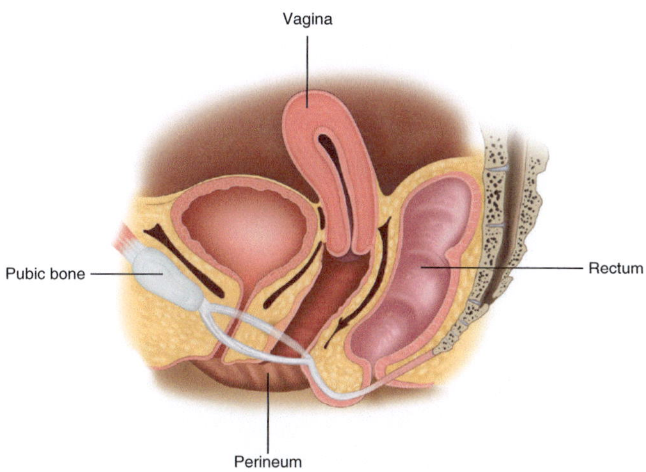

Fig. 3.156 In patients with perineal hernia, the normally flat perineum is weak with significant convexity, creating the bulging typical of a perineal hernia, with increased distance from the rectum to the posterior fourchette

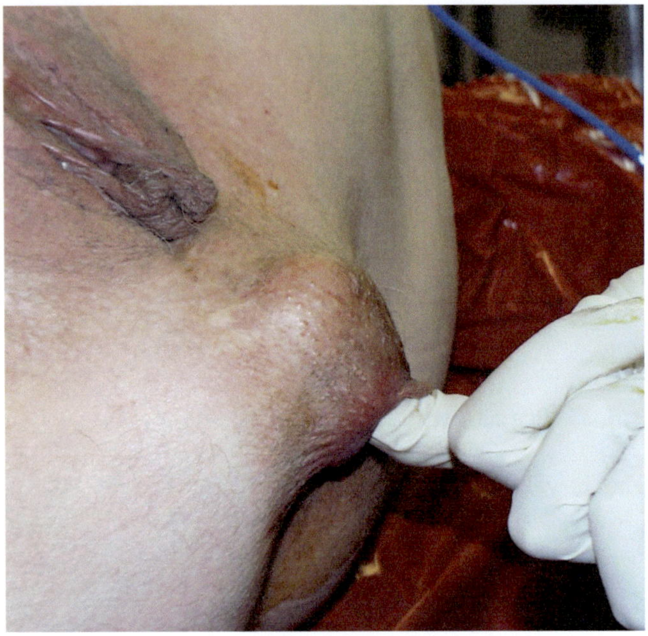

Fig. 3.157 Physical examination demonstrating the bulge of the perineum in a patient prior to surgery. The bulge may be spontaneous or induced by finger traction

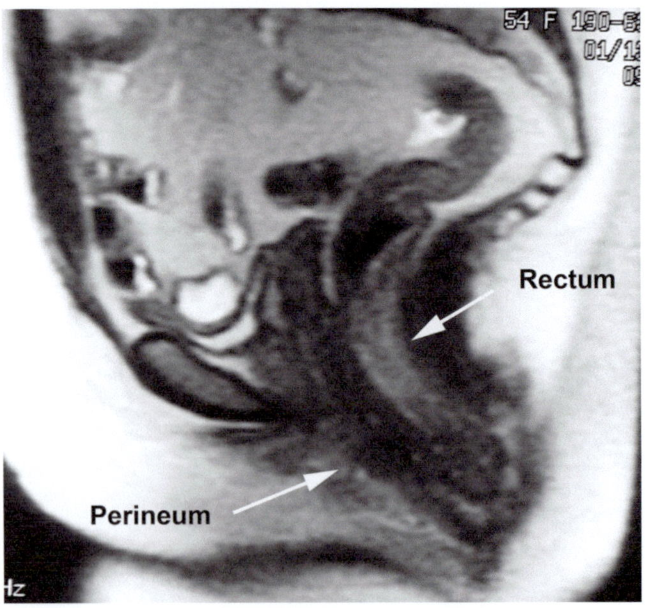

Fig. 3.158 Sagittal resting MRI of the midline pelvis showing the rectum, anal canal, and perineum

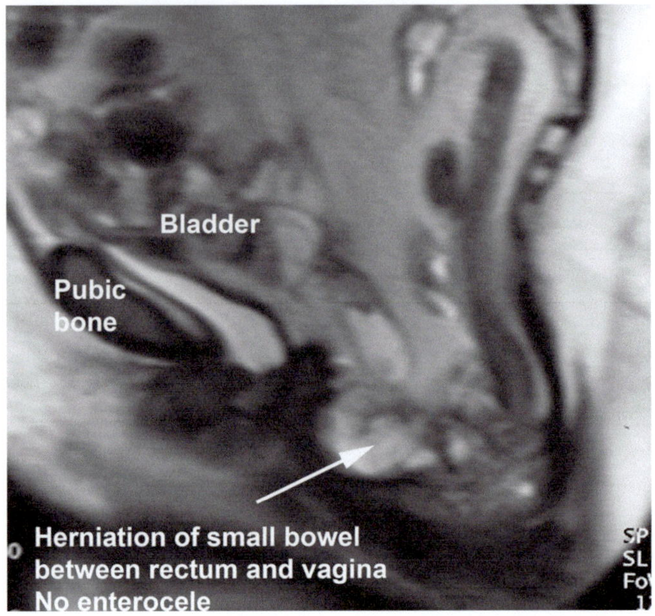

Fig. 3.159 Straining sagittal MRI of the pelvis showing significant herniation of the perineum. The patient has a normal vaginal examination after multiple reconstructive surgeries, but she complains of perineal pressure and severe constipation, with the need to apply perineal pressure in order to defecate

3.5.3 Surgical Technique

Figures 3.160, 3.161, 3.162, 3.163, 3.164, 3.165, 3.166, 3.167, and 3.168 illustrate the surgical technique for the repair of a perineal hernia.

3.5.4 Postoperative Care

A vaginal packing is inserted at the end of the procedure and left in place for 2 h. Long-acting local anesthesia is injected to improve postoperative pain. Ice packs, parenteral antibiotics, stool softeners, and pain medication are used in the perioperative period.

3.5.5 Postoperative Complications

Potential complications include pain, infection of the perineal and perirectal area, fistula, or recurrent hernia. Bowel changes should improve with a good anatomical repair, but patients can continue to have defecatory dysfunction in spite of a good repair.

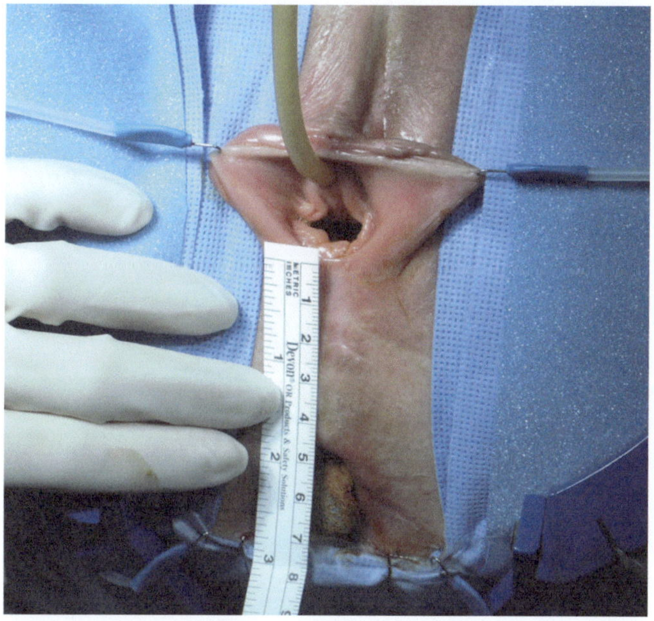

Fig. 3.160 Intraoperative photograph of the perineum of a patient suffering from a significant perineal hernia. The vaginal examination was unremarkable, but the distance between the posterior fourchette and the anal sphincter was 8 cm

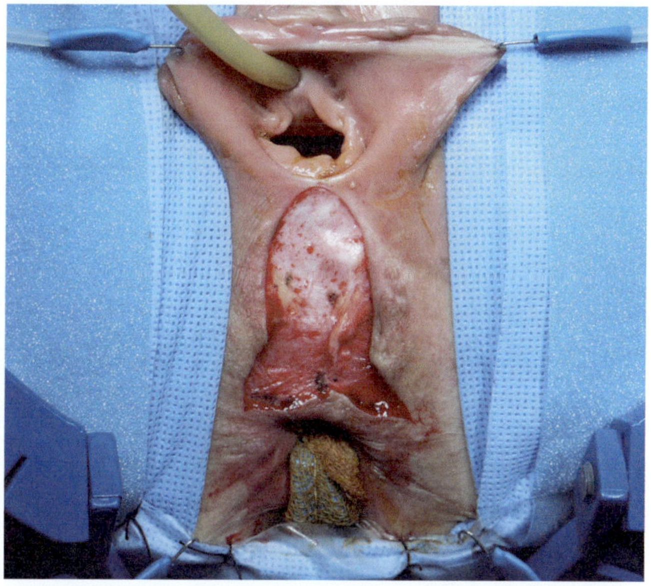

Fig. 3.161 A vertical incision is made in the perineum. The incision is extended as an inverted V around the anal canal

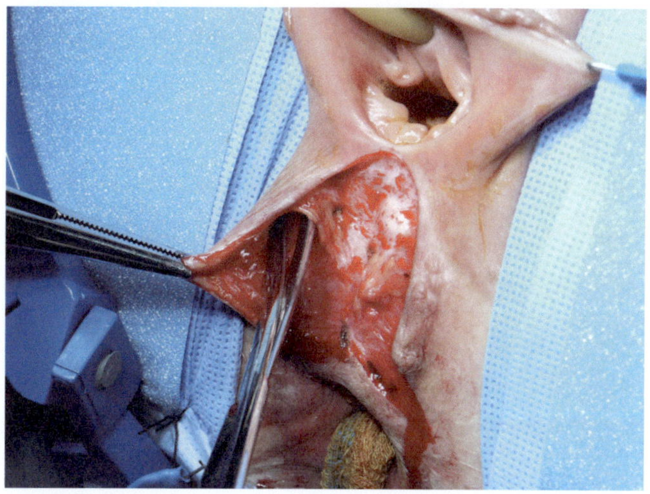

Fig. 3.162 Dissection is carried out laterally to expose the perineal musculature, including the transverse perineum and the external anal fibers

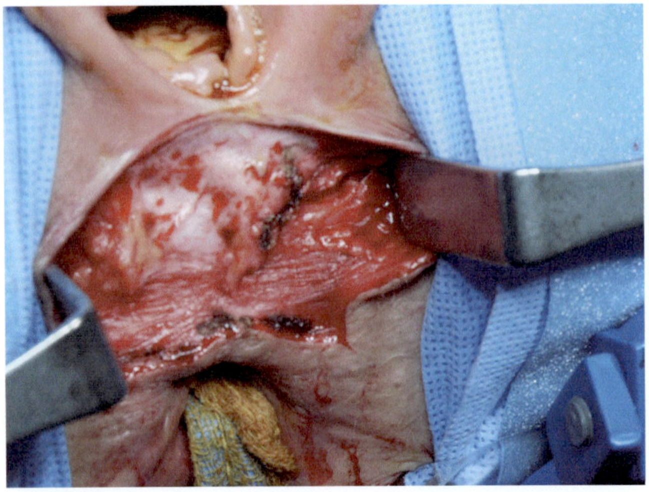

Fig. 3.163 In the posterior perineum, the ischiorectal fossa is entered on each side

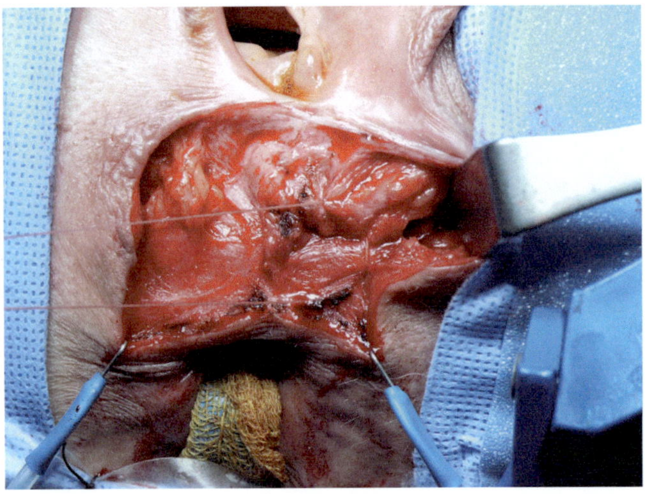

Fig. 3.164 The levator musculature in the posterior perineum is exposed. Horizontally placed mattress sutures using #2-0 delay absorbable sutures approximate the external anal sphincter and perirectal fascia to the transverse perineal musculature and fascia at the posterior fourchette. Strong bites of tissue are taken. A finger in the rectum may facilitate the placement of the sutures

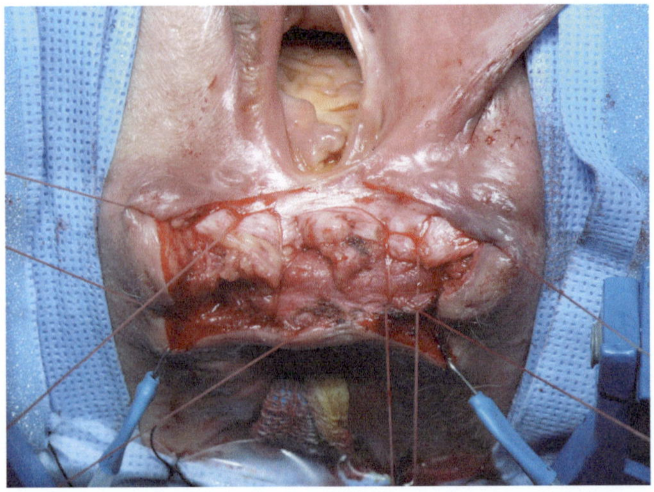

Fig. 3.165 Horizontal interrupted figure-of-eight sutures approximate the perirectal fascia at the anal canal to the posterior fourchette, closing the perineal defect and shortening the distance between the anal canal and posterior fourchette

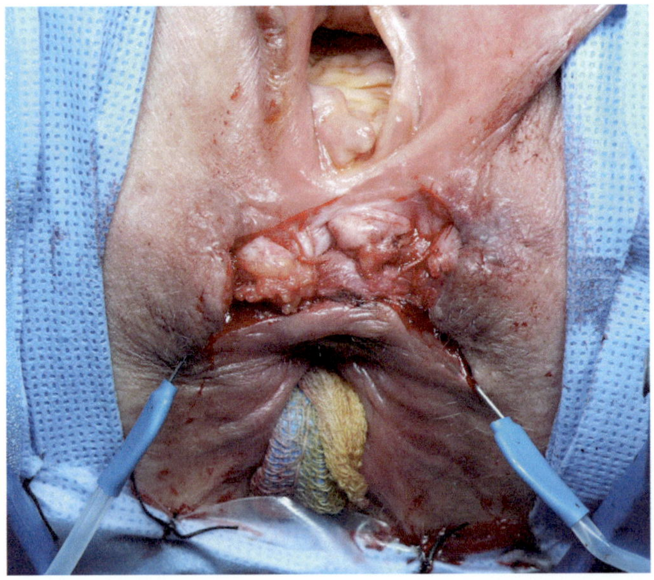

Fig. 3.166 The perineal sutures are tied, providing a shorter perineum and a strong perineal shelf. Rectal examination can confirm the strength of the repair

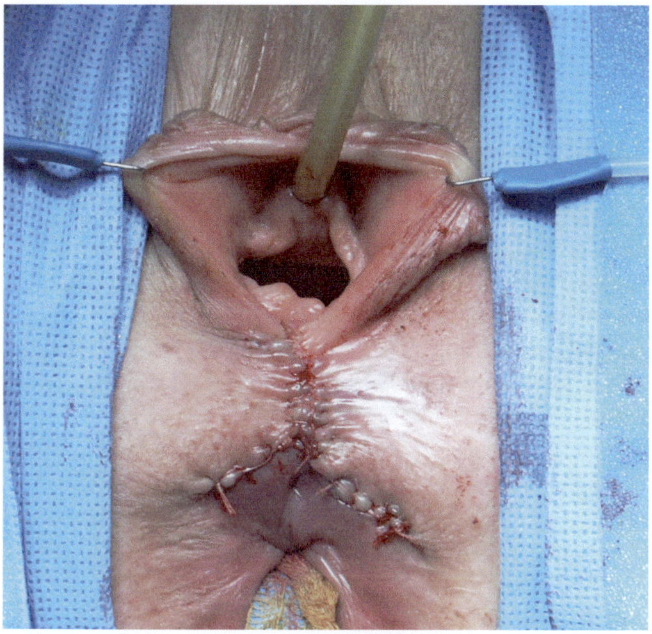

Fig. 3.167 The perineal skin is closed in two layers with delay absorbable sutures

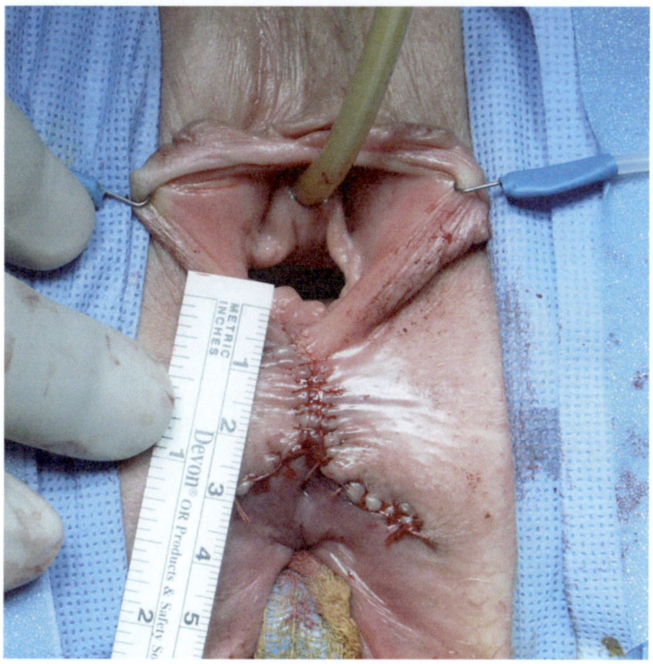

Fig. 3.168 The distance between the rectum and posterior fourchette is measured now to be only 3 cm

3.6 Transvaginal Pararectal Repair of Rectal Prolapse

3.6.1 Indications

Rectal prolapse is a disabling condition in which the rectal mucosa or the whole rectal wall protrudes through the anal canal. It can present with symptoms of constipation, loss of stool, rectal bleeding, or rectal pain. The prolapse may be minor, requiring only medical treatment, but if the protrusion is symptomatic or severe, surgical treatment is indicated. The main option for treatment is a rectopexy to the sacrum using sutures or mesh and, when indicated, concomitant colonic resection.

We have developed a minimally invasive transvaginal pararectal procedure to correct rectal prolapse. This operation restores the posterior rectal wall and vaginal axis to the normal 100-degree angulation with the horizontal line, helping to prevent further prolapse. The surgery is an outpatient procedure with 23-h stay. No complications (e.g., perirectal abscess, rectal fistula, or de novo defecatory dysfunction) have occurred. This kind of minimally invasive transvaginal procedure always can be tried prior to abdominal surgery.

3.6.2 Preoperative Considerations

Prior to preparation and draping, the rectum is irrigated with copious antibiotic solution until clear. Perioperative antibiotics are given.

3.6.3 Surgical Technique

The patient is placed in lithotomy position. After preparation and draping, a large Hegar dilator is inserted in the rectum and is fixed to the drapes with a Penrose drain to allow access and easy palpation of the rectal wall at the time of surgery (Fig. 3.169). After exposure of the posterior vaginal wall, two incisions are made laterally, and the pararectal space is entered (Figs. 3.170 and 3.171). A row of three to four delayed absorbable sutures is applied to the sacrospinous ligaments and the iliococcygeus muscle on each side (Fig. 3.172). After insertion of an Hegar dilator in the rectum, the preplaced sutures are applied to the posterolateral wall of the rectum in a sequential fashion, fixing the distal rectum for a distance of 10 cm to the lateral levator musculature (Figs. 3.173, 3.174, 3.175, and 3.176).

3.6.4 Postoperative Care

The surgery is done as an outpatient procedure. An overnight vaginal packing soaked with antibiotics is inserted in the vagina. The patient is allowed to resume normal activities except heavy lifting or straining. Stool softeners or laxatives are given as required. The Foley catheter is removed the day after surgery unless another anterior vaginal wall procedure was performed.

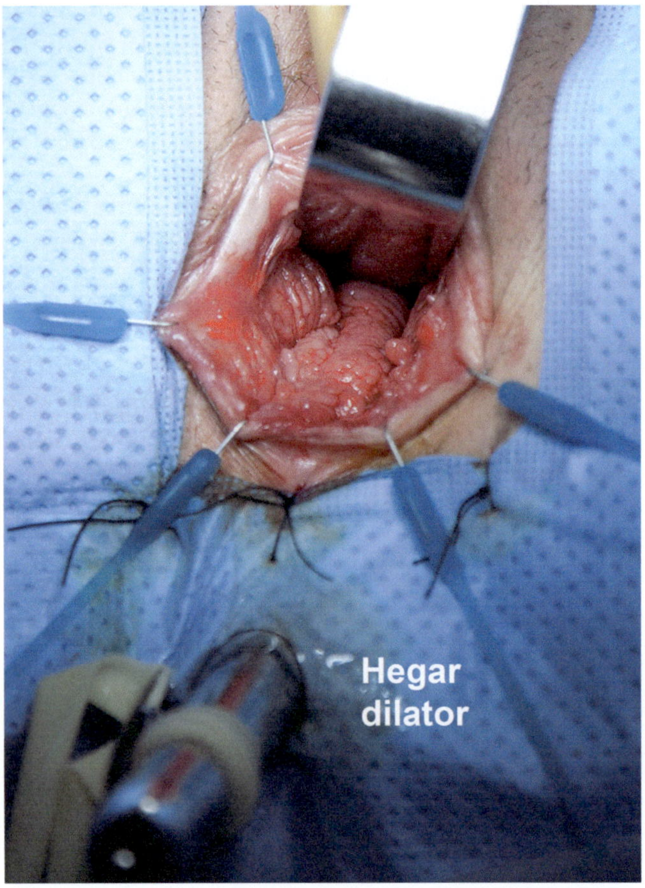

Fig. 3.169 Exposure of the posterior vaginal wall is obtained using an Heaney retractor. A ring retractor with hooks facilitates the exposure. A Hegar dilator is inserted in the rectum and fixed to the drapes using a Penrose drain

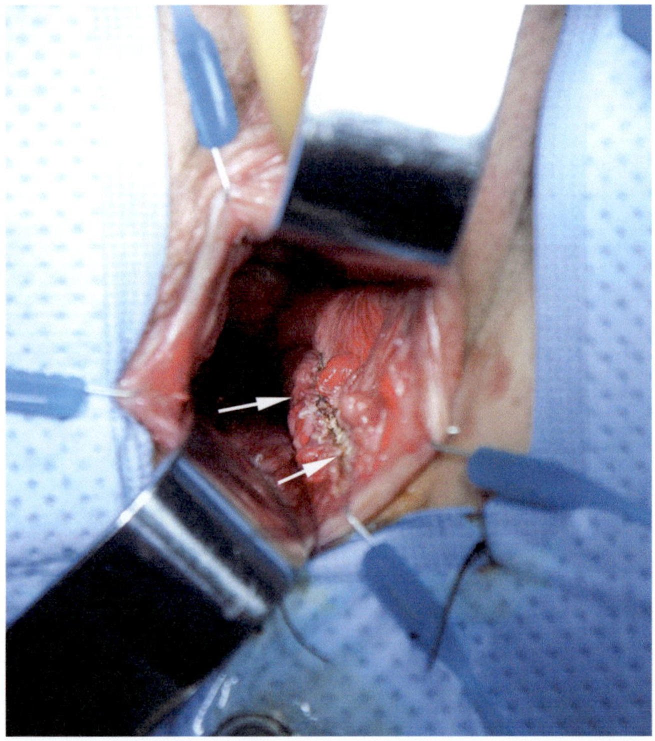

Fig. 3.170 Posterior lateral incisions are made in the vaginal wall at the 5 and 7 o'clock positions. The procedure is done in each pararectal space in a similar fashion

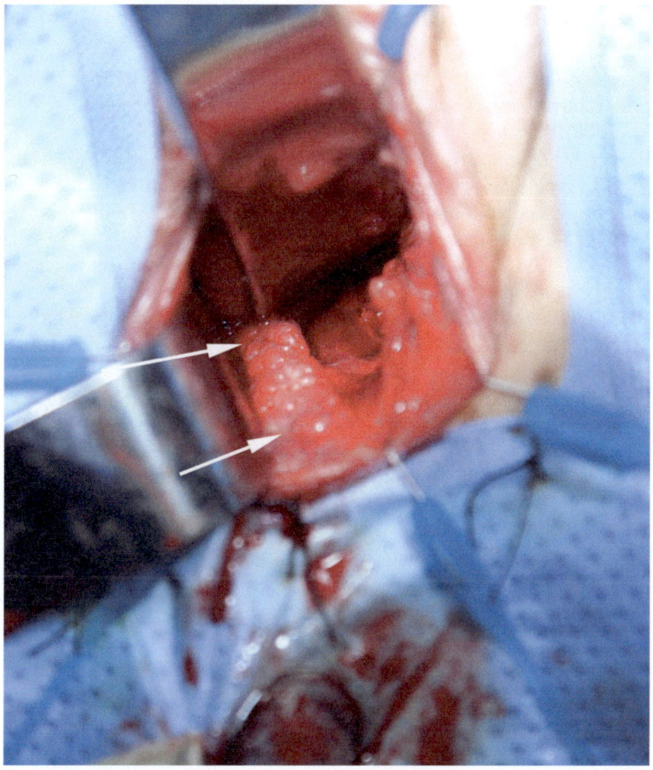

Fig. 3.171 The pararectal space is exposed, freeing the rectum from the iliococcygeus muscles up to the origin of the sacrospinous ligament

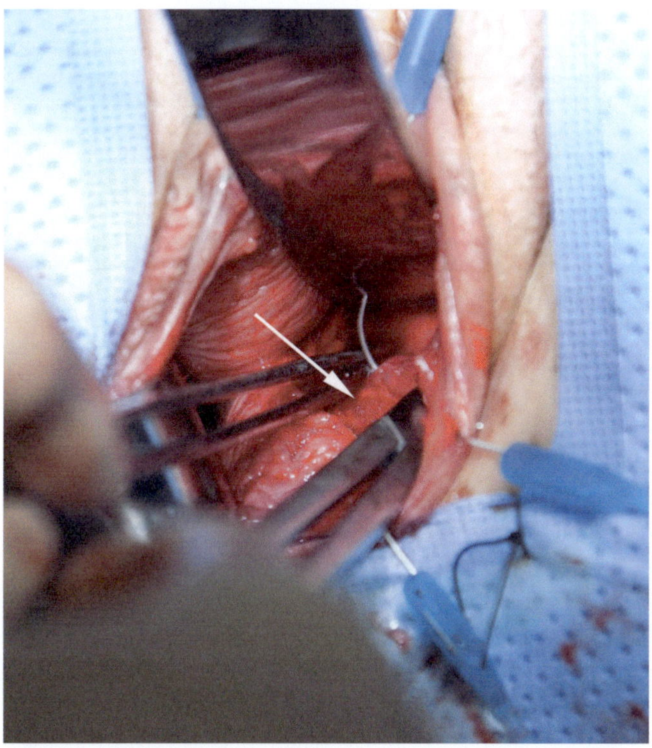

Fig. 3.172 With medial retraction of the rectum, multiple sequential #0 delayed absorbable sutures are applied to the levator musculature. The first suture is inserted just distal to the sacrospinous ligament, and two or three more sutures are inserted distally and sequentially, obtaining a strong anchor to the levator musculature

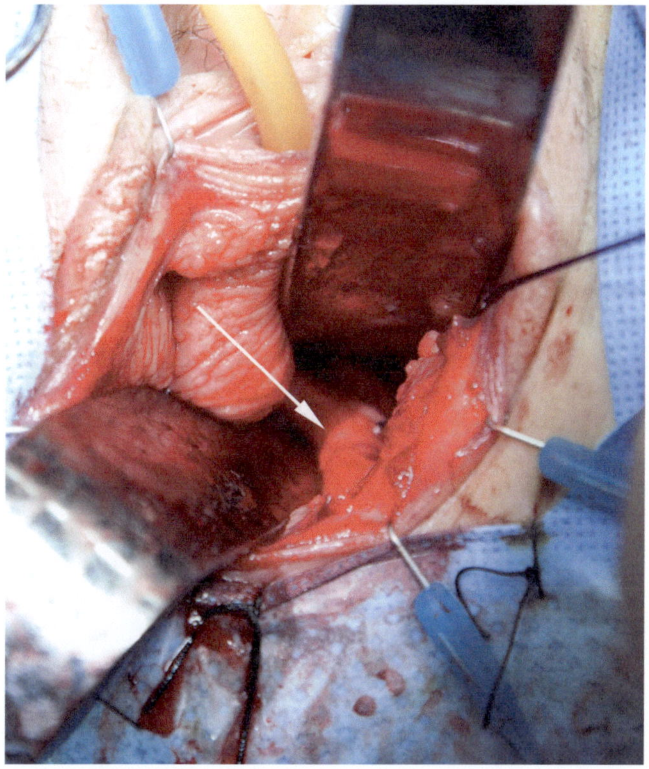

Fig. 3.173 The posterolateral rectal wall is exposed. The Hegar dilator helps in finding the rectal wall itself. The *arrow* is directed at the rectal wall elevated by the Hegar dilator

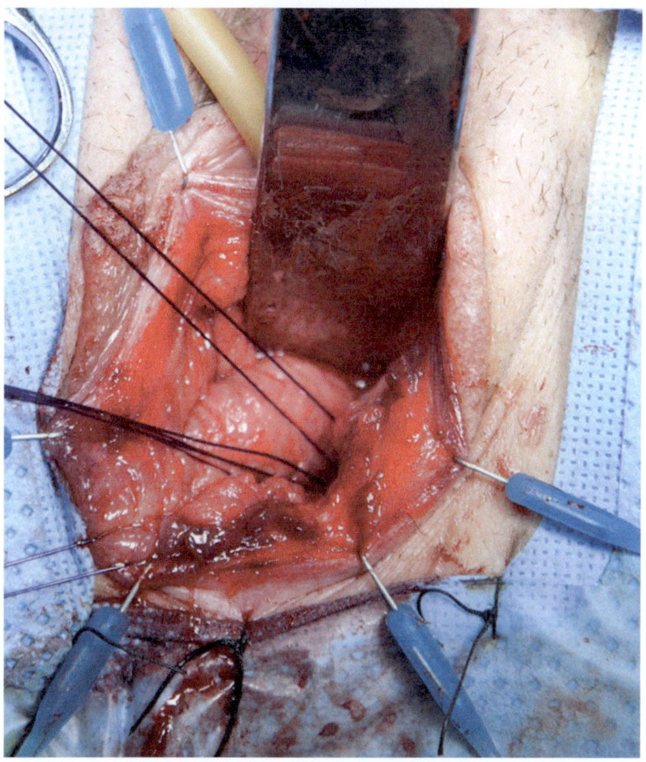

Fig. 3.174 The levator sutures are sequentially passed through the posterolateral rectal wall with guidance of the Hegar dilator in the rectal wall, taking care to incorporate the whole rectal wall. The sutures are tied. The rectal wall is now fixed to the lateral pelvic wall for a distance of more than 10 cm

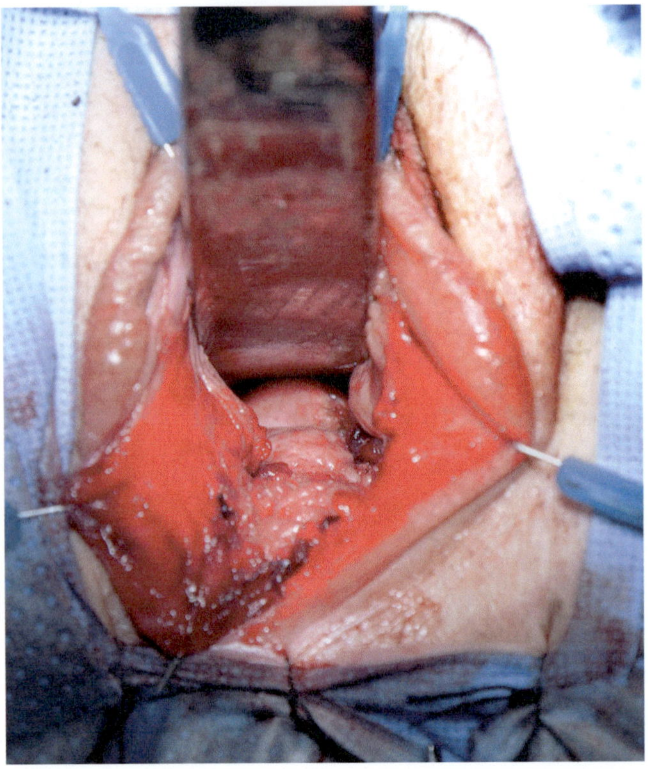

Fig. 3.175 After irrigations with antibiotic solution, the posterior vaginal wall is closed with multiple runs of #2-0 delayed absorbable sutures

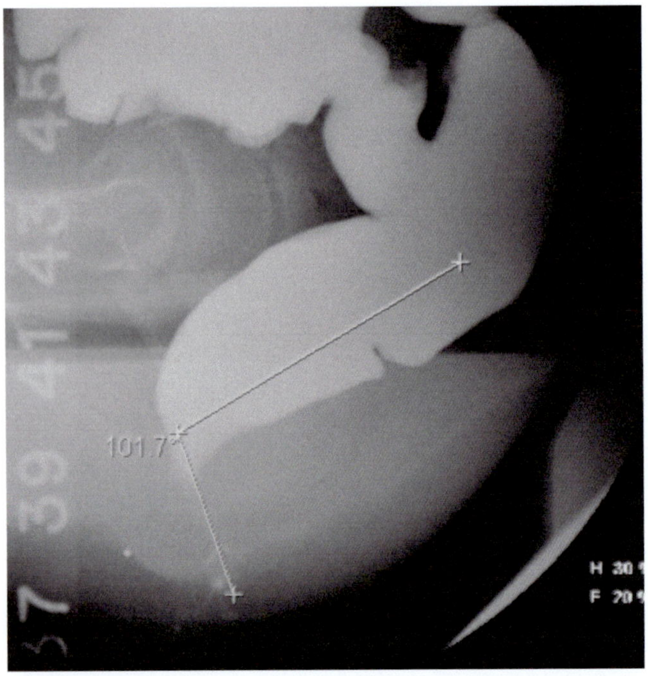

Fig. 3.176 A postoperative defecogram shows the restoration of the normal axis of the distal rectum without rectal prolapse

Suggested Reading

Baessler K, Maher CF. Mesh augmentation during pelvic-floor reconstructive surgery: risks and benefits. Curr Opin Obstet Gynecol. 2006;18:560–6.

Barber MD. Surgical correction of paravaginal defects. In: Vasavada SP, Appell RA, Sand PK, Raz S, editors. Female urology, urogynecology, and voiding dysfunction. New York: Marcel Dekker; 2005. p. 615–30.

Barber MD, Maher C. Epidemiology and outcome assessment of pelvic organ prolapse. Int Urogynecol J. 2013;24(11):1783–90.

Barber MD, Brubaker L, Burgio KL, Richter HE, Nygaard I, Weidner AC, Eunice Kennedy Shriver National Institute of Child Health and Human Development Pelvic Floor Disorders Network, et al. Comparison of 2 transvaginal surgical approaches and perioperative behavioral therapy for apical vaginal prolapse: the OPTIMAL randomized trial. JAMA. 2014;311(10):1023–34.

Birch C, Fynes MM. The role of synthetic and biological pros- theses in reconstructive pelvic floor surgery. Curr Opin Obstet Gynecol. 2002;14:527–35.

Bjelic-Radisic V, Aigmueller T, Preyer O, Ralph G, Geiss I, Müller G, Austrian Urogynecology Working Group, et al. Vaginal prolapse surgery with transvaginal mesh: results of the Austrian registry. Int Urogynecol J. 2014;25(8):1047–52.

Cervigni M, Natale F. The use of synthetics in the treatment of pelvic organ prolapse. Curr Opin Urol. 2001;11:429–35.

DeLancey JO. Structural anatomy of the posterior pelvic compartment as it relates to rectocele. Am J Obstet Gynecol. 1999;180(4):815–23.

DeLancey JOL. Fascial and muscular abnormalities in women with urethral hypermobility and anterior vaginal wall prolapse. Am J Obstet Gynecol. 2002;187:93–8.

Goldberg RP, Koduri S, Lobel RW, Culligan PJ, Tomezsko JE, Winkler HA, et al. Protective effect of suburethral slings on postoperative cystocele recurrence after reconstructive pelvic operation. Am J Obstet Gynecol. 2001;185:1307–13.

Hefni M, El-Toukhy T, Bhaumik J, Katsimanis E. Sacrospinous cervicocolpopexy with uterine conservation for uterovaginal prolapse in elderly women: an evolving concept. Am J Obstet Gynecol. 2003;188:645–50.

Huebner M, Hsu Y, Fenner DE. The use of graft material in vaginal pelvic floor surgery. Int J Gynaecol Obstet. 2006;92:279–88.

Jelovsek JE, Chagin K, Brubaker L, Rogers RG, Richter HE, Arya L, Barber MD, et al. A model for predicting the risk of de novo stress urinary incontinence in women undergoing pelvic organ prolapse. Obstet Gynecol. 2014;123(2 Pt 1):279–87.

Johnson N, Barlow D, Lethaby A, Tavender E, Curr E, Garry R. Surgical approach to hysterectomy for benign gynaecological disease. Cochrane Database Syst Rev. 2006;(2):CD003677.

Kahn MA, Stanton SL. Posterior colporrhaphy: its effects on bowel and sexual function. Br J Obstet Gynaecol. 1997;104:82–6.

Karram M, Maher C. Surgery for posterior vaginal wall prolapse. Int Urogynecol J. 2013;24(11):1835–41.

Lantzsch T, Goepel C, Wolters M, Koelbl H, Methfessel HD. Sacrospinous ligament fixation for vaginal vault prolapse. Arch Gynecol Obstet. 2001;265:21–5.

Maher C. Anterior vaginal compartment surgery. Int Urogynecol J. 2013;24(11):1791–802.

Maher C, Baessler K. Surgical management of posterior vaginal wall prolapse: an evidence-based literature review. Int Urogynecol J. 2005;17:84–8.

Maher C, Baessler K. Surgical management of anterior vaginal wall prolapse: an evidence based literature review. Int J Gynaecol Obstet. 2006;17:195–201.

Maher CF, Cary MP, Slack MC, et al. Uterine preservation or hysterectomy at sacrospinous colpopexy for uterovaginal prolapse? Int Urogynecol J. 2001;12:381–5.

Maher C, Baessler K, Glazener CM, Adams EJ, Hagen S. Surgical management of pelvic organ prolapse in women. Cochrane Database Syst Rev. 2007;(3):CD004014.

Maher C, Feiner B, Baessler K, Schmid C. Surgical management of pelvic organ prolapse in women. Cochrane Database Syst Rev. 2013;30:4.

Mallipeddi PK, Steele AC, Kohli N, Karram MM. Anatomic and functional outcome of vaginal paravaginal repair in the correction of anterior vaginal wall prolapse. Int Urogynecol J. 2001;12:83–8.

Meschia M, Bruschi F, Amicarelli F, Pifarotti P, Marchini M, Crosignani PG. The sacrospinous vaginal vault suspension: critical analysis of outcomes. Int Urogynecol J. 1999;10:155–9.

Miskry T, Magos A. Randomized, prospective, double-blind comparison of abdominal and vaginal hysterectomy in women without uterovaginal prolapse. Acta Obstet Gynecol Scand. 2003;82:351–8.

Nüssler E, Kesmodel US, Löfgren M, Nüssler EK. Operation for primary cystocele with anterior colporrhaphy or non-absorbable mesh: patient-reported outcomes. Int Urogynecol J. 2015;26:359–66.

Ottosen C, Lingman G, Ottosen L. Three methods for hysterectomy: a randomized, prospective study of short term outcome. Br J Obstet Gynaecol. 2000;107:1380–5.

Ramanah R, Berger MB, Parratte BM, DeLancey JO. Anatomy and histology of apical support: a literature review concerning cardinal and uterosacral ligaments. Int Urogynecol J. 2012;23(11):1483–94.

Richter LA, Carter C, Gutman RE. Current role of mesh in vaginal prolapse surgery. Curr Opin Obstet Gynecol. 2014;26(5):409–14.

Scarpero HM, Nitti VW. Anterior vaginal wall prolapse: mild/moderate cystoceles. In: Vasavada SP, Appell RA, Sand PK, Raz S, editors. Female urology, urogynecology, and voiding dysfunction. New York: Marcel Dekker; 2005. p. 575–94.

Shull BL, Capen CV, Riggs MW, Kuehl TJ. Bilateral attachment of the vaginal cuff to iliococcygeus fascia: an effective method of cuff suspension. Am J Obstet Gynecol. 1993;168:1669–77.

Sze EH, Karram MM. Transvaginal repair of vault prolapse: a review. Obstet Gynecol. 1997;89:466–75.

Tarr ME, Paraiso MF. Minimally invasive approach to pelvic organ prolapse: a review. Minerva Ginecol. 2014;66(1):49–67.

van der Ploeg JM, van der Steen A, Oude Rengerink K, van der Vaart CH, Roovers JP. Prolapse surgery with or without stress incontinence surgery for pelvic organ prolapse: a systematic review and meta-analysis of randomised trials. BJOG. 2014;121(5):537–47.

Walters MD, Muir TW. Surgical treatment of vaginal apex prolapse: transvaginal approaches. In: Vasavada SP, Appell RA, Sand PK, Raz S, editors. Female urology, urogynecology, and voiding dysfunction. New York: Marcel Dekker; 2005. p. 663–76.

Weber AM, Walters MD, Piedmonte MR, Ballard LA. Anterior colporrhaphy: a randomized trial of three surgical techniques. Am J Obstet Gynecol. 2001;185:1299–306.

Wu JM, Matthews CA, Conover MM, Pate V, Jonsson FM. Lifetime risk of stress urinary incontinence or pelvic organ prolapse surgery. Obstet Gynecol. 2014;123(6):1201–6.

Excision of Urethral Diverticula

4

Urethral diverticula result in most cases from inflammatory conditions of the periurethral glands. Most are the result of repeated infection and obstruction of the periurethral glands. Initially, a suburethral cyst is formed by both the inflammatory process of infection and by the pressures created within an obstructed periurethral gland. These cysts subsequently rupture into the urethral lumen. The resulting draining abscess cavity is eventually epithelialized, and thus a urethral diverticulum is formed. Very rarely, they are congenital or traumatic following urethroscopy or urethrotomy. Open surgical procedures such as anterior colporrhaphy or sling procedures surgery may damage the periurethral fascia and create a traction diverticulum.

Diverticula are usually posterior and lateral and are located in the mid or distal third of the urethra. They may be single or multiple, and the urethral communications may be wide or very narrow. Very rarely, urethral diverticula will occur in the anterior urethra or the proximal third. Distal urethral diverticula may originate from an obstructed Skene's gland draining into the urethral meatus. Circumferential diverticula are not uncommon and their excision requires a delicate and complex reconstruction.

4.1 Surgical Indications and Procedures

Surgery is indicated in patients with significant symptoms related to the presence of the diverticulum. These symptoms include recurrent urinary tract infections, severe pain, dyspareunia, frequency, urgency, and post-voiding dribbling. It is not uncommon to have stress urinary incontinence and urethral hypermobility in conjunction with urethral diverticula.

Surgical options include (1) transurethral incision of the diverticular communication, transforming a narrow mouth into a wide mouth; (2) marsupialization of the diverticular sac into the vagina by incision of the urethrovaginal septum; and (3) excision of the diverticula. In this chapter, we discuss only our technique for surgical excision of large urethral diverticula.

Electronic supplementary material The online version of this chapter (doi:10.1007/978-1-4939-2941-2_4) contains supplementary material, which is available to authorized users.

S. Raz, *Atlas of Vaginal Reconstructive Surgery*, DOI 10.1007/978-1-4939-2941-2_4

4.2 Diagnosis

On physical examination, the urethra may be tender, and manual compression may lead to the expression of purulent material from the external meatus. A cystic or soft mass of the anterior vaginal wall can be found (Fig. 4.1). The presence of urethral hypermobility and stress incontinence should be documented prior to surgery. The preoperative diagnosis of stress incontinence may warrant a combined operation to correct diverticula and the stress incontinence. In the presence of a large diverticulum, urine is commonly accumulated in the area, making the diagnosis of stress incontinence difficult. We prefer not to perform simultaneous anti-incontinence procedures at the time of removal of a large diverticulum.

Endoscopic evaluation of the urethra should be done routinely to assess the urethral coaptation and the location of the mouth of the diverticulum and to rule out any other pathology (such as tumors or stones) in patients with hematuria. Endoscopy is better done using a urethroscope with a zero-degree lens and a sheath with a very short beak, allowing the entire urethra to be distended for adequate visualization. Constant water flow and bladder neck occlusion at the time of urethroscopy enhance the yield of the test (Fig. 4.2). At the time of endoscopy, the urethra is compressed in order to look for the presence of any active drainage of pus from the mouth of the diverticulum.

The post-void film of a CT urogram will often reveal a collection of contrast in the subvesical area (Fig. 4.3). A voiding cystogram in the oblique position is often a reliable diagnostic tool (Fig. 4.4). This study will define the location, size, and number of diverticula. In the past, positive-pressure urethrography using a double-balloon catheter was used in difficult cases (Fig. 4.5). In some cases, direct injection of contrast material into a cystic mass in the anterior vaginal wall can help to better define a diverticular collection (Fig. 4.6). MRI is the gold standard for visualization of urethral diverticula (Figs. 4.7, 4.8, and 4.9). It will define without the use of radiation the location, the contents, the size, and the extension around the urethral mucosa. Ultrasound of the urethra can be a helpful tool to assess the extension and location of diverticula.

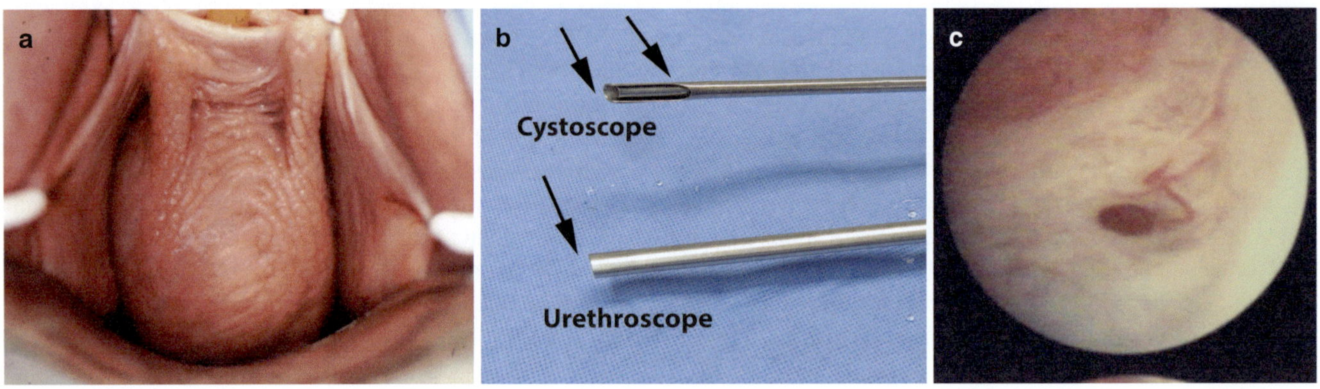

Fig. 4.1 (**a**) Large anterior cystic, tender mass present in a patient with pain and recurrent urinary tract infection resulting from a large, infected urethral diverticulum. (**b**) Comparison of a cystoscope and a urethroscope. As the arrows show in the cystoscope the optics are located at the end of the scope, and the inflow of fluid is a few centimeters behind the optics. In a urethroscope, the lens in the urethroscope are 15 degress and the inflow of fluid is at the same level as the lens, facilitating direct urethral observation and distension. (**c**) Cystoscopic view of a small urethral defect communicating with a large urethral diverticulum

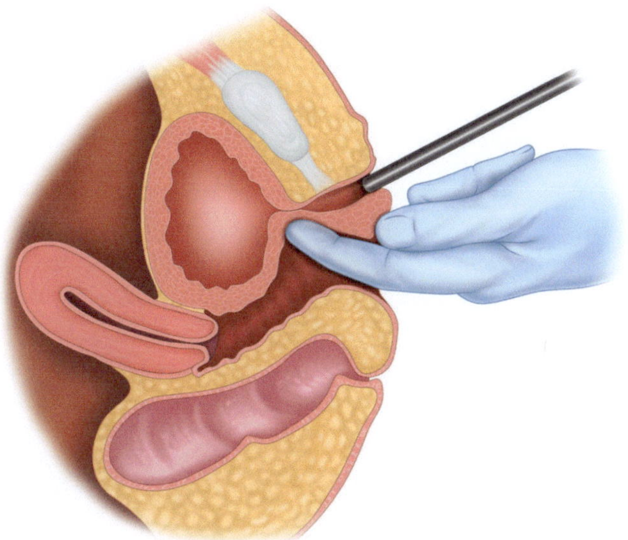

Fig. 4.2 Compression of the bladder neck at the time of urethroscopy facilitates urethral distension and direct observation

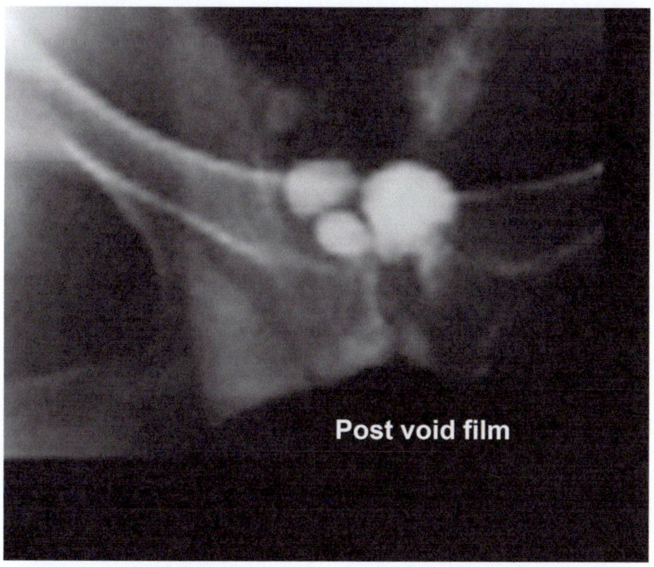

Fig. 4.3 Post-void film of a CT urogram shows several collections of contrast at the bladder base, representing multiple urethral diverticula

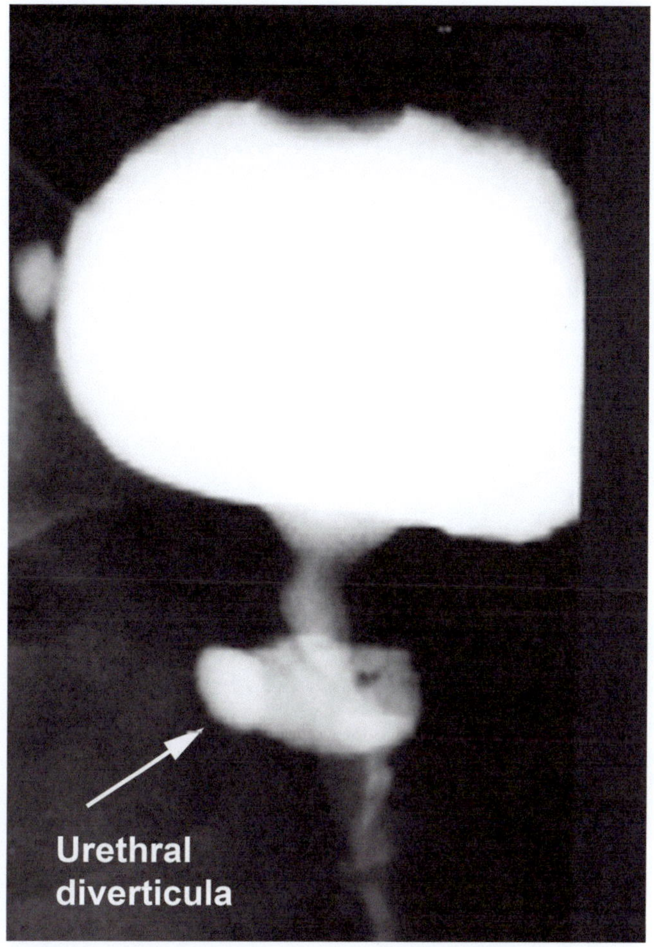

Fig. 4.4 Large diverticula seen during the voiding phase of a cystogram. A large collection of contrast in the mid- and distal urethra is seen

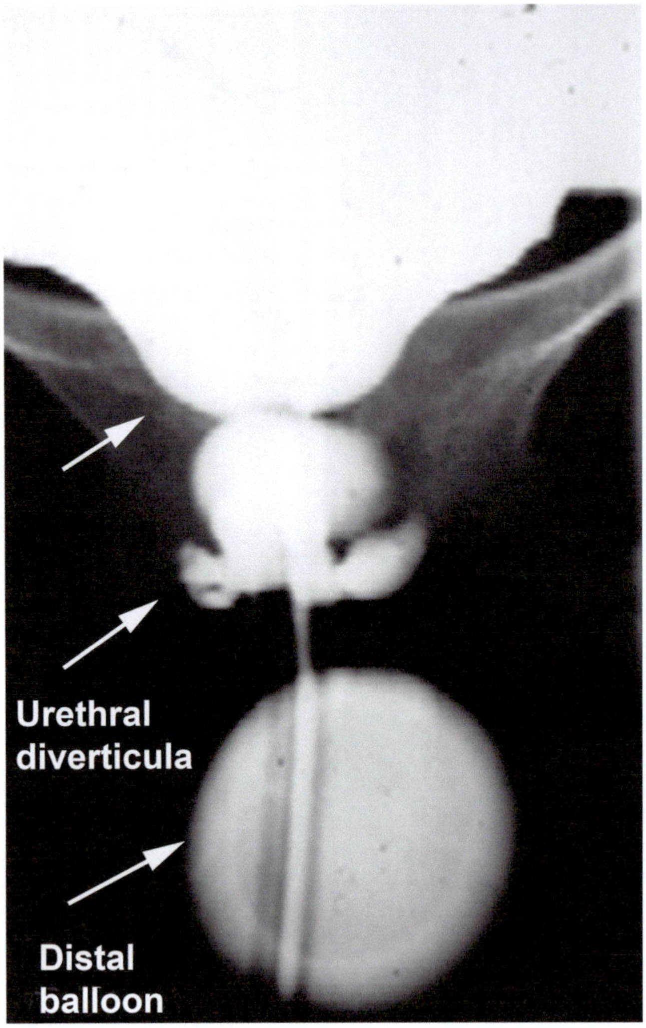

Fig. 4.5 A double-balloon positive-pressure urethrogram shows midurethral diverticula. This study is now rarely done

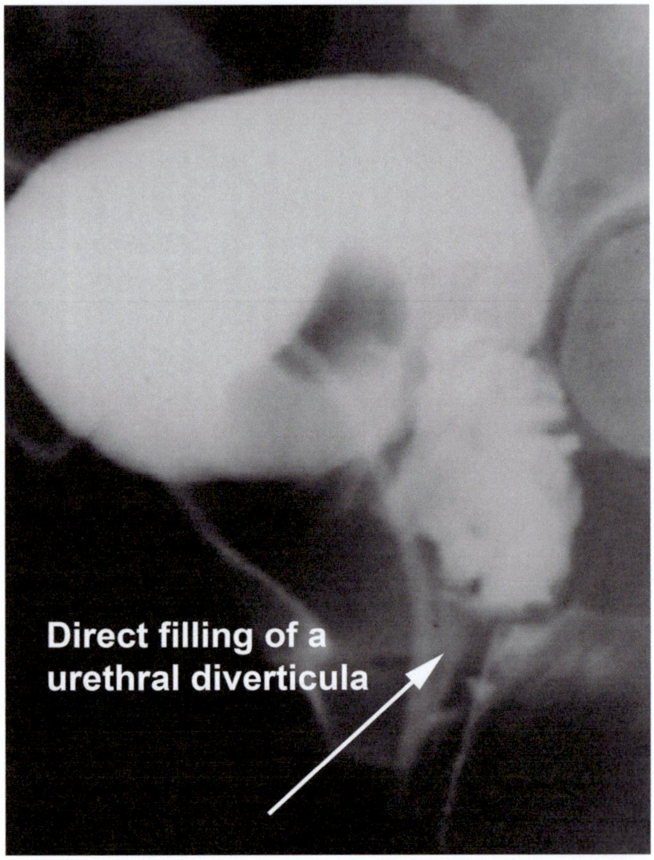

Fig. 4.6 Direct injection of contrast in a patient with a mass in the anterior vaginal wall makes it possible to drain and image a large anterior diverticulum

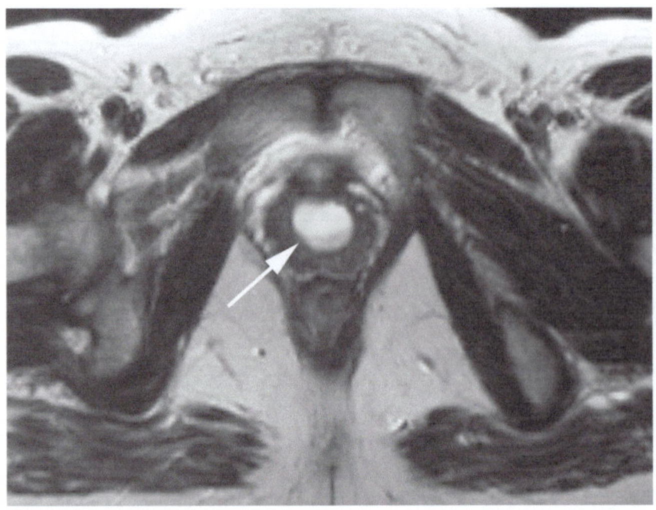

Fig. 4.7 Axial MRI of a patient with posterior urethral diverticula (*arrow*). The content of the diverticula has a darker fluid level owing to pus and an infected collection. The *arrow* point to the darker fluid level created by the pus collection

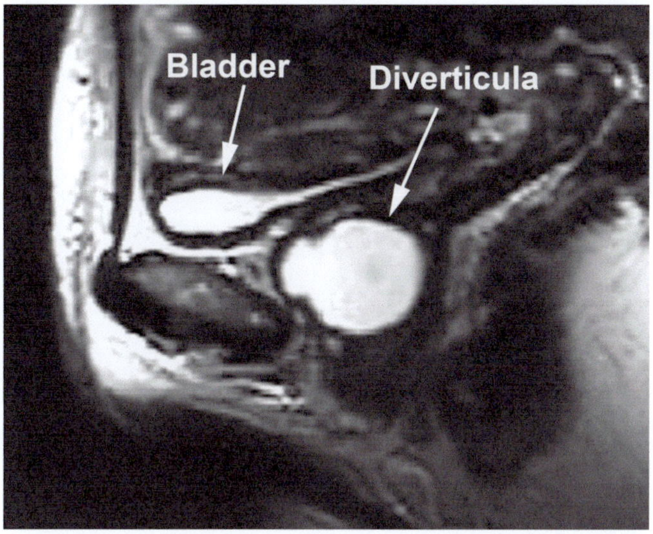

Fig. 4.8 Sagittal midpelvic T2 MRI in a patient with a large urethral diverticulum. The collection extends to the bladder neck and trigone

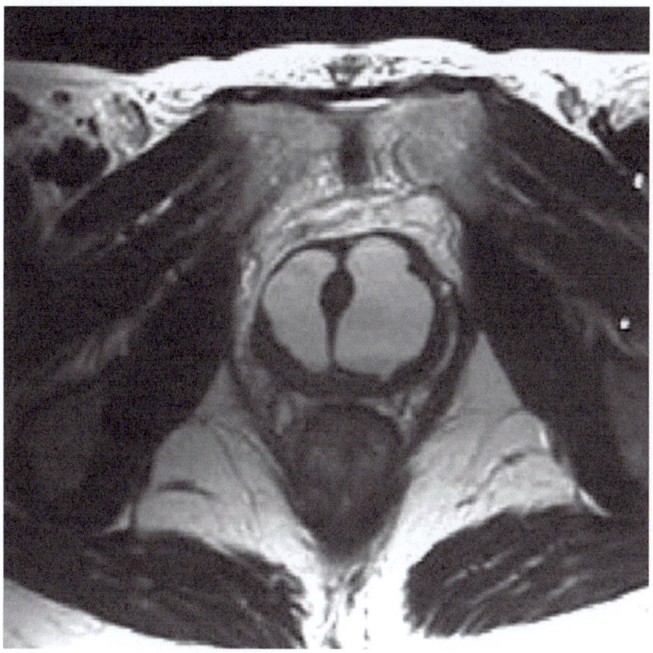

Fig. 4.9 Axial MRI of the pelvis showing a large, circumferential, urethral diverticulum. In the center of the diverticulum, the urethral sphincteric unit is seen with small residual attachments to the anterior and the posterior wall of the diverticulum

4.3 Surgical Technique

Figures 4.10, 4.11, 4.12, 4.13, 4.14, 4.15, 4.16, 4.17, 4.18, 4.19, 4.20, 4.21, 4.22, 4.23, 4.24, 4.25, 4.26, 4.27, 4.28, and 4.29 show the procedure used for surgical excision of a large urethral diverticulum. After the procedure is completed, a vaginal pack is placed and the Foley catheters are connected to a drainage bag.

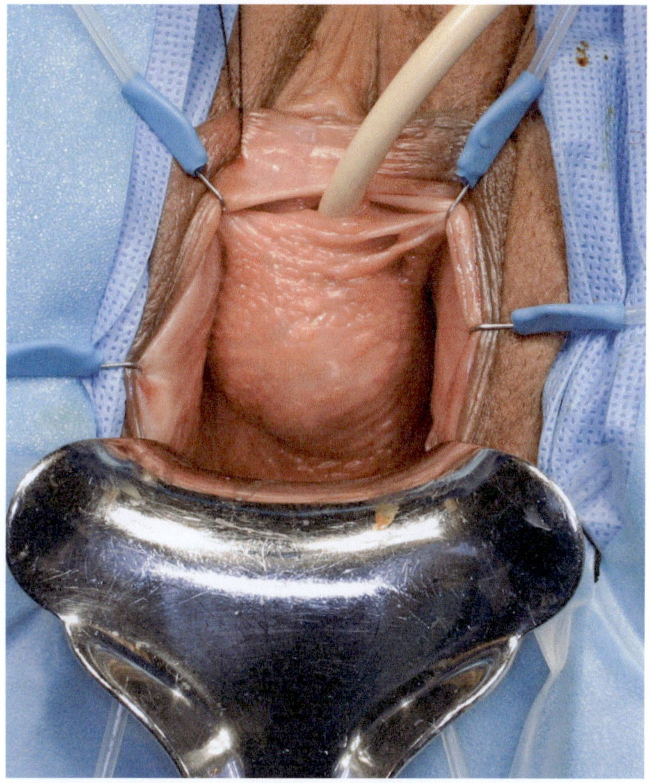

Fig. 4.10 Exposure of the anterior vaginal wall in a patient suffering from a diverticulum of the urethra. A large cystic mass is seen. A ring retractor and hooks help in the surgical exposure, and a Foley catheter has been placed

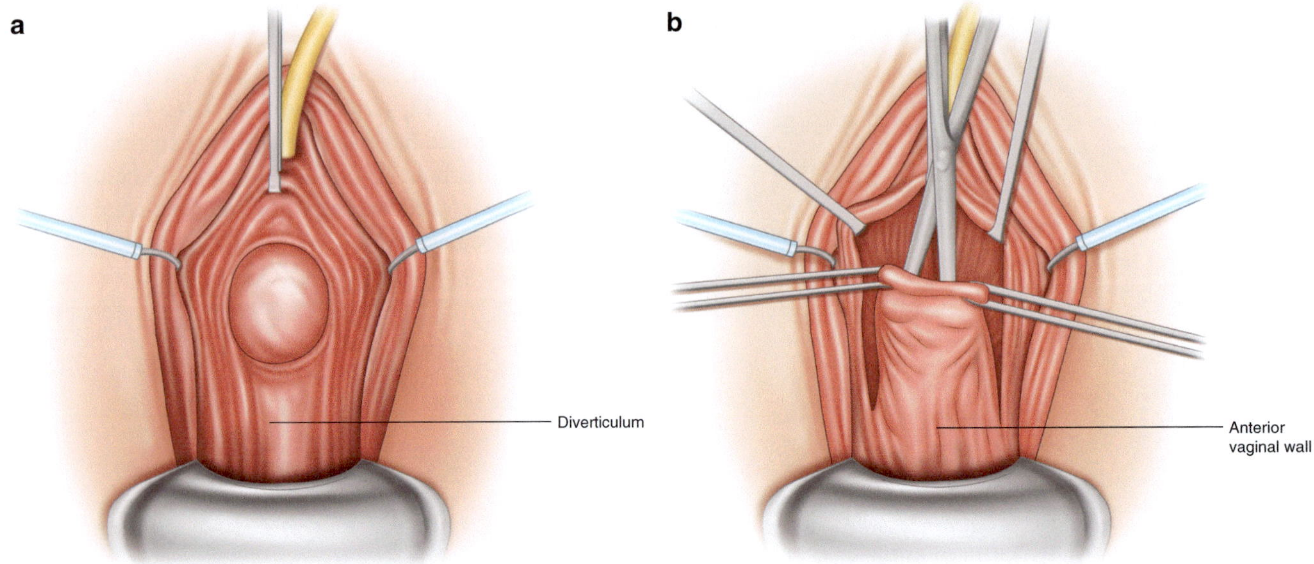

Fig. 4.11 (**a**) Diagram of the exposure of the anterior vaginal wall. (**b**) An inverted U incision is made and extended distally to the diverticulum so that normal vaginal tissue will cover the area of the reconstruction when the vaginal wall is closed

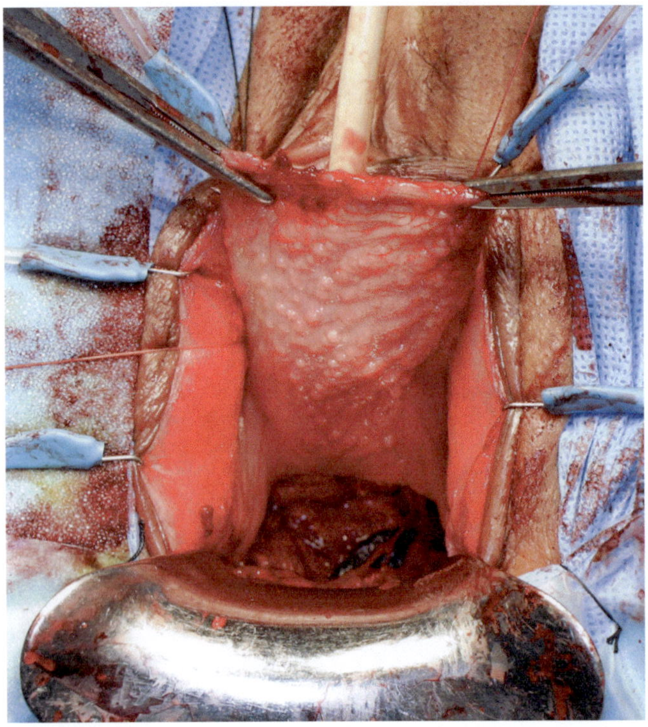

Fig. 4.12 An inverted U flap has been prepared, extending proximal to the bladder neck

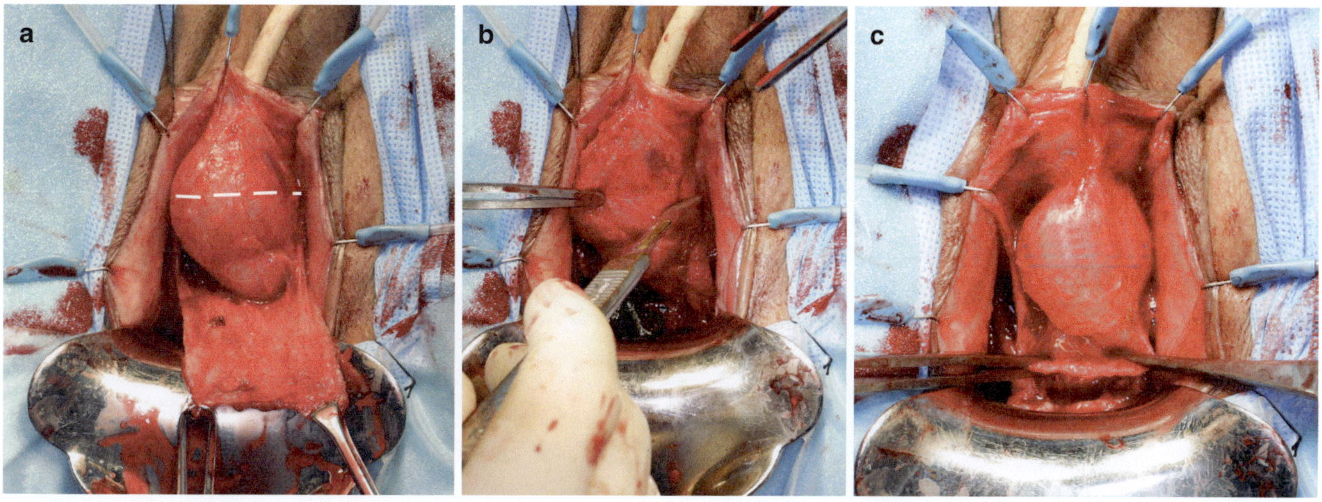

Fig. 4.13 (**a**) The anterior vaginal wall flap is reflected posteriorly, exposing the periurethral fascia. Care is taken to avoid any perforation or entry into this fascia. The *broken line* marks the site of incision of the periurethral fascia. (**b**) A transverse superficial incision of the periurethral fascia is initiated laterally and is extended to the contralateral side. Care is taken not to enter the wall of the diverticulum at this time. (**c**) The periurethral fascia has been reflected with one superior and one inferior flap, exposing the wall of the diverticulum

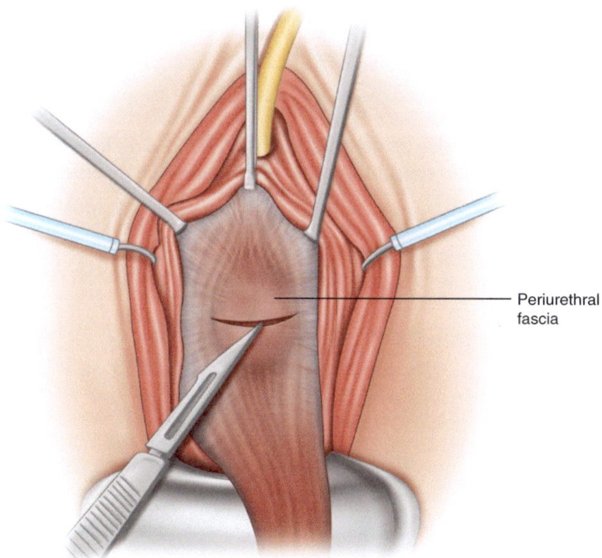

Fig. 4.14 Diagram showing the transverse incision of the periurethral fascia. Dissection of the periurethral fascia will expose the wall of the diverticulum

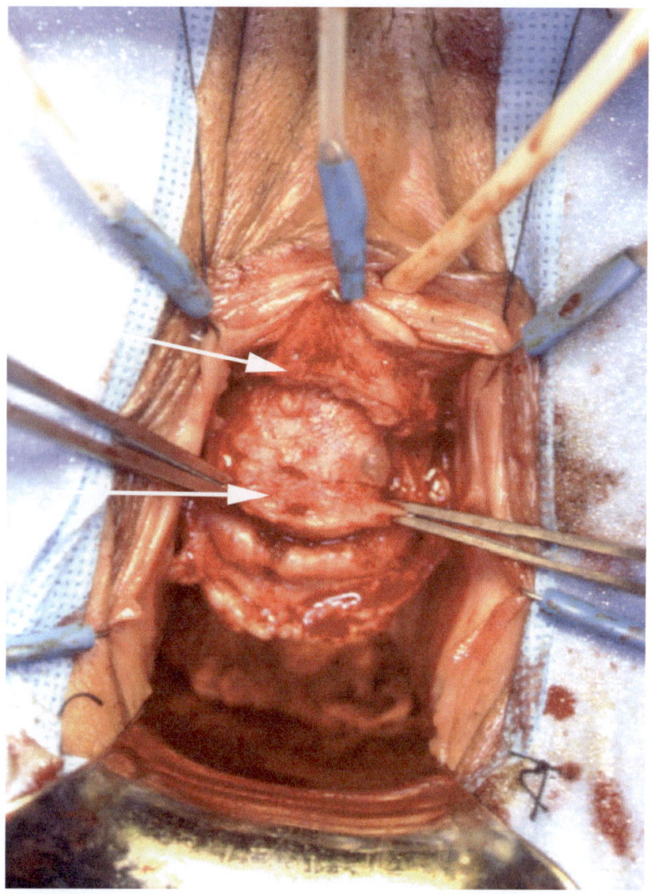

Fig. 4.15 The periurethral fascia is incised transversely over the area of the diverticulum. This fascia may be found to be very attenuated in patients with large diverticula. Two flaps (superior and inferior) are created by dissection of the periurethral fascia proximally and distally to the incision. The wall of the diverticulum is seen. The *arrows* point to the upper and lower edges of the incised periurethral fascia

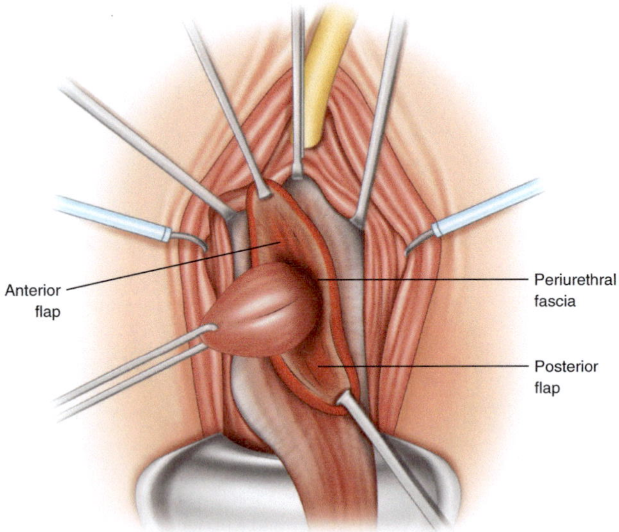

Fig. 4.16 Diagram showing the dissection of the diverticulum from the periurethral fascia and urethral wall

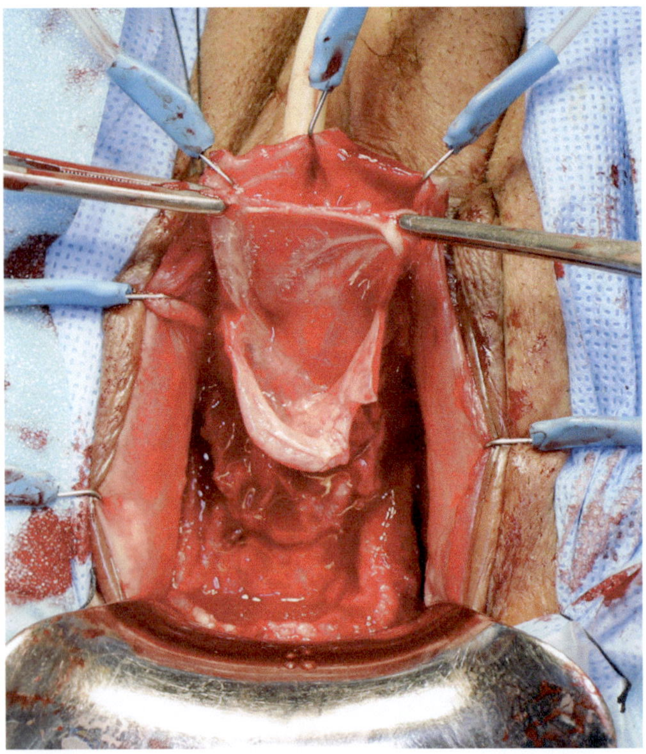

Fig. 4.17 The wall of the diverticulum is opened, and the inner wall of the diverticulum is exposed

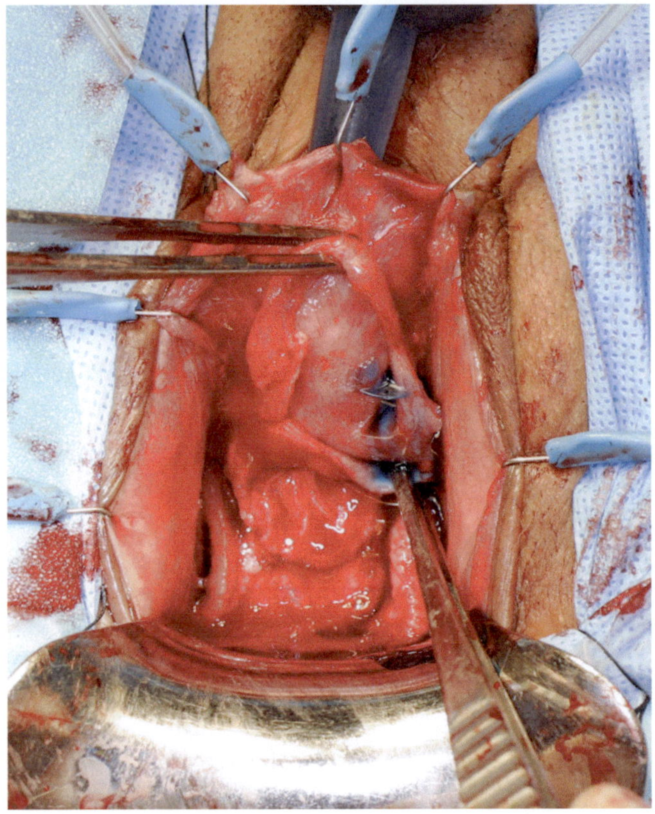

Fig. 4.18 After the catheter is removed, diluted indigo carmine is directly injected to reveal the communication of the diverticulum with the urethra

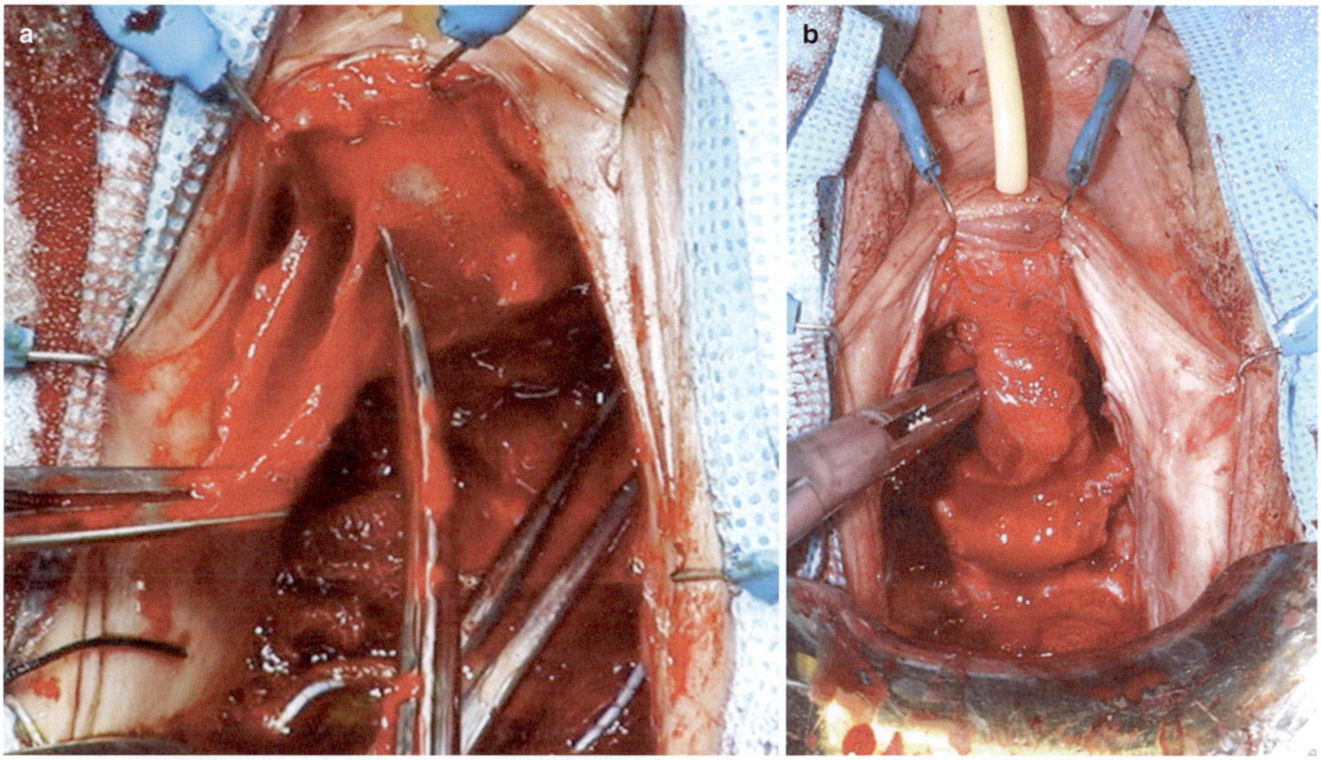

Fig. 4.19 (**a**) Using sharp dissection, the wall of the diverticular sac is freed from the surrounding structures. The communication to the urethral lumen is isolated and excised flush to the urethral wall. The lumen of the urethra and the indwelling catheter must be seen. In cases of severe inflammatory reaction, the sac may be very thin, adherent, and friable, requiring first the opening of the diverticulum and then the excision of the sac. It is important that all of the diverticular sac and the urethral communication be completely excised and that the urethral mucosa and the indwelling catheter are seen. (**b**) In cases of extensive or circumferential diverticula, it is best to divide the diverticulum in two, with each half dissected from the lateral and posterior wall to the urethra in order to remove the whole sac. A right-angle clamp is seen behind the urethral wall after excision of a circumferential diverticulum

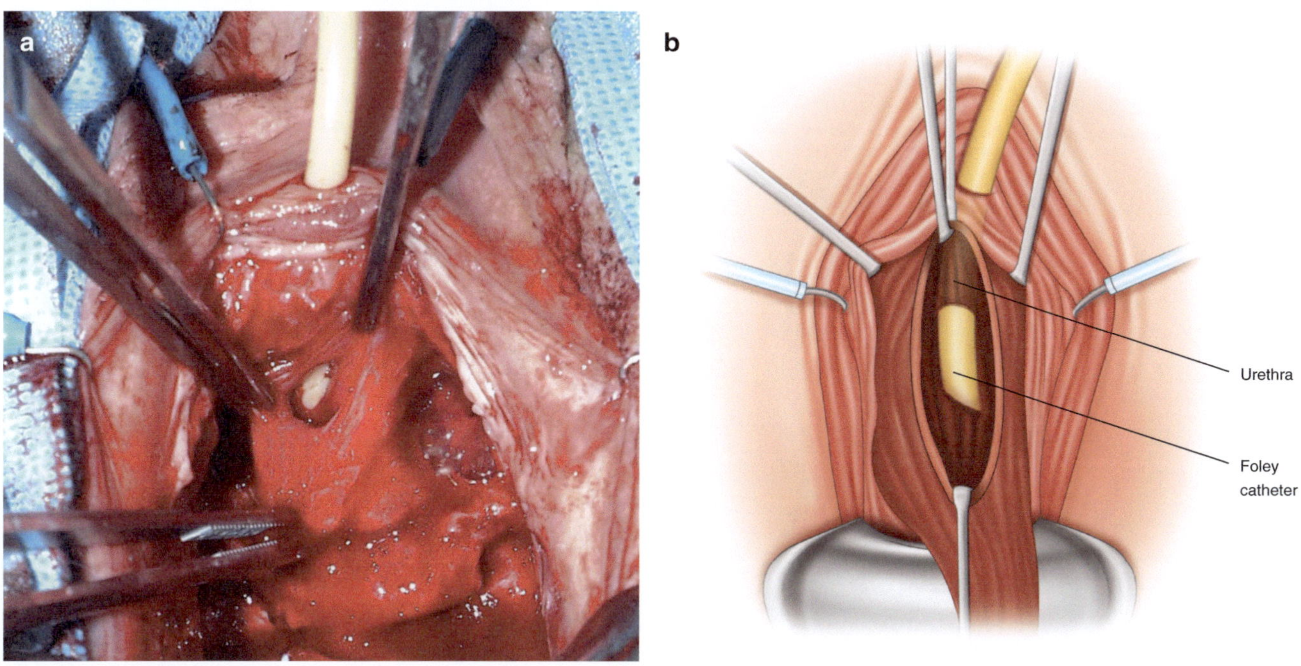

Fig. 4.20 (**a**) After excision of the wall of the diverticulum, the urethral communication and the Foley catheter are seen. (**b**) Diagram of the exposed urethral wall after excision of the diverticulum. The indwelling catheter is in place

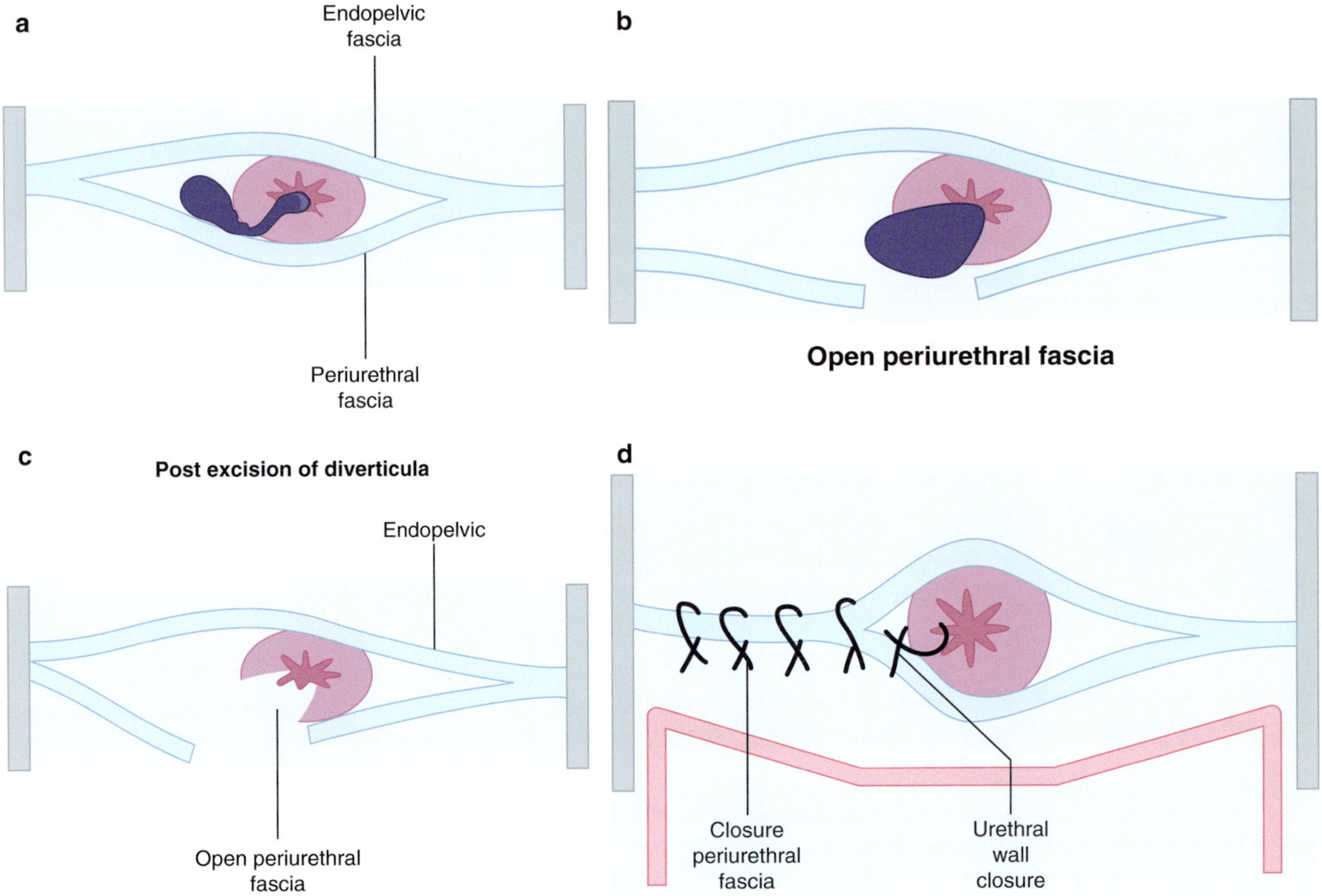

Fig. 4.21 (**a**) Diagram of the growth of a urethral diverticulum between the two layers (endopelvic and periurethral) of the urethropelvic fascia. (**b**) Opening the periurethral fascia exposes the wall of the diverticulum. (**c**) After excision of the urethral diverticulum, a defect of the urethral wall is seen. This defect will be closed with two layers of delayed absorbable sutures. (**d**) The wall of the urethra has been closed. Sutures will approximate the endopelvic and periurethral walls in order to seal completely the defect created by the removal of the diverticulum. All dead space is sealed in order to prevent urinary leakage and possible recurrence

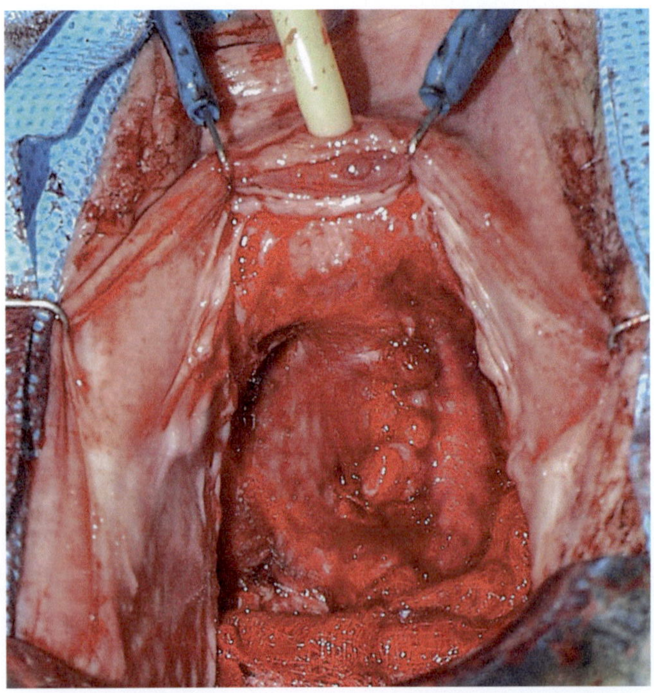

Fig. 4.22 The urethral wall has been closed with running and interrupted #4-0 delayed absorbable sutures in a vertical direction. The closure should be watertight and tension-free. A Foley catheter (14 Fr) is commonly used

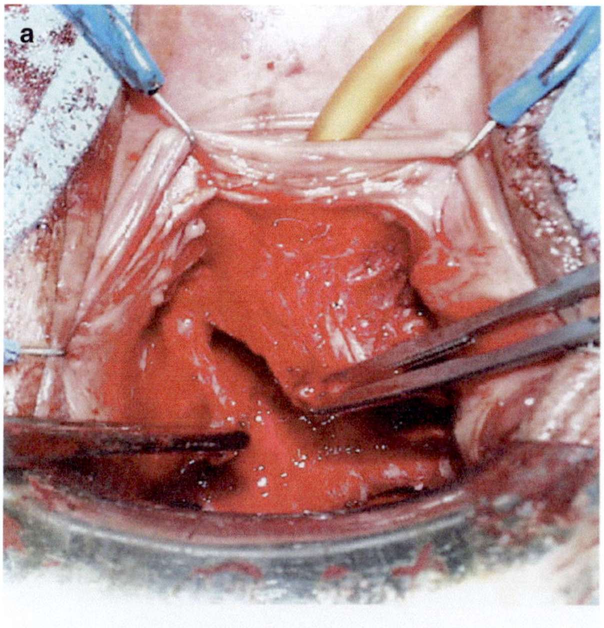

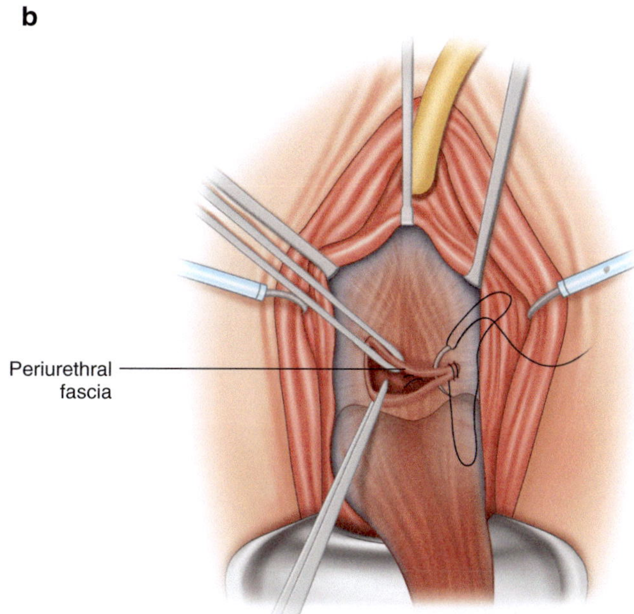

Fig. 4.23 (**a**) The superior and inferior edges of the incised periurethral fascia are exposed. (**b**) Diagram of the closure of the periurethral fascia. No dead space should be left in the periurethral area after the removal of the sac

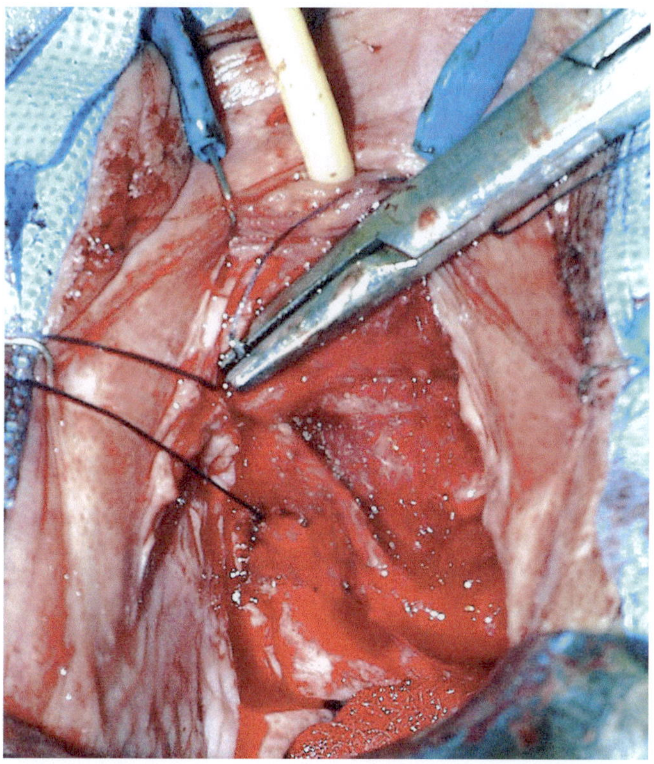

Fig. 4.24 Figure-of-eight delayed absorbable sutures incorporate the superior edge of the periurethral and endopelvic fasciae and the inferior edge of the endopelvic fascia. In cases of circumferential diverticula, a separate layer of closure is used. The figure-of-eight sutures will incorporate the endopelvic fascia posterior and lateral to the diverticulum so all the dead space is sealed, reducing the chances of leakage of urine and recurrence

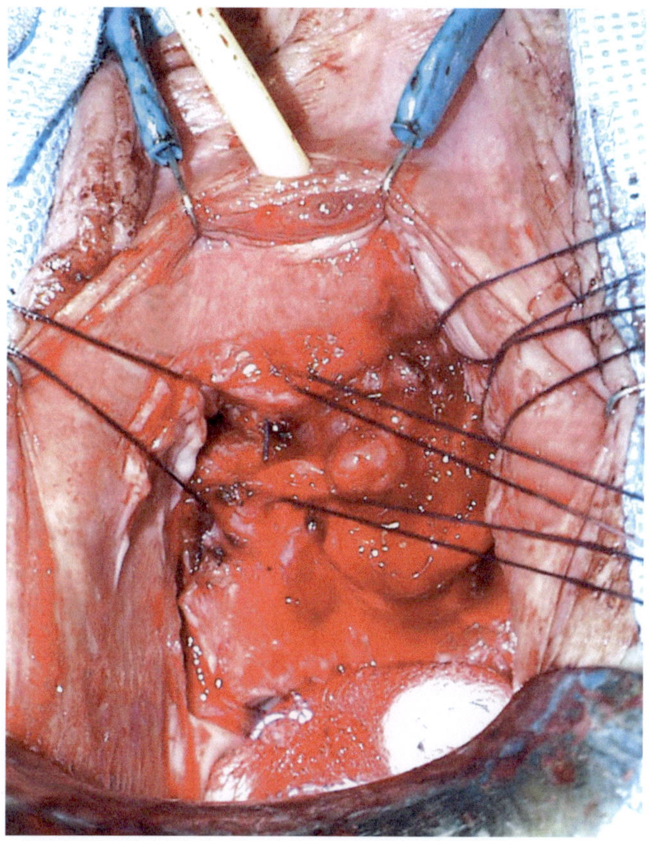

Fig. 4.25 The complete placement of the periurethral fascia sutures is seen. The sutures will include the urethral wall in the middle. With each application of the sutures, the catheter is moved back and forth to ensure that it is not included in the suture line

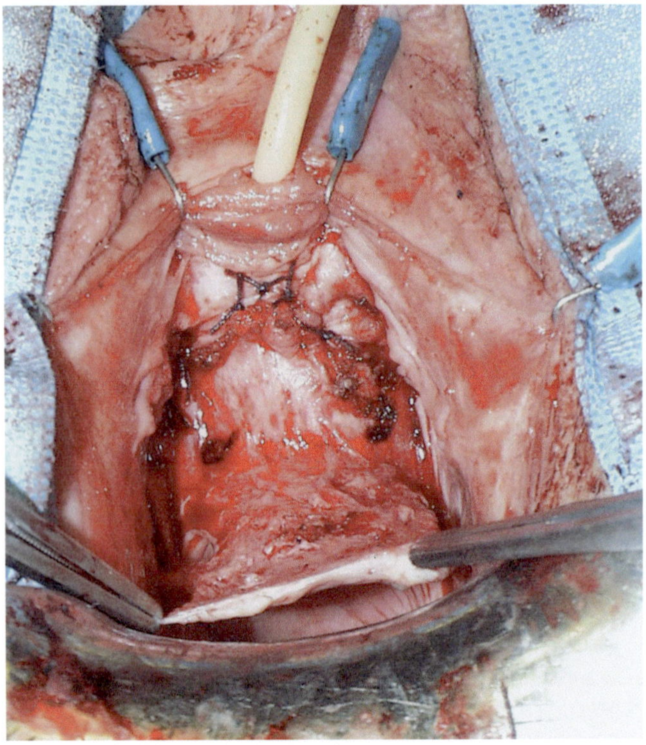

Fig. 4.26 The transverse closure of the periurethral fascia has been completed

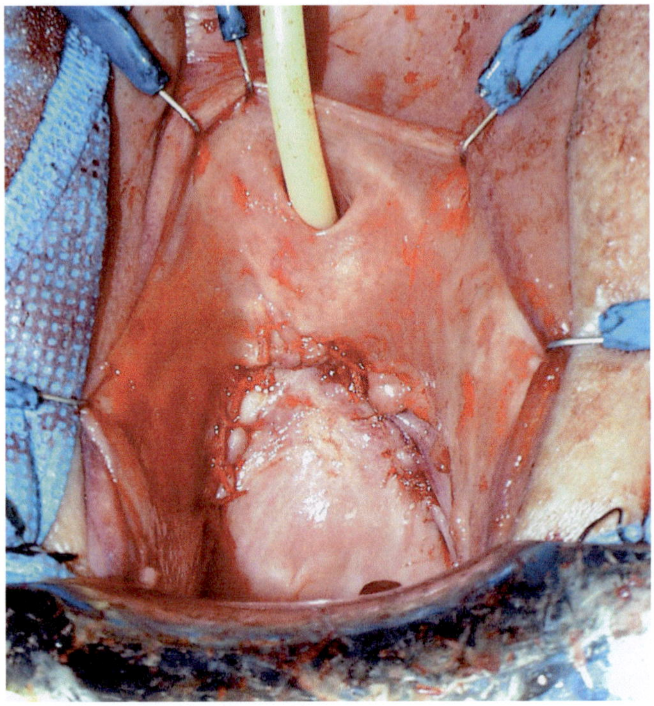

Fig. 4.28 The advancement of the vaginal flap has been completed, covering the area of the reconstruction

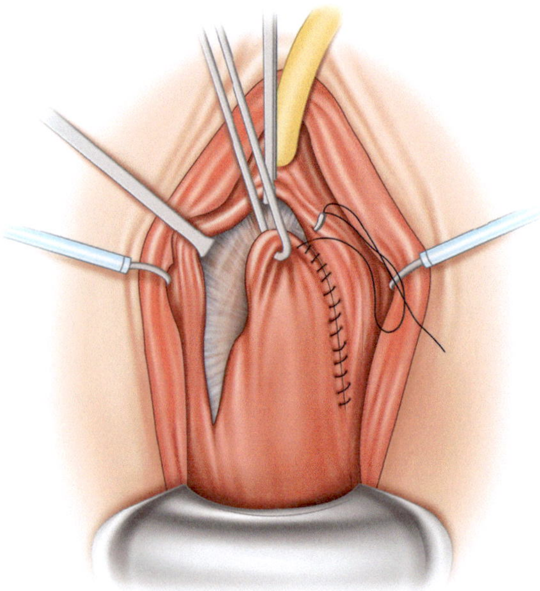

Fig. 4.27 Diagram of the advancement of the anterior vaginal flap covering distal to the area of the transverse closure of the periurethral fascia

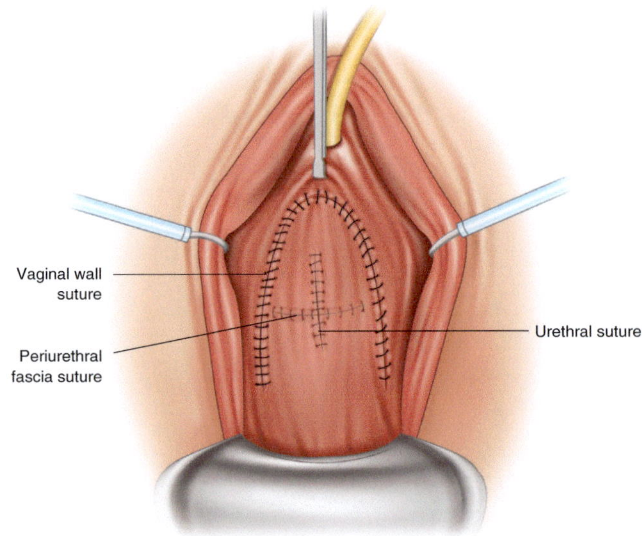

Fig. 4.29 Diagram of the three lines of sutures used in the procedure: vertical closure of the urethral wall, horizontal closure of the periurethral fascia, and the advancement of new vaginal tissue covering the area of reconstruction

4.4 Postoperative Care

The procedure is usually done as an outpatient surgery. Oral antibiotics are continued as indicated. The packing is removed 2 h after surgery. The patient may be discharged home after recovery from anesthesia. The urethral catheter is removed 2–3 weeks after surgery, and a voiding cystogram is performed through the suprapubic catheter. If the result is normal, the suprapubic catheter is removed.

4.5 Intraoperative Complications

Bleeding in the form of profuse oozing is not uncommon, particularly in patients with active infection and abscess formation. A vaginal packing should control this oozing.

Difficulty in closing the urethral mucosa because a large defect was created during the excision of the diverticulum may require further exposure of the urethral wall, with the closure performed over a 5–8-Fr feeding tube. We have not encountered urethral strictures following this procedure. An end-to-end anastomosis of the proximal urethral wall to the distal wall is rarely necessary.

If closure is difficult because of severely inflamed or poor-quality tissue, a fibro-fatty labial (Martius) flap can be used between the periurethral fascia and the vaginal wall. In this situation, a suprapubic catheter should be placed.

The finding of a large periurethral abscess may require a staged procedure in which the abscess is drained and the excision of the diverticulum is performed as a secondary procedure.

A large proximal urethral diverticulum may extend into the trigone, and bladder or ureteric injury may occur. Instillation of indigo carmine into the bladder will ensure bladder integrity, and cystoscopy after intravenous indigo carmine may be performed in selected cases to rule out ureteric injury.

4.6 Postoperative Complications

Proper antibiotic therapy before surgery is mandatory. Reconstructive surgery in patients with active urinary and diverticular infection may lead to fistula formation and recurrent diverticula.

Important factors in operative success and avoidance of fistula formation include a watertight closure, precise dissection, and anatomical closure of the urethral layers, avoiding overlapping lines of suture. Urethrovaginal fistula formation is the most difficult complication of diverticula surgery and should be treated after a reasonable period of healing.

Anterior vaginal infection is rare and responds well to antibiotics. If an abscess is formed, surgical drainage is required in spite of the potential damage to the repair.

Recurrent urethral diverticula may occur, especially in patients with active urethral infection, difficult dissection, tension of the suture lines, or postoperative difficulties with catheter drainage. Secondary surgery should be performed after a prudent period of observation.

Stress incontinence before surgery should be well documented and could be corrected (in selected cases) at the time of diverticula excision. Secondary stress urinary incontinence not present prior to surgery is rare, developing as a result of the dissection of the urethral structures. Severe incontinence due to a nonfunctional sphincter may arise after extensive dissection of the urethral wall. Surgery for this condition may require an autologous fascial sling.

Suggested Reading

Davis HJ, TeLinde RW. Urethral diverticula: an assay of 121 cases. J Urol. 1958;80:34–9.

Eilber KS, Raz S. Benign cystic lesions of the vagina: a literature review. J Urol. 2003;170(3):717–22.

Ganabathi K, Leach GE, Zimmern PE, Dmochowski R. Experience with the management of urethral diverticulum in 63 women. J Urol. 1994;152(5 Pt 1):1445–52.

Lee RA. Diverticulum of the urethra: clinical presentation, diagnosis, and management. Clin Obstet Gynecol. 1984;27(2):490–8.

Nickles SW, Ikwuezunma G, MacLachlan L, El-Zawahry A, Rames R, Rovner E. Simple vs complex urethral diverticulum: presentation and outcomes. Urology. 2014;84(6):1516–20.

Reeves FA, Inman RD, Chapple CR. Management of symptomatic urethral diverticula in women: a single-centre experience. Eur Urol. 2014;66:164–72.

5 Transvaginal Repair of Fistulae

There are three sections in the chapter on fistulae: vesicovaginal and urethrovaginal fistula, rectovaginal fistula, and repair of perineal fistula.

5.1 Vesicovaginal Fistula and Urethrovaginal Fistula

The appearance of a urinary fistula to the vagina is one of the most devastating complications after surgery. The emotional distress of the patient and the surgeon is high because of the little hope that conservative therapy offers and the need (in the majority of cases) for a second surgery to correct the problem. In developed countries, the most common cause of vesicovaginal fistulae is gynecologic surgery, specifically hysterectomy. Other causes include urologic surgery or manipulation, trauma, gastrointestinal surgery, and radiation therapy for pelvic malignancies. Obstetric trauma resulting in fistulae is more common in underdeveloped nations.

5.1.1 Diagnosis

The suspicion of a fistula should lead one to diagnostic maneuvers to confirm or deny its presence. The clinical history and pelvic examination will aid in diagnosis. An unaccounted increase in vaginal drainage and the occurrence of bloody urine immediately after hysterectomy may be suggestive of fistula formation. Most vesicovaginal fistulae classically present as continuous day and night incontinence following a recent pelvic operation, but a watery vaginal discharge accompanied by normal voiding may be the only sign of a small fistula.

Fistulae related to radiation therapy may develop months after therapy or up to 20 years later, and recurrent tumor must be considered. Ureterovaginal fistulae may present as both continuous leakage from the vagina and normal voiding.

Distending the bladder with saline dyed with methylene blue or indigo carmine can identify the site of leakage in the vagina. Cystoscopy and vaginoscopy may demonstrate the size, location, and relation to the ureteric orifices, as well as collateral fistulae. A biopsy of the site is mandatory in any patient with a history of pelvic neoplasm. Performing these studies under anesthesia may aid in diagnosis.

Up to 10 % of patients with a vesicovaginal fistula may have a second fistula, especially a ureterovaginal fistula. CT urogram may demonstrate partial or complete obstruction suggesting a ureterovaginal fistula, but many times it can be perfectly normal. Retrograde pyelograms are more likely to demonstrate the exact location of a ureterovaginal fistula.

A cystogram or voiding cystourethrogram may demonstrate the extent of the fistula, the presence of vesicoureteral reflux, and associated urethral or vesical prolapse or stress incontinence, which may require simultaneous repair (Fig. 5.1).

Electronic supplementary material The online version of this chapter (doi:10.1007/978-1-4939-2941-2_5) contains supplementary material, which is available to authorized users.

S. Raz, *Atlas of Vaginal Reconstructive Surgery*, DOI 10.1007/978-1-4939-2941-2_5

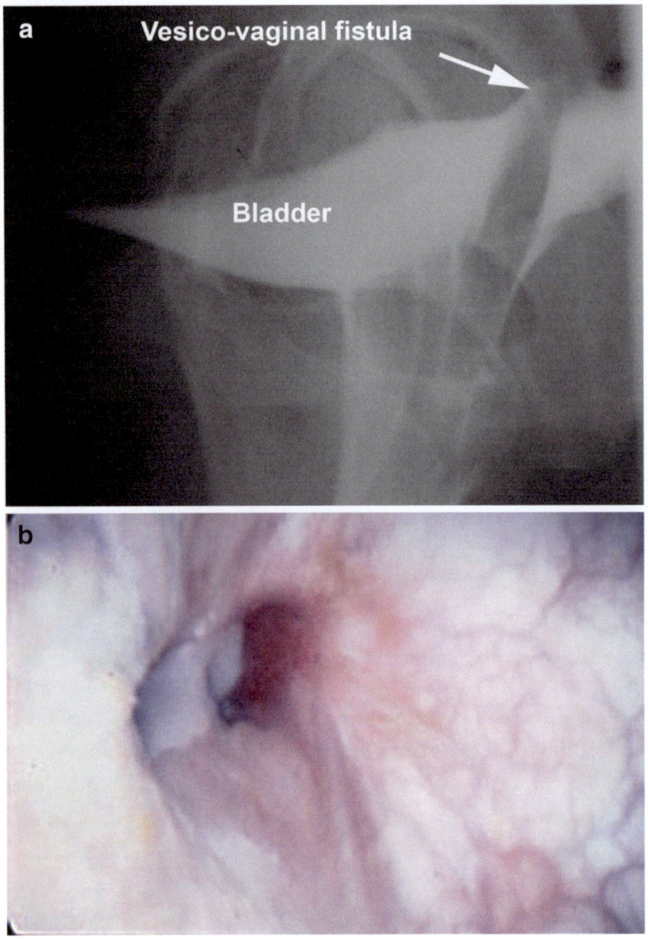

Fig. 5.1 (**a**) Lateral cystogram of a patient suffering from a high vesicovaginal fistula after hysterectomy. (**b**) Cystoscopic findings in a patient with a recurrent vesicovaginal fistula at the vaginal cuff

5.1.2 Indications for Surgery

As soon as the diagnosis of fistula is made, a trial of conservative therapy should be started. These measures include proper and undisturbed bladder drainage and antibiotics when indicated. If the fistula is extremely small (1 mm), coagulation of the fistulous tract may occasionally be successful. Only 5–10 % of small iatrogenic fistulae will close spontaneously with continuous bladder drainage and antibiotics. If the fistula has not closed after 3 weeks of catheter drainage, it is unlikely that it will close without surgical intervention. When conservative treatment has failed and the fistula is large enough that most of the urine passes per vagina in spite of continuous bladder drainage, immediate surgical repair is indicated.

5.1.3 Preoperative Considerations

Sound surgical principles should be used in the treatment of this condition. The blood supply to the tissues must be adequate to support the area of repair. The tissues must be in optimal condition for repair. That is, tissue should be free of infection, excessive inflammation, and cancer. A layered, tension-free closure, and tissue interposition should be used, avoiding overlapping suture lines. Suture material must be absorbable and cause little tissue reaction.

Continuous, uninterrupted postoperative urinary drainage is critical to prevent extravasations and distention with breakdown of suture lines. A urethral catheter and, if required, suprapubic catheter drainage are highly recommended.

In planning the treatment of vesicovaginal fistula, several important issues should be addressed: the timing of surgery; the surgical approach (abdominal, vaginal, or combined); the use of estrogens or antibiotics; the decision whether to excise the fistulous tract; and the use of adjuvant surgical measures to improve the repair, such as flaps from the labia (Martius fibro-fatty flaps), vagina, peritoneum, or skin.

5.1.3.1 Timing of Surgery

The timing of surgery remains controversial. It is obvious that infection of the vaginal cuff or pelvic infection after abdominal hysterectomy requires prolonged antibiotic therapy before any attempted repair is made. The classic opinion regarding timing of repair is to wait 3–6 months to allow the surgical inflammatory reaction to subside, particularly if an abdominal approach is contemplated and the etiology of the fistula was a complicated abdominal hysterectomy. Shortening the waiting period is socially very important for these "totally wet" patients, who are already distressed; early surgery would be of great psychological help. Nevertheless, one should not trade social convenience for compromised surgical success.

We favor early repair in the properly selected patient. Early surgery is not indicated for patients with ischemia (obstetric fistula), cuff infection, or poor general condition. For others, we do not feel that the short wait period has added extra risks to the surgical results. The patients are very satisfied with this early transvaginal repair, which prevents the emotional distress of long months of constant wetting.

5.1.3.2 Abdominal or Vaginal Approach?

The selected route of repair depends mostly on the surgeon's training and experience. The best approach is probably the one with which the surgeon feels most experienced and comfortable. We personally favor the vaginal approach because we can avoid a laparotomy and the splitting of the bladder. With the advances in robotic and laparoscopy surgery, repair of vesico vaginal fistulae can be done also in a minimal invasive approach. The vaginal repair is done as an outpatient procedure, providing a quicker recovery with less morbidity. We reserve the abdominal approach for rare patients with intra-abdominal pathology that requires simultaneous care. The most common case is radiation cystitis and fistula with a small contracted bladder capacity requiring cystoplasty and fistula repair. Radiation fistula per se does not preclude the vaginal approach if the bladder capacity is appropriate.

5.1.3.3 Use of Estrogens and Antibiotics

Estrogen replacement in the postmenopausal or post-hysterectomy patient may improve the tissue quality and vascular supply of the vaginal wall, aiding in healing, so it is strongly recommended. Broad-spectrum antibiotics are required in any fistula repair, particularly if an early approach is used.

5.1.3.4 Excision of the Fistulous Tract

The classic approach to the repair of vesicovaginal fistula or any other fistula includes the wide excision of the fistulous tract in order to freshen the margins and provide a better repair. We have challenged this dogma and have not excised the fistulous tract in our last 210 cases of early transvaginal repair of vesicovaginal fistula, without apparent adverse effects. In our view, not excising the fistulous tract has many advantages: (1) During repair, a small fistula stays small if it is not excised, whereas excising a fistulous tract makes a small opening into one that is very large. (2) Bleeding of the freshly excised margins may require coagulation of the edges and compromise the closure. (3) The fistulous tract provides a ring of protection against postsurgical bladder spasms that, if severe, may compromise the healing. If the fistulous tract is removed, this protective ring is lost and the fresh repair may be at higher risk from severe bladder spasms. (4) Excision of a fistulous tract that is very close to the ureteric orifices will necessitate open surgery and reimplantation of the ureters, whereas if the fistula is not excised, the ureter can be catheterized with a stent, and a safe transvaginal closure of the fistula can be performed under direct vision of the ureteric catheter, avoiding ureteric reimplantation. We have found this to be the greatest advantage of not excising the fistulous tract.

5.1.3.5 Adjuvant Measures

In most patients, uncomplicated vesicovaginal fistula requires only multilayer tension-free repair of the fistula. But when complicating factors such as prior radiation, prior failed surgery, or poor quality of tissues are present, adjuvant measures are required, including the techniques listed below.

In short, our technique of transvaginal repair of vesicovaginal fistula includes no excision of the fistulous tract, multilayer tension-free closure of the fistula, and the advancement of a vaginal flap to cover the area of the repair with healthy tissue. Very often, however, it is desirable or necessary to reinforce a routine closure. Several measures are available in these cases:

- The use of fibro-fatty tissue from the labia (Martius flap), used mainly in cases of urethral or trigonal fistula
- The use of rotation flaps of the entire labia, inner thigh skin, or both to cover large vaginal wall defects
- The use of myocutaneous gracilis muscle flaps for unusual radiation injury
- The use of peritoneum flaps in the repair of high fistulae (repair of a high vesicovaginal fistula after hysterectomy is the most common repair)

5.1.3.6 Repair of Post-hysterectomy Vesicovaginal Fistula Using a Peritoneal Flap

The patient is placed in the lithotomy position. In a narrowed vaginal vault, increased exposure can be obtained by posterolateral relaxing incisions prior to insertion of the posterior-weighted vaginal retractor. If the fistula is close to the ureteral orifices, cystoscopy and ureteral catheterization should be performed. A urethral catheter and optionally a suprapubic catheter can be placed by means of a Lowsley retractor. Figures 5.2, 5.3, 5.4, 5.5, 5.6, 5.7, 5.8, 5.9, and 5.10 illustrate the technique for transvaginal repair of the fistulous tract using a flap of vaginal tissue.

Figure 5.11 shows the use of omentum.

In patients with high fistula after hysterectomy, we routinely use a peritoneal flap to cover the fistulous tract. This simple maneuver (Figs. 5.12, 5.13, 5.14, 5.15, 5.16, and 5.17) will result in a multilayer closure of the fistula with tissue that is easy to harvest and is found in the vicinity of the surgical area.

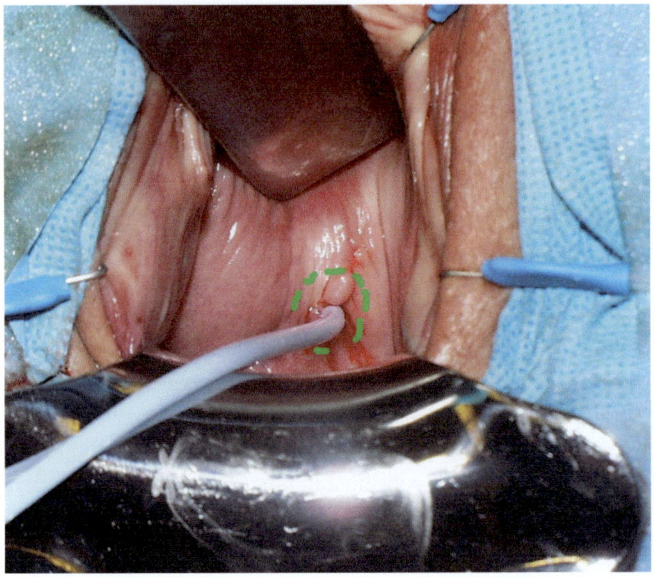

Fig. 5.2 To facilitate the exposure (in particular, exposure of a high fistula after hysterectomy), the fistulous tract is dilated to 12 Fr and a small 8–10-Fr Foley catheter is inserted into the fistula. This catheter will facilitate retraction and exposure at the time of initial preparation of the vaginal flaps. A *green line* marks the area of the circumferential incision around the fistula

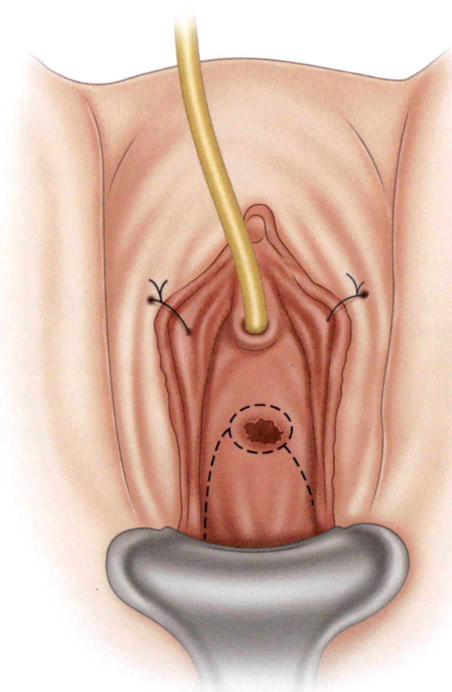

Fig. 5.3 Diagram of the vaginal incisions. An inverted J shaped incision is made in the anterior vaginal wall circumscribing the fistula. The long end of the incision is extended toward the apex of the vagina. The convex portion of the incision circumscribes the fistulous tract. This asymmetric incision allows for the later advancement and rotation of the posterior flap over the fistula repair

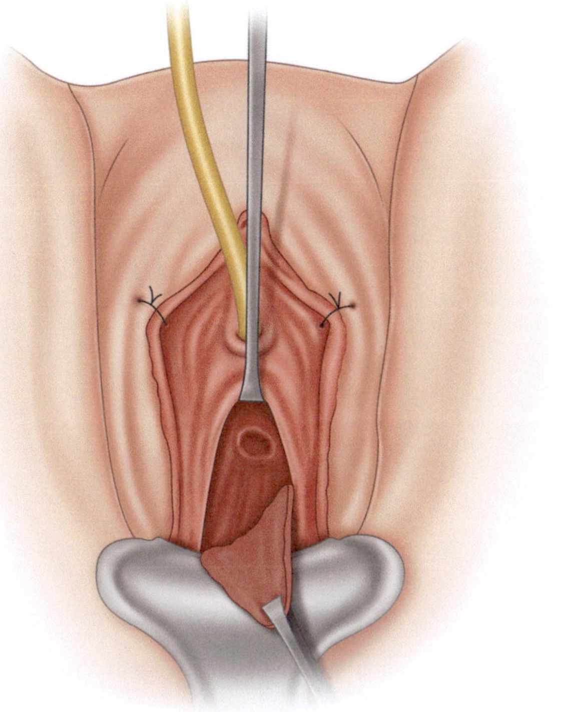

Fig. 5.4 Diagram of the two flaps created anterior and posterior to the fistula

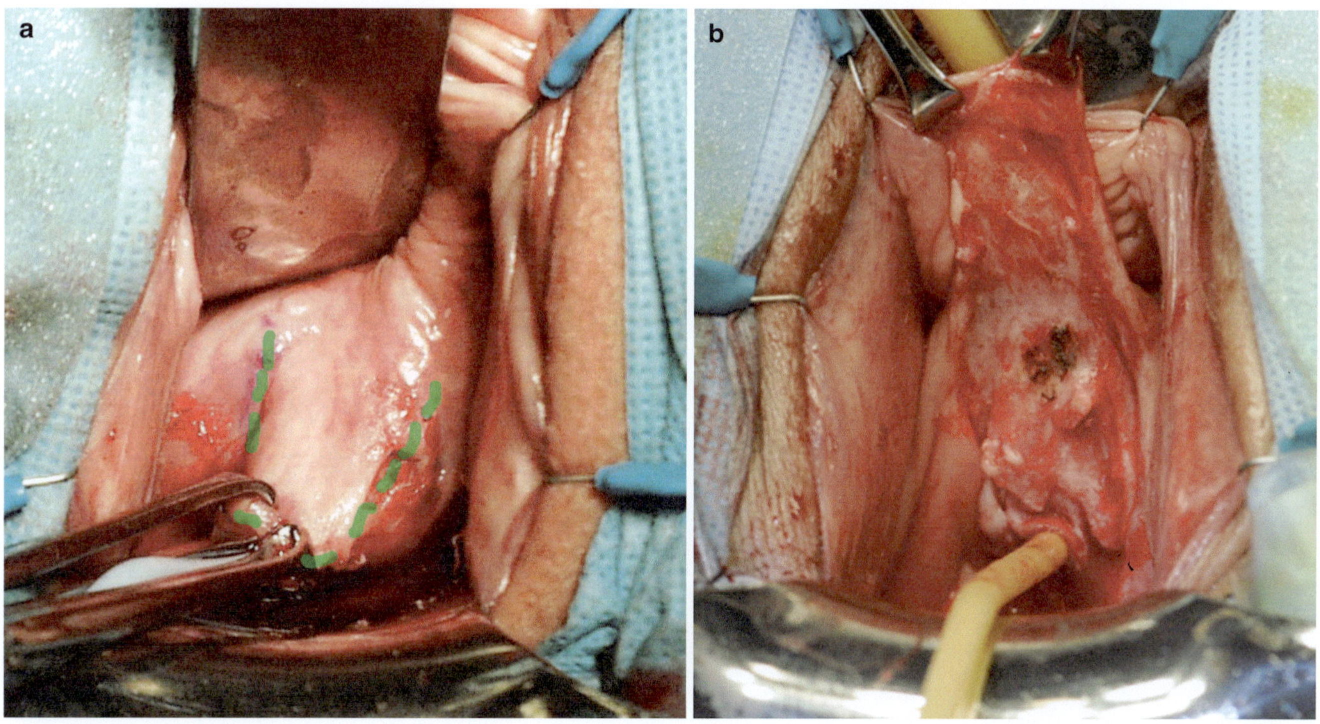

Fig. 5.5 (**a**) A U-shaped anterior vaginal wall flap is prepared. Creation of the flaps is begun in healthy tissue away from the fistulous tract. This maneuver aids in the dissection of proper tissue planes without perforating the bladder or increasing the size of the fistulous tract. The scarred margin of the fistula is left in place, and no attempt is made to dissect the thin layer of the vaginal wall overlying the fistula. The *green line* indicate the outline of the anterior flap preparation. (**b**) The flap of the vaginal wall is retracted superiorly. The dissection of the flaps is extended at least 2–4 cm from the fistulous tract, exposing the perivesical fascia

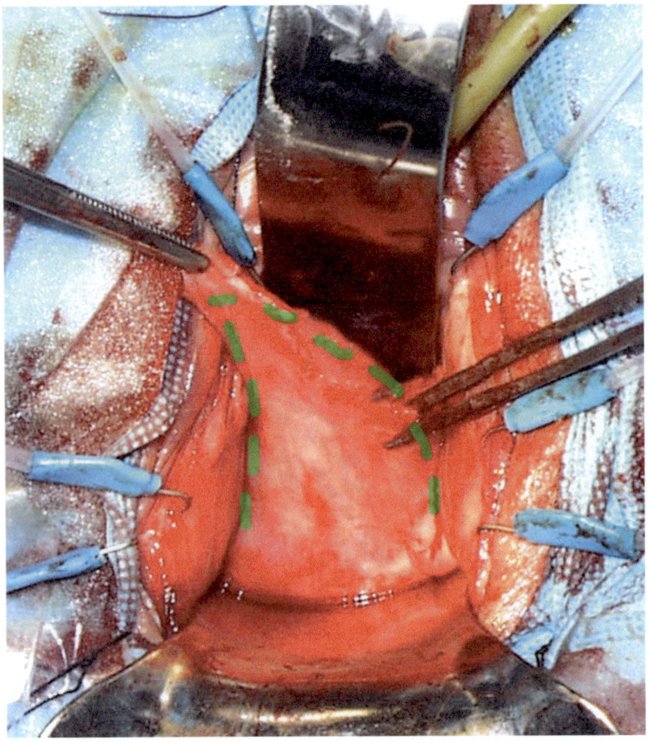

Fig. 5.6 A wide posterior vaginal flap is prepared. The dissection is carried out for a distance of at least 4–5 cm from the fistula. It is directed toward the bladder base without incorporating the margins of the fistula. The flap is retracted posterior

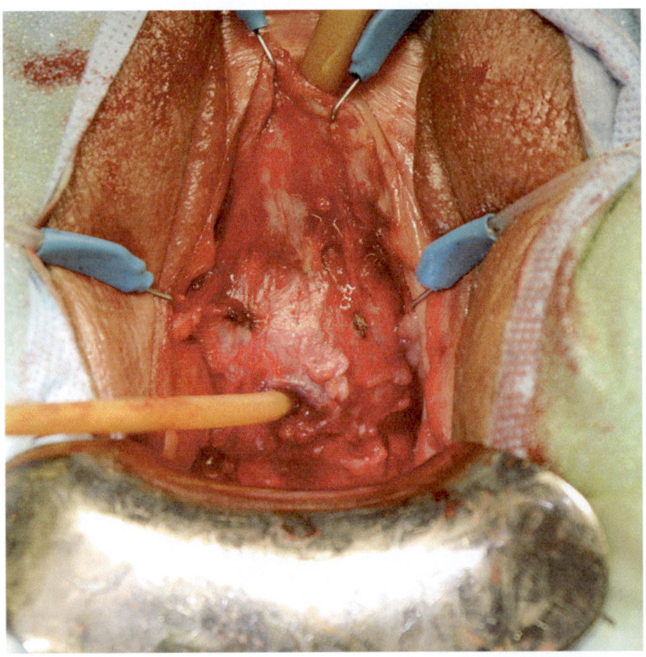

Fig. 5.7 Exposure of the fistulous tract with the catheter in place is seen. Further lateral dissection has been performed to expose the fistulous tract for at least a distance of 3–4 cm around the fistula. The cuff of the vagina is often involved and can be excised

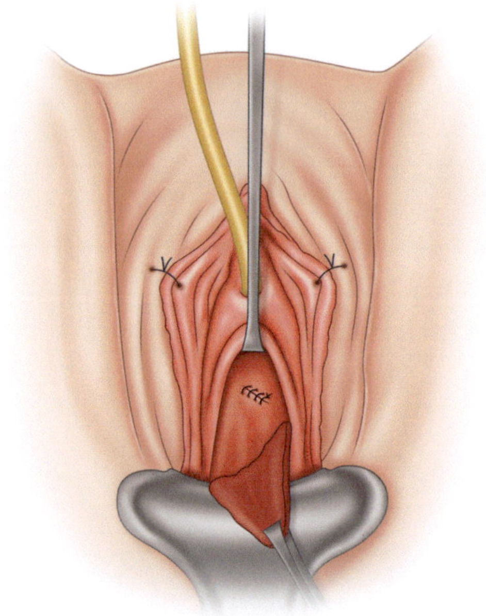

Fig. 5.8 Diagram of the closure of the fistulous tract with the superior and inferior vaginal flaps retracted

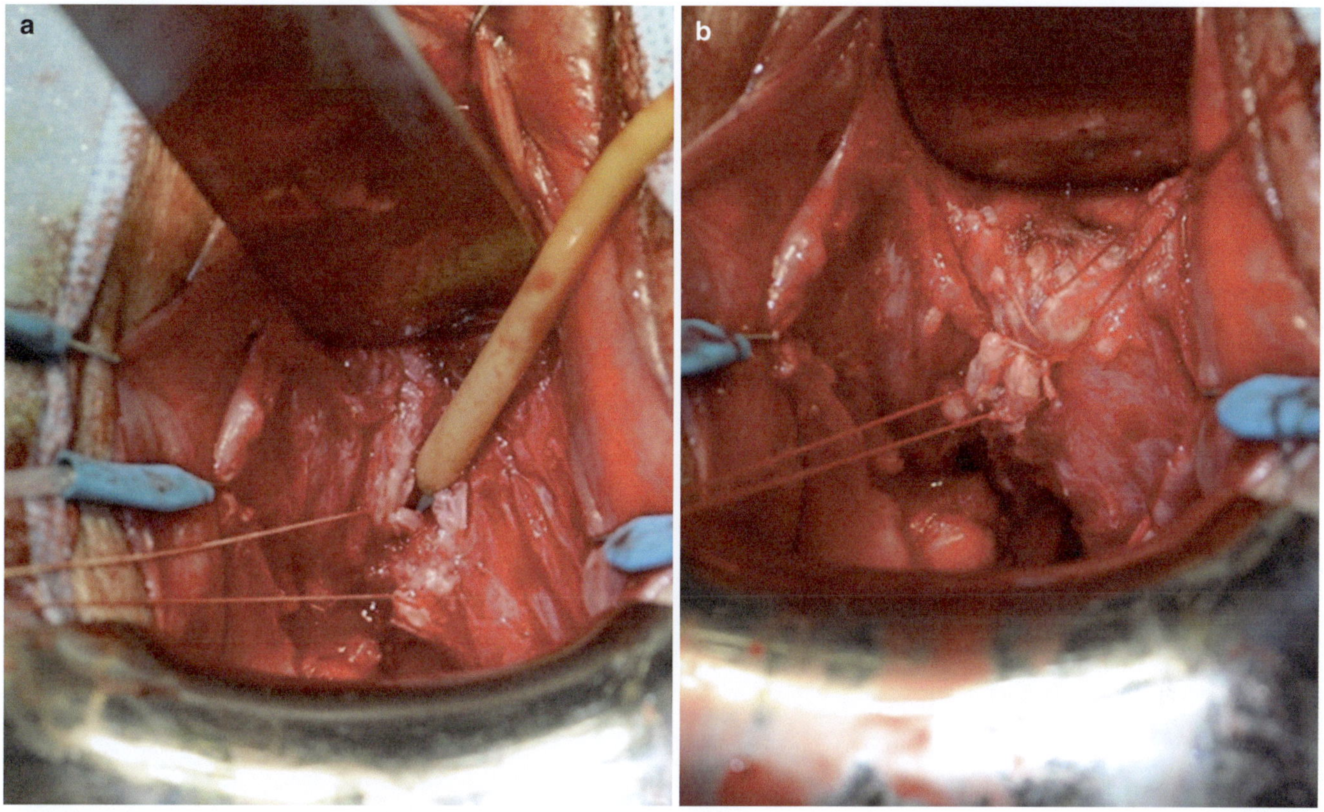

Fig. 5.9 (**a**) Interrupted sutures of #2-0 delayed absorbable sutures are used to close the first layer of the repair. Included in this suture line is the whole thickness of the bladder and the vaginal wall, which has remained connected to the fistulous tract. A strong bite of tissue 2–3 mm from the margin of the fistula is obtained. (**b**) After application of the sutures, the intra-fistula catheter is removed and the sutures are tied, closing the fistulous tract. The bladder is irrigated with diluted indigo carmine solution to ensure that no extravasations are seen after the sutures are tied

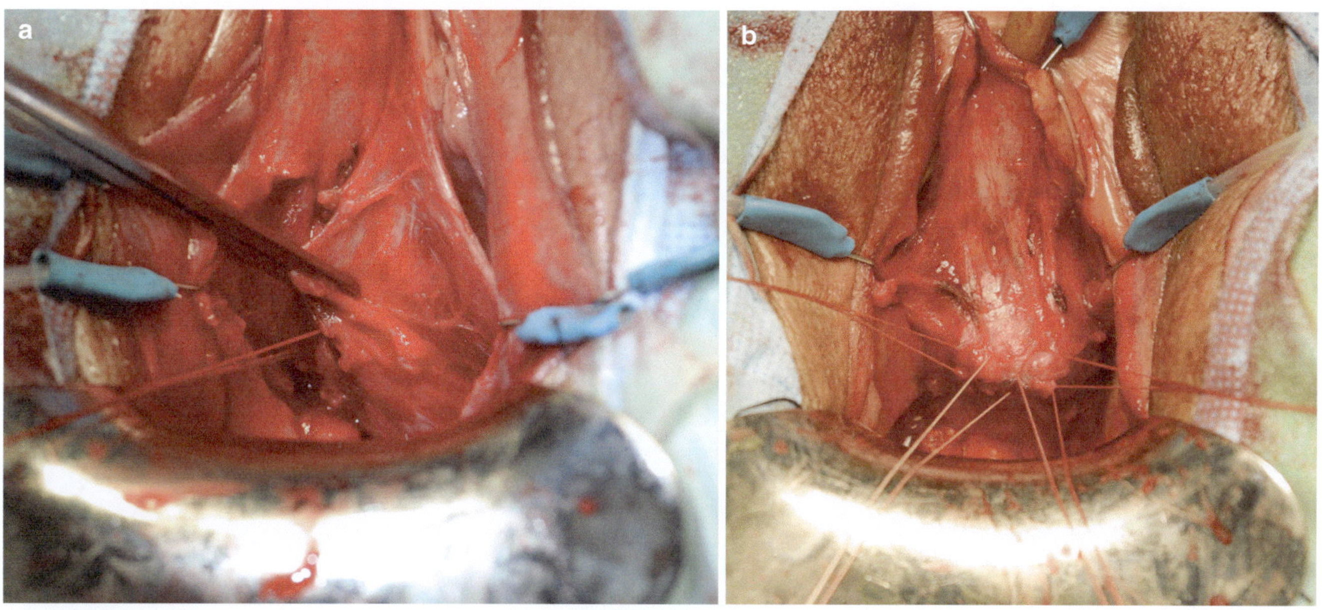

Fig. 5.10 (**a**) The perivesical fascia is dissected free and mobilized around the fistulous tract. (**b**) A second layer of interrupted absorbable sutures is used to invert and cover the prior layer. These sutures include the perivesical fascia and deep musculature of the bladder. The sutures should be applied at least 1 cm from the prior line of sutures and should be tied free of tension. The first layer of the repair remains invaginated and is covered by the second layer of sutures. At this time, the bladder again is filled with diluted indigo carmine solution to test the integrity of the repair. In a simple repair, the operation can now be completed. The previously raised anterior flap is partially resected, allowing the posterior (proximal) flap to rotate and extend beyond the closure of the fistula in order to cover the fistulous tract with fresh vaginal tissue and to avoid adjacent and overlapping suture lines. A running suture of #2-0 absorbable material is used to complete this layer

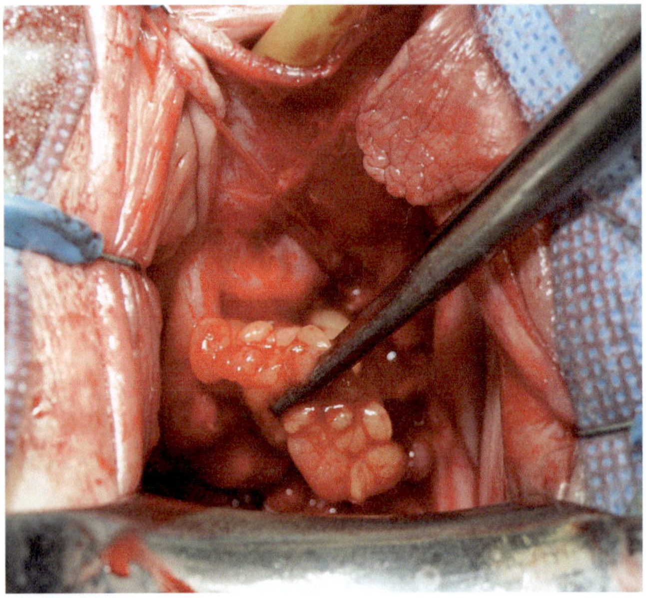

Fig. 5.11 In cases of prior failed surgery with the use of omentum, a peritoneal window is made. The omentum is freed and advanced with interrupted sutures to cover the fistula repair

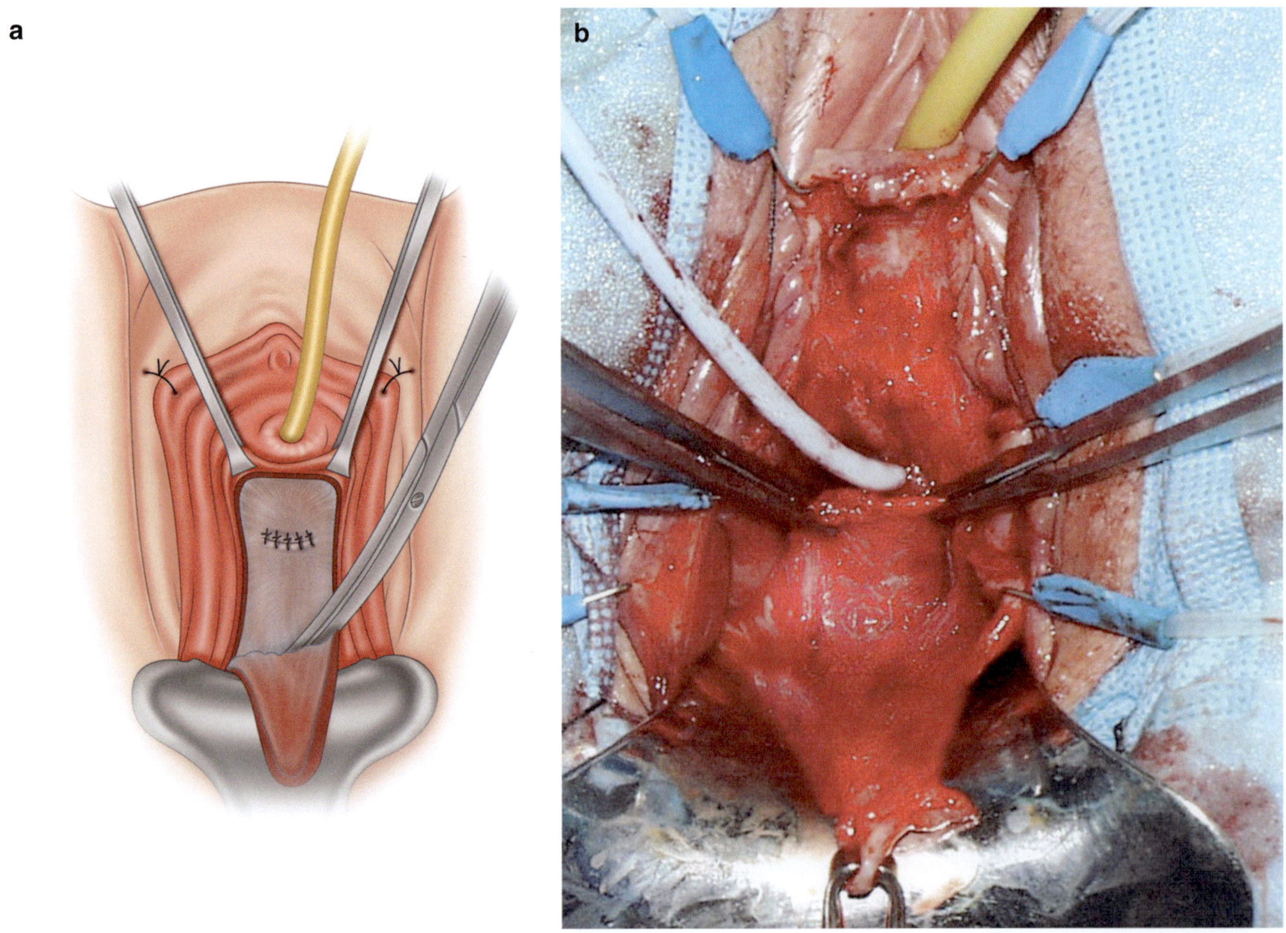

Fig. 5.12 (**a**) Diagram of the dissection of the perivesical fascia, extended more proximally toward the prerectal fascia to expose the peritoneal fold. (**b**) Allis clamps retract the double-fold peritoneal flap, helping its dissection and mobilization. (**c**) The peritoneal flap is advanced 2 cm distal to the fistula repair so a double layer of peritoneum covers the fistula repair. If the peritoneum is open during this maneuver, it is not necessary to close because the advancement of the flap against the posterior bladder wall will close it.

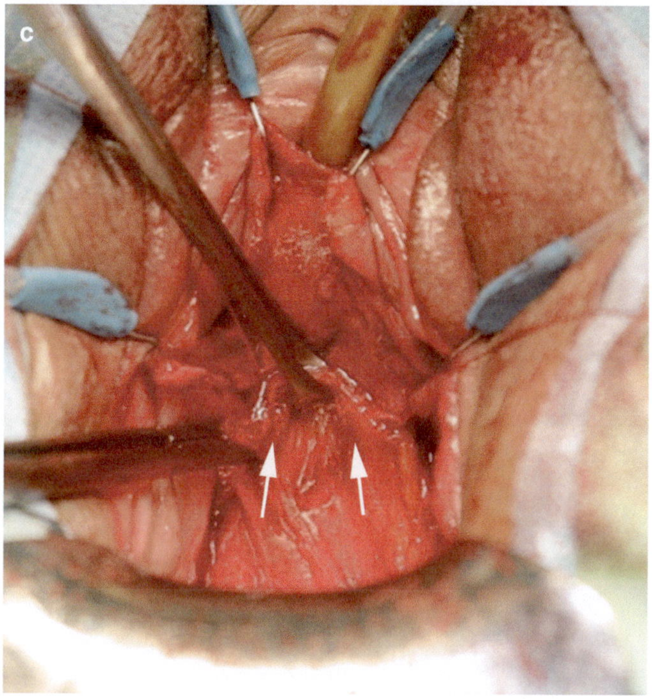

Fig. 5.12 (continued) The peritoneal flap is extensively mobilized to allow a tension free advancement to cover the fistula repair

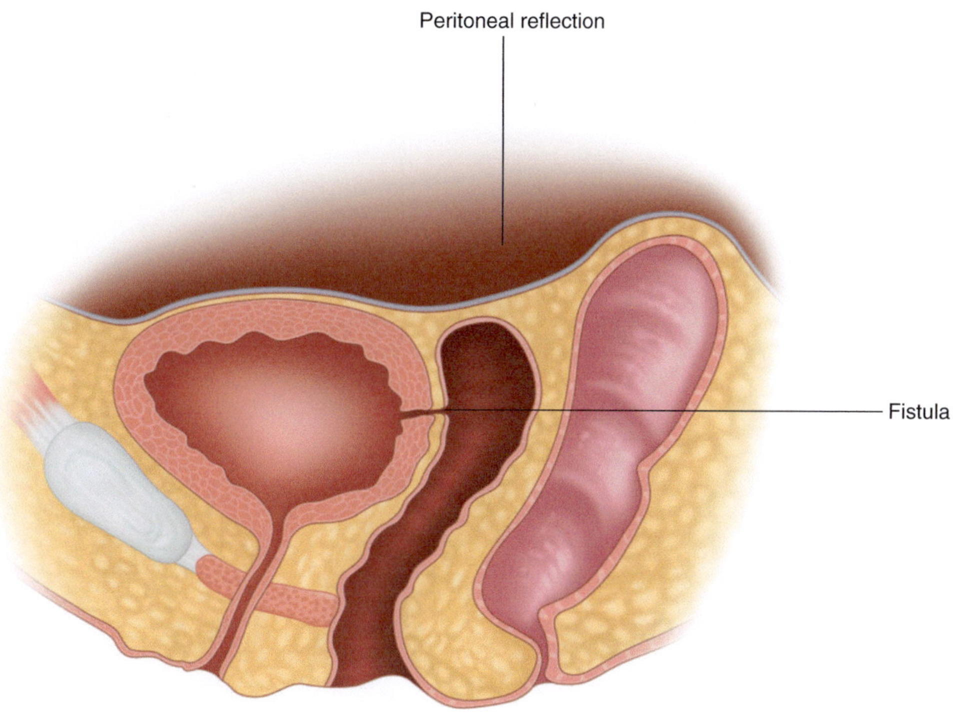

Fig. 5.13 Diagram of the anatomical location of a high vesicovaginal fistula and its relationship to the surrounding peritoneum

Fig. 5.14 Diagram of the interposition of the peritoneal flap between the vagina and bladder

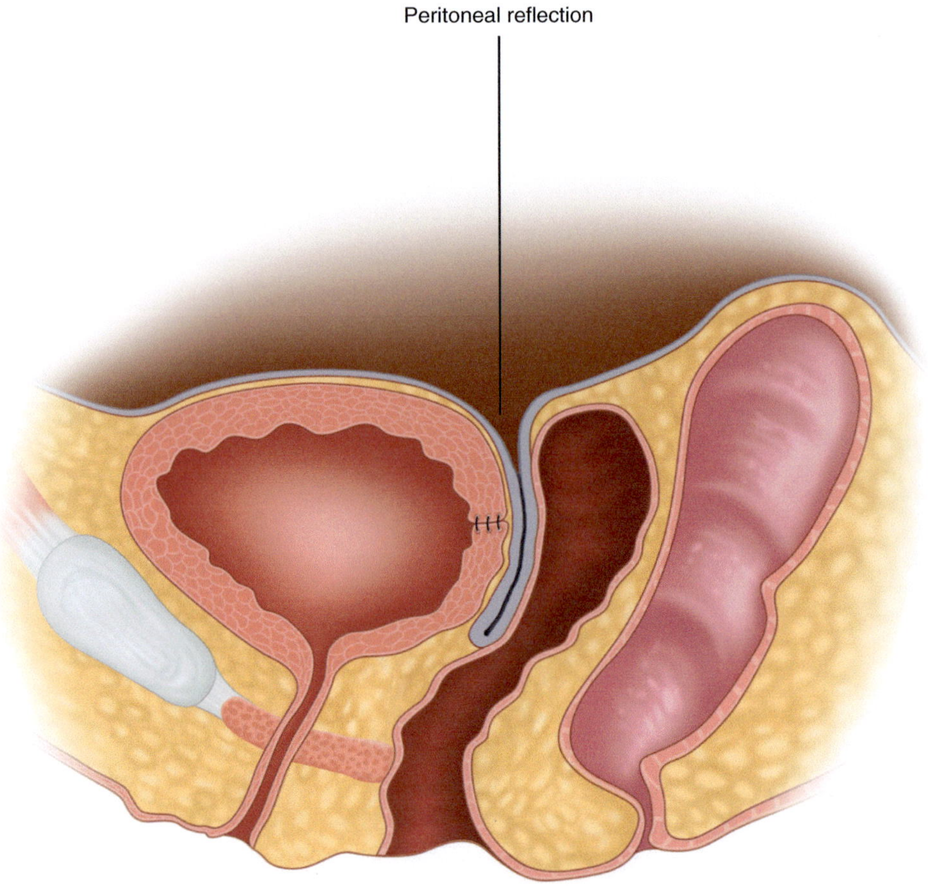

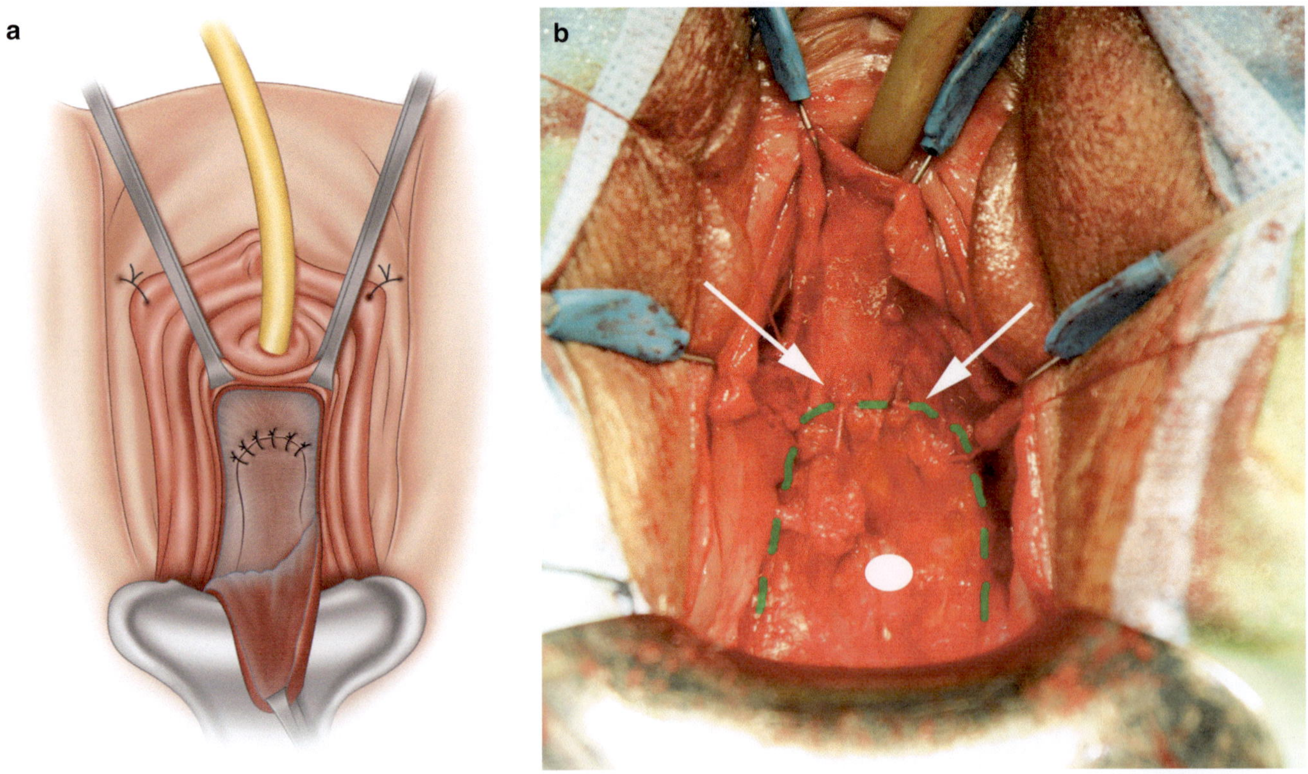

Fig. 5.15 (**a**) Diagram of the peritoneal flap advancement a few centimeters distal to the suture line of the fistula repair. (**b**) Interrupted absorbable sutures are used to advance the peritoneal flap. The sutures are applied over the perivesical fascia several centimeters distal of the original line of closure of the fistulous tract. *Green line* depicts the peritoneal flap advancement. *Arrows* indicated the line of sutures of the peritoneal flap to cover the area of the fistula repair. The *white dot* marks the area of the fistula closure

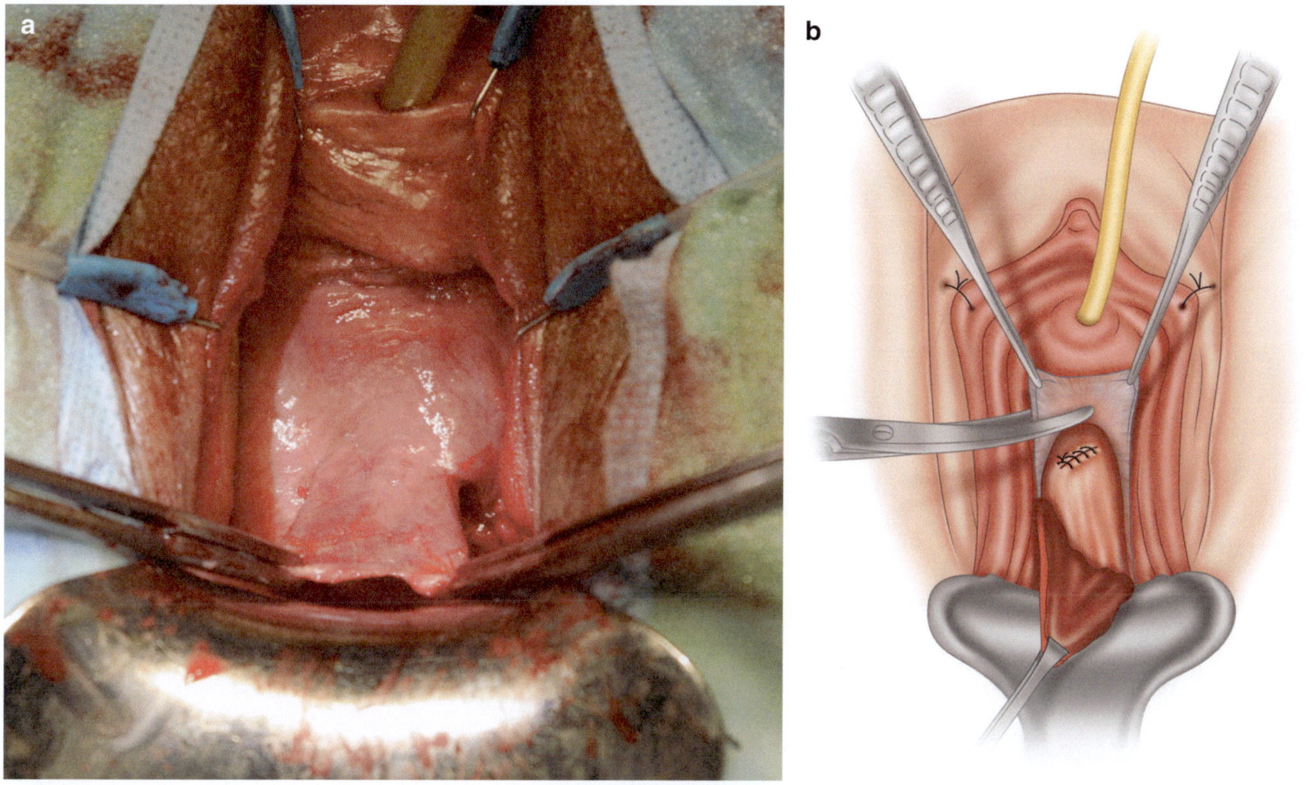

Fig. 5.16 (**a**) The anterior vaginal wall flap created at the beginning of the surgery is exposed. (**b**) Diagram of the excision of the distal vaginal flap that will allow to cover the fistula repair with new tissue from the posterior flap

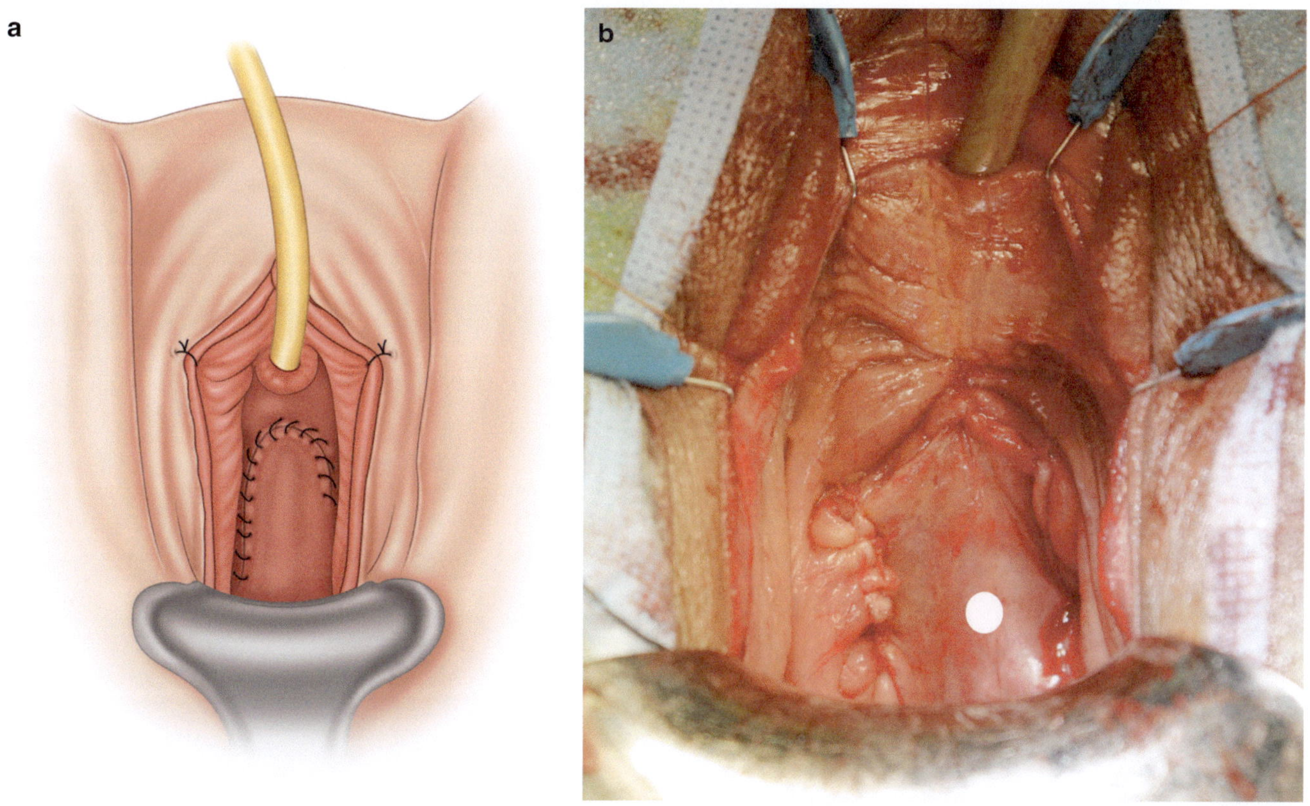

Fig. 5.17 (**a**) Diagram of the advancement of the vaginal wall to cover the area of the reconstruction. (**b**) Final closure of the vagina: #2-0 absorbable sutures are used to advance the posterior flap over the freshly excised margin of the anterior flap to cover far distal the area of the repair of the fistula (*white dot*)

5.1.3.7 Repair of Urethrovaginal Fistula Due to Radiation: Use of a Martius Flap

The patient shown in Figs. 5.18, 5.19, 5.20, 5.21, 5.22, 5.23, 5.24, 5.25, 5.26, and 5.27 presented with a recurrent vesicovaginal fistula located at the proximal urethra, 1 cm distal to the bladder neck. There was no hydronephrosis.

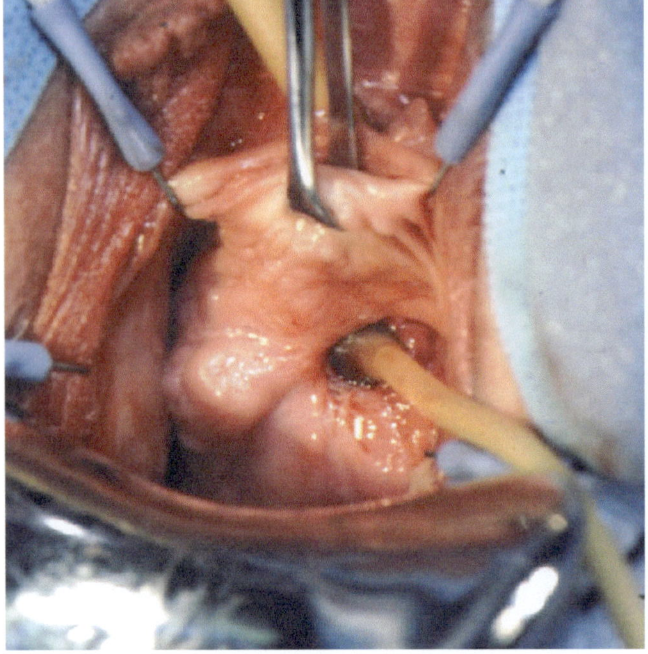

Fig. 5.18 A Foley catheter is inserted in the large fistulous tract

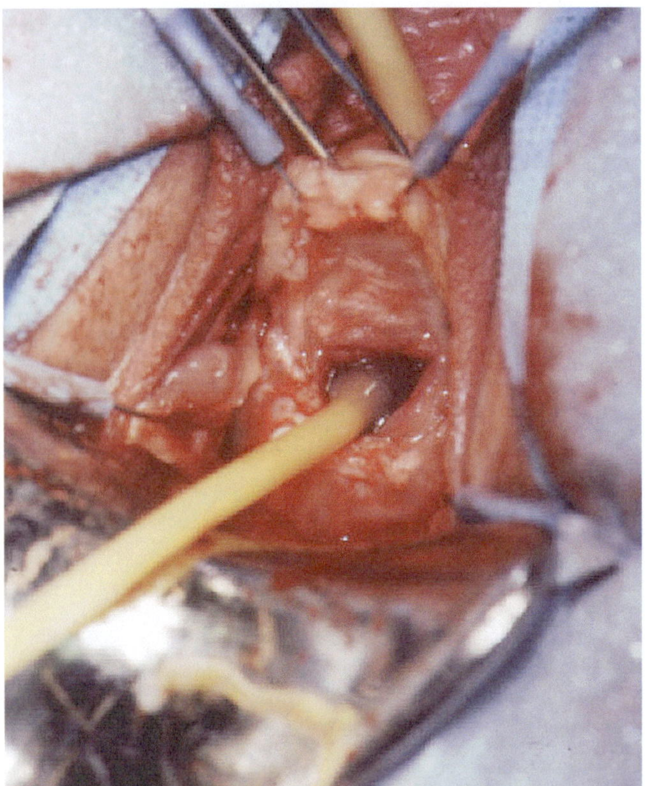

Fig. 5.19 A circular incision is made around the fistula, and superior and inferior flaps of the vaginal wall are created. The fistulous tract itself is not excised

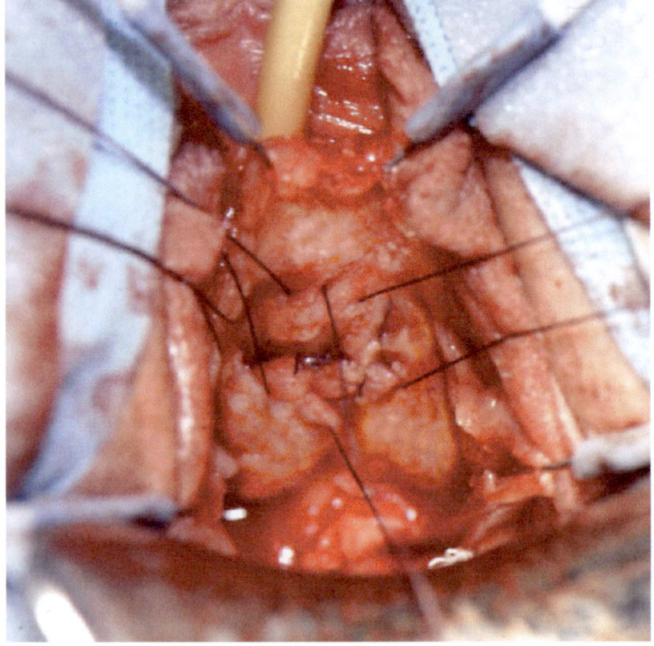

Fig. 5.20 Two layers of delayed absorbable sutures are used to close the fistulous tract. The first layer includes the whole fistulous tract, and the second layer uses the perivesical fascia to cover the first layer

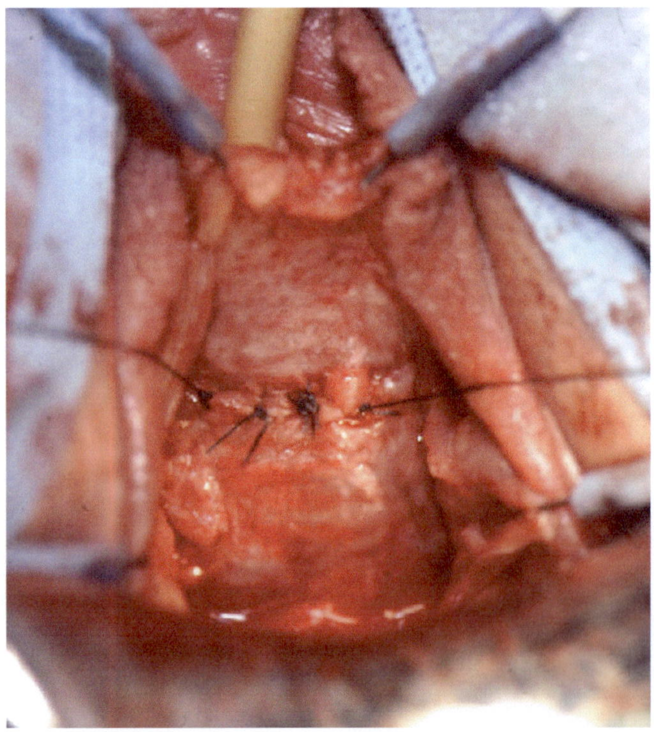

Fig. 5.21 The sutures over the perivesical fascia have been tied. The Foley catheter is irrigated with diluted indigo carmine solution to ensure proper closure of the fistula. Tying the sutures over the periurethral fascia will imbricate and cover the first line of sutures

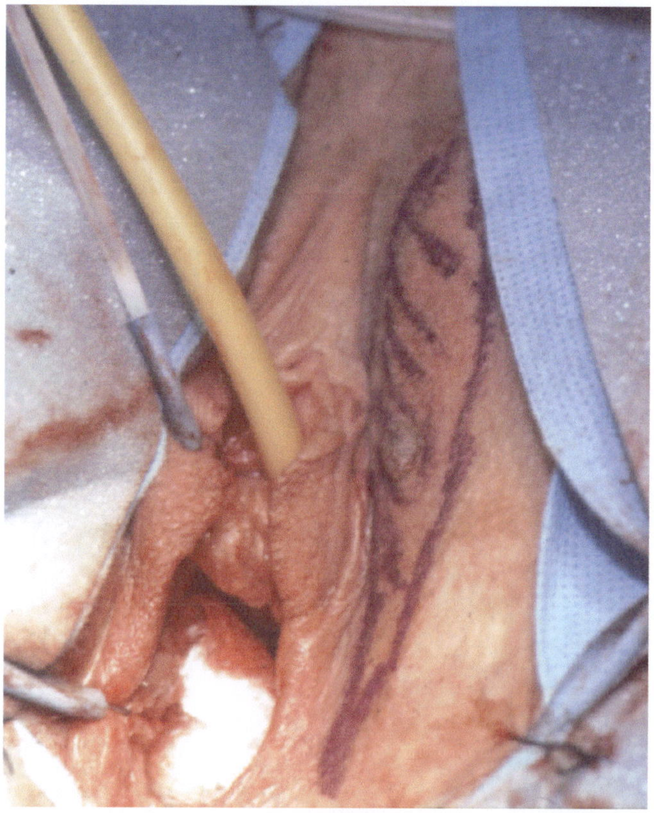

Fig. 5.22 The left labia majora is exposed

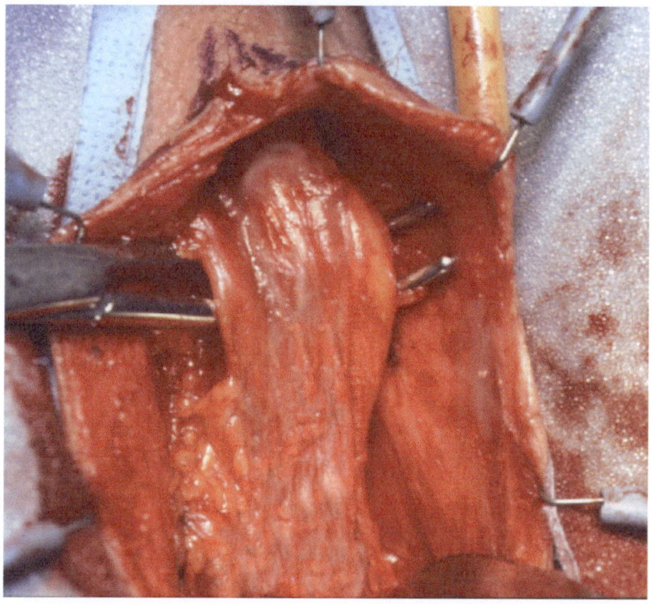

Fig. 5.23 The fibro-fatty tissue of the labia is dissected free from the underlying adductor fascia and is isolated over a retractor. A Penrose drain will be placed under the flap to facilitate the dissection

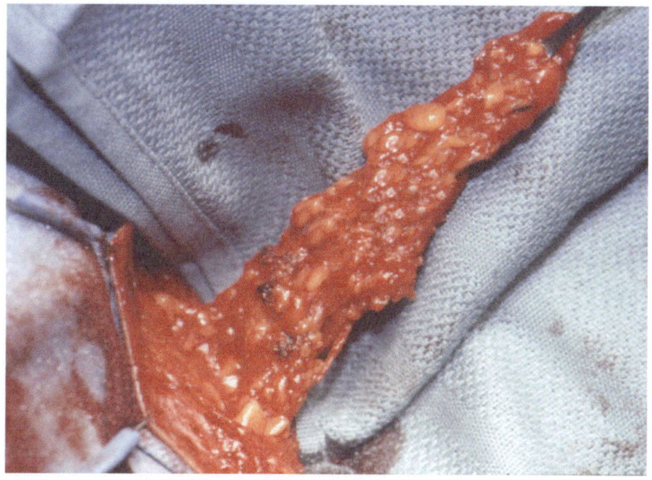

Fig. 5.24 The Martius flap is dissected superiorly toward the anterior pubic bone and transected. The flap is mobilized proximal toward the base of the labia majora. A tunnel will be made under the labia toward the left vaginal wall incision

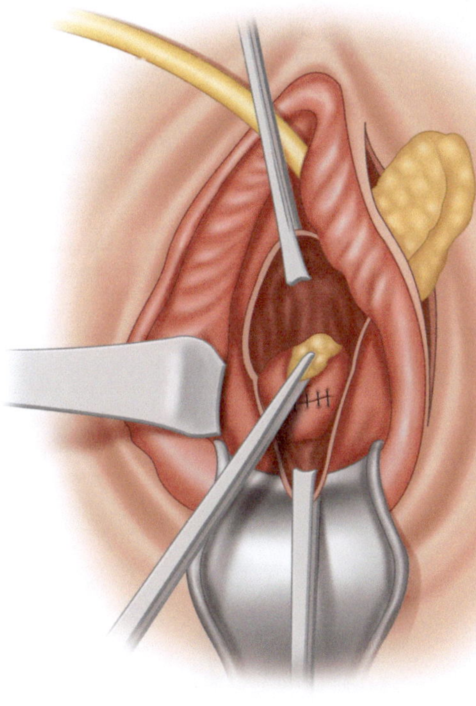

Fig. 5.25 Diagram of the transfer of the Martius flap under the labia toward the anterior vaginal wall

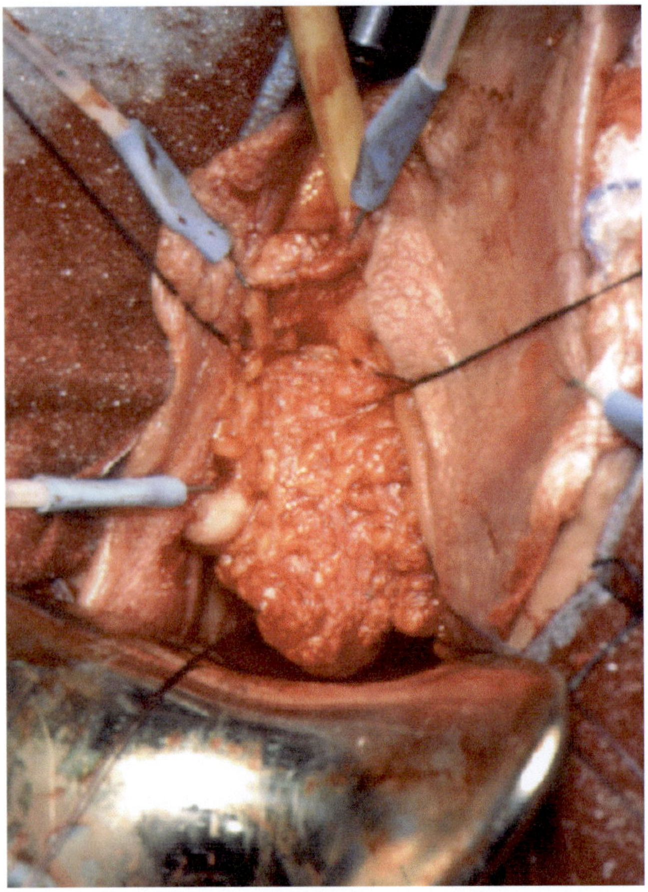

Fig. 5.26 The flap has been transferred and interrupted sutures are used to expand the flap and widely cover the area of the repair

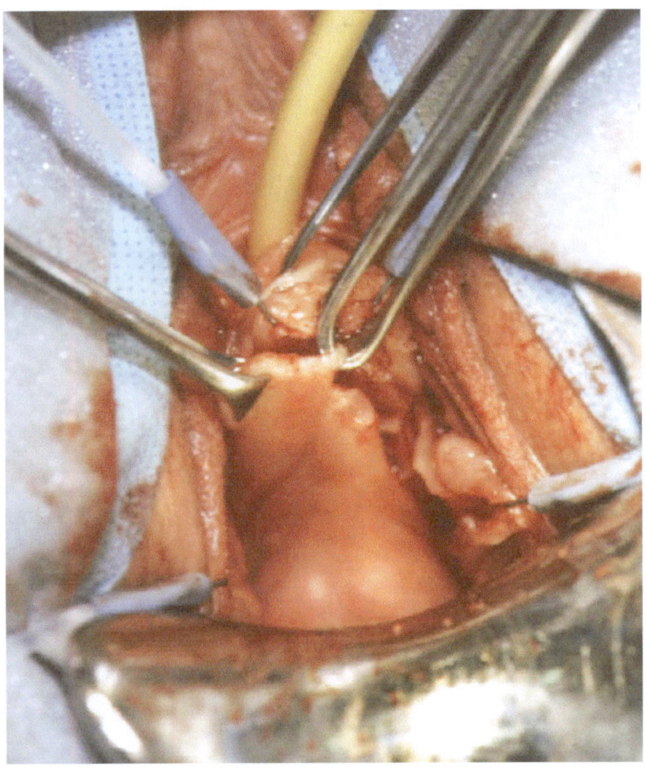

Fig. 5.27 The anterior vaginal wall is advanced distally to cover the fistula repair and the underlying Martius flap

5.1.3.8 Repair of Urethrovaginal Fistula After Anterior Repair: Use of a Martius Flap

The etiology of a urethrovaginal fistula and the principles of its repair are slightly different from those of a vesicovaginal fistula. The etiology of urethral fistula is mainly obstetric or surgical, especially as a complication of anterior colporrhaphy, repair of urethral diverticula, or transvaginal surgery for incontinence using mesh. The urethra is a high-pressure system during voiding, and with the inherent weakness of the traumatized urethral wall, a fibro-fatty flap of the labia (Martius flap) is strongly recommended in most cases.

The patient shown in Figs. 5.28, 5.29, 5.30, 5.31, 5.32, and 5.33 presented with a large urethral defect after complications of the excision of a urethral diverticulum.

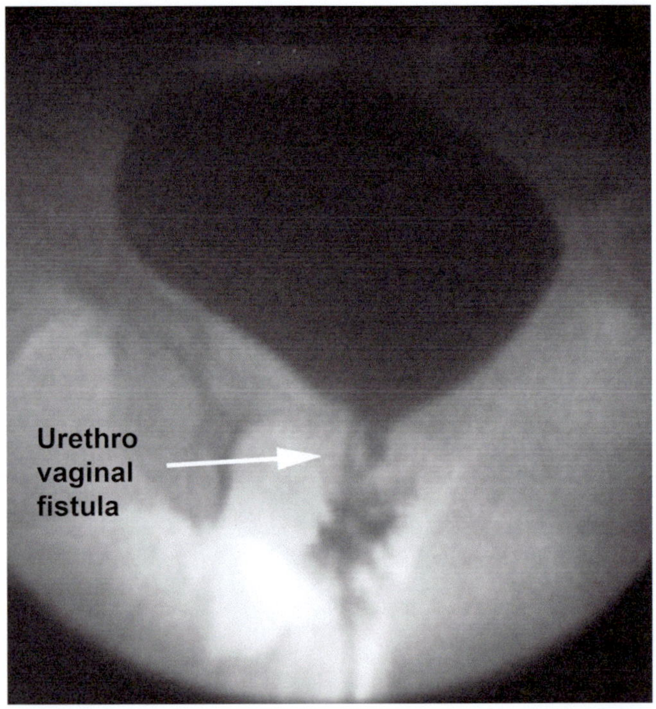

Fig. 5.28 Voiding cystogram of the patient. Urine leaks into the vagina through the midurethral fistula

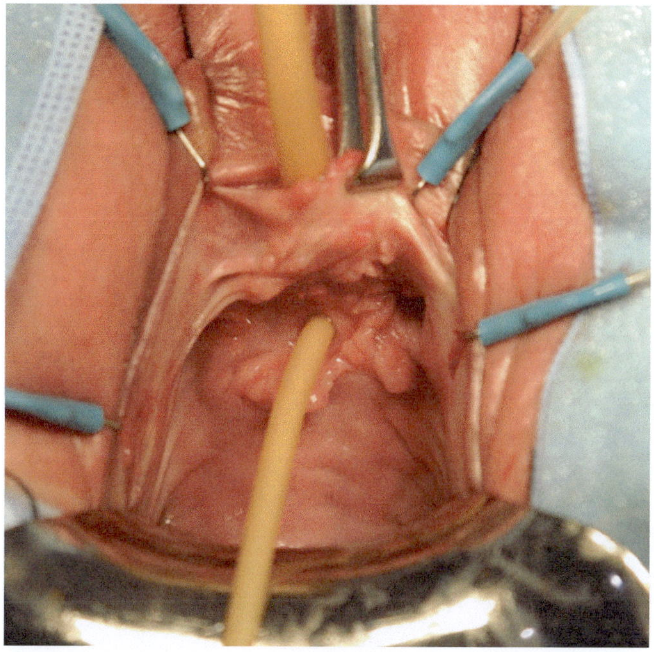

Fig. 5.29 Exposure of the anterior vaginal wall shows the urethral defect. A small Foley catheter is inserted into the fistula

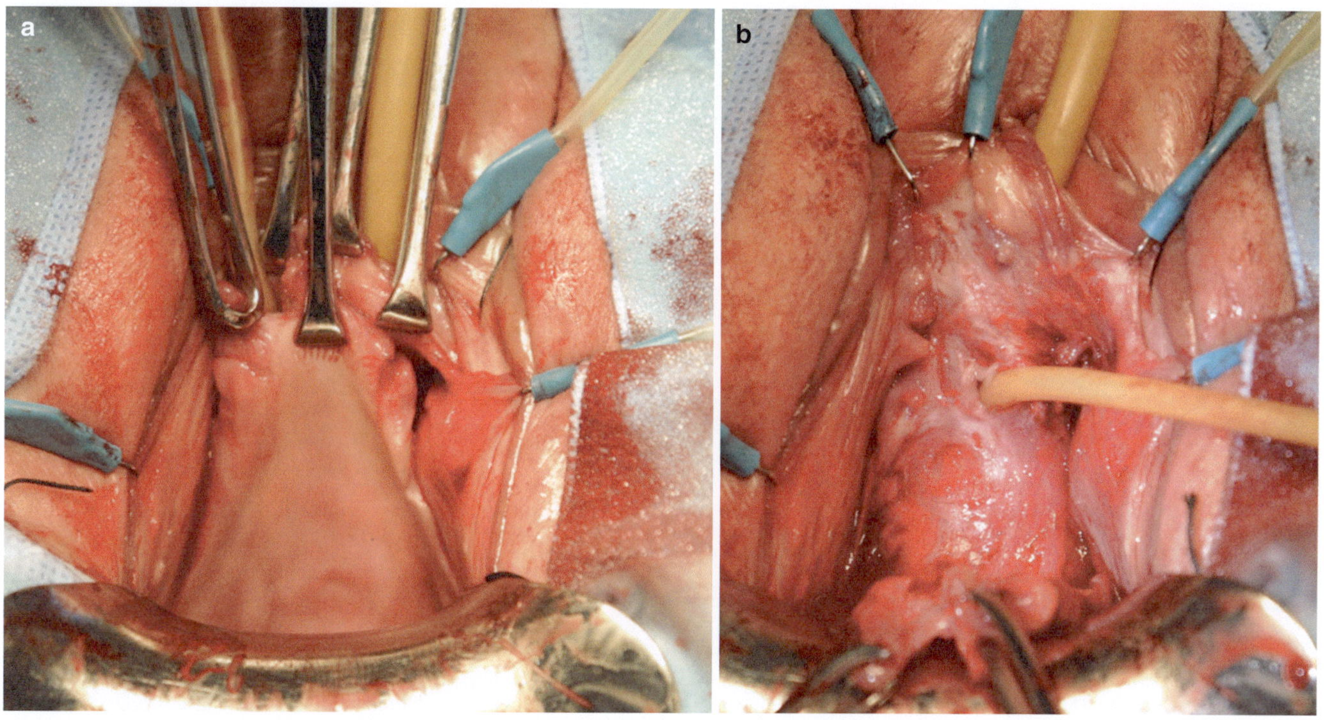

Fig. 5.30 (**a**) An inverted U incision is made posterior to the fistula, and an anterior vaginal wall flap is created. It is extended toward the bladder neck. A distal vaginal wall is also created to expose the length of the urethra. (**b**) The anterior vaginal flap is retracted inferiorly to expose the urethral fistula and a few centimeters around it

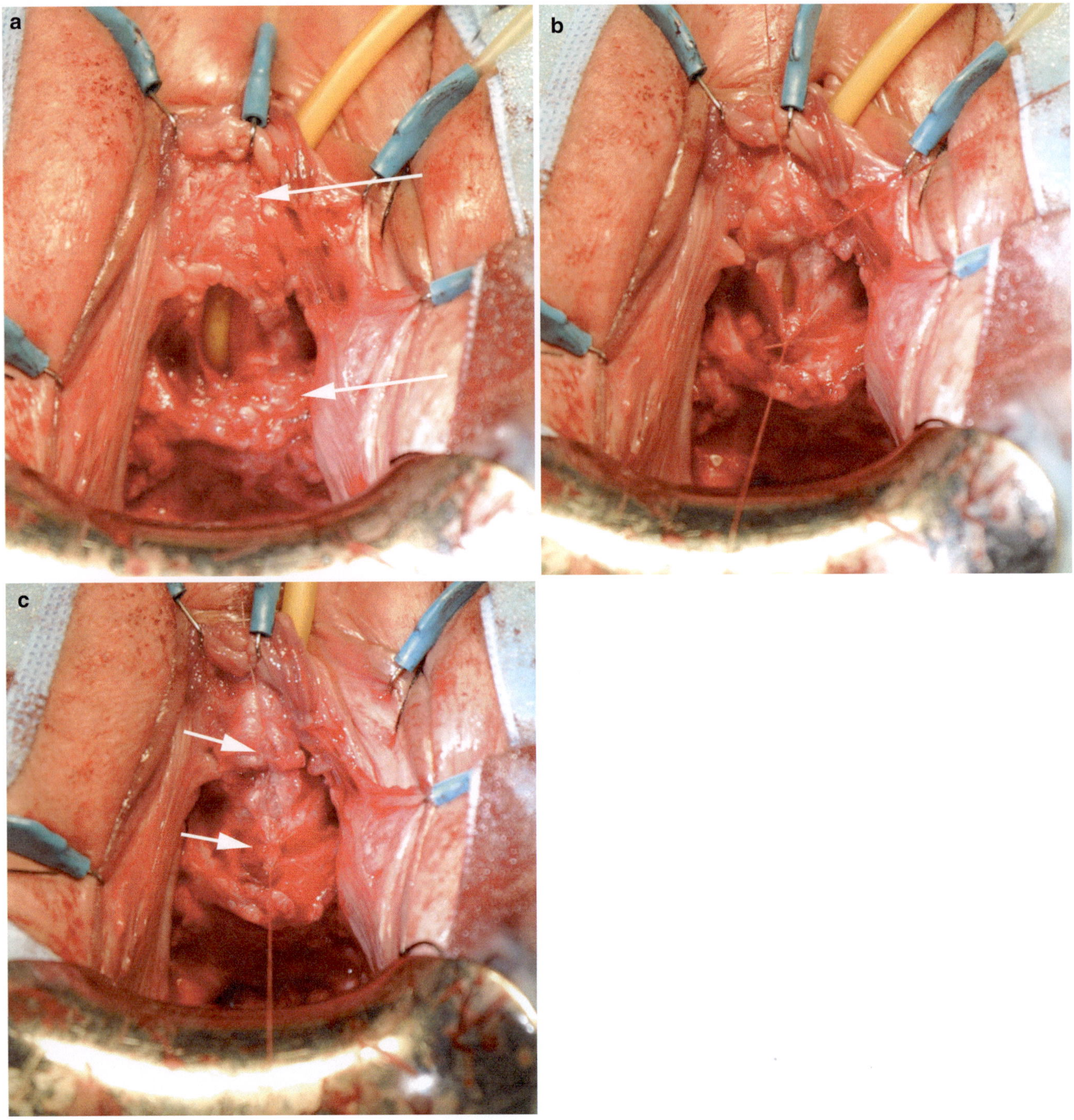

Fig. 5.31 (**a**) A transverse incision is made over the periurethral fascia, and two flaps of periurethral fascia (*arrows*) are dissected superior and inferior to the fistula. (**b**) The urethral wall is closed with running, locking #3-0 delayed absorbable sutures and a second layer of interrupted figure-of-eight sutures to reinforce the closure. (**c**) The urethral wall is closed and the integrity of the closure is tested by the injection of diluted indigo carmine solution through the urethral meatus. *Arrows* indicate the line of sutures closing the urethral wall

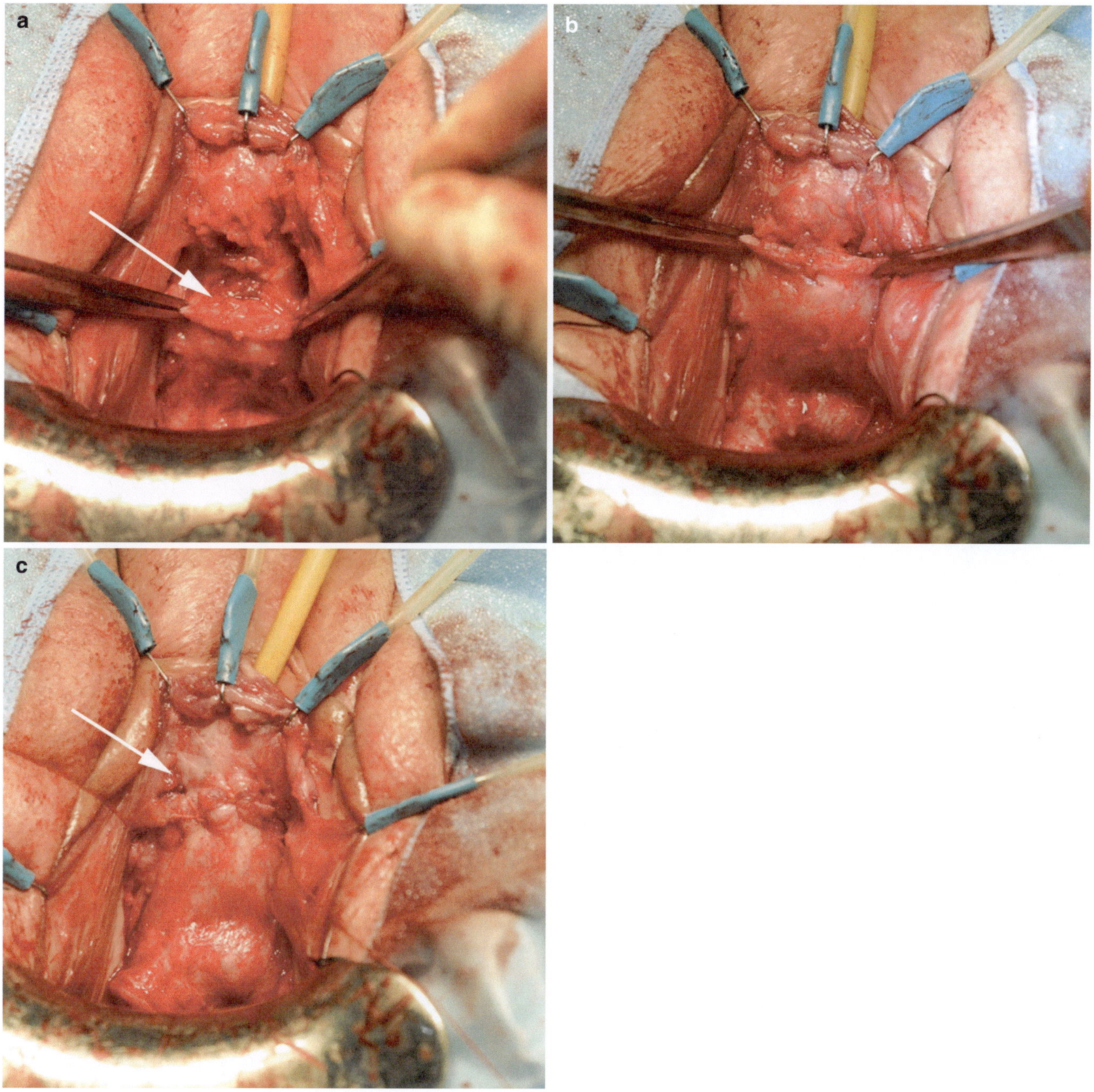

Fig. 5.32 (**a**) The inferior margin of the transversely incised periurethral fascia (*arrow*) is elevated and mobilized as required to reach the distal segment of the incision. (**b**) The inferior margin of the periurethral fascia is advanced distally to cover the area of the fistula. (**c**) The periurethral fascia is closed in a transverse fashion with interrupted figure-of-eight #3-0 delayed absorbable sutures, providing support and cover to the area of the fistula

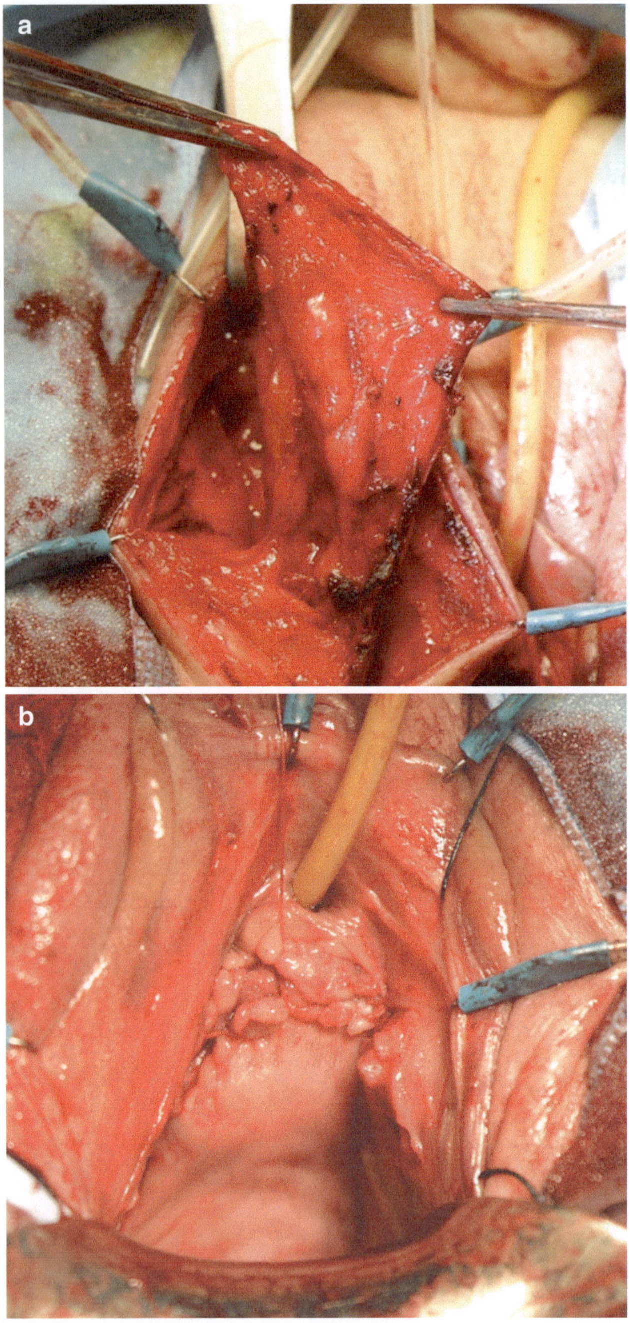

Fig. 5.33 (**a**) A Martius flap is prepared and mobilized in the right labia. It will be transferred toward the anterior vaginal wall, covering the reconstructed periurethral fascia. Sutures are applied to spread the flap a few centimeters distal, proximal, and lateral to the line of sutures. (**b**) The flap of the anterior vaginal wall is advanced distally, covering the Martius flap and the reconstructed urethra

5.1.3.9 Repair of Urethrovaginal and Urethral Reconstruction After Mesh and Urethral Transection: Use of an in-situ Martius Flap

Four months after an obturator sling procedure, the patient in Figs. 5.34, 5.35, 5.36, 5.37, 5.38, 5.39, 5.40, 5.41, 5.42, and 5.43 presented with pain, urinary infections, and severe incontinence due to a urethrovaginal fistula. The arms of the mesh were already removed in another surgery.

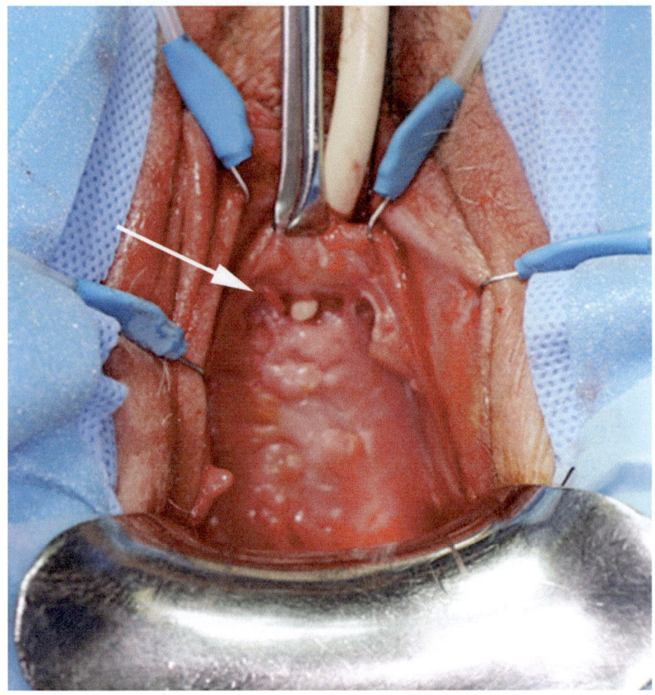

Fig. 5.34 Exposure of the anterior vaginal wall showing a midurethral fistula (*arrow*). A Foley catheter is in place

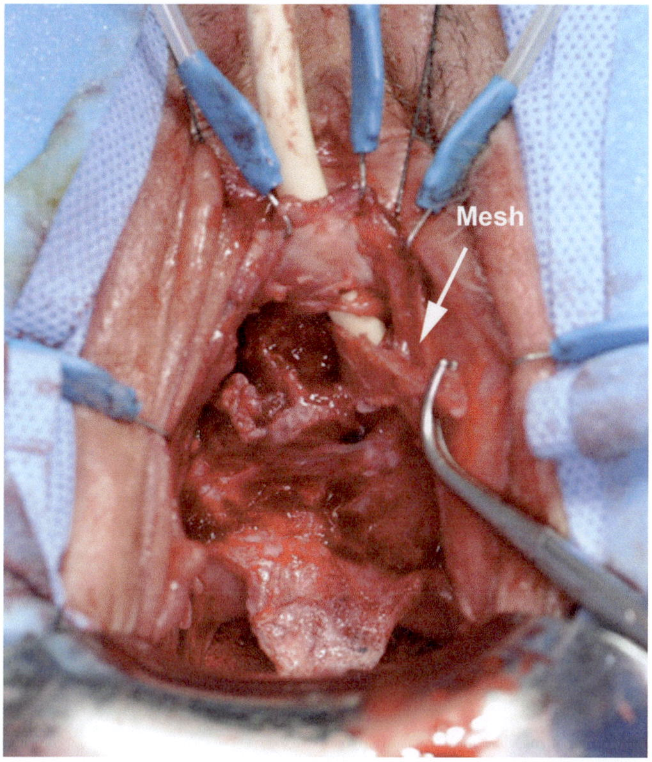

Fig. 5.35 An inverted U anterior vaginal flap is created and dissected toward the bladder neck area. The mesh surrounding the urethra has been excised in the right urethral wall

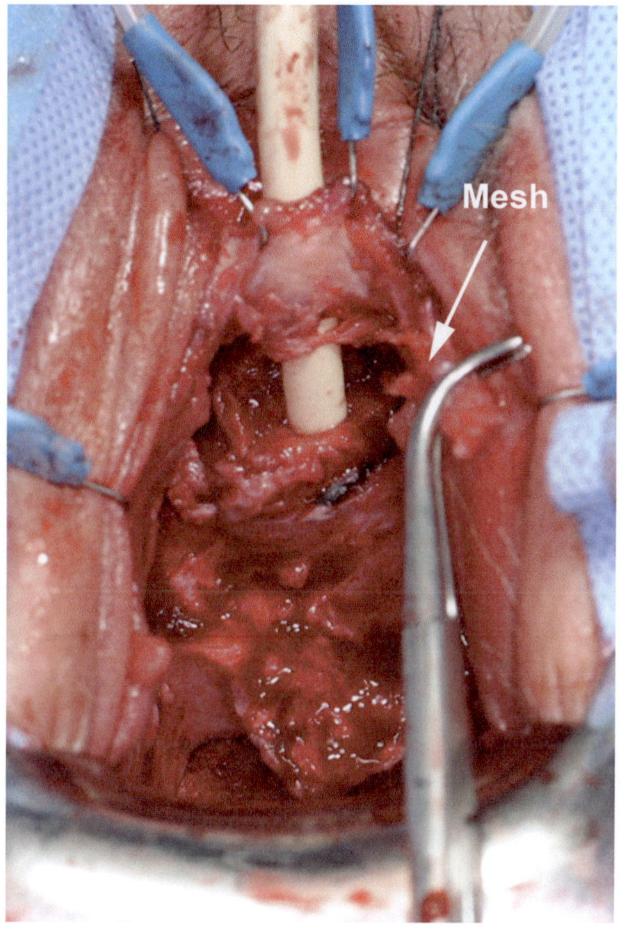

Fig. 5.36 The mesh is dissected free from the urethral wall and removed lateral to the urethra toward the obturator fossa

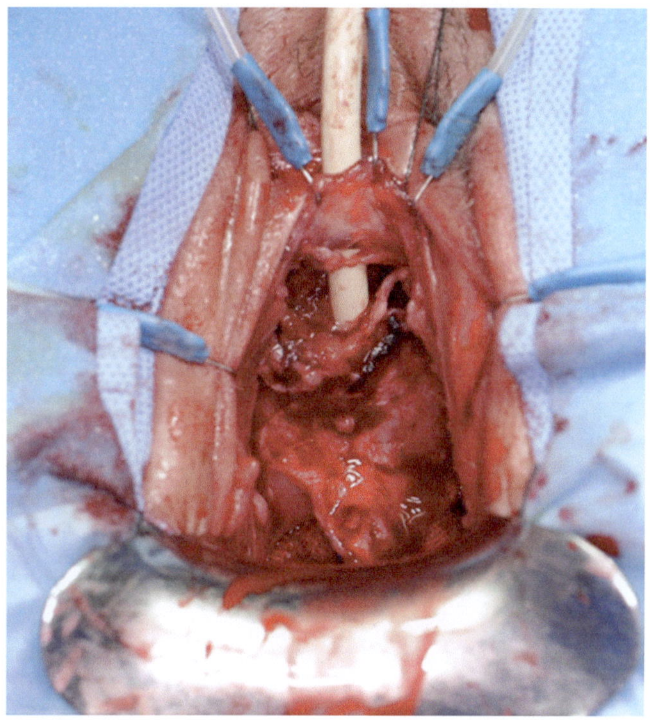

Fig. 5.37 The mesh is removed and the large circular defect of the urethra is seen

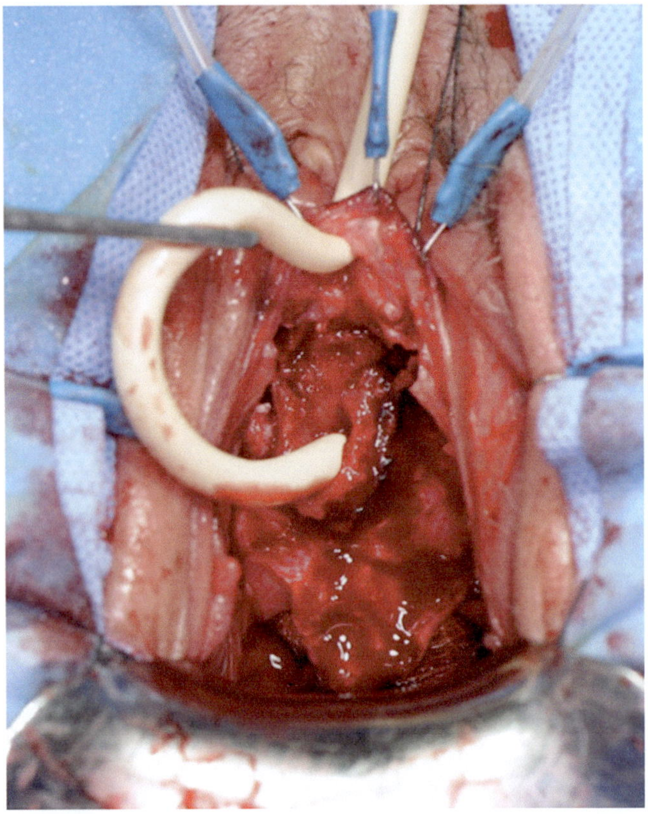

Fig. 5.38 The Foley catheter is retracted to expose the large urethral defect and the small bridge of posterior urethral wall

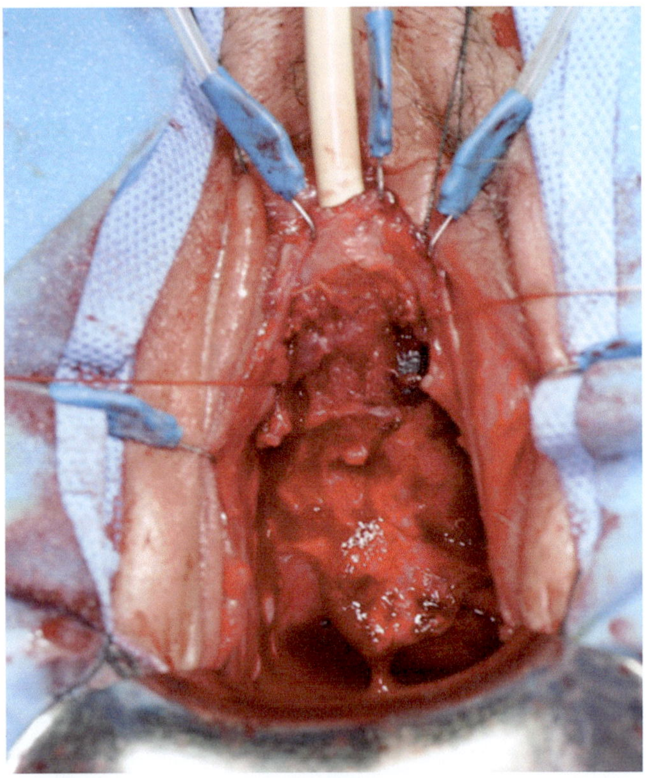

Fig. 5.39 An end-to-end anastomosis of the urethra has been performed in two layers of #3-0 delayed absorbable sutures

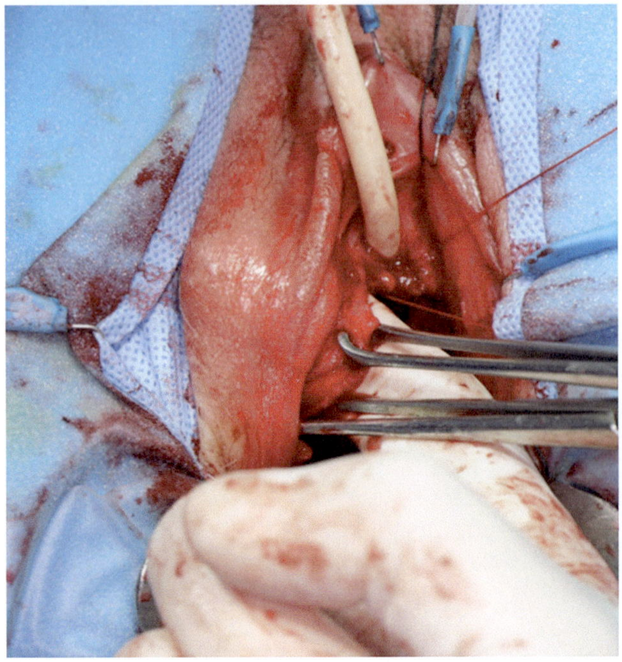

Fig. 5.40 A tunnel is made under the right labia to expose the fibro-fatty tissue of the labia. An in situ Martius flap will be used to cover the urethral defect

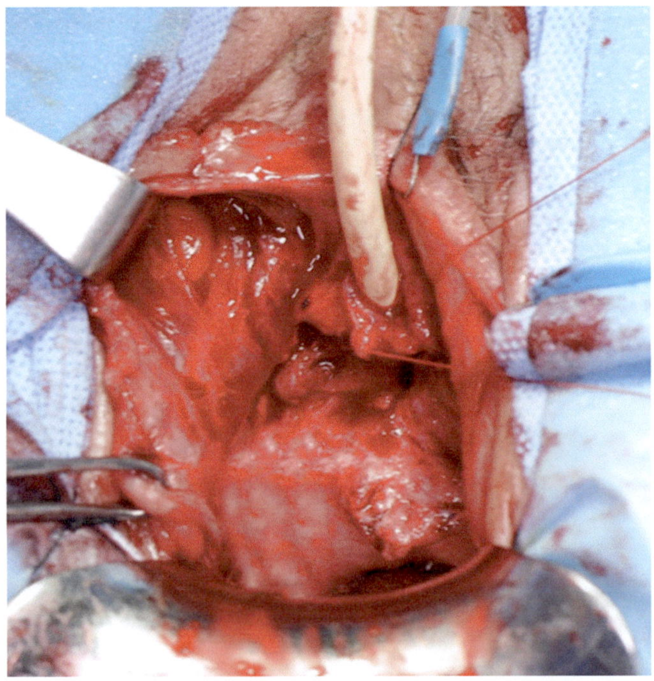

Fig. 5.41 Exposure of the inner aspect of the labia showing the fibro-fatty tissue that will be used for the in situ Martius flap

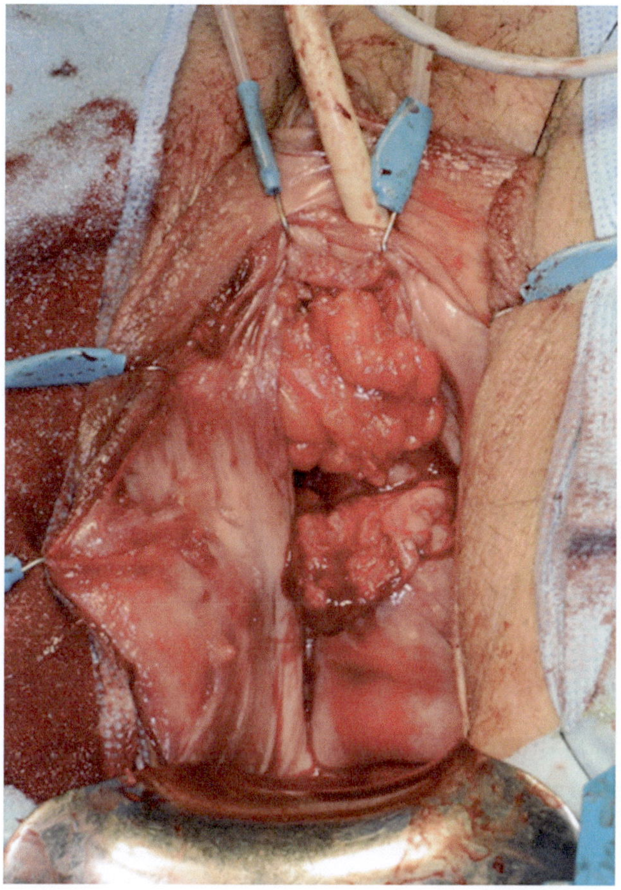

Fig. 5.42 After dissection and exposure of the right labial fatty tissue, the upper segment is freed and transected. The Martius flap is transferred toward the anterior urethral wall and sutured to the periurethral fascia, forming a wide area of cover

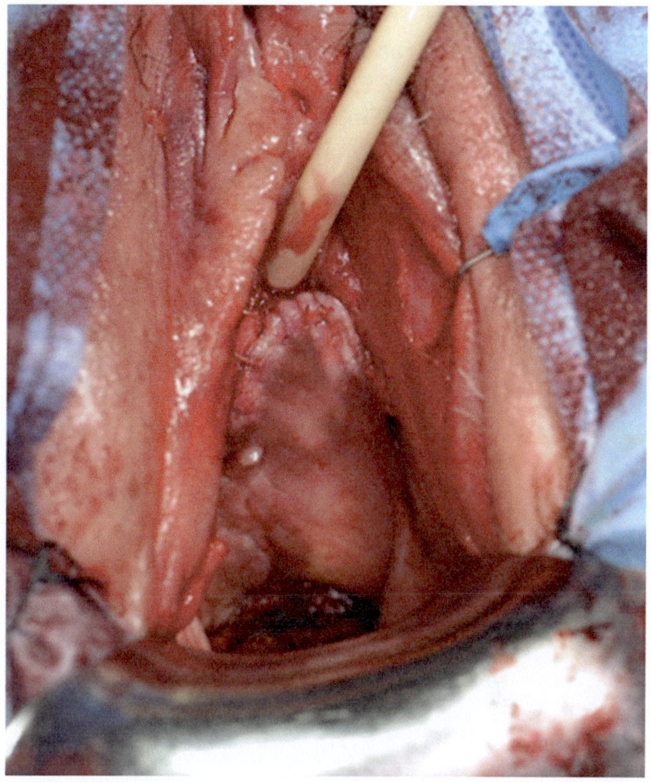

Fig. 5.43 The anterior vaginal wall flap is advanced to cover the area of the reconstruction

5.1.3.10 Repair of Urethral Fistula with Total Urethral Transection as Complication of Hymeneal Excision: Use of a Martius Flap

An 18-year-old woman had a surgical procedure to excise the hymeneal ring. As a complication, the whole urethra was transected from the external meatus to the bladder neck, resulting in total urinary incontinence. Figures 5.44, 5.45, 5.46, 5.47, 5.48, and 5.49 illustrate the reconstructive procedure.

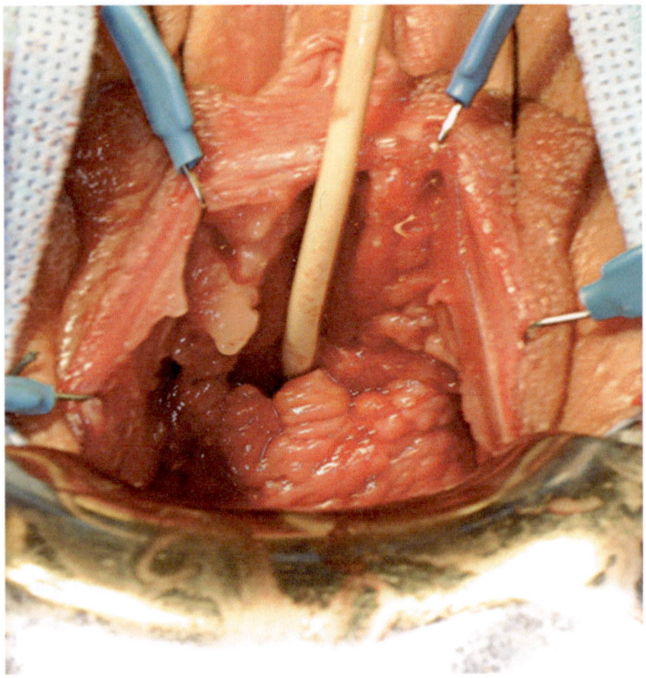

Fig. 5.44 Exposure of the anterior vaginal wall shows the open urethral wall from the meatus to the bladder neck. The tissues have healed at the margin of the incision

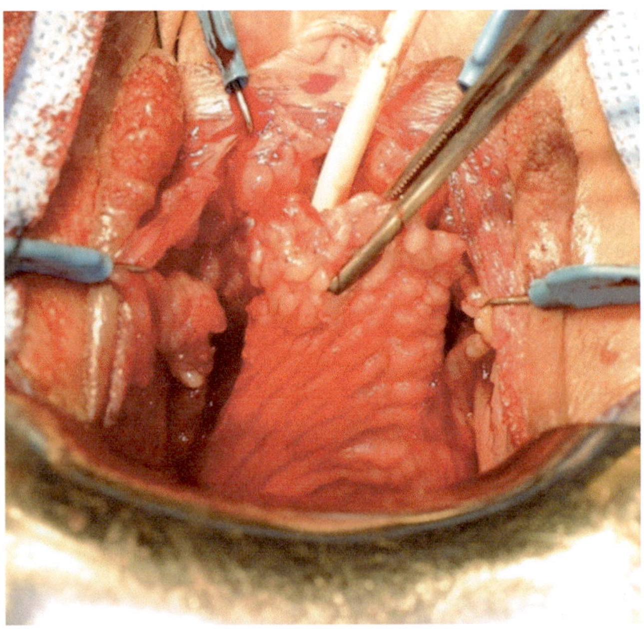

Fig. 5.45 An inverted U flap of the anterior vaginal wall is created proximal to the fistula. The flap is mobilized to reach the external meatus

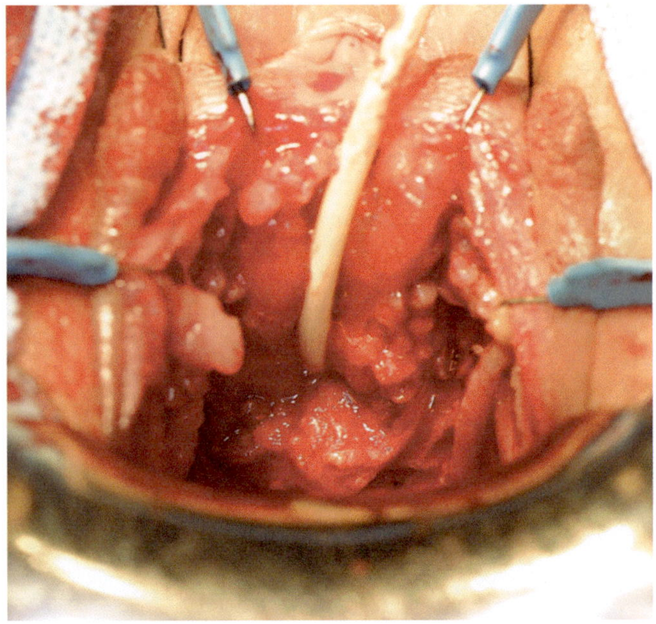

Fig. 5.46 Two parallel incisions are made between the open urethral mucosa and the vaginal wall. The lateral vaginal flaps and the medial urethral wall are mobilized

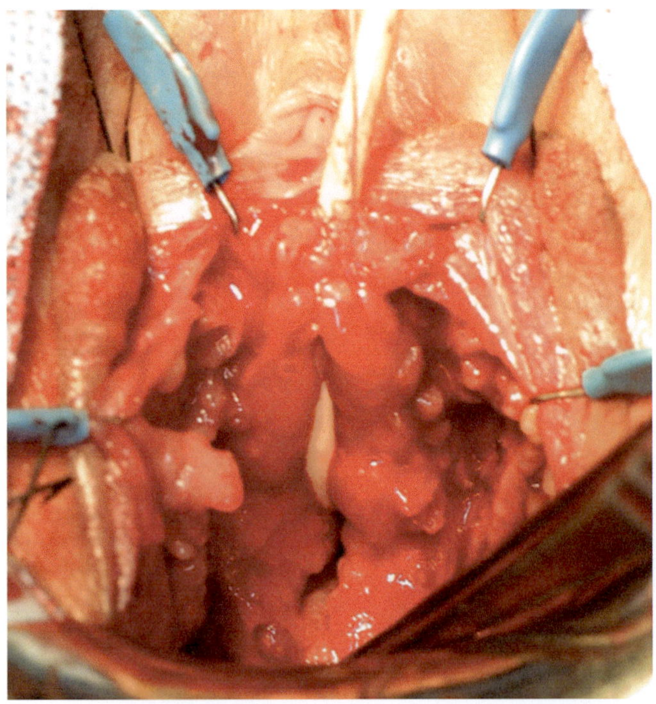

Fig. 5.47 The mucosa and the whole urethral wall are approximated using two layers of #3-0 delayed absorbable sutures

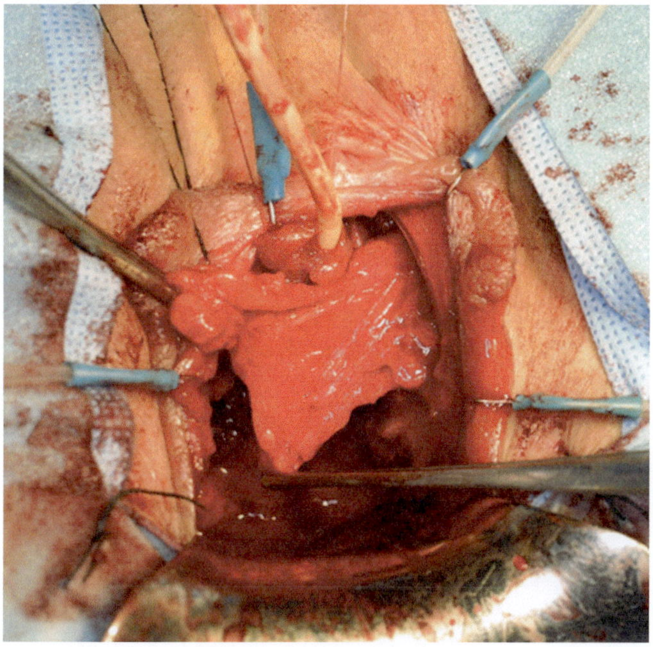

Fig. 5.48 An in situ Martius flap is prepared and transferred to cover the urethral defect. Multiple sutures are used to anchor the flap over the area of urethral reconstruction

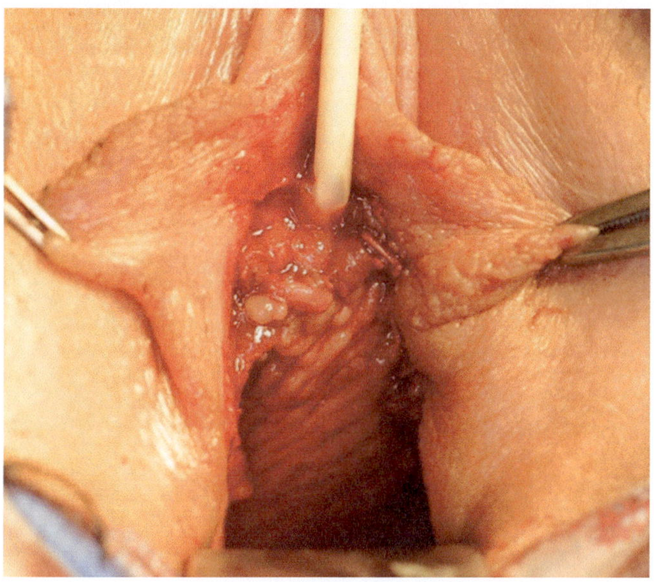

Fig. 5.49 The anterior vaginal flap is advanced to cover the Martius flap. The Foley catheter was left indwelling for 3 weeks. The patient regained full continence after the procedure because the midline 6 o'clock surgical incision did not damage the lateral or anterior segments of the urethra

5.1.3.11 Repair of Recurrent Radiation Vesicovaginal Fistula in a Patient with Prior Colpocleisis: Use of a Rotational Labial Flap

The patient shown in Figs. 5.50, 5.51, 5.52, 5.53, 5.54, 5.55, and 5.56 developed a vesicovaginal fistula of the bladder base after pelvic radiation. Three prior surgeries, including colpocleisis, failed to correct the problem.

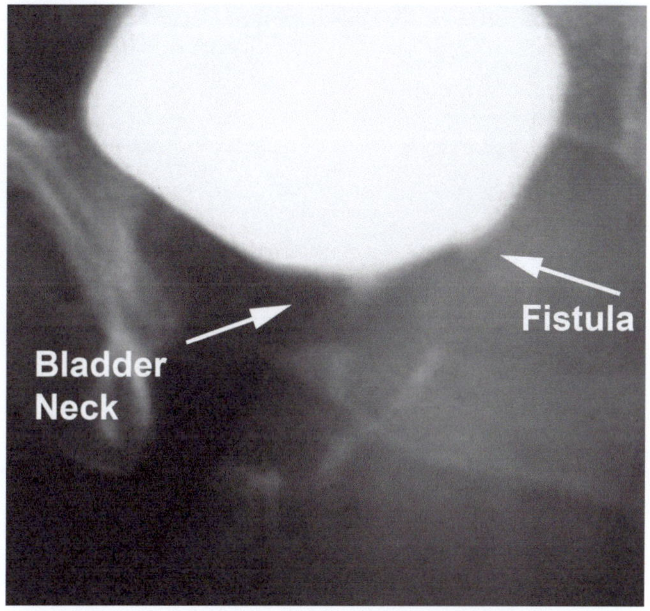

Fig. 5.50 Voiding cystogram showing the recurrent fistula of the bladder next to the trigone

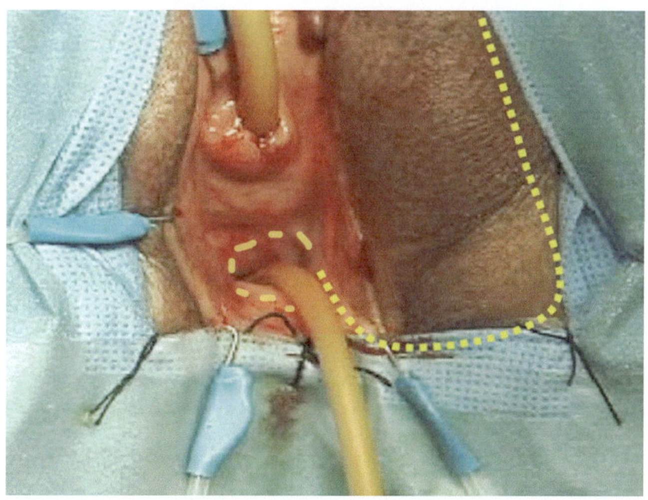

Fig. 5.51 Exposure of the anterior vaginal wall shows the short vaginal canal, with a Foley catheter in the bladder and a second one in the fistulous tract. A circular incision is made over the fistula. The incision is extended as an inverted U incision of the left labia. The skin and subcutaneous tissues are incised, elevated, and dissected free to allow rotation of the labial flap. The vascular supply of the labia will be from the superior pudendal pedicle, coming from the femoral artery

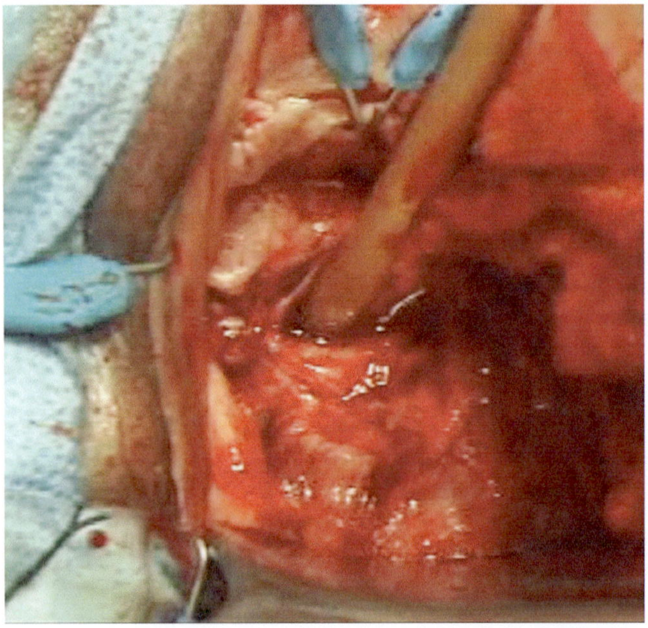

Fig. 5.52 After exposure of the anterior bladder wall, a catheter is inserted into the fistulous tract

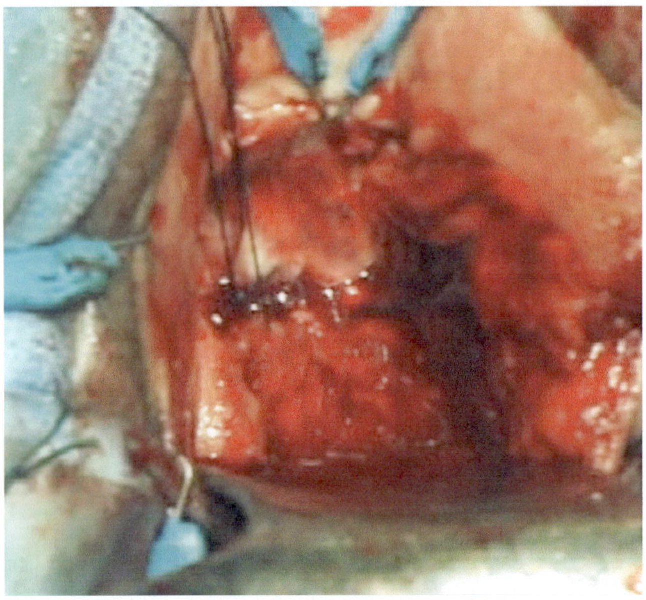

Fig. 5.53 The labial flap was rotated toward the left, exposing the bladder wall and the fistula. The fistula is closed in two layers of delayed absorbable sutures. The bladder is irrigated with diluted indigo carmine solution to ensure the integrity of the fistula closure

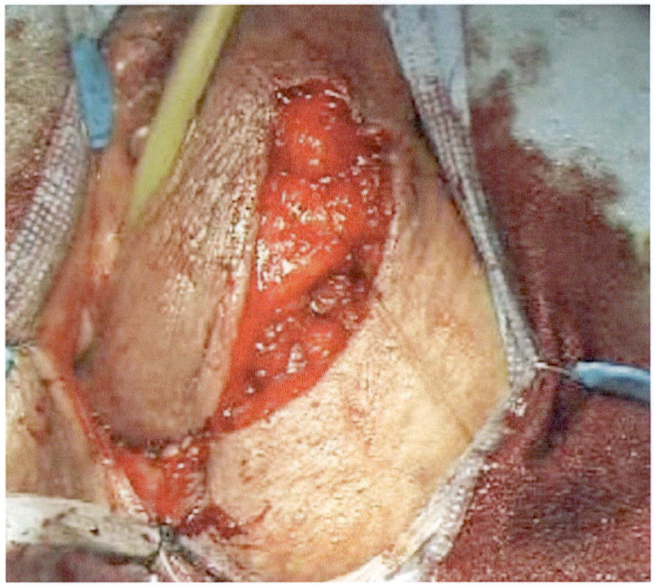

Fig. 5.54 After closure of the fistula, the labial flap is rotated medially. The medial segment of the flap covers the area of the fistula closure so new, thick fat pad and vascularized tissue cover the fistula repair

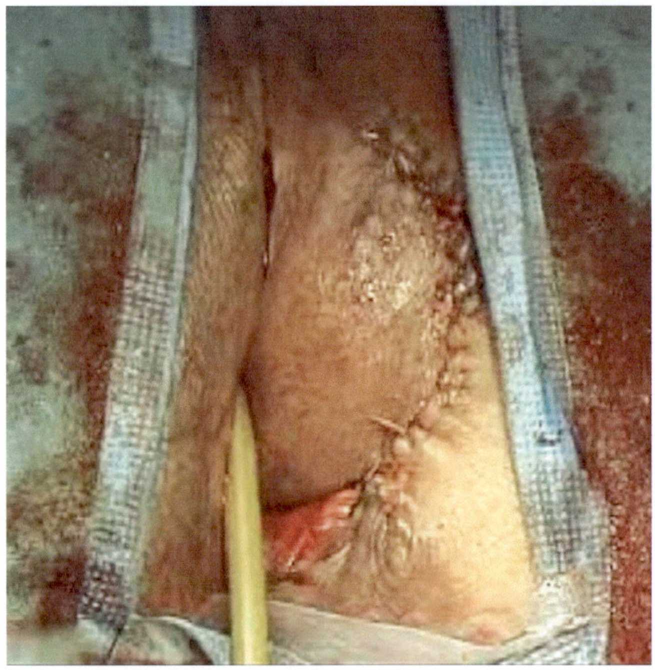

Fig. 5.55 The rotational flap transfer has been completed and new labial flap tissue covers the area of the fistula. After removal of the catheter 4 weeks after surgery, the fistula was cured

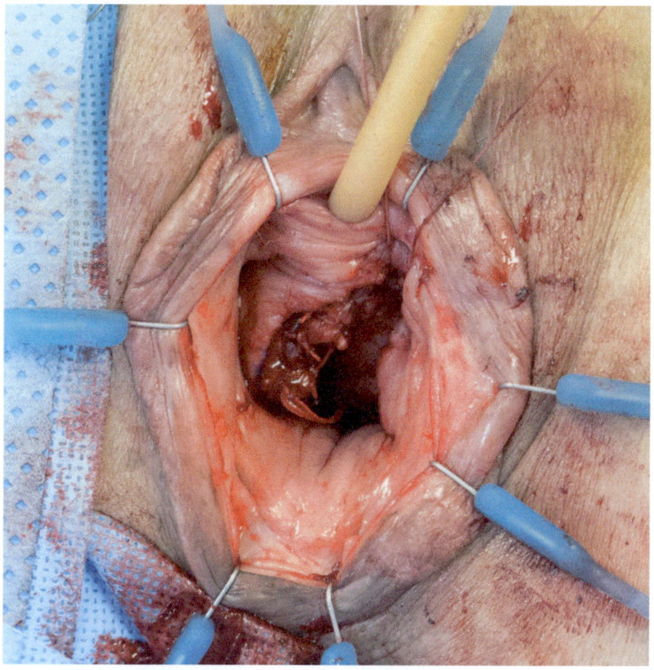

Fig. 5.56 Exposure of the vaginal wall shows a large defect after closure of a recurrent radiation vesicovaginal fistula. The fistula was closed in layers. The patient had a wide introitus. Two layers of delayed absorbable sutures were used to close the fistula. After closure of the fistula the inner thigh is exposed in the left side

5.1.3.12 Repair of Recurrent Radiation Vesicovaginal Fistula: Use of a Pudendal Artery-Based Inner Thigh Island Flap

Inner thigh flaps provide great versatility and excellent vascularized skin and fatty tissue to cover large vaginal defects. For patients with a wide introitus and radiation fistula, this island flap is our preferred technique (Figs. 5.57, 5.58, 5.59, 5.60, 5.61, 5.62, 5.63, 5.64, 5.65, 5.66, 5.67, and 5.68). In patients with a narrow introitus due to prior surgery or radiation, a rotational inner thigh flap will be used after a lateral episiotomy, as demonstrated in the next case.

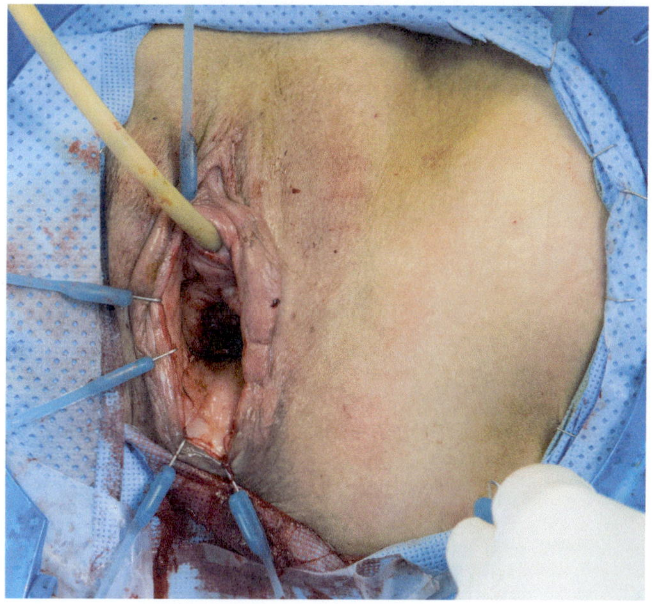

Fig. 5.57 The area of the inner thigh lateral to the left labia is exposed

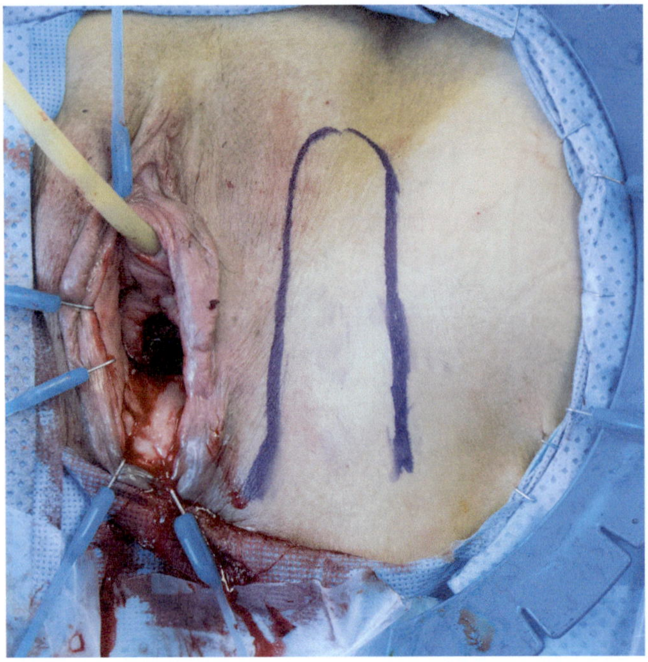

Fig. 5.58 The area of the incision is marked. It will be an inverted U flap with a wide base just lateral to the labia majora

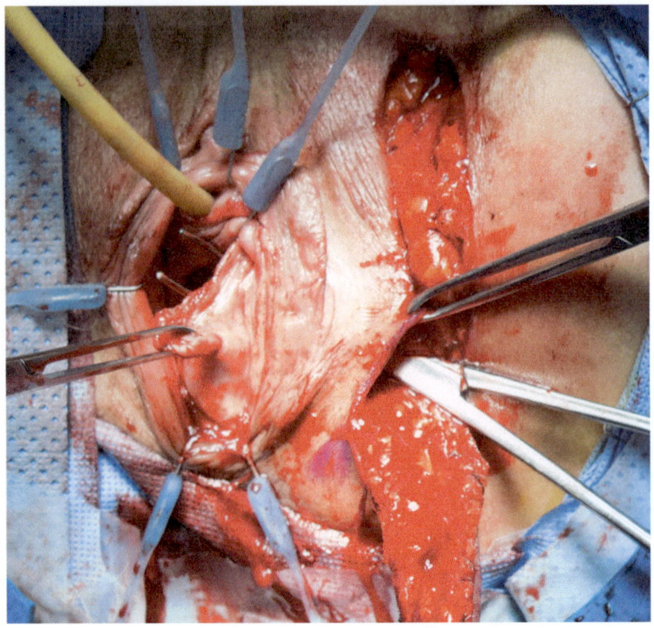

Fig. 5.60 A tunnel is made under the left labia toward the vaginal canal and the area of the closed fistula. A wide tunnel is created to allow the passage of the inner thigh flap

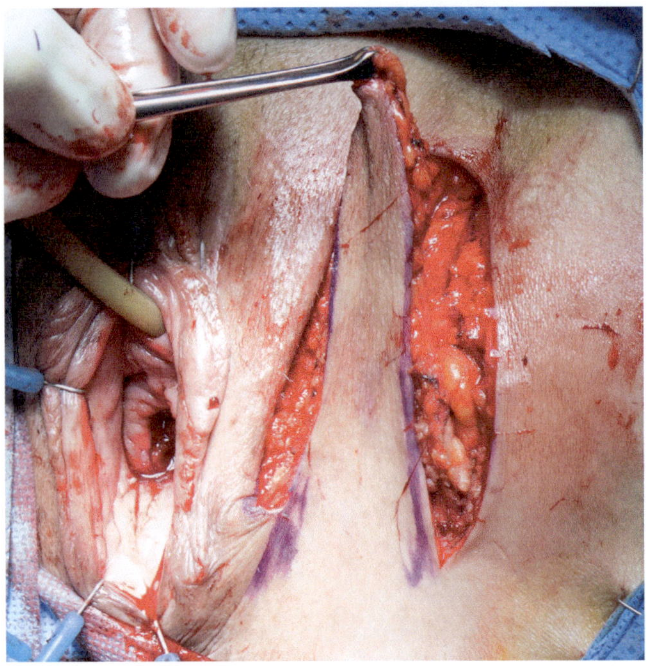

Fig. 5.59 The incision has been made and the flap is mobilized from the underlying adductor fascia

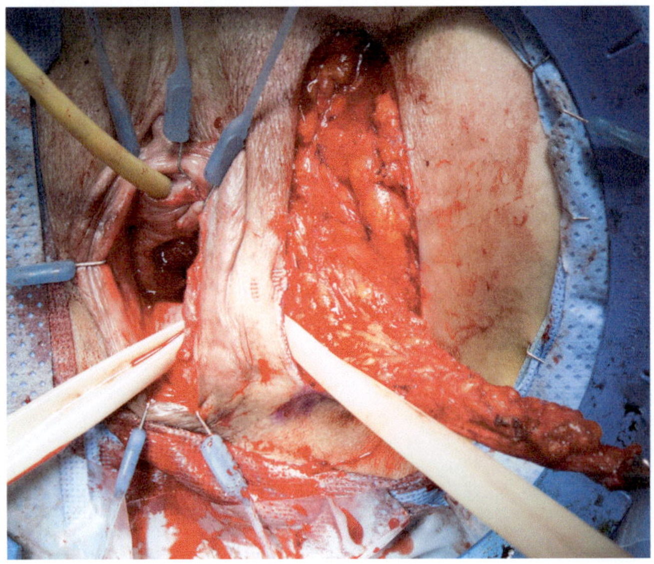

Fig. 5.61 A Penrose drain is inserted at the labial flap for retraction

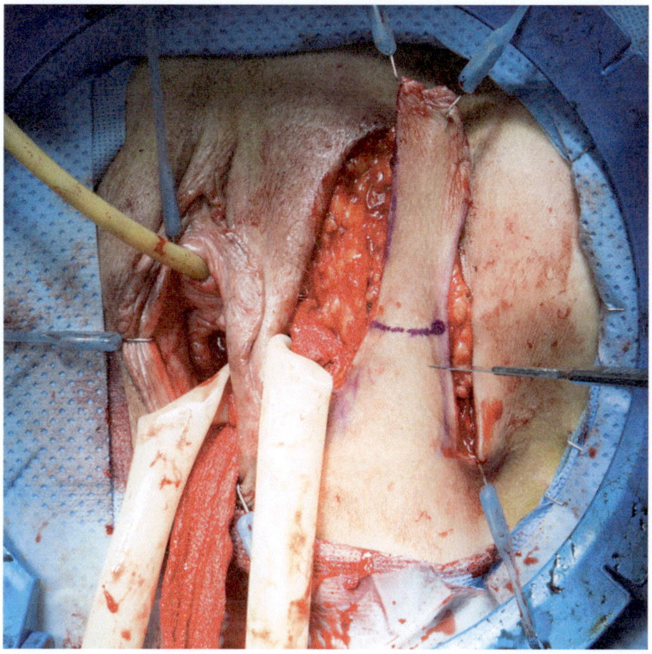

Fig. 5.62 An incision will be made at the distal flap and a rectangle of skin will be isolated. The size of the rectangle will depend on the size of the vaginal defect

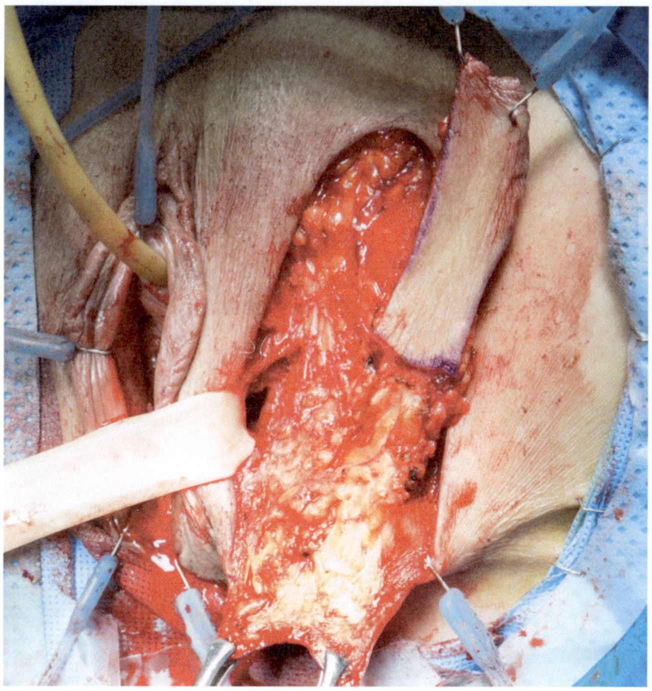

Fig. 5.63 The skin at the base of the inner thigh flap is excised, taking care to remain superficial to avoid damaging the vascular supply to the flap

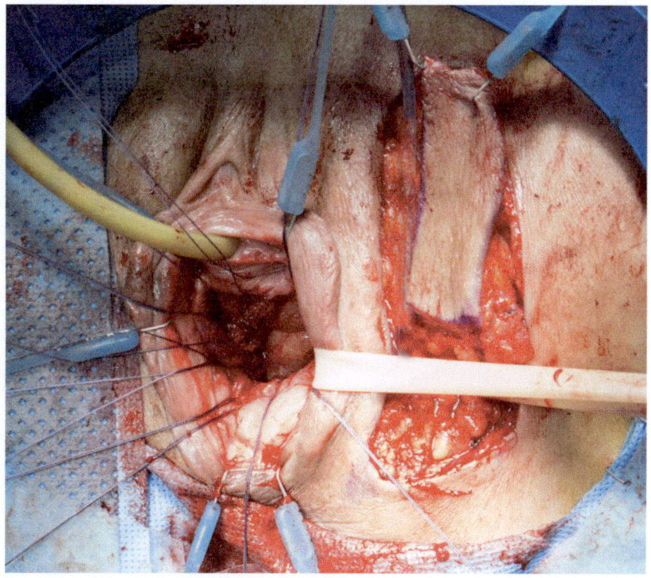

Fig. 5.64 Before transferring the flap, interrupted sutures are applied to the margins of the vaginal defect. The needles are left in place and will be used to suture the vaginal margins to the island flap

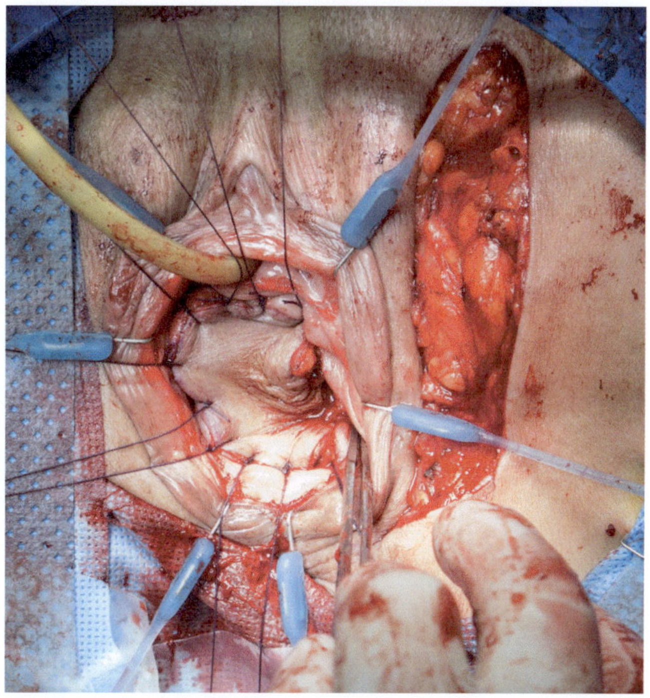

Fig. 5.65 The rectangular flap has been transferred, and the preplaced vaginal sutures are incorporated to the flap in a sequential fashion

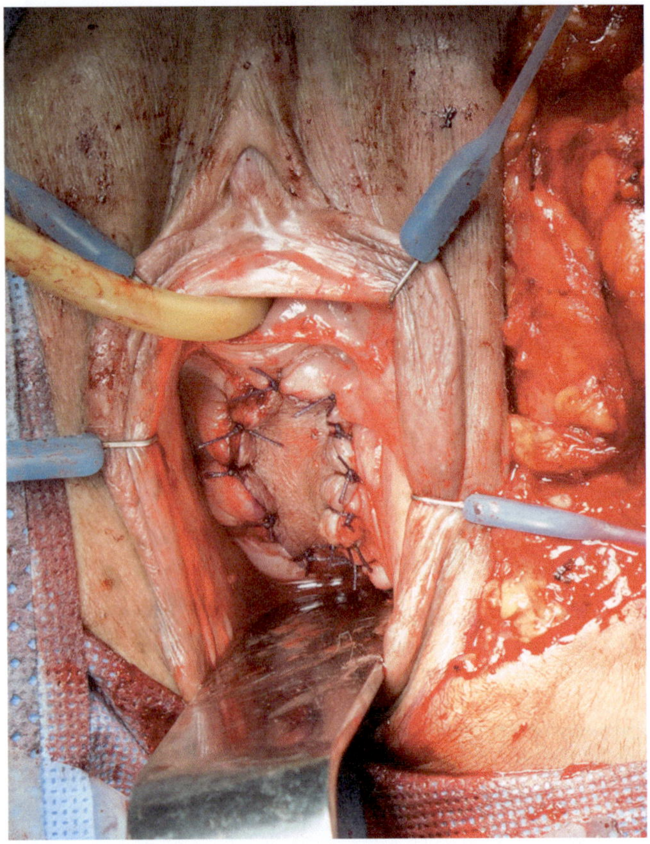

Fig. 5.66 The vaginal sutures are sequentially tension-free. The fistula is now covered by the flap of well-vascularized skin and fatty tissue

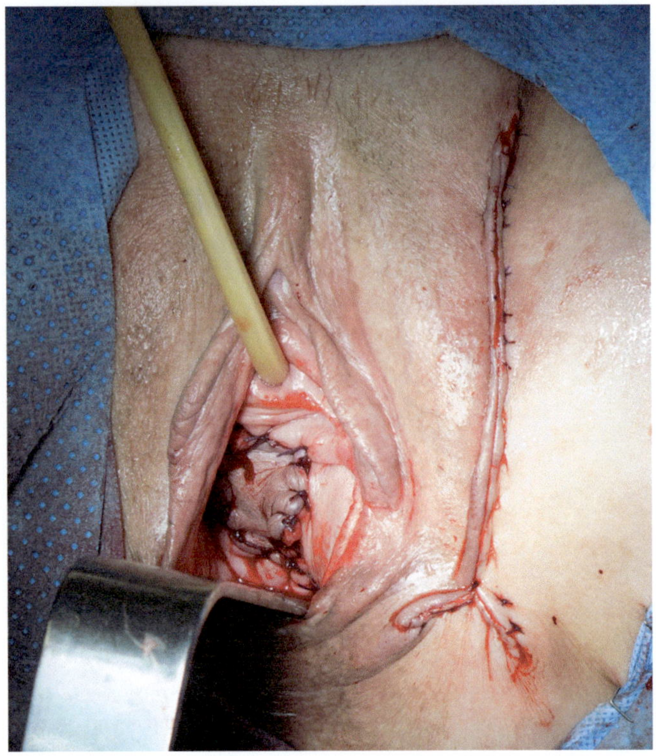

Fig. 5.67 The skin defect of the inner thigh is closed with interrupted sutures after undermining the medial and lateral margins of the donor site

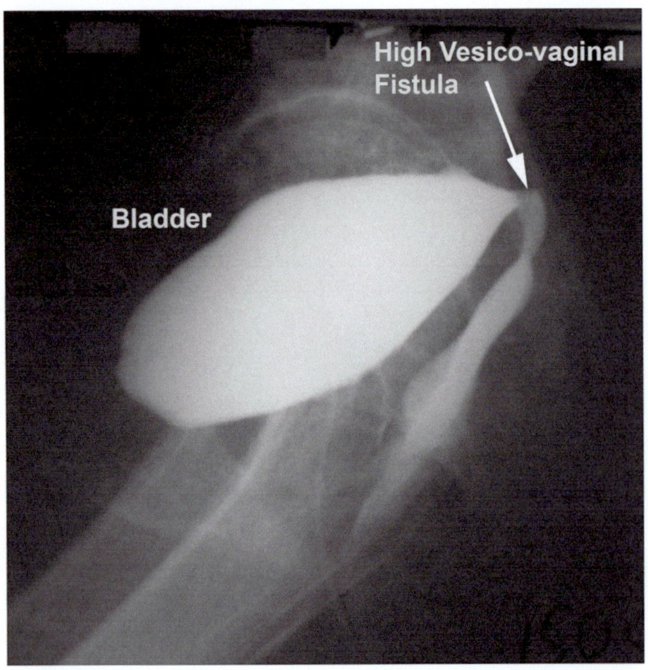

Fig. 5.68 Voiding cystogram in a patient suffering from recurrent radiation vesicovaginal fistula. The fistula is at the cuff of the hysterectomy, in a very high position. The vaginal canal is narrow and stenotic

5.1.3.13 Repair of Recurrent Radiation Vesicovaginal Fistula: Use of Rotational Inner Thigh Flap in a Patient with Vaginal Stenosis

The patient in Figs. 5.69, 5.70, 5.71, 5.72, 5.73, 5.74, 5.75, 5.76, 5.77, 5.78, and 5.79 suffers from a recurrent vesicovaginal fistula after radiation for cancer of the uterus. The introitus is very narrow and fibrotic, making access to the vaginal cuff practically impossible. A lateral episiotomy at the 5 o'clock position will be done to obtain access to the fistula. A rotational inner thigh flap will be used to widen the vaginal canal and cover the fistula repair with a flap of well-vascularized skin and fatty tissue.

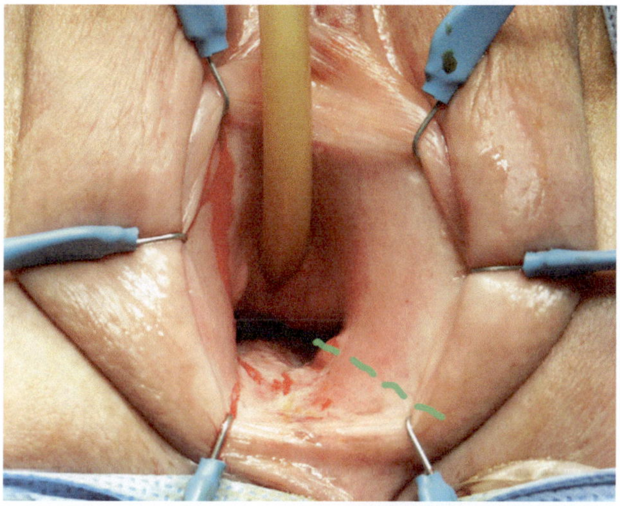

Fig. 5.69 Exposure of the vaginal area shows a very narrow, fibrotic introitus not allowing the passage of deep instruments or retractors. A line marks the site of the lateral episiotomy

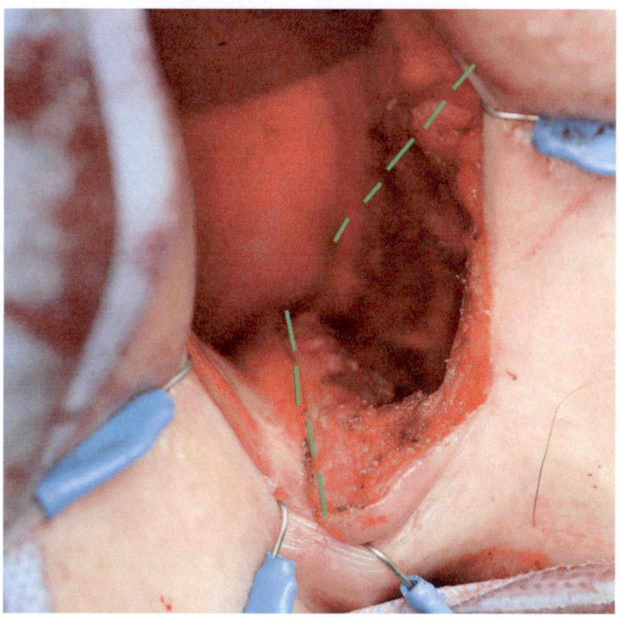

Fig. 5.70 A lateral 5 o'clock episiotomy is performed by transecting the lateral vaginal wall, levator hiatus, and labial skin. The dissection is carried out toward the pararectal space, which is dissected free and reaches the vaginal cuff at the area of the fistula. The incisions have widened the vaginal canal, creating a superior incision at the 2 o'clock position and a second incision at the 7 o'clock position. The fistula will be repaired in multiple layers, and diluted indigo carmine solution will be used to irrigate the bladder to ensure the integrity of the closure. *Green line* shows the margins of the vagina after the incision

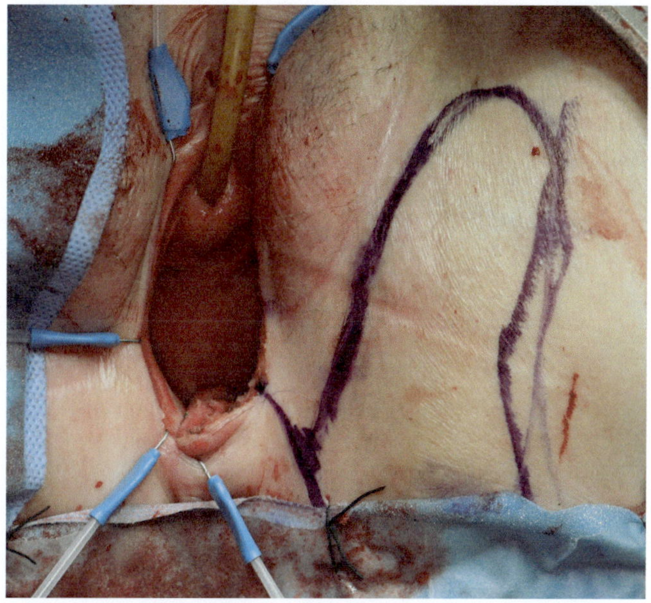

Fig. 5.71 An inverted U flap with a wide base will be created lateral to the labia, reaching the anterior pubic bone

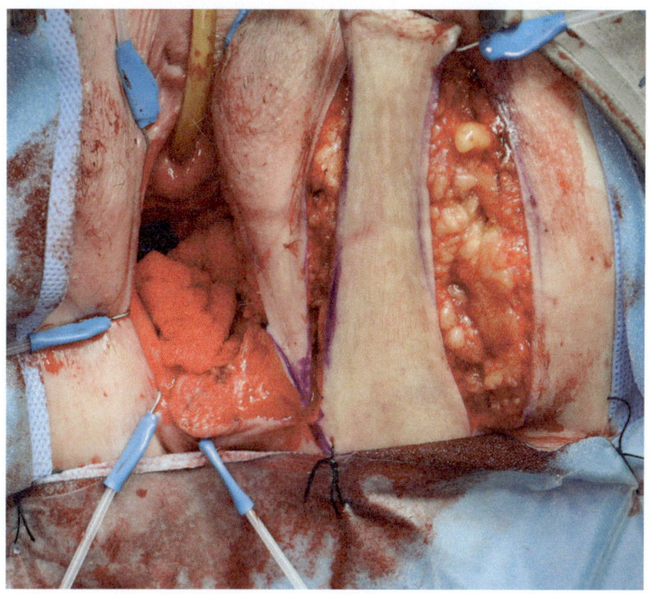

Fig. 5.72 The inverted U flap is created deep to the adductor fascia medial and lateral. The flap is extended to the line of incision of the labia at the site of the episiotomy

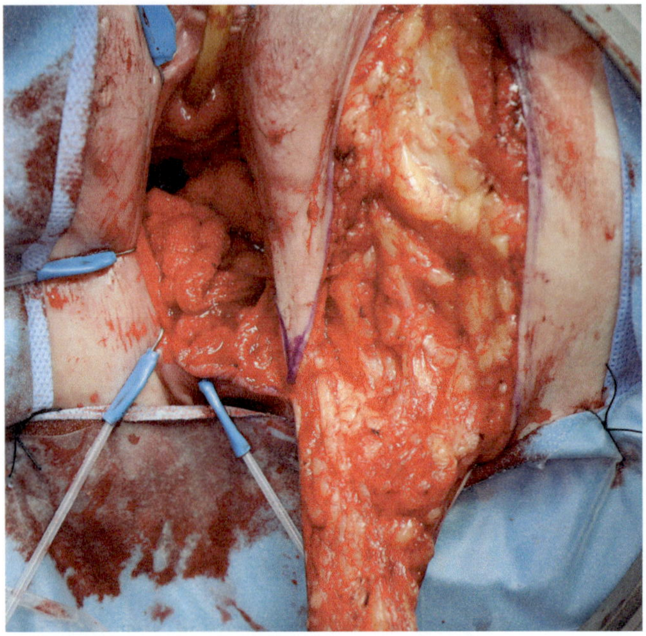

Fig. 5.73 The tight flap has been mobilized and retracted inferiorly

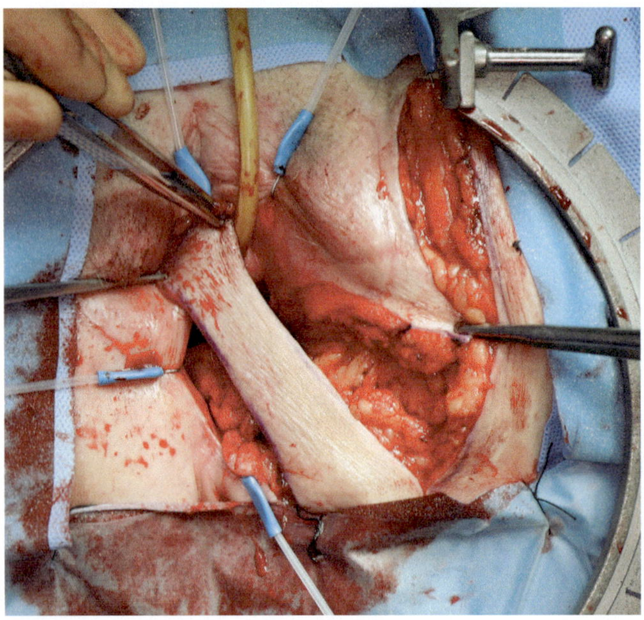

Fig. 5.74 The base of the labia is grasped with Allis clamps, elevated, and detached from the lateral vaginal fascia and the underlying pubic bone and obturator fascia. The labial flap is mobilized lateral toward the left

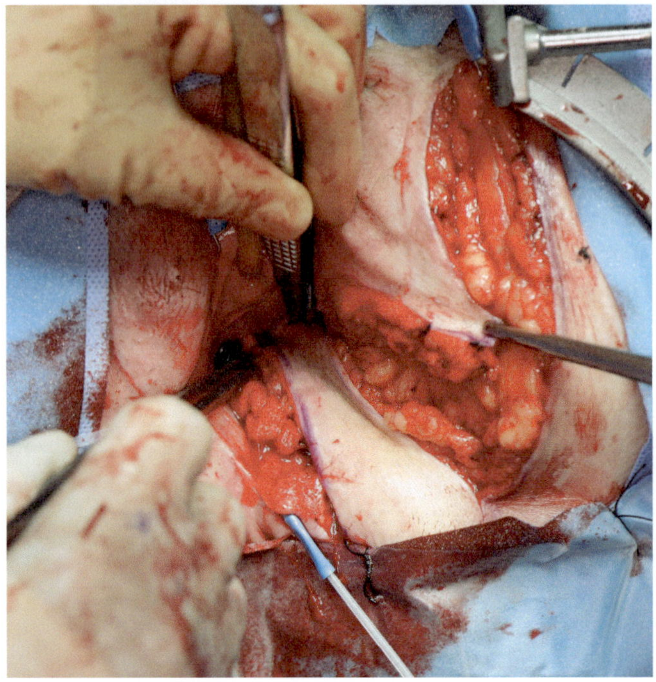

Fig. 5.75 The flaps will be crossed over. The inner thigh flap is rotated medially toward the vaginal canal and the labial flap is rotated laterally toward the lateral thigh incision

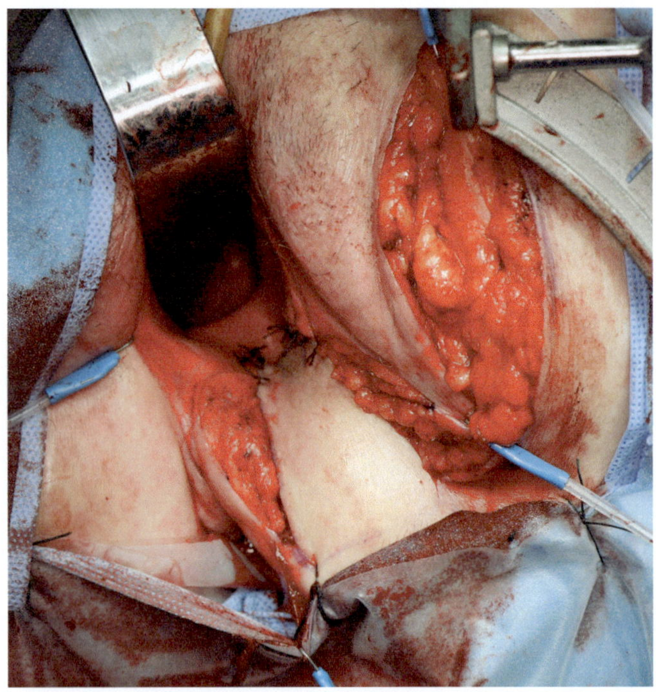

Fig. 5.76 The inner thigh flap is transferred to the vaginal cuff to cover the area of the fistula repair. Preplaced sutures facilitate the advancement and suturing of the flap to the vaginal wall margins

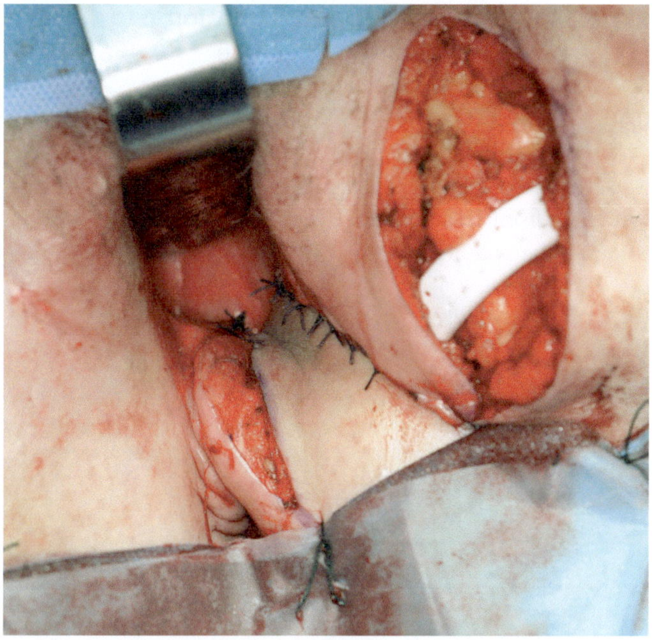

Fig. 5.77 Interrupted delay absorbable sutures have completed the anastomosis of the flap to the vaginal incision at the 2 o'clock position

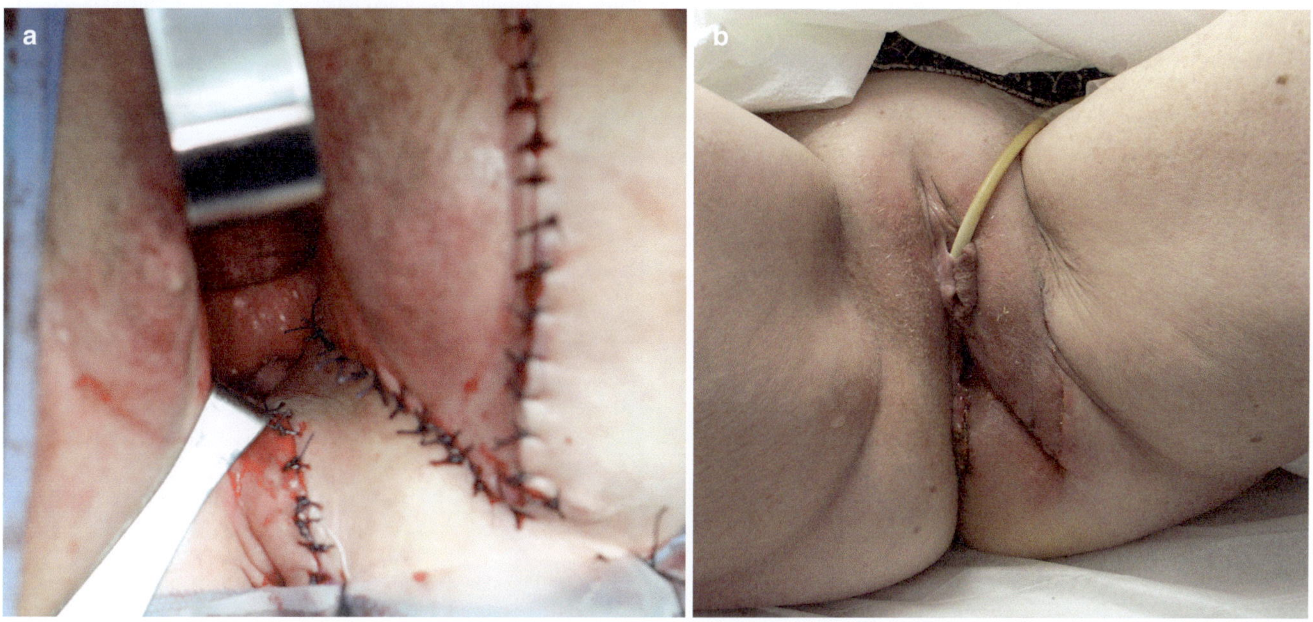

Fig. 5.78 (a) The anastomosis of the medial segment of the flap and the medial vaginal incision at the 7 o'clock position have been completed. The incision of the inner thigh is also completed, using interrupted delay absorbable sutures. The lateral aspect of the labia flap is easily approximated to the lateral donor site incision. (b) Postoperative picture 5 months after surgery, showing good take of the flap. The patient has good vaginal depth, the fistula was cured, and the patient was able to resume sexual relations

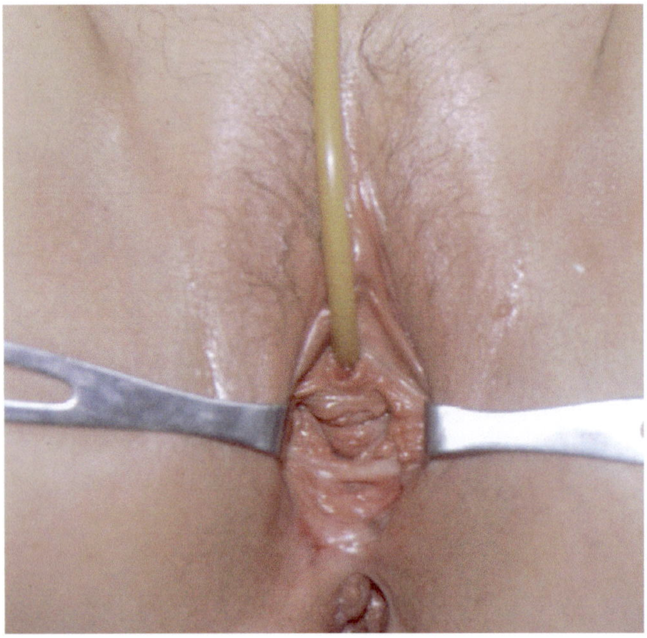

Fig. 5.79 Exposure of the vaginal wall showing a short, fibrotic vagina with a high vesicovaginal fistula

5.1.3.14 Repair of Recurrent Radiation Vesicovaginal Fistula: Use of a Myocutaneous Gracilis Flap

The patient in Figs. 5.80, 5.81, and 5.82 presented with a recurrent vesicovaginal fistula due to pelvic radiation. She was treated with the use of a myocutaneous gracilis flap, which is used less frequently in very selected cases as an alternative to an inner thigh flap.

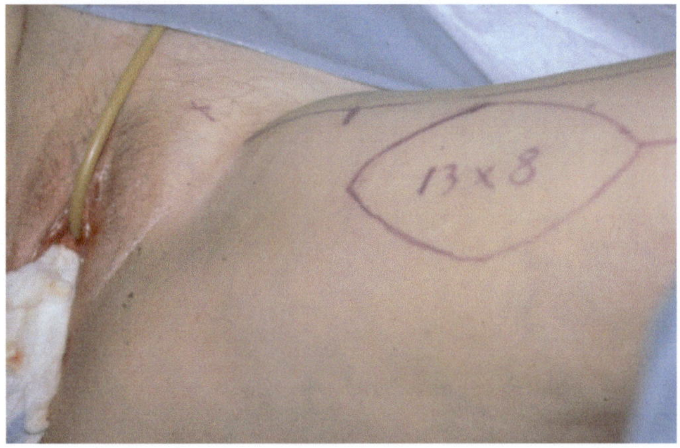

Fig. 5.80 The inner thigh and inner aspect of the leg are exposed. The size and location of the donor site are marked

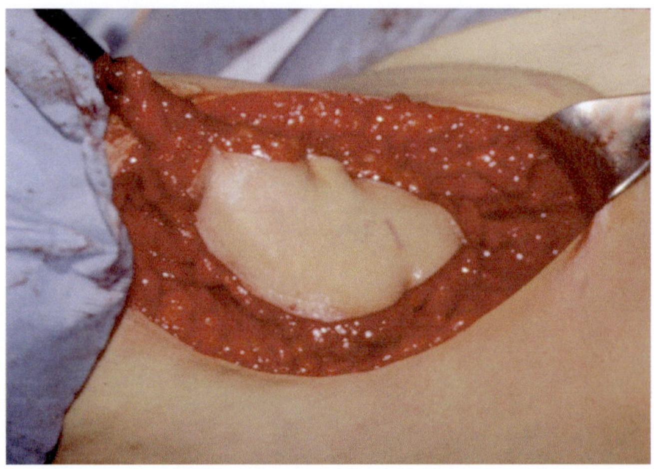

Fig. 5.81 The skin, the subcutaneous tissue, and the detached gracilis muscle are mobilized free

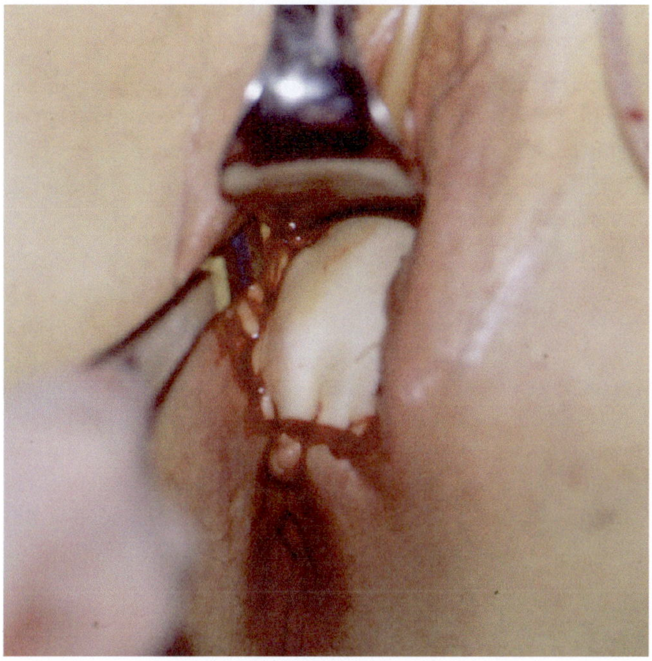

Fig. 5.82 The myocutaneous gracilis flap is transferred through a tunnel under the thigh to the vaginal canal, where it is anastomosed to the margins of the excised vaginal wall after closure of the fistula

5.1.4 Intraoperative Complications

Bleeding can be a problem during the dissection of the vaginal flaps and should be controlled with fine absorbable sutures. Apical fistulae generally do not require ureteric catheterization, but this maneuver is recommended for fistulae close to the trigonal area because of the higher risk of ureteric injury. If there is doubt, cystoscopy after injection of indigo carmine and ureteric catheterization should be performed to ensure the integrity of the ureters. The strength of the first and second lines of closure is crucial for a successful outcome. Excessive dissection of the fistulous tract may turn a small opening in a large tract and compromise the quality of the repair, so we advocate not excising the fistulous tract, avoiding the thinning of the surgical margins, and providing a strong anchor to the line of suture. When in doubt, adjunctive procedures such as the fibro-fatty labial flap (Martius flap) or the other techniques described should be used.

5.1.5 Postoperative Care

The vagina is packed with an antibiotic-impregnated gauze, which may be removed after several hours. The suprapubic and urethral catheters are joined to a Y connector and left in place for 10 days. An oral cephalosporin or fluoroquinolone is continued until the catheters are discontinued, and cholinolytics are given to minimize bladder spasms. Prior to catheter removal, a voiding cystogram is performed to evaluate the integrity of the repair. Sexual relations may resume after 12 weeks.

Postoperatively, the patient receives antibiotics until the Foley catheter is removed and anticholinergics to avoid bladder spasms. Most of the procedures described above can be performed as outpatient surgery. The patient is discharged after surgery, with the only restriction being instructions to avoid strenuous exercise. The most important aspect of postoperative care is uninterrupted catheter drainage. The urethral catheter is removed on days 10–14 after surgery and a suprapubic cystogram is performed. If the outpatient cystogram documents vesical integrity, the suprapubic catheter is removed. Patients should abstain from sexual intercourse for 3 months.

5.1.6 Postoperative Complications

Immediate complications such as vaginal infection, bladder spasms, or vaginal bleeding should be treated aggressively to avoid fistula recurrence. Perioperative antibiotics are important to avoid vaginal wall infection and should be continued as required. Bladder spasms may lead to breakage of the repair and should be treated with cholinolytic agents, as well as local anesthetics if required. Secondary vaginal bleeding should be treated with bed rest and vaginal packing if necessary.

Vaginal stenosis and shortening may result from unnecessary excessive resection of the vaginal wall and may require secondary vaginoplasty. Unrecognized ureteric injury (leak or, more commonly, obstruction) may require percutaneous nephrostomy and a cooling-off period. Endoscopy procedures such as retrograde catheterization or transurethral ureteroscopy should be avoided in the immediate postoperative period; antegrade procedures are more acceptable.

The most important complication is recurrence of the fistula. The repair will succeed in more than 95 % of cases with adherence to the basic principles of wide mobilization and tension-free closure, with multiple non-crossing layers. If the fistula does recur, it can be repaired through the vagina again after a proper waiting period, but a flap of fibro-fatty labial tissue or peritoneum should be used.

5.2 Repair of Rectovaginal Fistula

Rectovaginal fistula may occur spontaneously (as in immune-suppressed patients), but most commonly they result from radiation, perirectal or intra-abdominal infections, or traumatic injury of the rectovaginal area (obstetric, instrumental, or external).

5.2.1 Indications

Corrective surgery is indicated in medically fit patients. Diverting colostomy is required in some cases, depending on the size and etiology of the fistula and whether the patient has a history of prior failures or inflammatory conditions such as ulcerative colitis. Colostomy may be avoided if the fistula is small, well defined, and distal.

5.2.2 Diagnosis

The diagnosis is obvious, as stool material is seen flowing into the vagina. Physical examination reveals the location, size, and number of fistulous tracts. It is important to determine the function and tone of the anal sphincter and the integrity of the rest of the rectal wall and distal colon. Rectosigmoidoscopy, pelvic CT scans, and radiological evaluation of the gastrointestinal tract should be performed when indicated.

5.2.3 Preoperative Considerations

The use of adjuvant measures like proper antibiotic cover, estrogen replacement, and complete bowel preparation are important. The decision to perform simultaneous or initial diverting colostomy is based on the extent of the fistula, its size, its etiology (radiation fistula requires colostomy), and the general condition of the patient.

Tissue flaps to cover the fistulous area with fresh vascularized tissue should be used routinely. The most common alternatives are fibro-fatty tissue of the labia (Martius flap), labial skin, inner thigh skin, or gracilis muscular flaps. Prior to preparation and draping, copious irrigation of the rectum is performed to clear any residual stool matter.

5.2.4 Surgical Technique

Figures 5.83, 5.84, 5.85, 5.86, 5.87, 5.88, 5.89, 5.90, 5.91, 5.92, 5.93, 5.94, 5.95, and 5.96 illustrate the surgical treatment of a patient with a small, distal rectovaginal fistula.

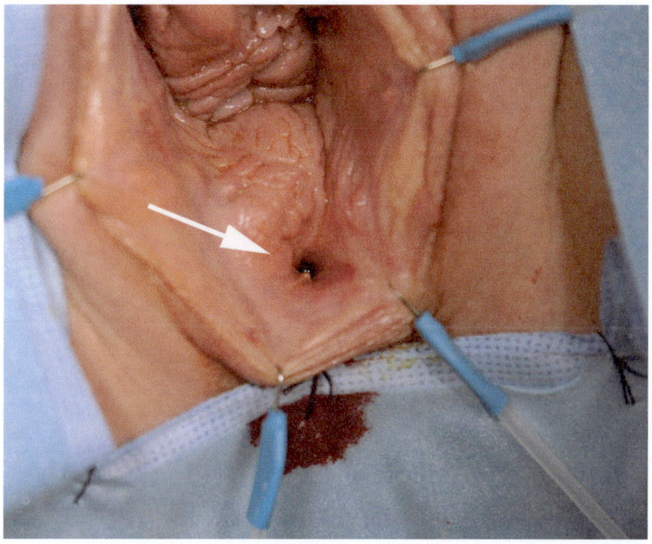

Fig. 5.83 Vaginal examination showing a small, distal rectovaginal fistula (*arrow*)

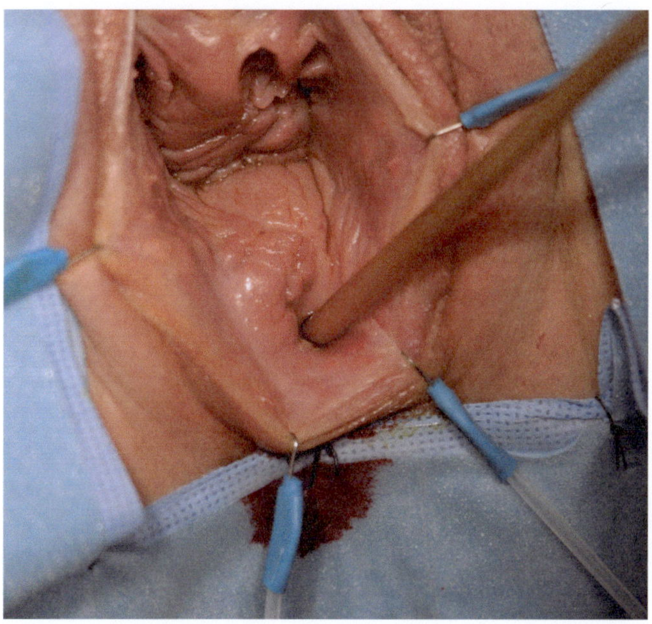

Fig. 5.84 A Foley catheter is inserted into the fistulous tract. The catheter will facilitate the dissection and isolation of the fistulous tract

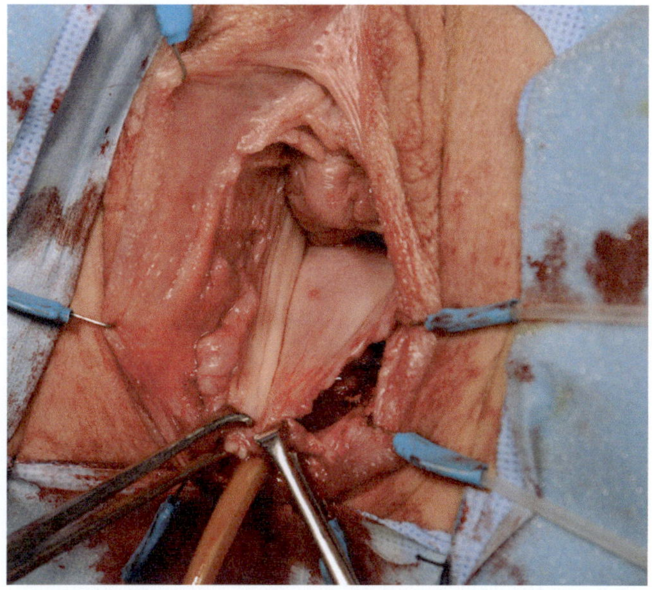

Fig. 5.85 A U incision in the posterior vaginal wall is created with the distal tip in the area of the fistula. The flap is extended 5–8 cm toward the proximal vagina. A flap to the prerectal fascia (if present) will be developed and used later to reinforce the closure of the fistula. A flap of the vaginal wall is created distally to the fistula, reaching the posterior fourchette or distal vagina 3–4 cm from the fistula

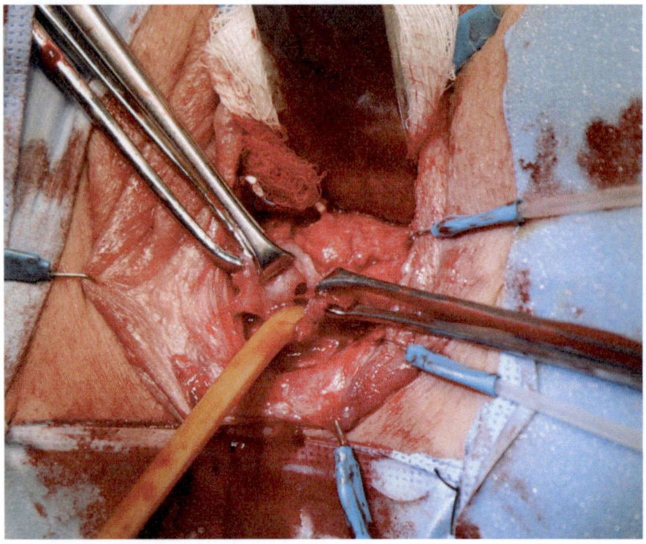

Fig. 5.86 The fistulous tract and the anterior rectal wall are exposed while the Foley catheter is in place

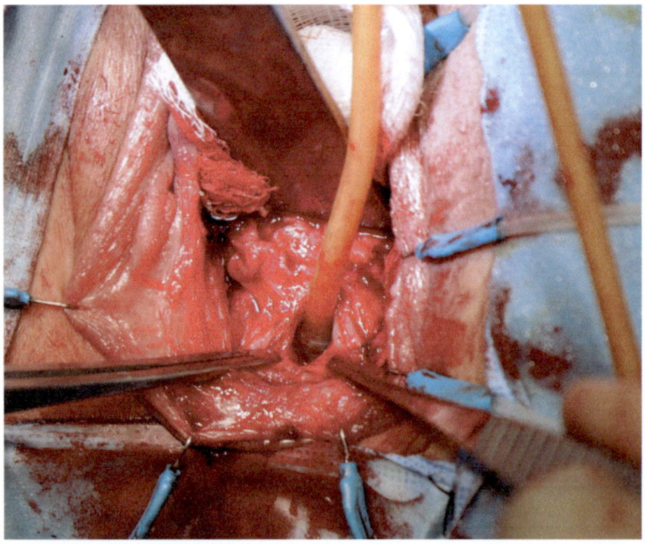

Fig. 5.87 The fistulous tract has been leaving a small ring of the fistulous tract. Wide exposure of the fistula is obtained for several centimeters around the fistula

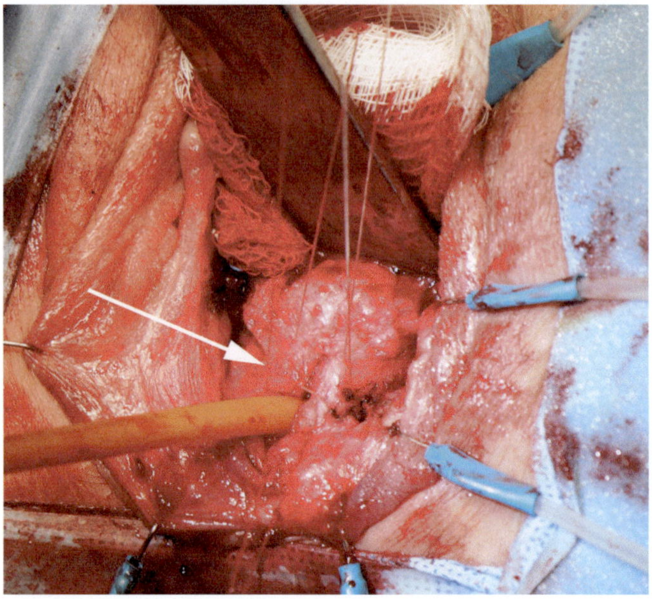

Fig. 5.88 The fistulous tract is closed, incorporating the whole rectal wall and the margins of the fistulous tract

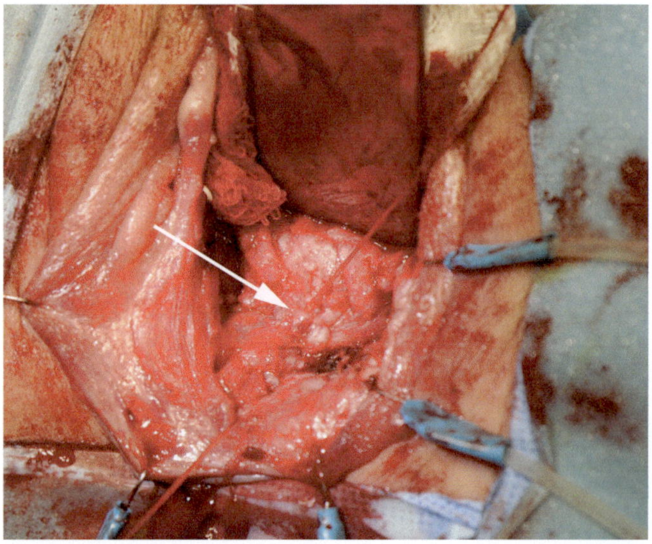

Fig. 5.89 The fistulous tract (*arrow*) is closed with two layers of delayed absorbable sutures. Irrigation of the rectum with a diluted iodine solution confirms that there is no extravasation

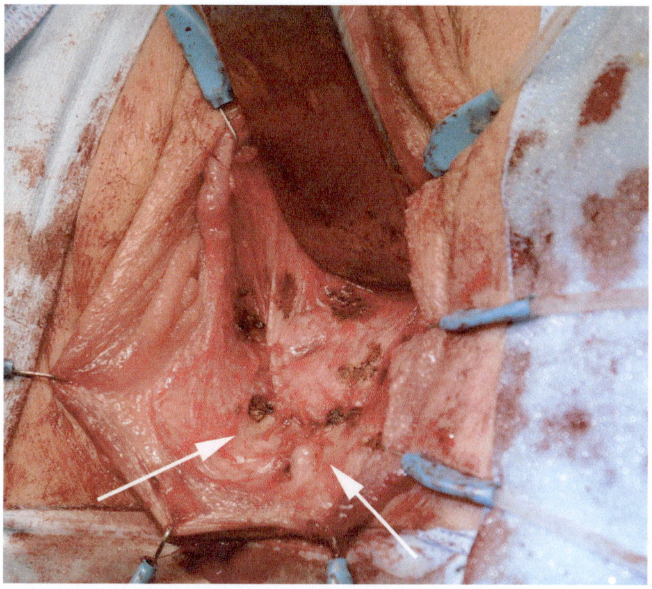

Fig. 5.90 The prerectal flap created at the beginning of the posterior flap creation is advanced distally to cover the area of the fistula repair

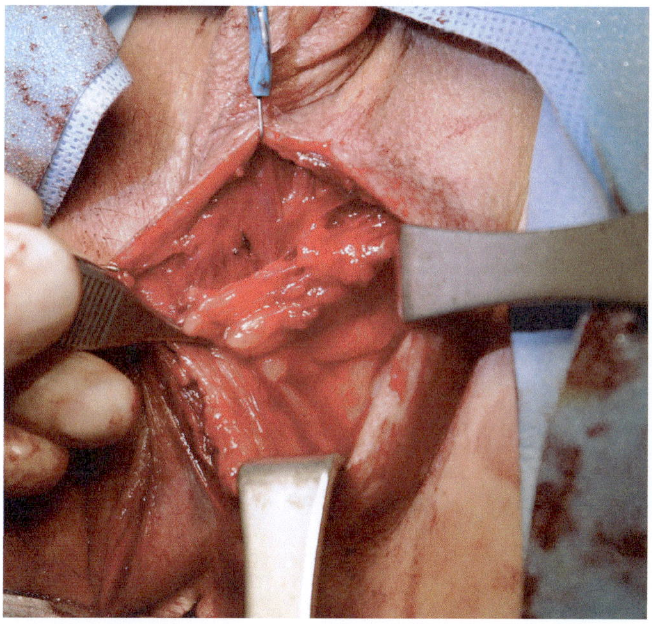

Fig. 5.91 A vertical incision is made over the left labia majora. The fibro-fatty (Martius) flap is isolated, preserving its inferior pedicle

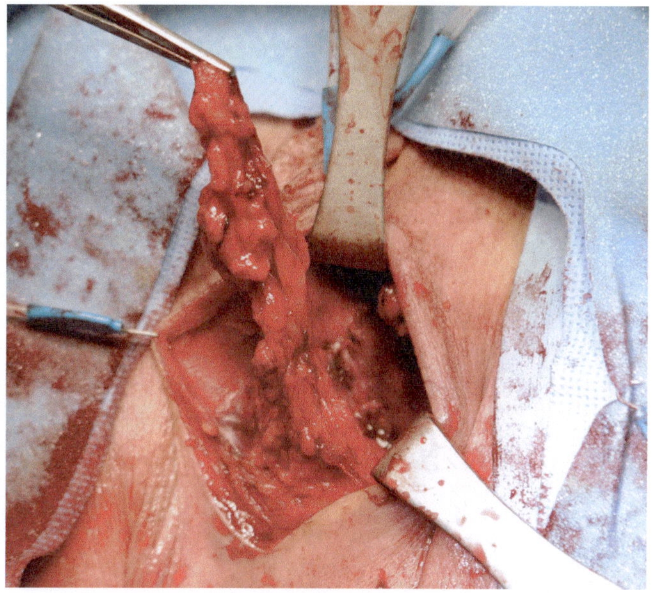

Fig. 5.92 The Martius flap has been mobilized and the superior segment tied and cut anterior to the pubic bone

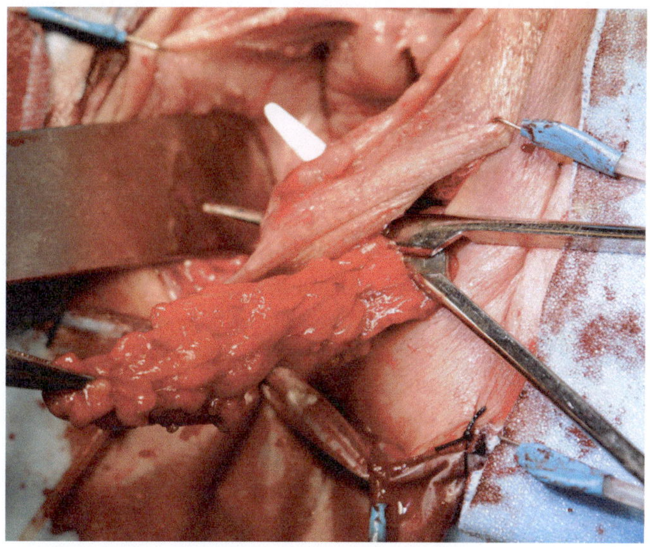

Fig. 5.93 A tunnel is made under the labia toward the anterior rectal wall

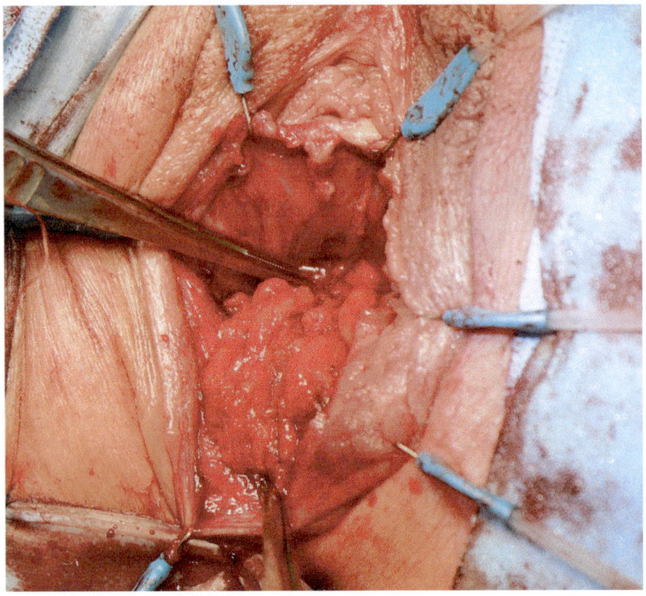

Fig. 5.94 The fibro-fatty tissue (Martius flap) is transferred over the anterior rectal wall in the vaginal canal. Interrupted absorbable sutures are used to fix the flap to the rectal wall and prevent displacement. The flaps should cover at least 3 cm around the closed fistulous tract

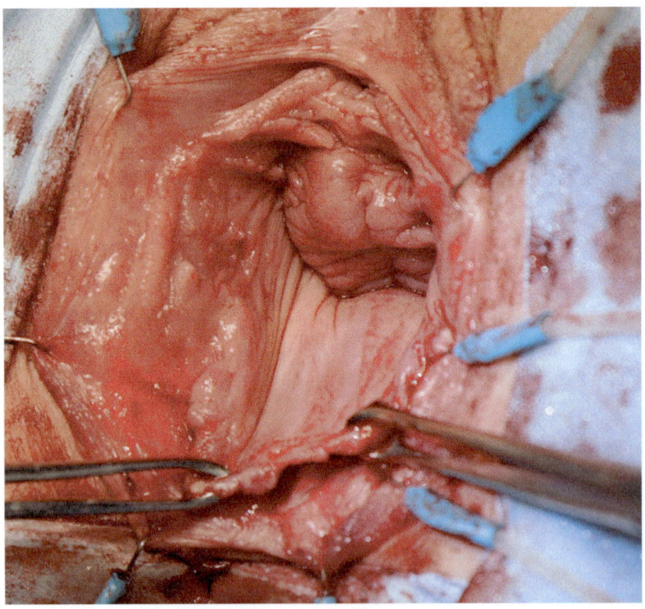

Fig. 5.95 The posterior vaginal wall flap is advanced distally so new tissue covers the area of the reconstruction

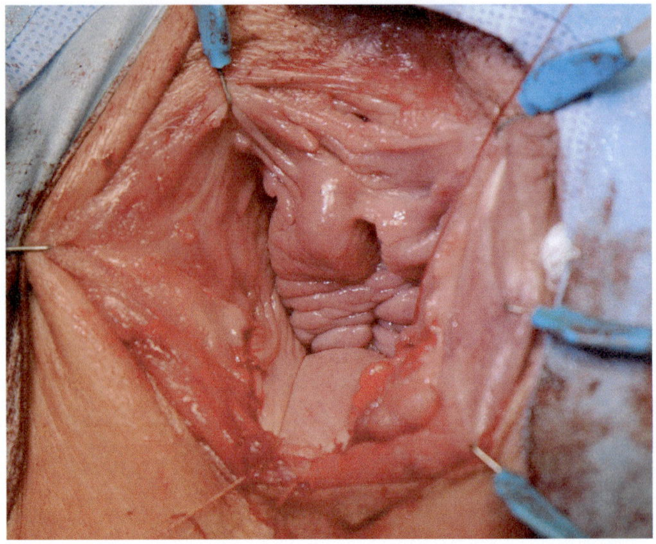

Fig. 5.96 Final view of the posterior vaginal wall. The posterior vaginal wall flap extends to the introitus

5.2.5 Intraoperative Complications

Complications are rare and common to other rectal surgery. An inability to bring together the edges of the fistula may be caused by poor quality of the tissues owing to radiation or infection. In these cases, the surgery should be performed with a concomitant diverting colostomy.

5.2.6 Postoperative Care

The vaginal packing is removed after a few hours. Regular diet can be resumed immediately. Broad-spectrum antibiotic coverage should be continued for at least 1 week. If a diverting colostomy is performed, a waiting period of 3–6 months is recommended before a takedown. Direct and radiological examination should be performed to confirm the healing of the fistula.

5.2.7 Postoperative Complications

Recurrent fistula requires re-exploration and a diverting colostomy, if it was not performed in the first surgery. Contributing to this complication is undue tension of the suture line or wound infection. Abscess formation requires incision and drainage. Vaginal or rectal stenosis is a rare complication.

5.3 Repair of Rectoperineal Fistula

Traumatic delivery, perineal surgery, or direct trauma to the vaginal area may cause a fistula from the rectum to the perineum. On occasion, a perirectal or perineal abscess may drain into the rectum and create a fistulous tract to the perineum.

5.3.1 Diagnosis

This condition is clinically manifested with the appearance of stool contents in the perineal or vaginal area. On physical examination, the open fistula is seen in the perineum or vagina. The rectal examination will help to characterize the size and location of the communication. A probe or catheter in the fistula will help to better define the fistulous tract. Assessment of anal function and sphincter tone should be documented preoperatively. Radiological or endoscopic examinations are usually not necessary; they are performed only to rule out conditions like cancer, ulcerative colitis, or Crohn's disease.

5.3.2 Preoperative Considerations

A 48-h full bowel preparation should be performed prior to any surgery. Diverting colostomy is recommended in most cases but is not always necessary. Rotational flaps of fibro-fatty tissue from the labia or the gluteal or perineal area are usually performed to provide a thick, vascular layer of tissue interposition.

5.3.3 Surgical Technique

This section describes the surgical technique for three cases. First is a simpler case of rectoperineal fistula due to ulcerative colitis, in which a subcutaneous flap of fat from the perineum is used for the reconstruction (Figs. 5.97, 5.98, 5.99, 5.100, 5.101, 5.102, 5.103, 5.104, 5.105, and 5.106). The second case has stool incontinence due to poor sphincter function and a rectoperineal fistula requiring anal sphincter repair and repair of the fistula (Figs. 5.107, 5.108, 5.109, 5.110, 5.111, 5.112, 5.113, 5.114, 5.115, 5.116, 5.117, 5.118, and 5.119). The third, more complex case had a rectoperineal fistula, rectovaginal fistula, and anal sphincter incompetence due to traumatic delivery. After multiple failed repairs, this patient required repair of the rectovaginal fistula, reconstruction of the anal sphincter (internal and external), and repair of the rectoperineal fistula (Figs. 5.120, 5.121, 5.122, 5.123, 5.124, and 5.125).

5.3.3.1 Repair of Recurrent Rectoperineal Fistula with Interposition of Perineal Fat

Prior to preparation and draping, the rectum is irrigated with a copious amount of antibiotic solution. Broad-spectrum antibiotics are given intravenously. A Foley catheter is inserted and a ring retractor with hooks is used to facilitate the surgical exposure. Figures 5.98, 5.99, 5.100, 5.101, 5.102, 5.103, 5.104, and 5.105 show the technique used.

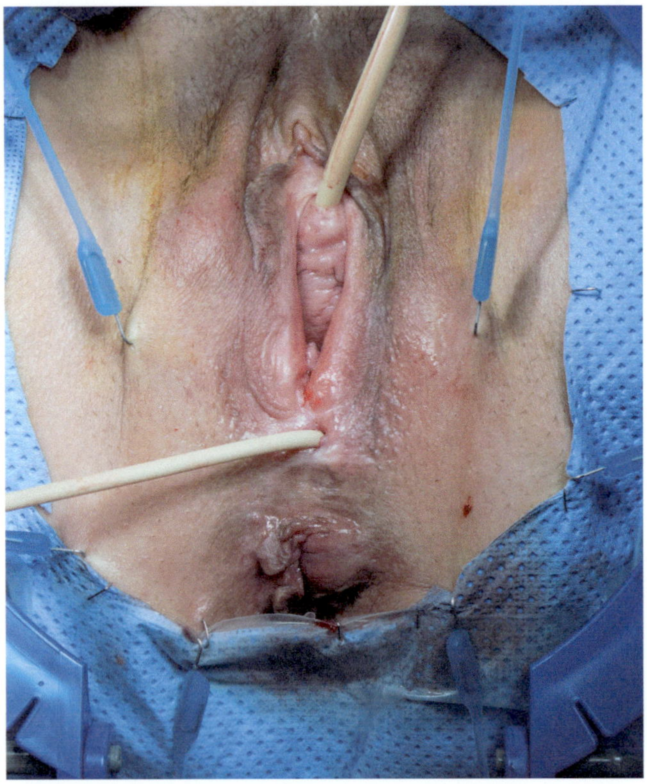

Fig. 5.97 Exposure of the perineum is obtained. A small Foley catheter is inserted through the fistula into the rectum and placed under slight traction

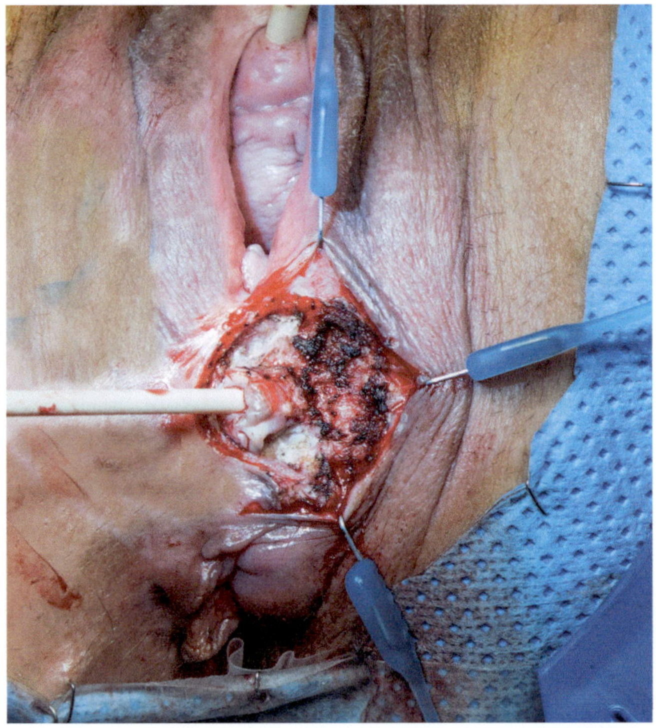

Fig. 5.98 A circular incision is made in the perineum around the fistula, and lateral dissection is done at least 3–4 cm from the fistula

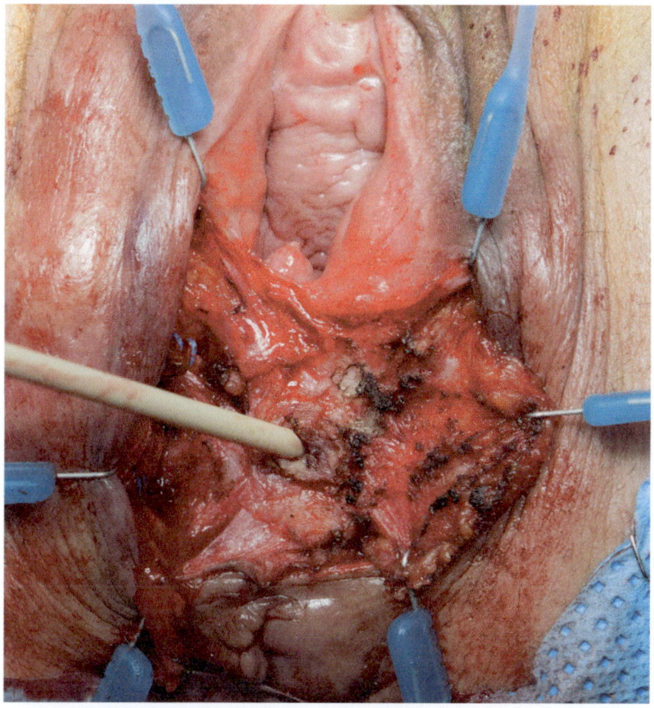

Fig. 5.99 After the dissection, the trans-anal fistulous tract is isolated

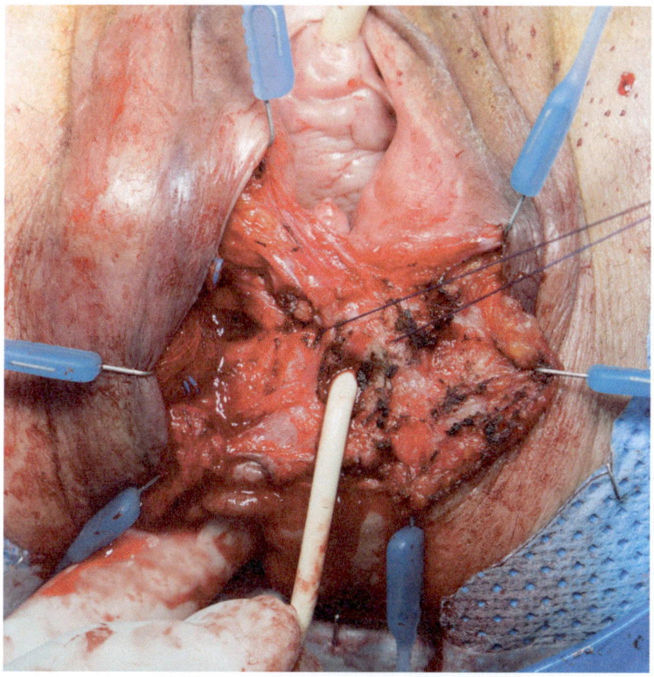

Fig. 5.100 Under finger control in the rectum, multiple figure-of-eight delayed absorbable sutures are used to approximate the fistulous tract

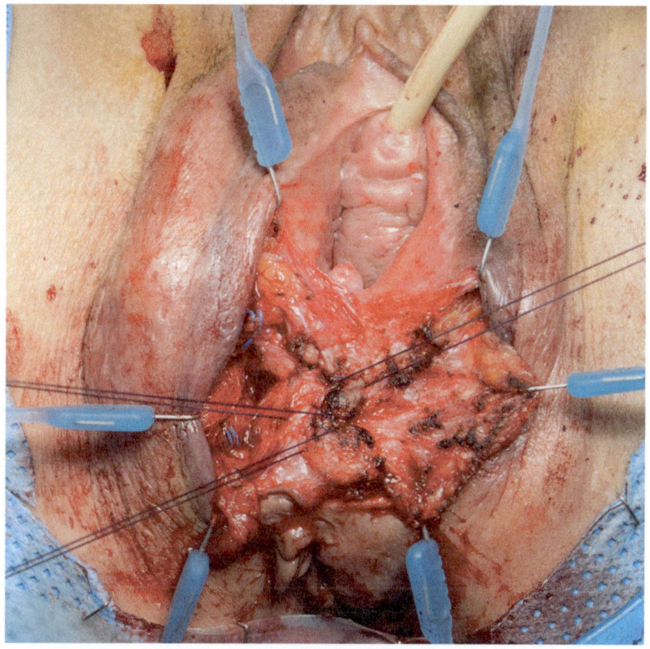

Fig. 5.101 A second layer of mattress sutures 5 mm from the fistula is applied to cover the first layer of closure. Rectal irrigation with a diluted iodine solution will confirm that there is no leakage from the fistula

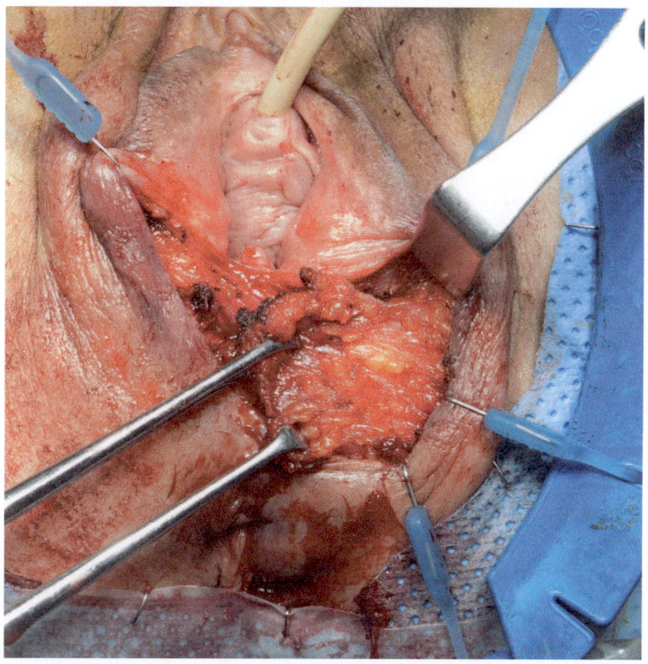

Fig. 5.102 On the left side, the skin is undermined and the perineal fat is mobilized. The dissection will often include the incision of the lower margin of the fat flap to allow mobility and rotation. The flap must reach the contralateral side of the skin incision and cover the rectal repair without tension

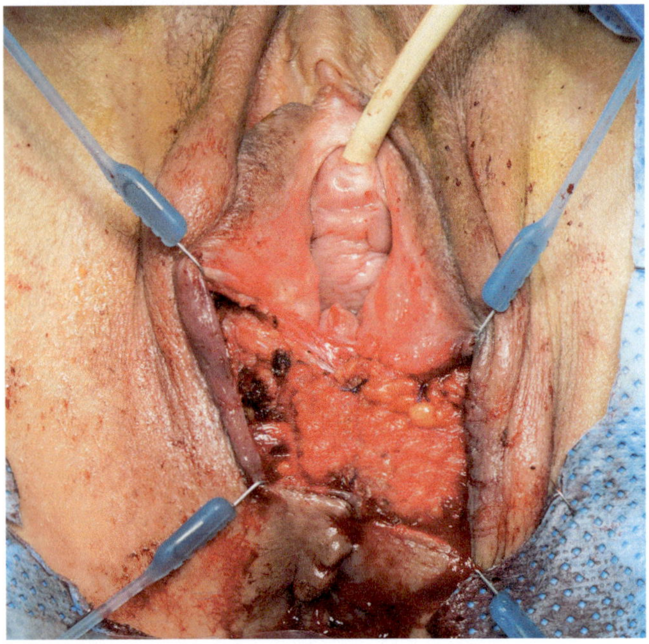

Fig. 5.103 The free margins of the perineal fat flap are transferred to the contralateral side and sutured medial, superior, and inferior to the perineal tissues, covering the area of the fistula repair

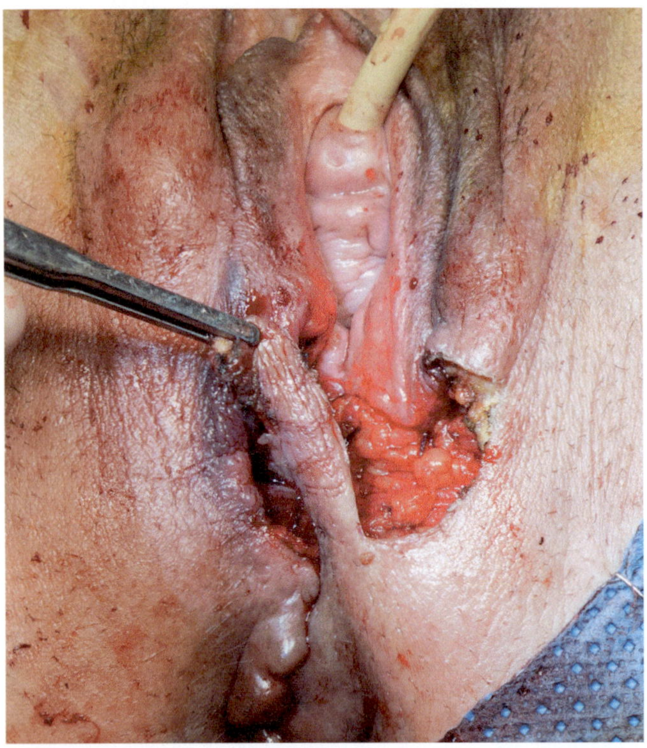

Fig. 5.104 A strip of the superficial skin of the left lateral incision is excised, exposing the subcutaneous tissue

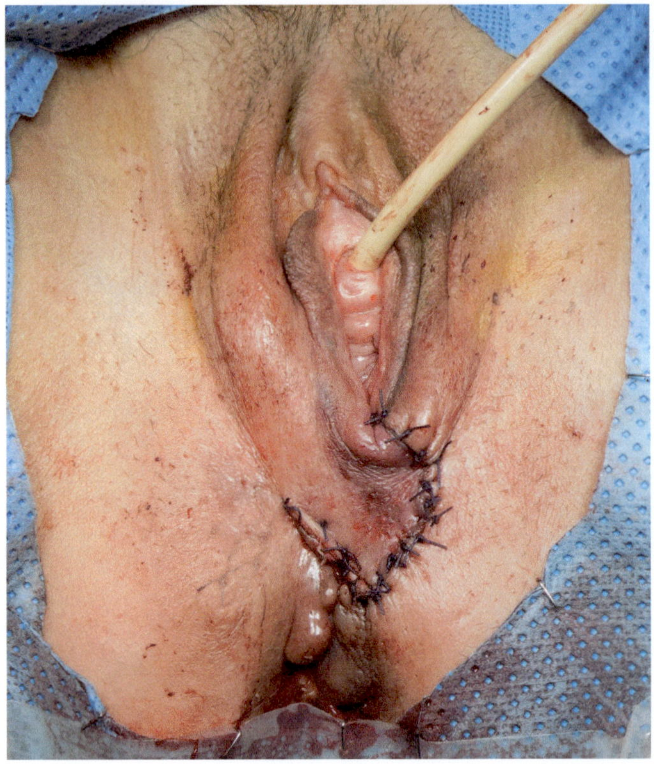

Fig. 5.105 The lower segment of the labia majora (with its subcutaneous fat) and the right skin incision are transferred to the left and sutured to the left skin margin. This segment of skin and subcutaneous tissue covers the reconstructed area, preventing overlapping lines of sutures

5.3.3.2 Repair of Rectoperineal and Rectovaginal Fistula with Concomitant Anal Sphincter Reconstruction

The patient in Figs. 5.106, 5.107, 5.108, 5.109, 5.110, 5.111, 5.112, 5.113, 5.114, 5.115, 5.116, 5.117, and 5.118 had a traumatic delivery resulting in an extensive rectal and perineal tear. Multiple repairs have failed, and the patient remains with a perineal rectal fistula, rectovaginal fistula, and an open, incompetent anal sphincter. Most stools come from the vagina and perineum.

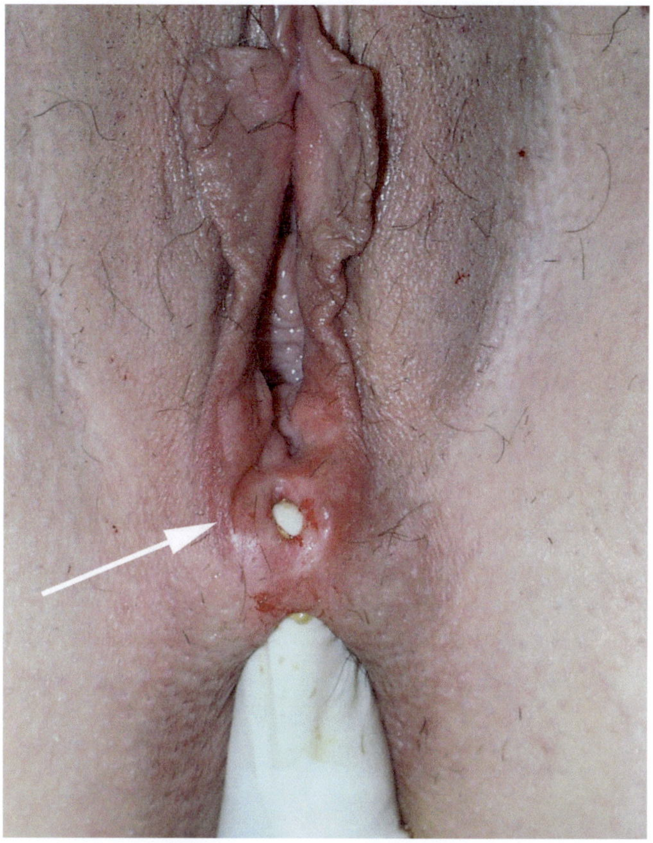

Fig. 5.106 Perineal examination of the patient who has a perineal fistula (*arrow*). A finger in the rectum is seen through one of the multiple fistulous tracts

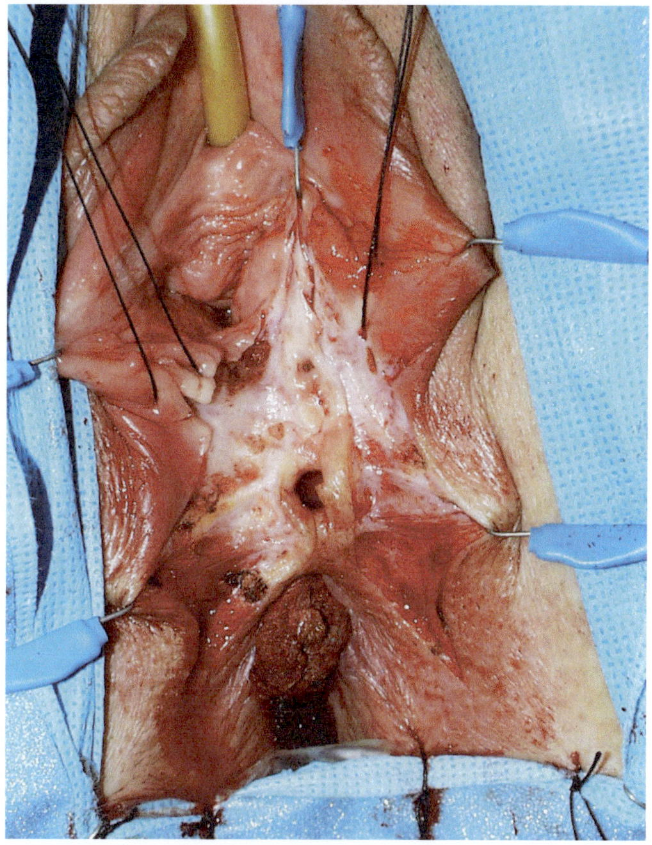

Fig. 5.107 A vertical incision is made from the distal vagina to the perineum. The perineal and vaginal skin is excised, exposing the fistulous area

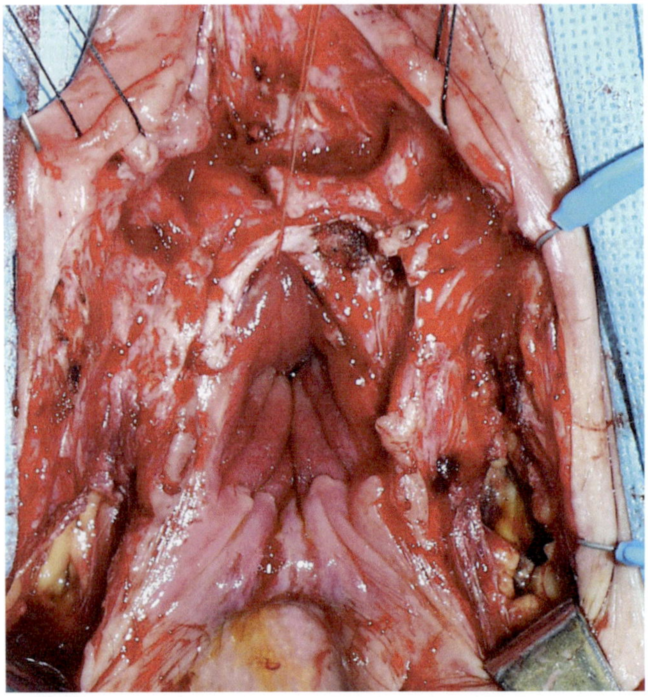

Fig. 5.108 After excision of the perineal and vaginal scar, the distal rectum and the anal canal are fully exposed. The anal sphincter was incompetent and damaged, and the musculature retracted laterally

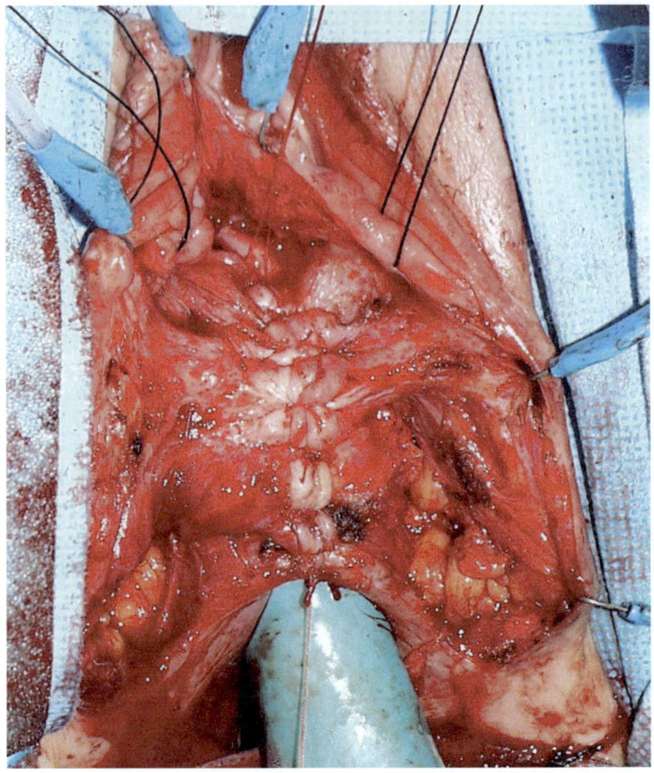

Fig. 5.110 With a finger in the rectum, the complete closure of the recto-anal mucosa and internal sphincter can be seen

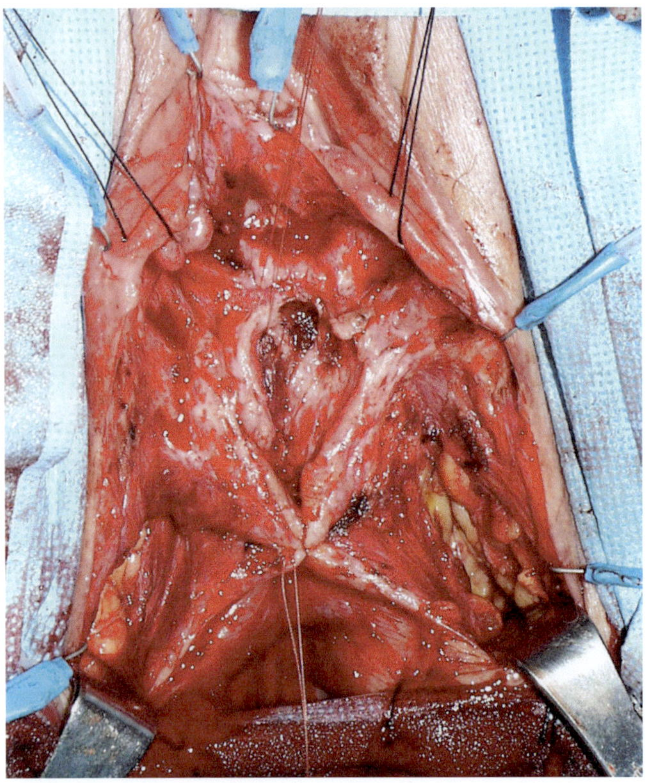

Fig. 5.109 The rectal wall and the mucosa of the anal canal are closed with running and interrupted #3-0 delay absorbable sutures

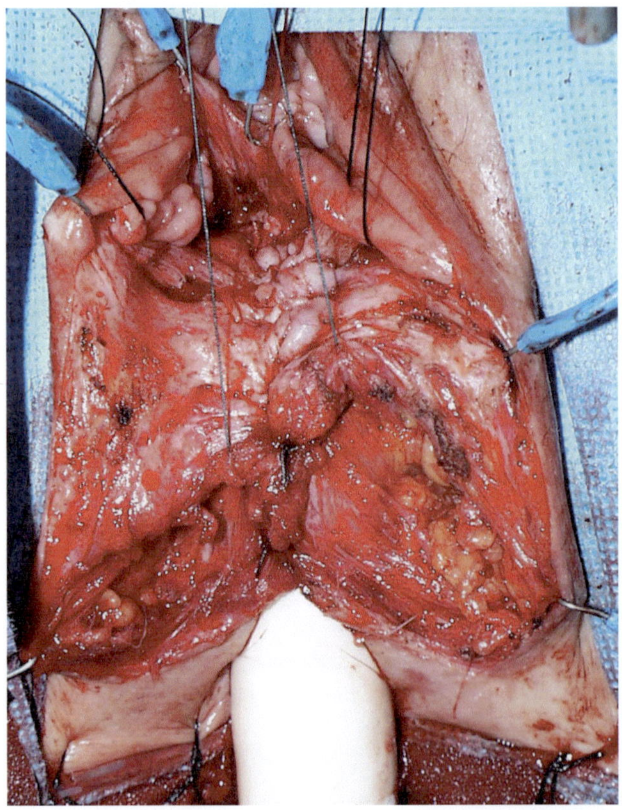

Fig. 5.111 The external anal sphincter and perineal musculature are approximated with figure-of-eight delay absorbable sutures to rebuild the anal canal and the perineal musculature

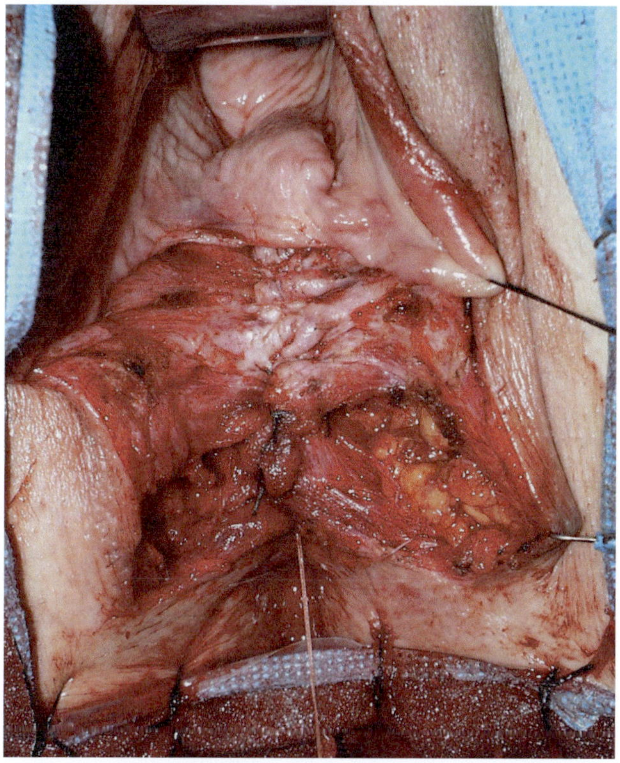

Fig. 5.112 Exposure of the posterior vaginal wall after the reconstruction of the anterior rectal wall and the anal sphincter

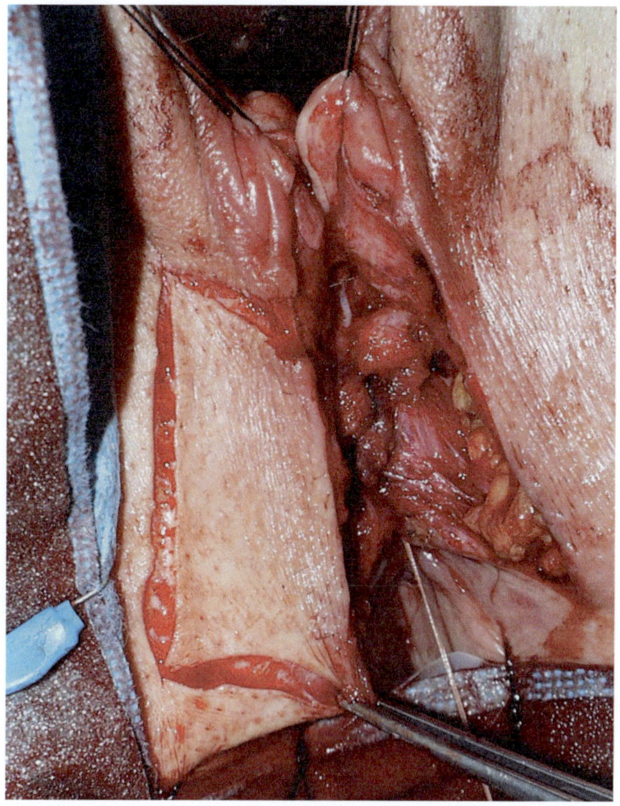

Fig. 5.114 A rectangle of superficial skin incision is made on the right margin of the perineal incision

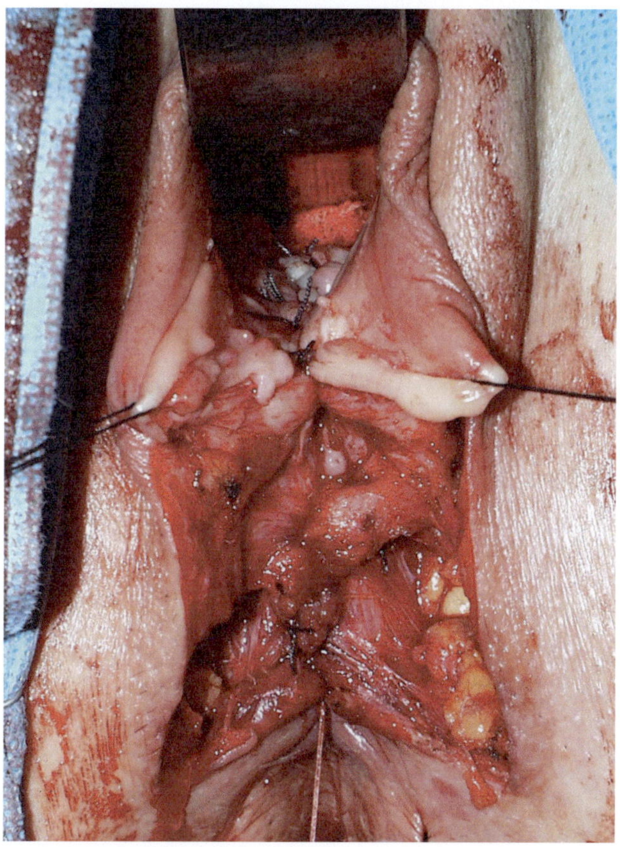

Fig. 5.113 The posterior vaginal wall is closed with running #2-0 delay absorbable sutures

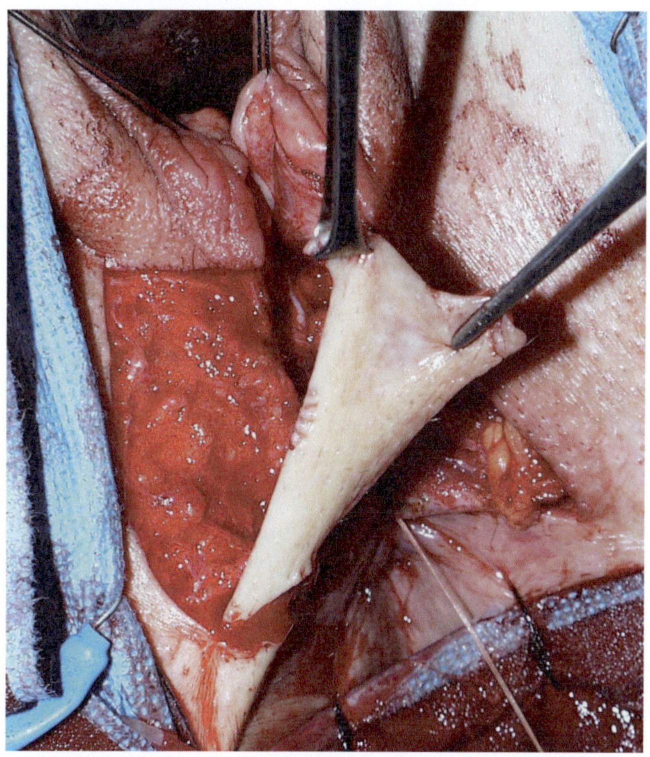

Fig. 5.115 The rectangle of skin is excised to expose the subcutaneous fatty tissue of the perineum on the right. The skin lateral to the right margin of the incision is mobilized

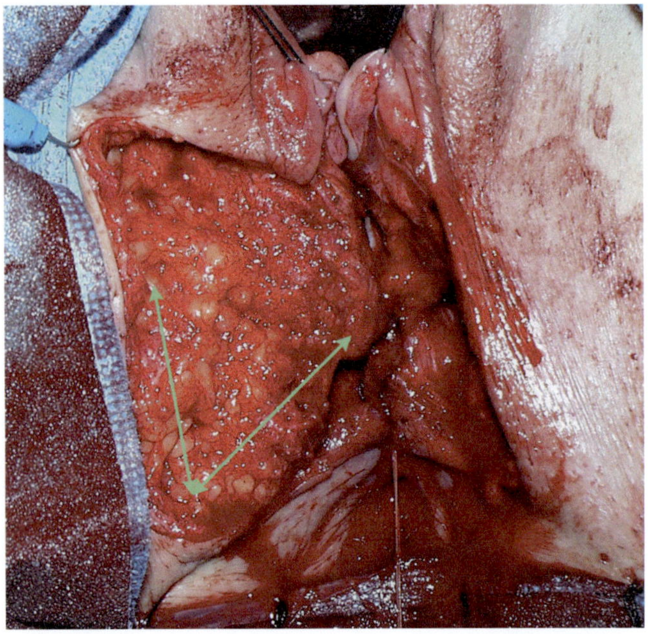

Fig. 5.116 An incision of subcutaneous fat is made at the inferior and lateral segments (*arrows*) to help mobilize a large flap of subcutaneous fat

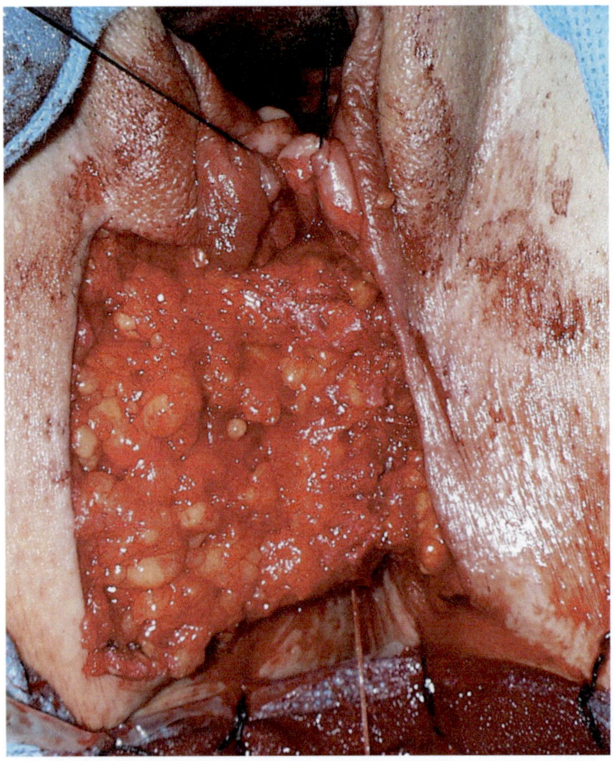

Fig. 5.117 The right subcutaneous flap of fat is rotated, transferred toward the left side of the perineum, and anchored with delayed absorbable sutures. The flap completely covers the perineal reconstruction

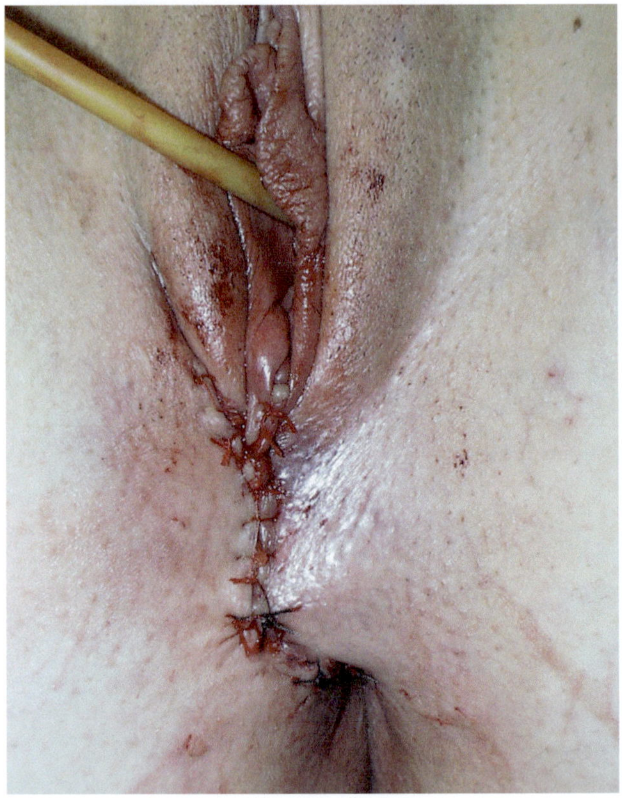

Fig. 5.118 The skin closure is done with multiple delayed absorbable sutures. The line of suture is asymmetric and crosses toward the right, where the rectangular skin flap was excised

5.3.3.3 Repair of Rectoperineal Fistula and Anal Sphincter Reconstruction

The patient in Figs. 5.119, 5.120, 5.121, 5.122, 5.123, 5.124, and 5.125 had a traumatic delivery resulting in a low-output perineal fistula and severe stool incontinence due to anterior anal sphincter damage.

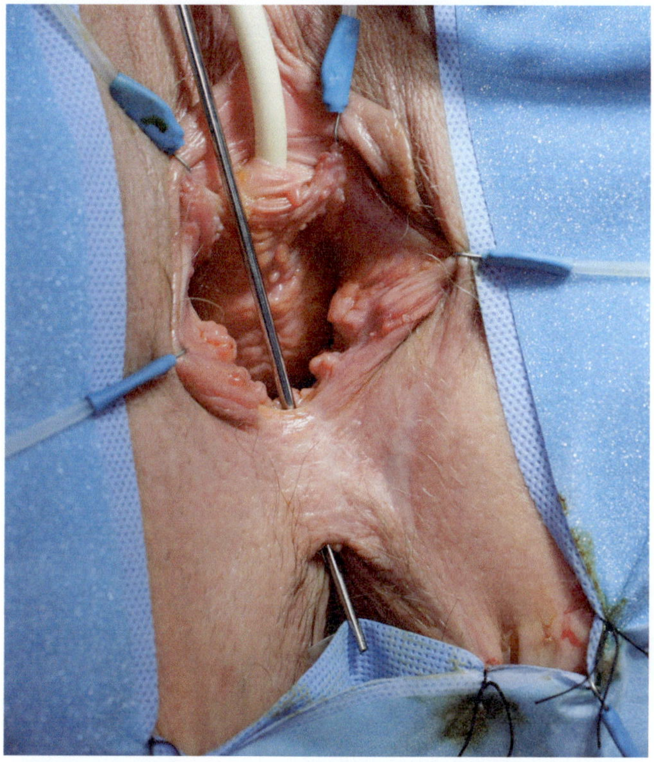

Fig. 5.119 With exposure of the perineum, a small probe inserted into the fistula can be seen coming out from the rectum

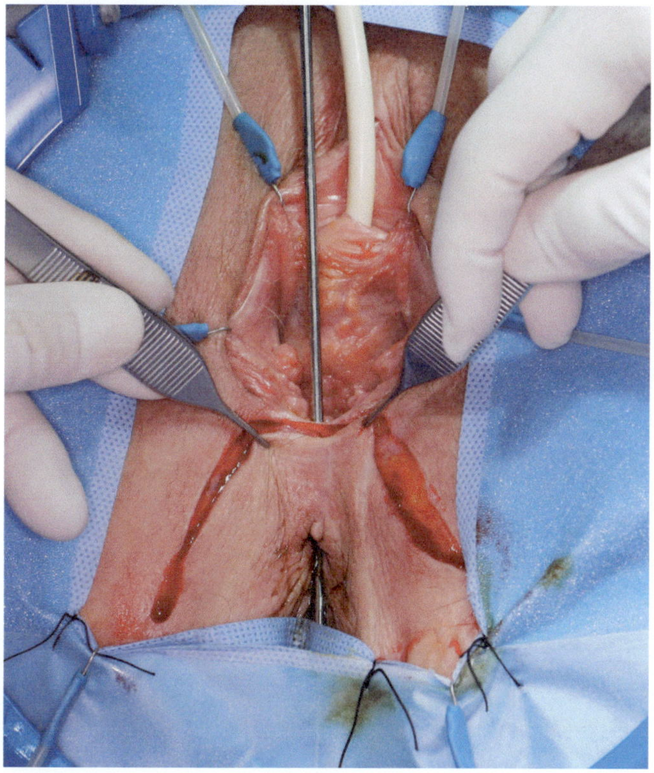

Fig. 5.120 An inverted U incision is made in the perineum, extending to the ischial tuberosities and distally toward the fistulous tract

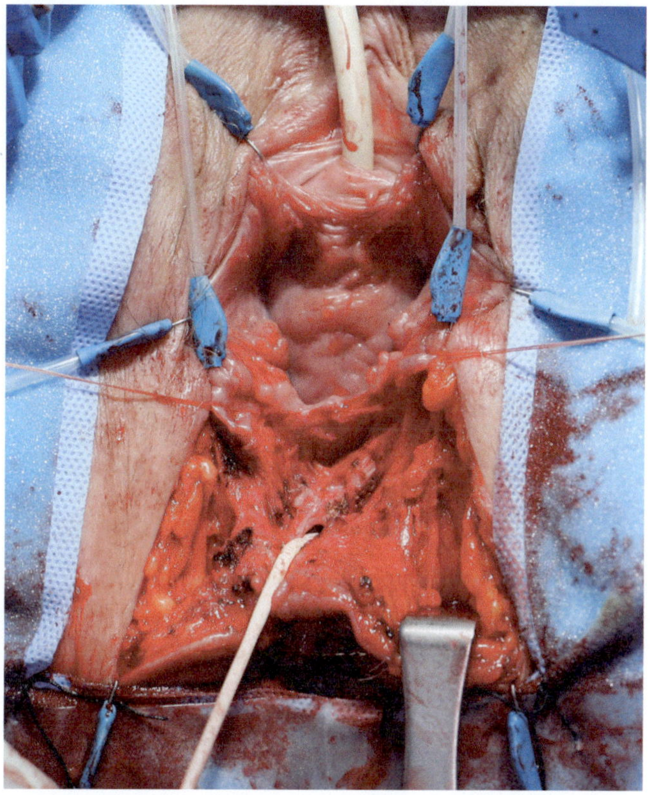

Fig. 5.121 The posterior perineum is exposed by entering the ischial fossa and exposing the levator (puborectalis and pubococcygeus). The perineal fistula will be closed in two layers of delayed absorbable sutures

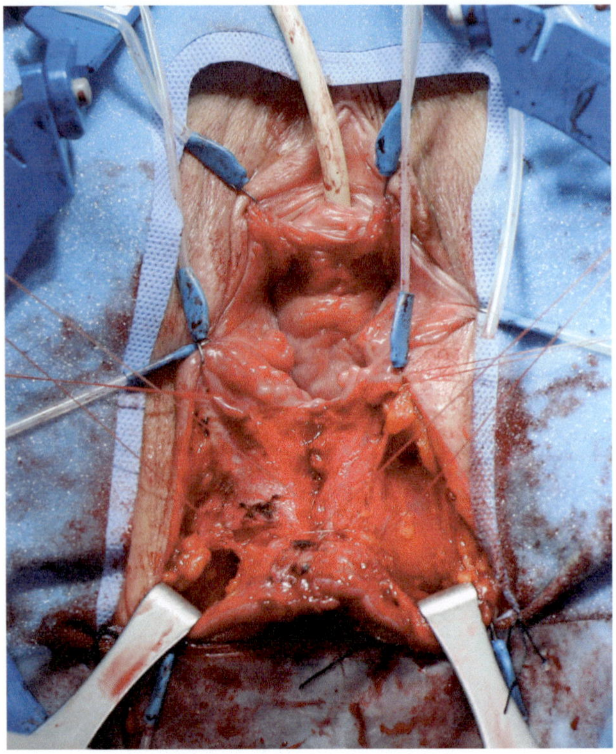

Fig. 5.122 Multiple figure-of-eight #0 delayed absorbable sutures are used to approximate the external anal sphincter musculature to the midline. The sutures are placed with a finger in the rectum to prevent mucosal penetration of the sutures. The sutures should avoid the inverted U flap of the perineum in order to allow for maximal mobility of the flap

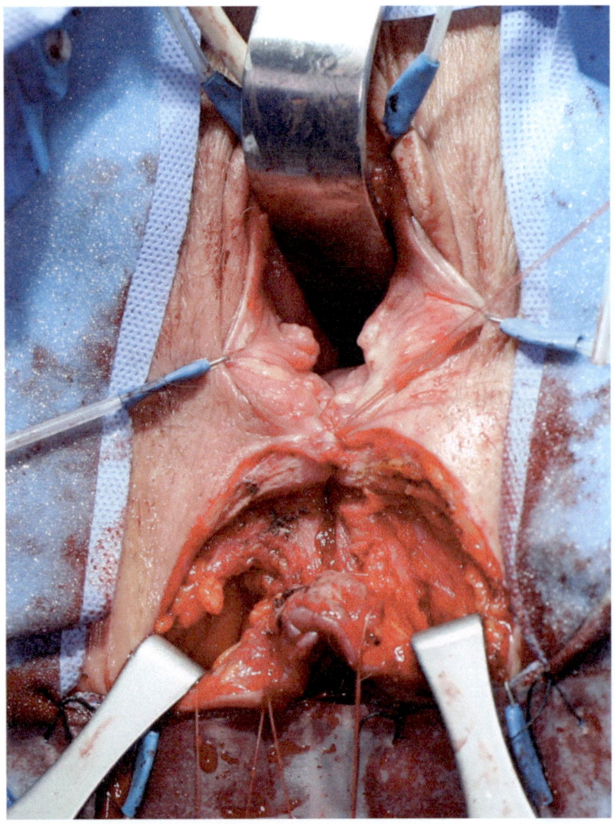

Fig. 5.123 The sutures are tied and the reconstructed perineum is seen

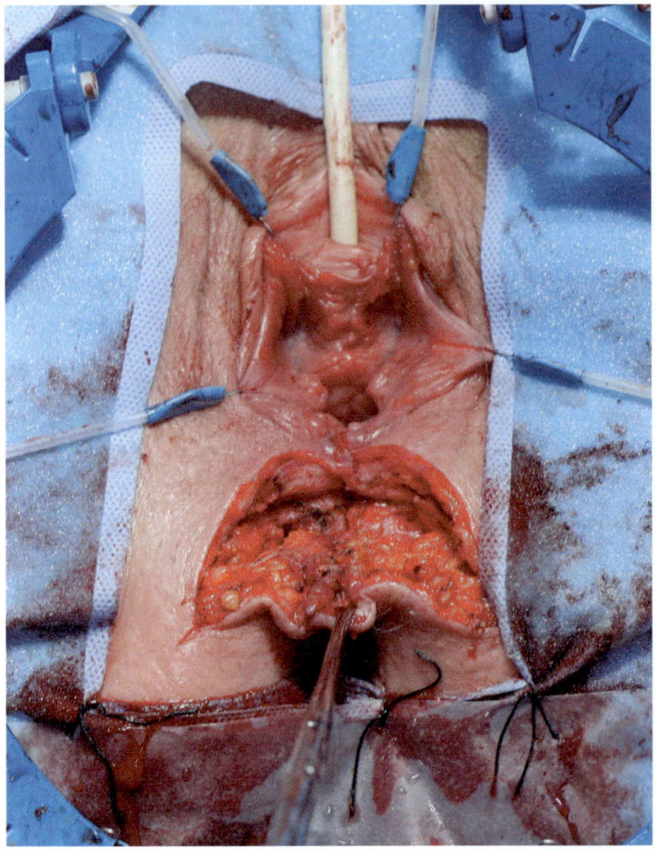

Fig. 5.124 The perineal skin flap is mobile and will be advanced distally to cover the area of reconstruction

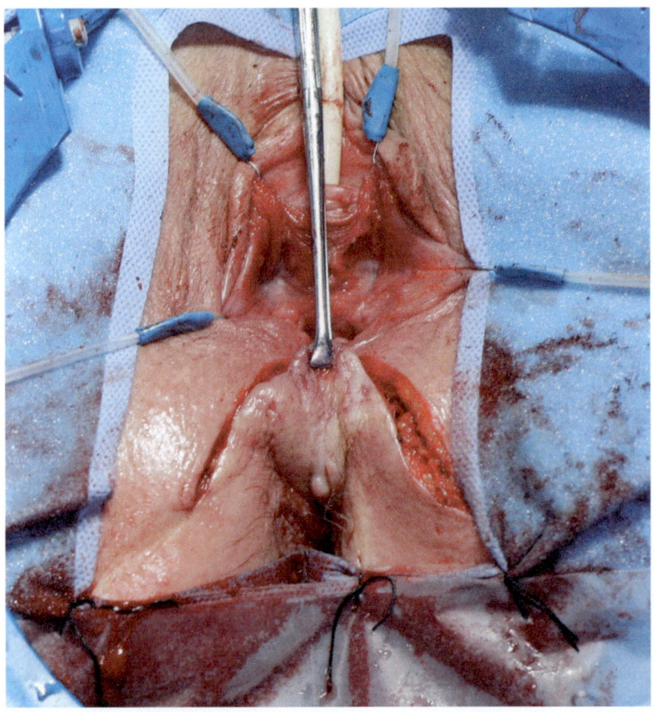

Fig. 5.125 The perineal flap is advanced distally, covering with new skin the fistula and the reconstructed anal sphincter

5.3.4 Intraoperative Complications

Intraoperative complications are rare. They include bleeding or an inability to close the rectal or perineal wounds. Wide tissue mobilization may be required in these cases. A temporary diversion of stool is indicated in recurrent cases and in patients with poor-quality tissues, a history of radiation, or other inflammatory conditions.

5.3.5 Postoperative Care

The packing is removed the next day after surgery. The Foley catheter is removed as soon as the patient is ambulating freely. Broad-spectrum antibiotics should be used in the perioperative area. If a diverting colostomy is performed, it should be closed 3–6 months after the closure of the fistula is ensured.

5.3.6 Postoperative Complications

Infection of the perineal and vaginal wound or tension of the suture lines may lead to recurrent fistula formation. Stool incontinence may be the result of surgery, or it may have existed prior to surgery but could not be demonstrated at that time. Wound infection and perineal abscess may require incision and drainage.

Suggested Reading

Arrowsmith S, Hamlin EC, Wall LL. Obstructed labor injury complex: obstetric fistula formation the multifaceted morbidity of maternal birth trauma in the developing world. Obstet Gynecol Surv. 1996;51(9):568–74.

Blaivas JG, Heritz DM, Romanzi LJ. Early versus late repair of vesicovaginal fistulae: vaginal abdominal approaches. J Urol. 1995;153(4):1110–2.

Blandy JP, Badenoch DF, Fowler CG, Jenkins BJ, Thomas NW. Early repair of iatrogenic injury to the ureter or bladder after gynecological surgery. J Urol. 1991;146(3):761–5.

Cass AS, Odl M. Ureteroarterial fistula: case report review of literature. J Urol. 1990;143(3):582–3.

Eilber KS, Kavaler E, Rodríguez LV, Rosenblum N, Raz S. Ten-year experience with transvaginal vesicovaginal fistula repair using tissue interposition. J Urol. 2003;169(3):1033–6.

Falk HC, Tancer ML. Vesicovaginal fistula; an historical survey. Obstet Gynecol. 1954;3(3):337–41.

Gerber GS, Schoenberg HW. Female urinary tract fistulae. J Urol. 1993;149(2):229–36.

Kim J, Smith A, Raz S. Urinary fistulae: what does the evidence say? Curr Bladder Dysfunct Rep. 2008;3:208–13.

Lee D, Dillon BE, Zimmern PE. Long-term morbidity of Martius labial fat pad graft in vaginal reconstruction surgery. Urology. 2013;82(6):1261–6.

Lee RA, Symmonds RE, Williams TJ. Current status of genitourinary fistula. Obstet Gynecol. 1988;72(3 Pt. 1):313–9.

Margolis T, Mercer LJ. Vesicovaginal fistula. Obstet Gynecol Surv. 1994;49(12):840–7.

McConnell DB, Sasaki TM, Vetto RM. Experience with colovesical fistula. Am J Surg. 1980;140(1):80–4.

O'Conor Jr VJ, Sokol JK, Bulkley GJ, Nanninga JB. Suprapubic closure of vesicovaginal fistula. J Urol. 1973;109(1):51–4.

Tenggardjaja CF, Goldman HB. Advances in minimally invasive repair of vesicovaginal fistulas. Curr Urol Rep. 2013;14(3):253–61.

6 Reconstructive Surgery

6.1 Anal Sphincter Reconstruction

The etiology of anal sphincter incompetence can be multifactorial. Traumatic delivery can cause tearing of the internal and external anal sphincter musculature, particularly in the anterior segment. Repair immediately after delivery usually is highly effective, but some patients will develop significant stool incontinence. Pudendal nerve damage after traumatic delivery or other injury can cause sphincter neuropathy and poor sphincteric function. Posterior or lateral episiotomy can be another factor in anal sphincter damage. Surgery, inflammation, traumatic injury, or radiation can directly damage the anal sphincter, and neurogenic disease (e.g., paraplegia with sacral arc lesion) is often associated with anal incompetence.

6.1.1 Indications

Anal sphincter reconstruction is indicated in very selected symptomatic patients for whom medical therapy has failed. Patients with severe neurogenic paralysis of the anal sphincter will not improve after surgery. Factors controlling surgical success include the integrity of the anal skin tissues, the innervation, the anal sphincter musculature, the location of the damage (segmental or circular, external or internal sphincter, or both), and prior surgeries (Figs. 6.1, 6.2, and 6.3).

Electronic supplementary material The online version of this chapter (doi:10.1007/978-1-4939-2941-2_6) contains supplementary material, which is available to authorized users.

S. Raz, *Atlas of Vaginal Reconstructive Surgery*, DOI 10.1007/978-1-4939-2941-2_6

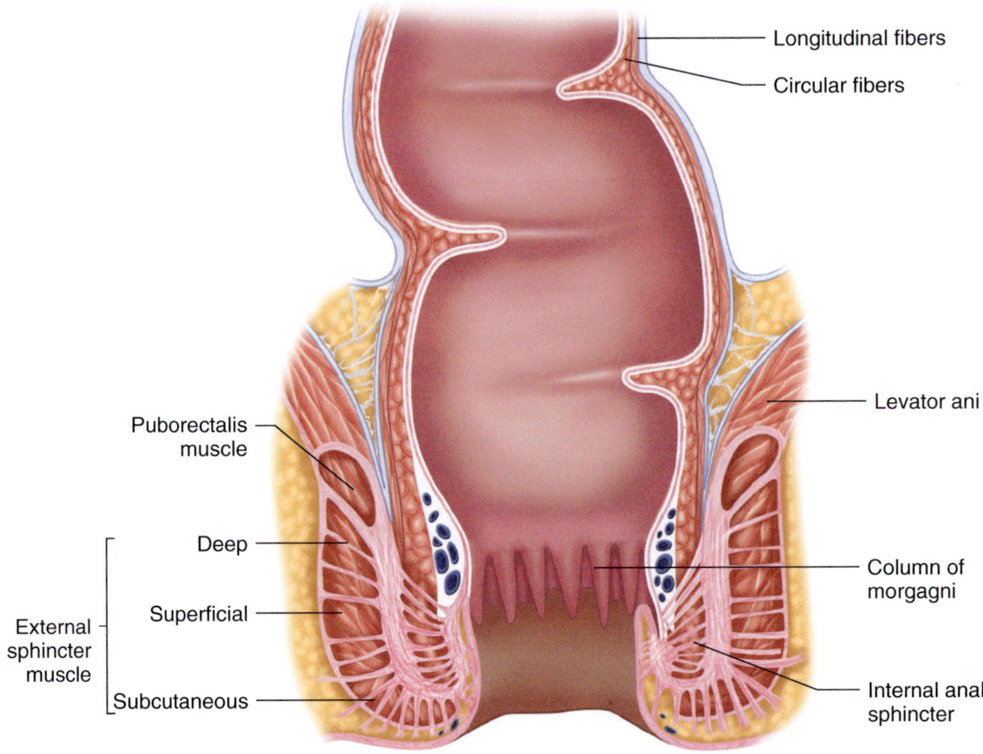

Fig. 6.1 Anatomical diagram of the distal rectum and anal sphincter. The internal sphincter is a continuation of the circular and longitudinal fibers of the rectum. The most medial segment of the levators is the puborectalis muscle, which forms a posterior sling or notch at the posterior rectal wall

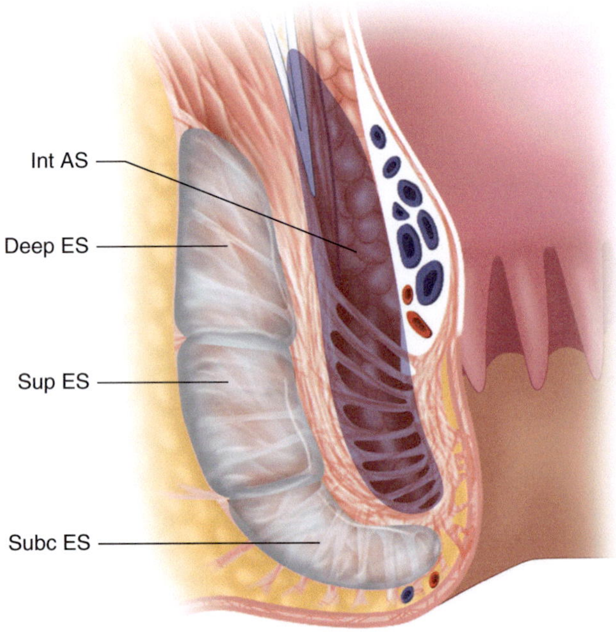

Fig. 6.2 The external anal sphincter (ES) is divided into deep, superficial (Sup), and subcutaneous (Subc) sections and surrounds the internal anal sphincter (Int AS)

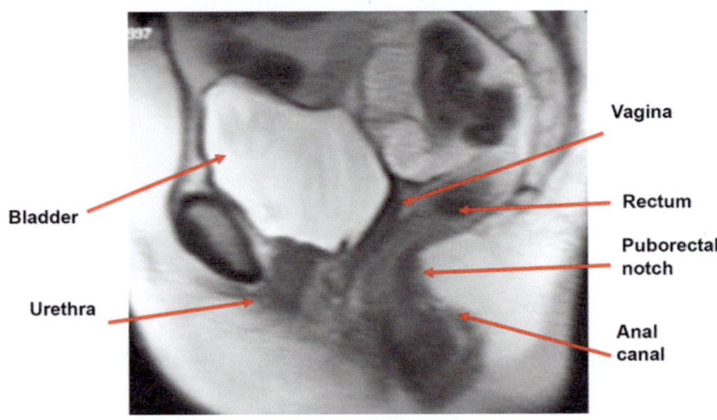

Fig. 6.3 Sagittal MRI cut of the midpelvis showing the elevation and angulation created by the levator plate on the distal posterior rectum, above the anal canal

6.1.2 Diagnosis

Most patients present with differing degrees of intermittent or daily episodes of stool incontinence or inability to control flatus. In some patients, the loss of stool occurs only with liquid stool, with good control of solid matter. The incontinence can be continuous or it can be intermittent, occurring with stress maneuvers such as cough, strain, or exercise. Physical examination should include perianal sensations, rectal tone, voluntary activity of the sphincter, sensations of the genitalia, and observation of any perianal scars or lesions. Anal manometry and transrectal ultrasound will confirm the diagnosis and better define the lesions (Figs. 6.4 and 6.5).

6.1.3 Surgical Technique

Prior to surgery a bowel preparation should be done. After anesthesia but before beginning surgery, the rectum is irrigated with copious amount of diluted antibiotic solution to clean any residual stool matter from the rectum.

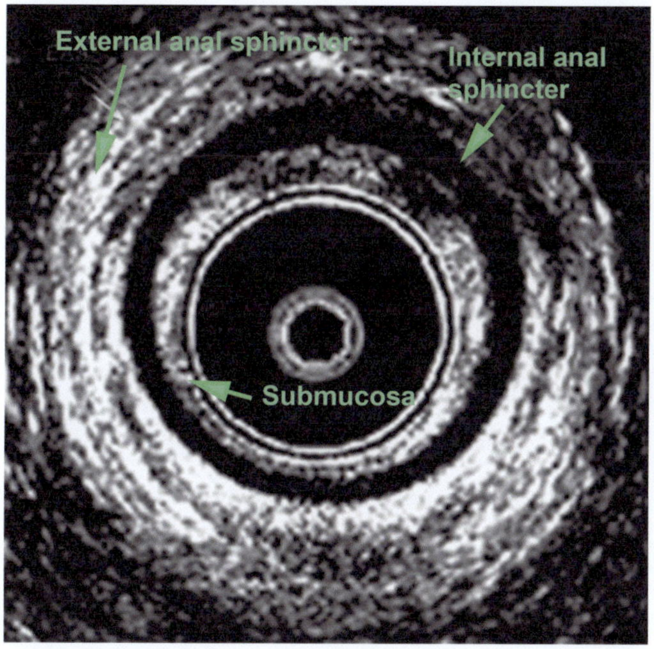

Fig. 6.4 Endorectal ultrasound showing the layers of the anal canal: submucosa and internal and external sphincter

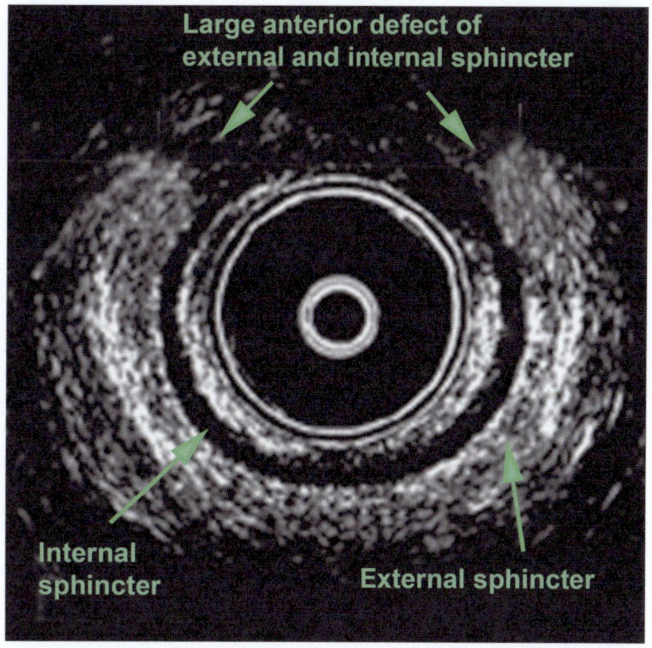

Fig. 6.5 Endorectal ultrasound of a patient with extensive anterior external and internal sphincter damage after traumatic delivery and perineal tear

6.1.3.1 Anterior anal Sphincter Repair

Figures 6.6, 6.7, 6.8, 6.9, 6.10, 6.11, 6.12, 6.13, 6.14, and 6.15 illustrate the surgical technique for anterior anal sphincter repair.

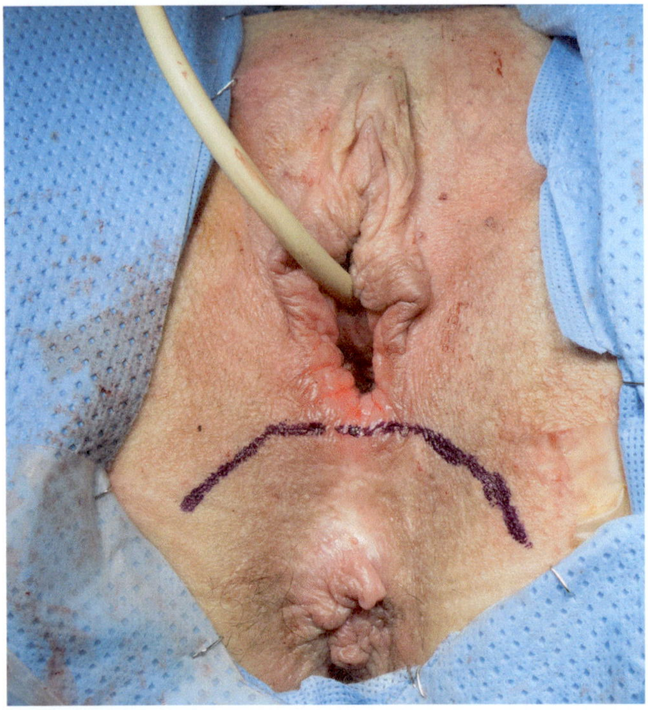

Fig. 6.6 The perineum, the vaginal area, and the rectum are exposed. An inverted U incision will be performed around the anal sphincter, extending superiorly to the posterior fourchette and laterally to the medial aspect of the ischial tuberosities

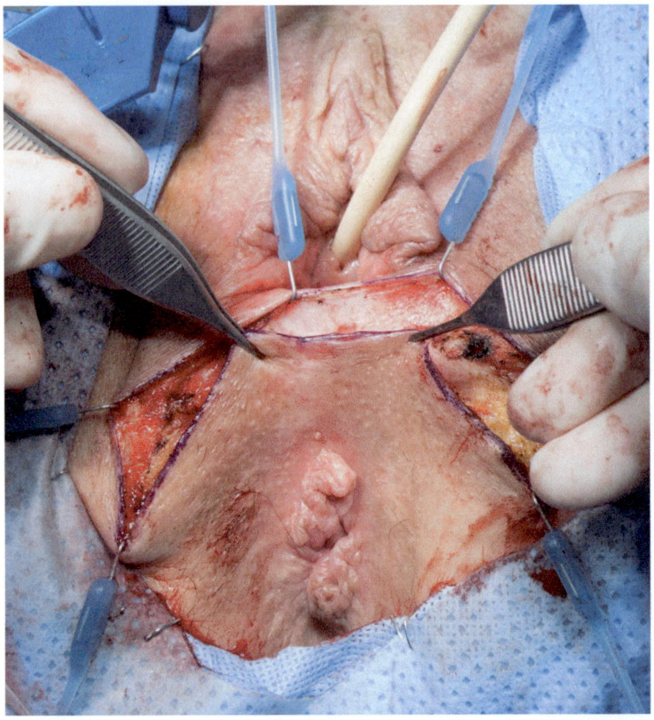

Fig. 6.8 A flap of the perineal skin will be created. The skin is dissected toward the anal canal to expose the superficial anal sphincter fibers, the ischial fossa, and the transverse perineal musculature

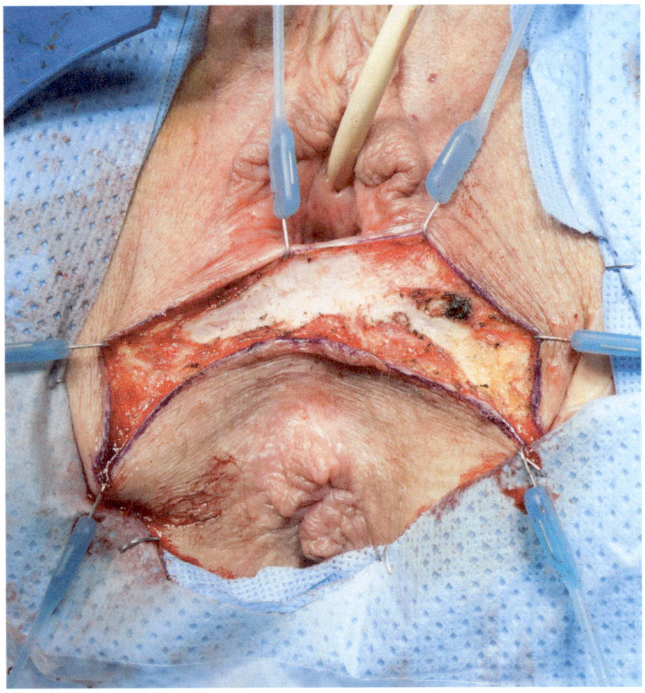

Fig. 6.7 The incision is made, and the margins are retracted using a ring retractor and hooks

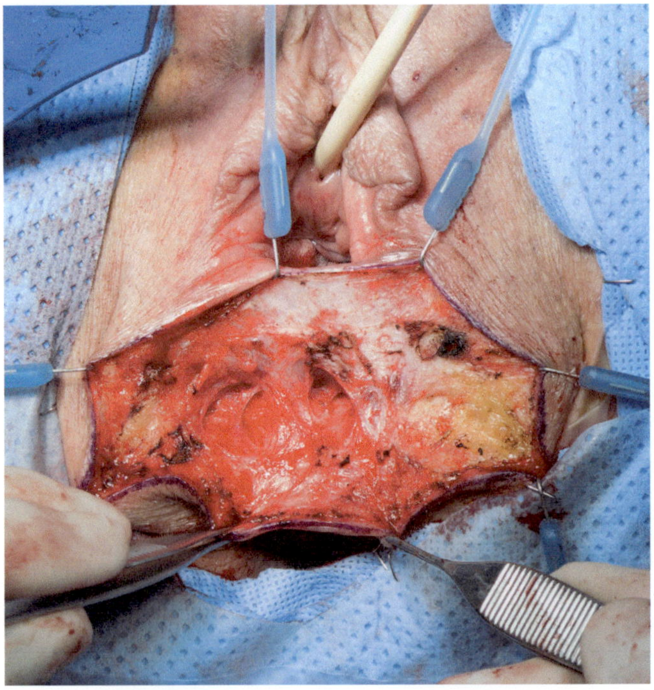

Fig. 6.9 The skin flap is retracted inferiorly, exposing the posterior perineum, the external anal sphincter, and the ischial fossa

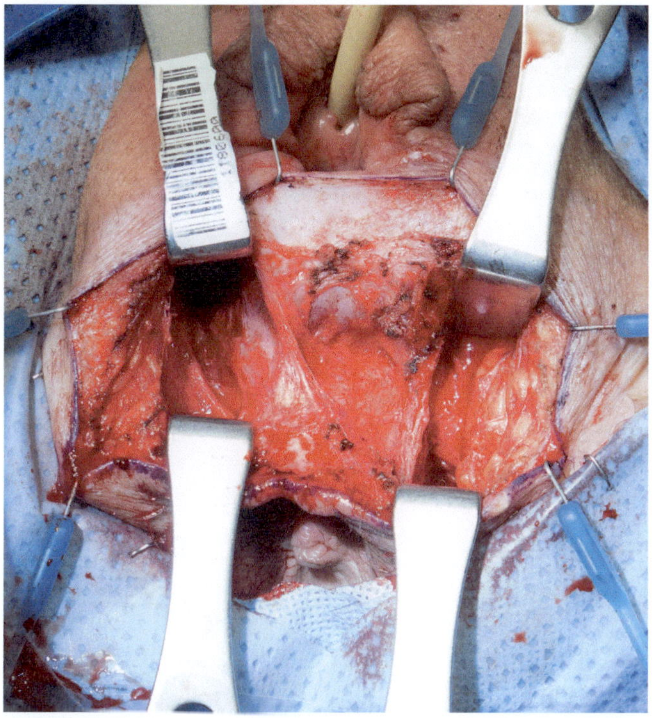

Fig. 6.10 Dissection is carried out just lateral to the anal sphincter toward the ischial fossa, exposing the external anal sphincter fibers. An anterior defect is present due to traumatic delivery and perineal tear

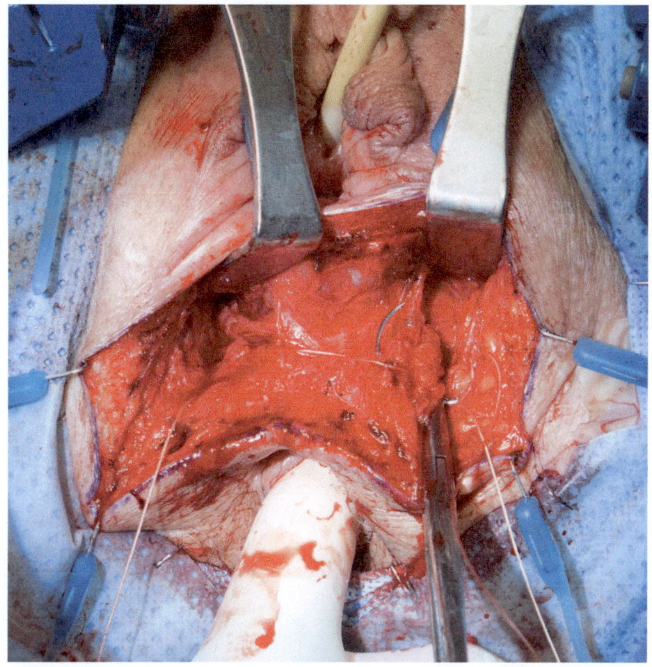

Fig. 6.12 The sutures include the 3 o'clock, 12 o'clock, and 9 o'clock portions of the anal sphincter. Care should be taken not to perforate the rectal wall and to include only rectal musculature without the fatty tissue

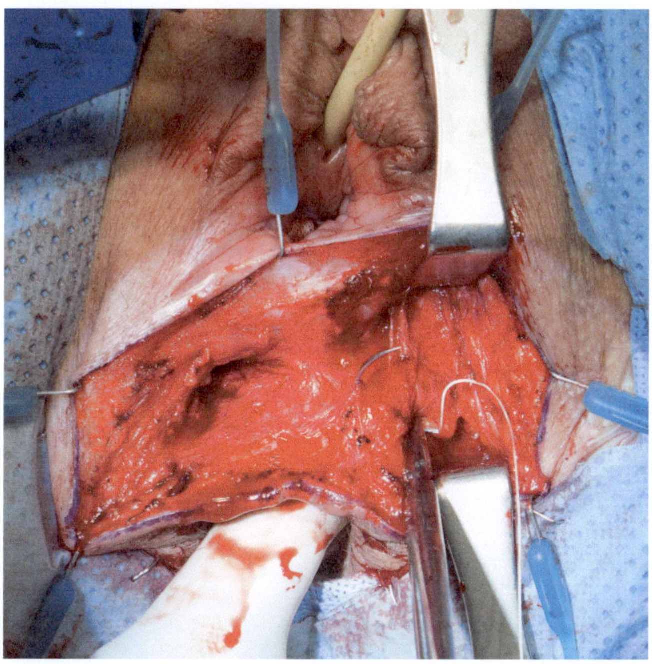

Fig. 6.11 Exposure of the ischial fossa and perirectal area is obtained. With a finger in the rectum to prevent passage of sutures through it, figure-of-eight sutures of #0 delayed absorbable sutures are applied

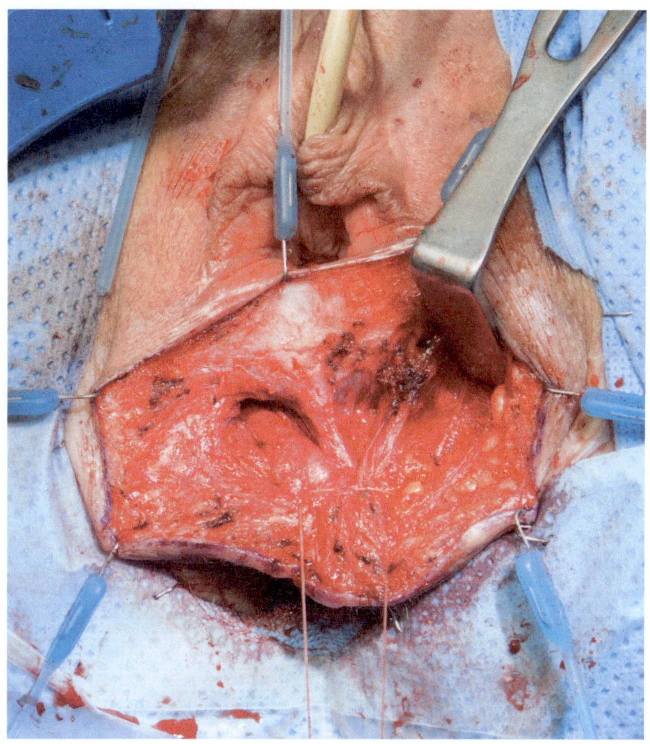

Fig. 6.13 After application of the sutures, traction is applied to ensure approximation and tightening of the open rectal canal

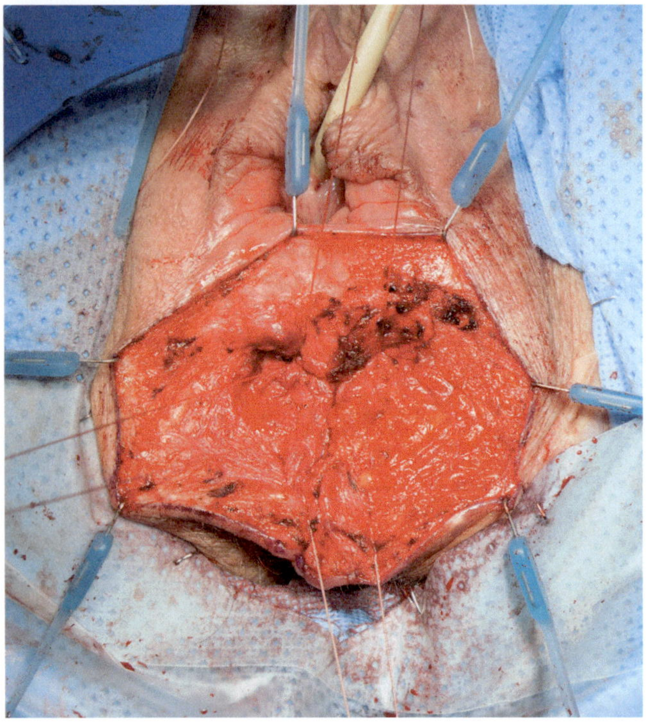

Fig. 6.14 A series of three or four sutures are applied sequentially, with the most superior sutures incorporating the transverse perineal musculature. Care should be taken not to incorporate the skin flap. Again it is important that all the sutures are applied with a finger in the vagina to ensure that no sutures are in the rectum and that elevation of the sutures tightens the anal sphincter. The sutures will be tied

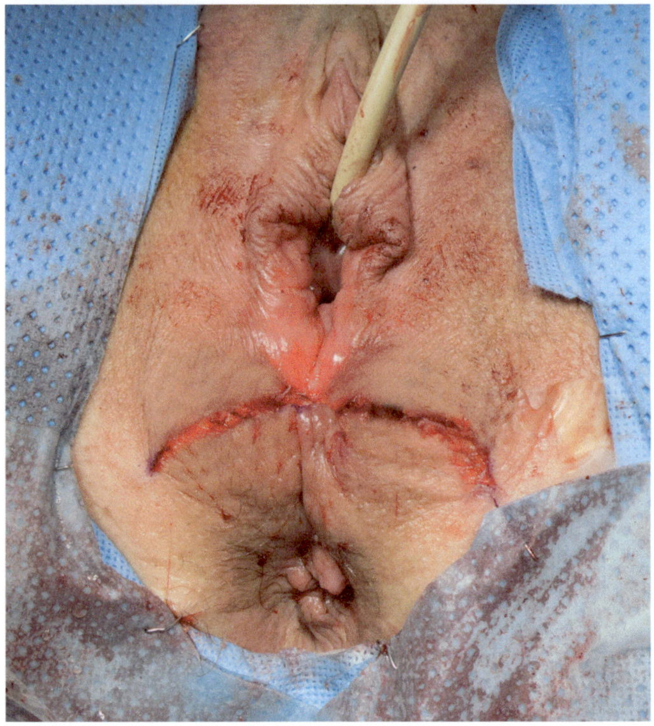

Fig. 6.15 Throughout the surgery and prior to closure, the area is irrigated with copious amounts of antibiotic solution. The inverted U flap is advanced to cover the area of the reconstruction. A two-layer closure is done with delayed absorbable sutures. A local anesthetic agent is injected to improve postoperative pain control

6.1.3.2 Combined Anterior and Posterior Anal Sphincter Repair

In selected cases of circular defect of the anal sphincter, both anterior and posterior plications of the anal sphincter may be indicated (Figs. 6.16, 6.17, 6.18, 6.19, 6.20, and 6.21).

6.1.4 Postoperative Care

The surgery is done as an outpatient procedure. Postoperative antibiotics, stool softeners and laxatives, and pain medications are given. The patient starts in sitz baths soon after surgery. Injection of long-acting local anesthetic at the end of surgery will help with pain control. No particular restrictions of activities are required.

6.1.5 Intraoperative Complications

The most important intraoperative complication is rectal wall injury, which can lead to fistula formation, wound infection, and dehiscence. Bleeding can occur from injury to the internal pudendal branches in the ischial fossa. Dissection close to the pubococcygeus and external anal sphincter fibers will avoid this complication. If the tissues have damage from prior trauma, surgery, or radiation, proper approximation of the anal sphincter structures may not be possible. In cases with difficult reconstruction, bleeding, or rectal injury, bilateral JP drains can be inserted in each ischial fossa and the end transferred superiorly, lateral to the labia.

6.1.6 Postoperative Complications

The most important postoperative complication is wound infection, which is reported in 5–25% of patients. Some surgeons prefer to leave the skin open after surgery. Opening the wound in one or more areas can be required for drainage.

In spite of good surgical technique and anatomical reconstruction, some patients continue to suffer from sphincter incompetence, which probably is due to neuropathic damage (anatomy does not correlate with function). It is also possible that the sutures may have become dislodged, broken, or detached owing to sudden strain or cough episodes. The patient may feel a pop in the perineum at the time of the sudden event.

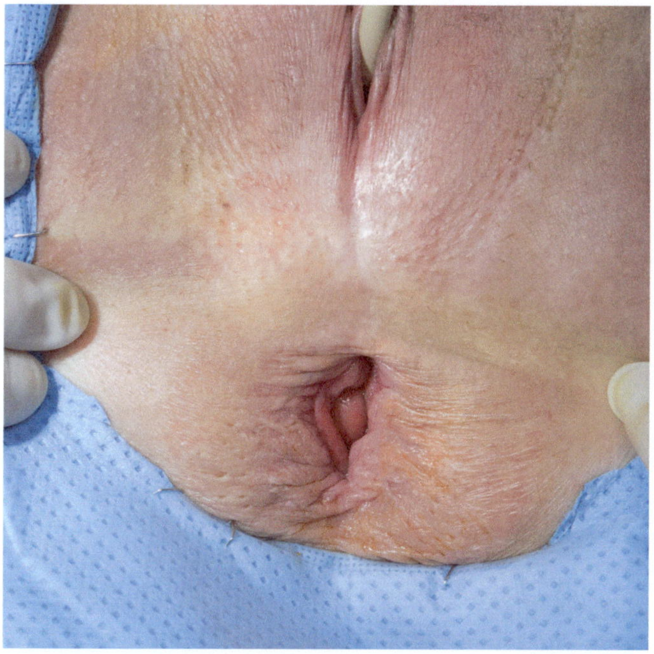

Fig. 6.16 Wide-open anal sphincter with mild rectal mucosal prolapse in a patient with severe stool incontinence and a wide circular open anal sphincter

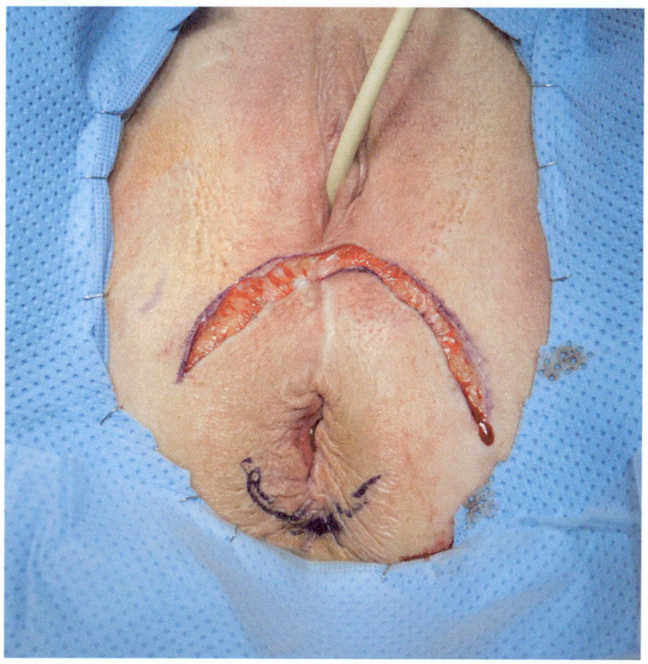

Fig. 6.17 A semicircular inverted U incision is made in the perineum

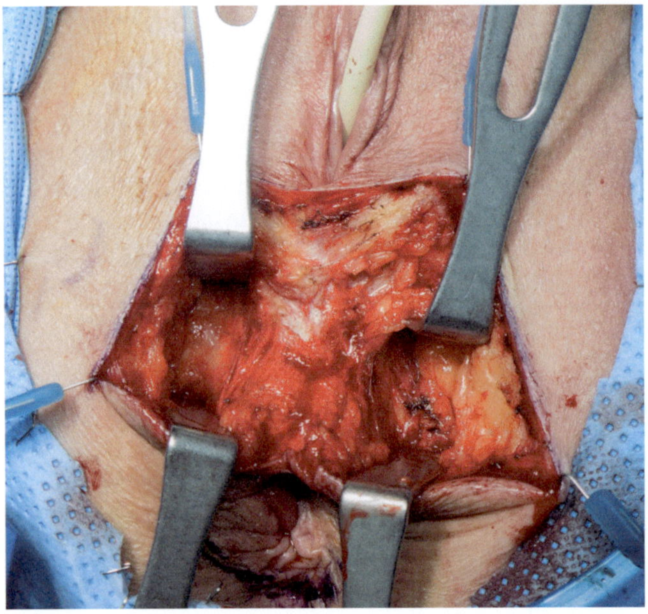

Fig. 6.18 Similar to the previously described procedure, the anterior anal sphincter musculature is exposed and will be repaired with a sequence of delayed absorbable sutures. Tying these sutures does not produce adequate anal sphincter approximation

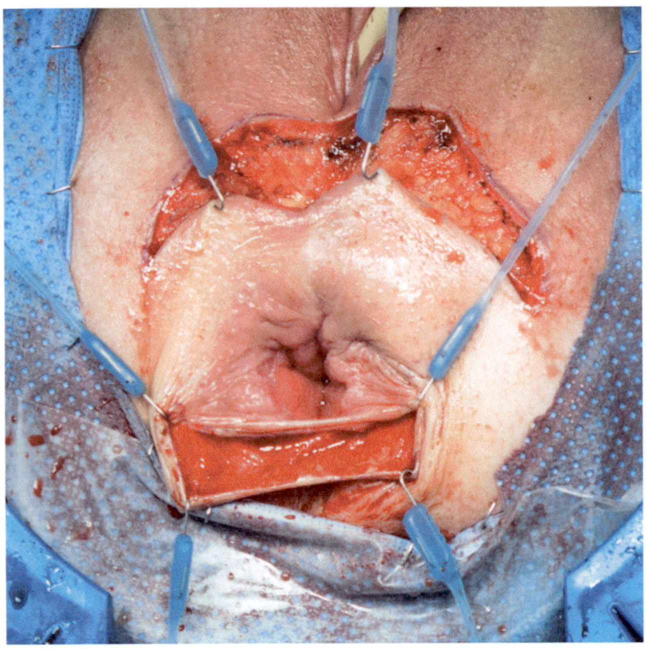

Fig. 6.19 A transverse semicircular incision is made posterior to the anal sphincter. Dissection is carried out laterally to expose the puborectalis and pubococcygeus muscles and the posterior structures of the anal sphincter

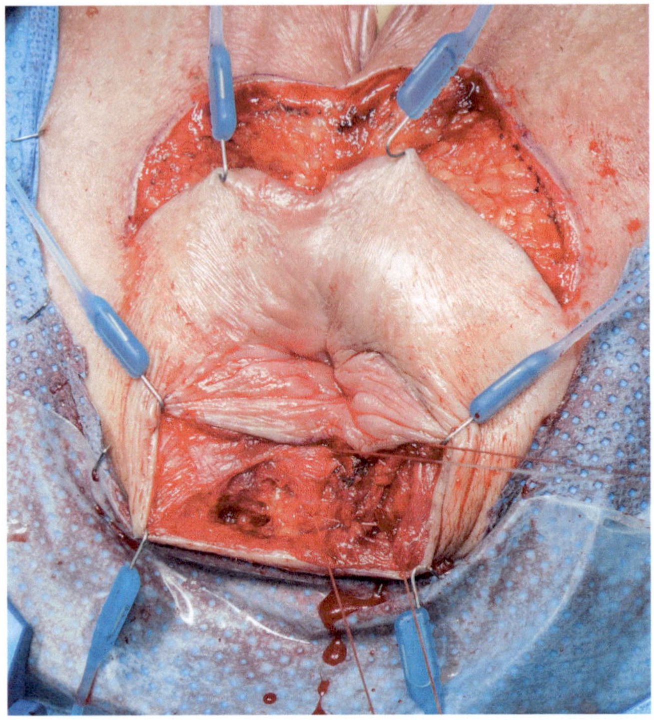

Fig. 6.20 Under finger control in the rectum, figure-of-eight sutures approximate the posterior fibers of the anal sphincter. Care is taken not to penetrate the rectal wall. Traction of the sutures produces tightening and further closure of the anal sphincter

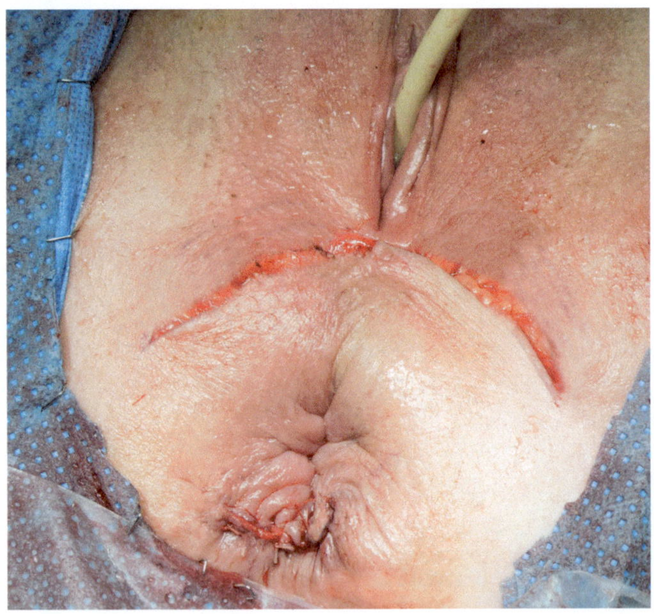

Fig. 6.21 The posterior anal sphincter area is irrigated with copious amounts of antibiotic solution and closed in layers with delayed absorbable sutures

6.2 Closure of the Bladder Neck

6.2.1 Indications

Closure of the bladder neck and urethra is indicated in patients with severe urinary incontinence due to serious damage to the urethra from trauma, radiation, surgery, or a chronic indwelling catheter. In patients with indwelling catheters, the presenting symptoms are generally severe incontinence with leakage around a Foley catheter and the need to progressively increase of the size of the catheter to maintain continence.

Closure of the bladder neck is also indicated in patients with paraplegia and urinary retention who are unable to perform self-catheterization, even if they have an intact urethra.

Closure of the bladder neck requires a concomitant procedure for urinary diversion. The simplest is the placement of a suprapubic catheter. Patients with severe frequency or bladder spasms due to an overactive detrusor may not be good candidates for this procedure because the spasms and pain can be exacerbated by the indwelling catheter.

Patients with paraplegia and neurogenic bladder suffering from incontinence in whom other treatments have failed are candidates for placement of a suprapubic catheter, continent or incontinent augmentation cystoplasty, and closure of the bladder neck.

In patients with pelvic radiation, the urethra and the bladder are usually affected, and augmentation procedures are required at the time of bladder neck closure.

6.2.2 Diagnosis

The findings on physical examination depend on the etiology of the condition. The urethra may be intact, as in paraplegic patients, or it may be a totally open channel with constant leakage of urine. Sometimes the whole urethral length has necrosed and only the bladder neck and trigone are seen on examination.

Before any surgery, it is important to assess the quality of the surrounding vaginal tissues and labial tissues because it is necessary to cover the area of the closed bladder neck with rotational or advancement flaps.

The ability of the patient or a family member to perform self-catheterization via an abdominal stoma will indicate the use of a continent or an incontinent bladder diversion.

Cystoscopy should be performed prior to surgery to rule out any intravesical pathology. Upper tract evaluation by ultrasound or CT urogram is indicated to rule out any upper tract condition such as stones or obstruction, which may change the surgical procedure.

6.2.3 Surgical Technique

Figures 6.22, 6.23, 6.24, 6.25, 6.26, 6.27, 6.28, 6.29, 6.30, 6.31, 6.32, 6.33, 6.34, 6.35, 6.36, 6.37, 6.38, 6.39, 6.40, and 6.41 illustrate the technique for bladder neck closure, including the optional use of a Martius flap.

At the end of the procedure, vaginal packing will be inserted and a bladder diversion procedure will be performed. In cases of placement of a suprapubic catheter, only the catheter should be inserted prior to the closure of the bladder neck.

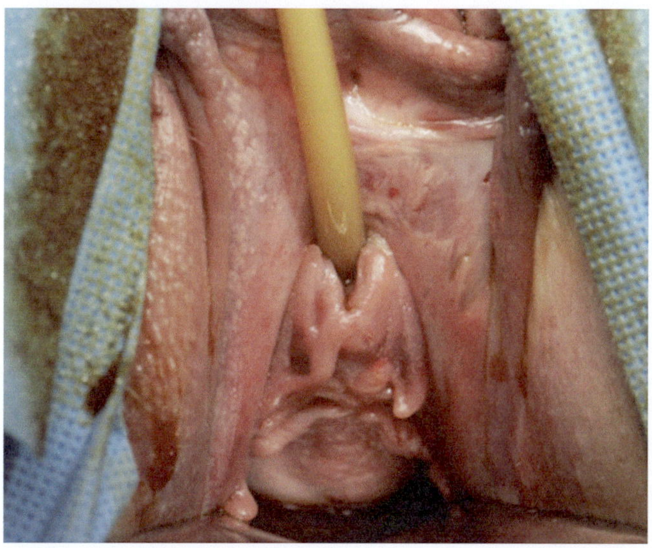

Fig. 6.22 Exposure of the anterior vaginal wall is obtained. A Foley catheter is inserted, and a ring retractor with hooks will help with the exposure

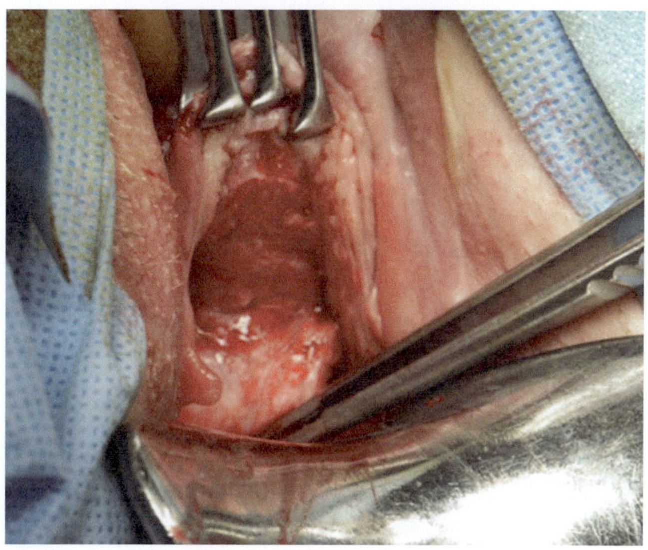

Fig. 6.23 An anterior inverted U vaginal flap is created and dissected free from the periurethral tissues down to the bladder neck area

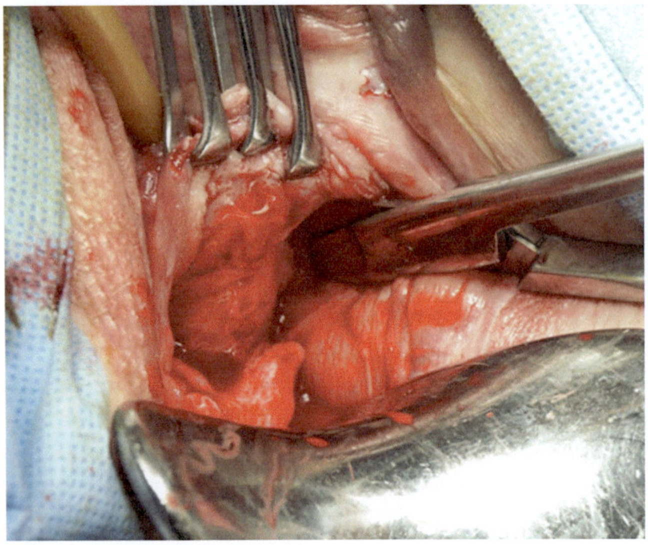

Fig. 6.24 Dissection is carried out laterally around the periurethral fascia to enter the retropubic space, detaching the urethropelvic fascia from the arcus tendineus fascia pelvis. Sharp and blunt dissection is performed in the retropubic space to free any adhesions of the bladder or urethra from the lateral and posterior pubic bone

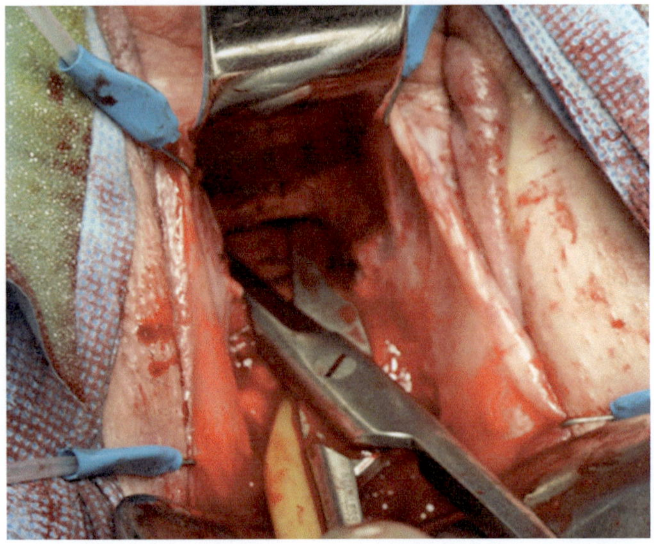

Fig. 6.26 A circular incision is made around the urethra toward the anterior rami of the pubic bone

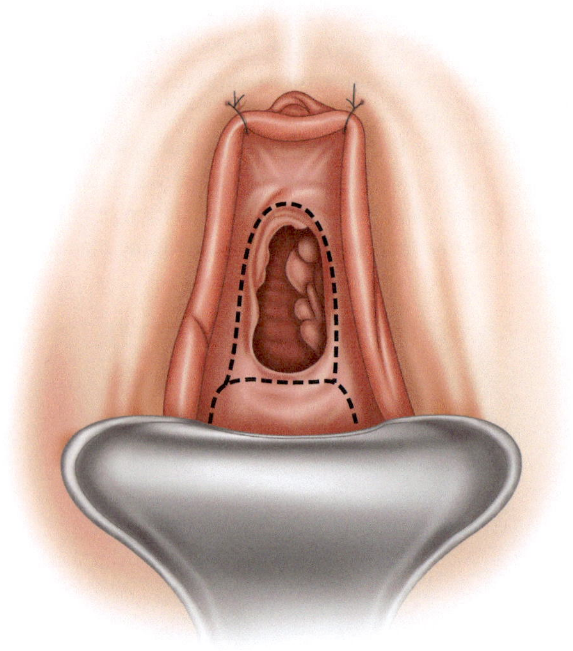

Fig. 6.25 Diagram of the incisions used for the bladder neck closure. An anterior vaginal flap and a circular incision around the urethra will be made. The incision is begun 5–10 mm lateral to the remnant of the urethral meatus and is extended superiorly to the mid-anterior rami of the pubic bone

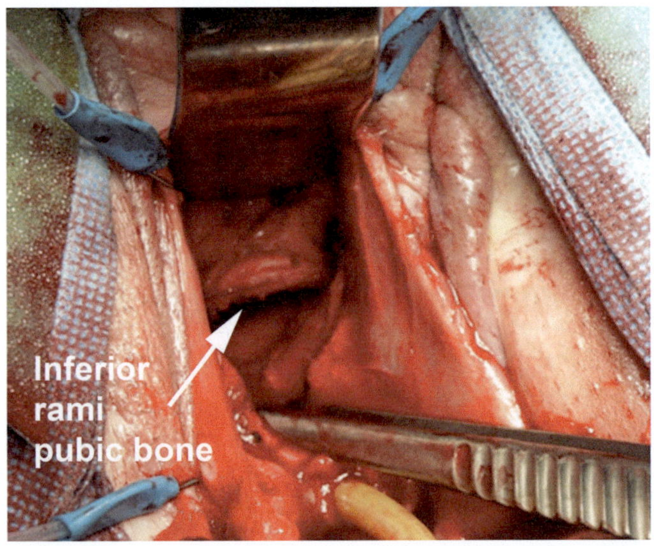

Fig. 6.27 Dissection is carried out toward the anterior pubic bone. The periosteum of the anterior pubic bone is exposed. The urethra is pushed inferiorly, and with sharp dissection the pubourethral fascia is detached, allowing entrance into the retropubic space

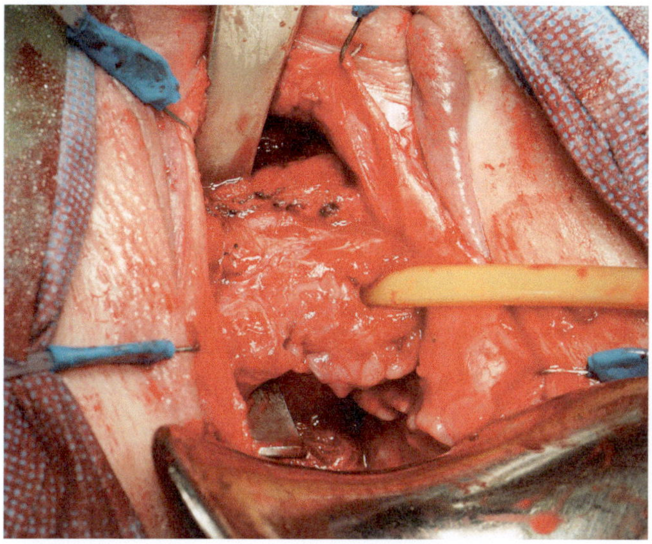

Fig. 6.28 All adhesions of the retropubic space are freed to expose the anterior bladder wall and the lateral attachments of the urethra. A finger is inserted in the retropubic space from the vaginal periurethral incision. Under finger control in the vagina, a right-angle retractor is inserted anterior and lateral to the bladder neck. This maneuver will isolate all the remaining tissue that supports the urethra to the lateral pelvic wall

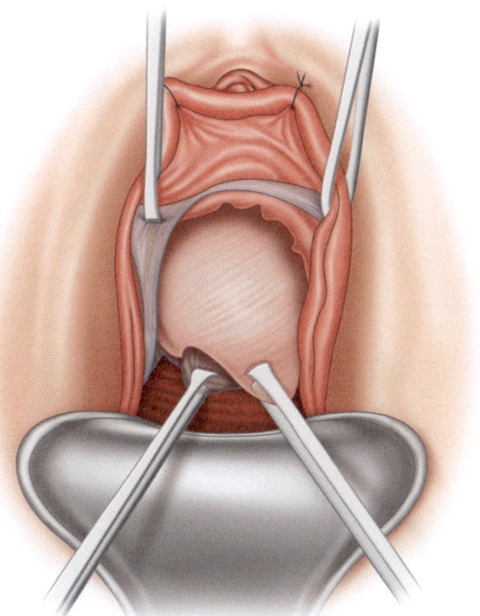

Fig. 6.29 Diagram of the exposure of the anterior bladder wall after detaching the pubourethral fascia from the inferior rami of the pubic bone

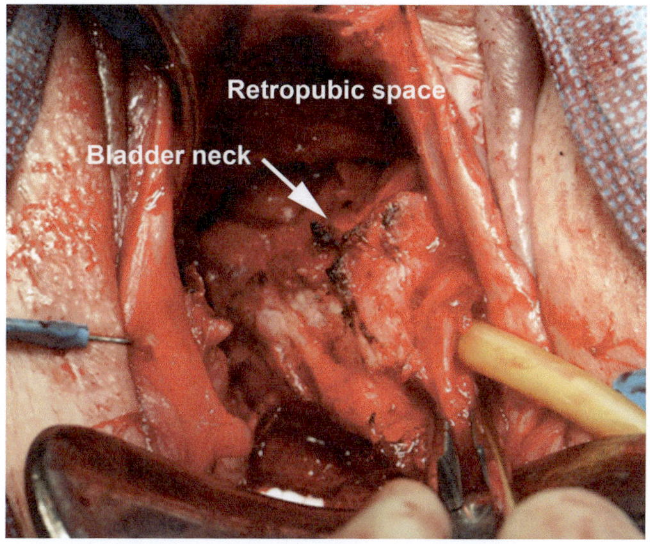

Fig. 6.30 Using a coagulation knife, all the lateral supporting tissue of the urethra to the lateral pelvic wall is transected. The urethra, the bladder neck, and the bladder are totally free in the retropubic space. The same maneuver is performed on the contralateral side

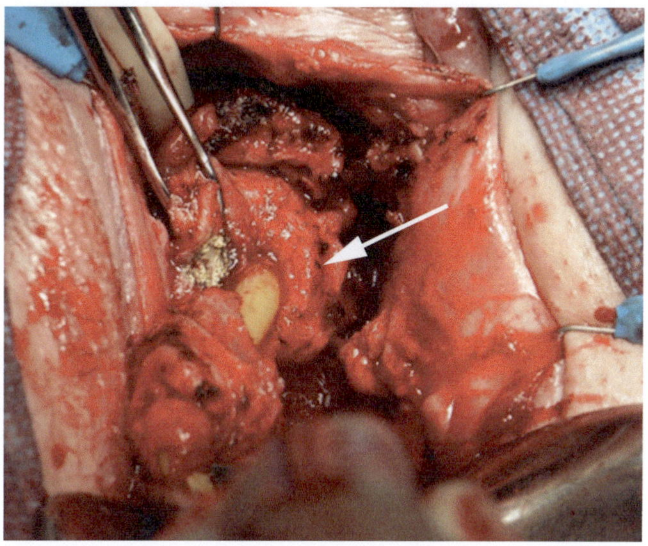

Fig. 6.31 The urethra is transected at the level of the bladder neck (*arrow*) over the Foley catheter

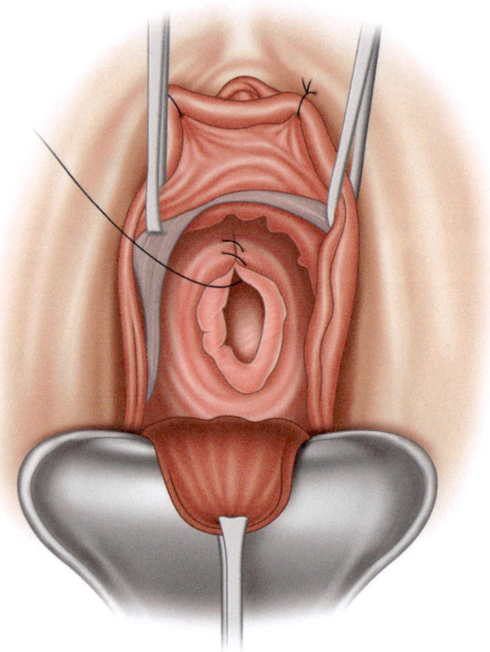

Fig. 6.32 Diagram of the closure of the bladder neck. A two-layer closure is performed using delayed absorbable sutures

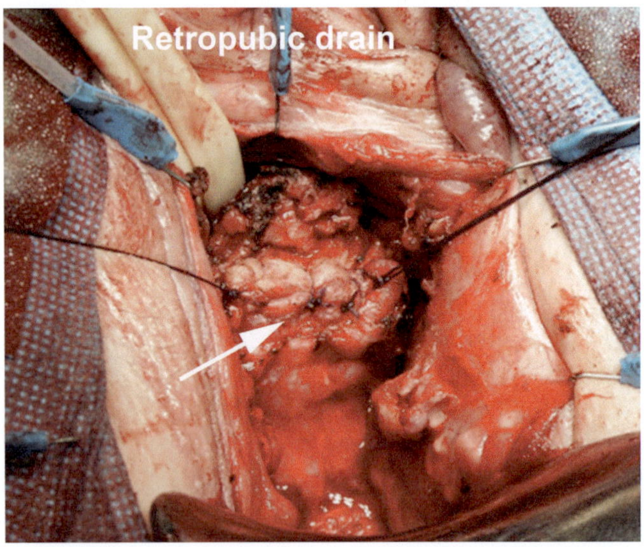

Fig. 6.33 The bladder neck has been closed with a first layer of running, locking delayed absorbable sutures and a second layer of imbricating sutures to cover the first layer of closure. Electively, a retropubic drain can be inserted under finger control in the retropubic space, using a small suprapubic puncture. If a suprapubic catheter is present, it should be irrigated with diluted indigo carmine solution to ensure the integrity of the closure. The *arrow* indicates the stump of the closed bladder neck

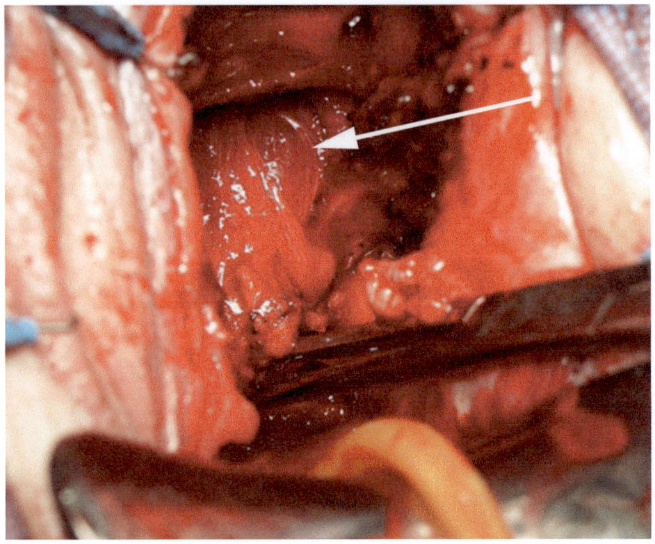

Fig. 6.34 Wide exposure of the anterior bladder wall is obtained. Several delayed absorbable sutures are applied to the anterior bladder wall and posterior to the line of sutures at the closed bladder neck, to advance it toward the retropubic space and away from the vagina. *Arrow* indicates bladder neck closure

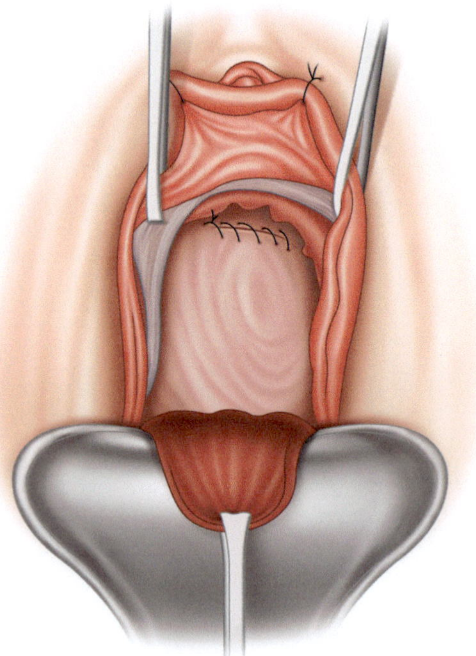

Fig. 6.35 Diagram of the anterior bladder wall showing the advancement of the closed bladder neck toward the retropubic space. The closed bladder neck will be away from the vaginal area

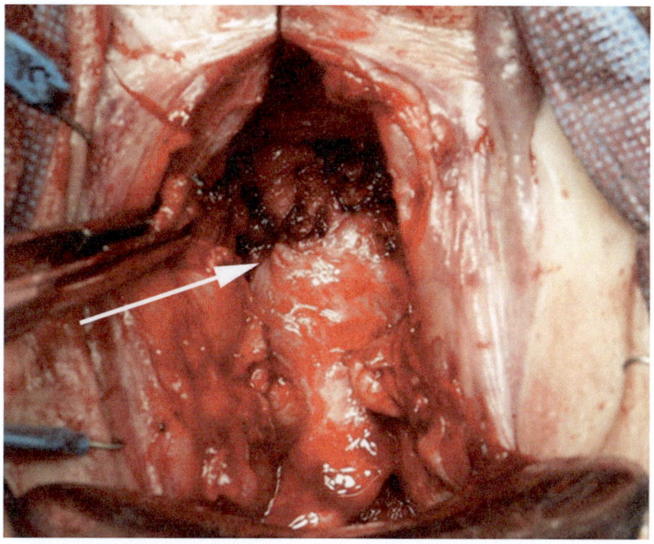

Fig. 6.36 The sutures from the closed bladder neck to the anterior bladder have been tied, showing the repositioning of the closed bladder neck (*arrow*) into the retropubic space

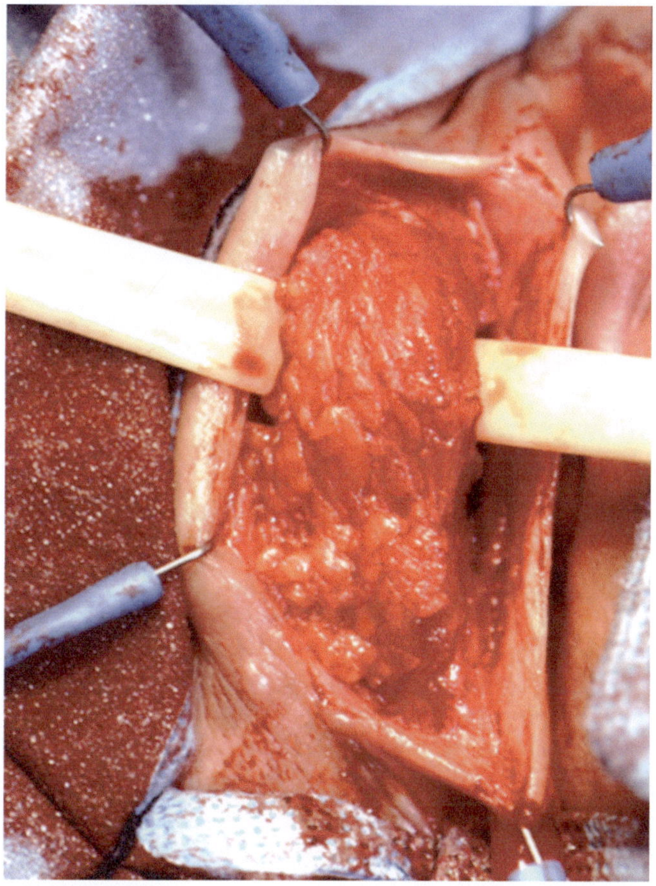

Fig. 6.37 In cases of severe urethral necrosis, radiation, or difficult closure of the bladder neck due to poor tissue quality, the use of a Martius flap is an option. An incision is made over the labia majora and the fibro-fatty tissue is isolated over a drain

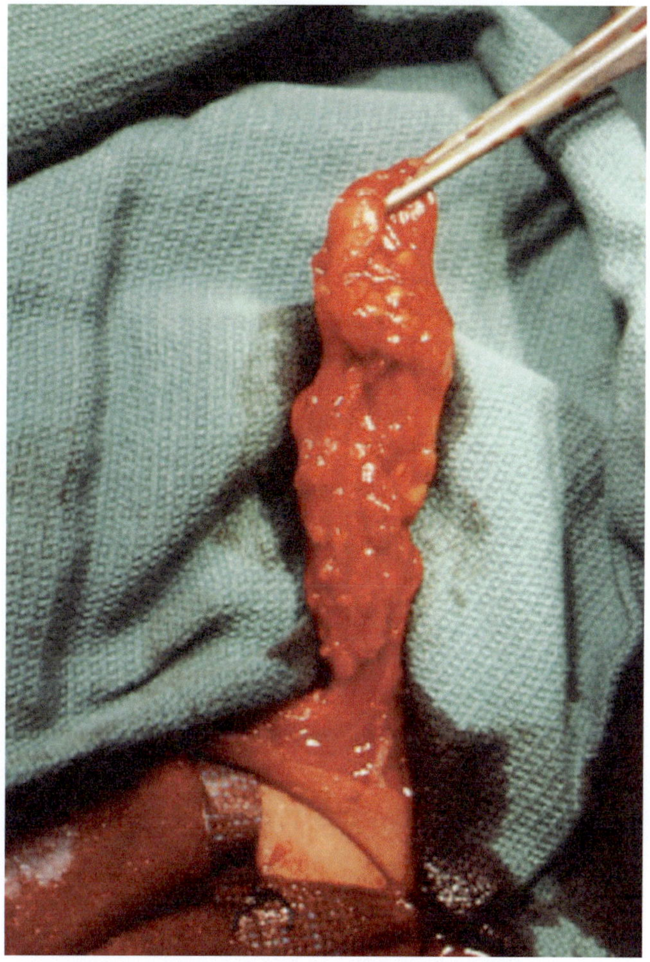

Fig. 6.38 The superior pedicle of the flap is transected and a tunnel is created under the skin of the labium to transfer the flap toward the anterior vaginal wall

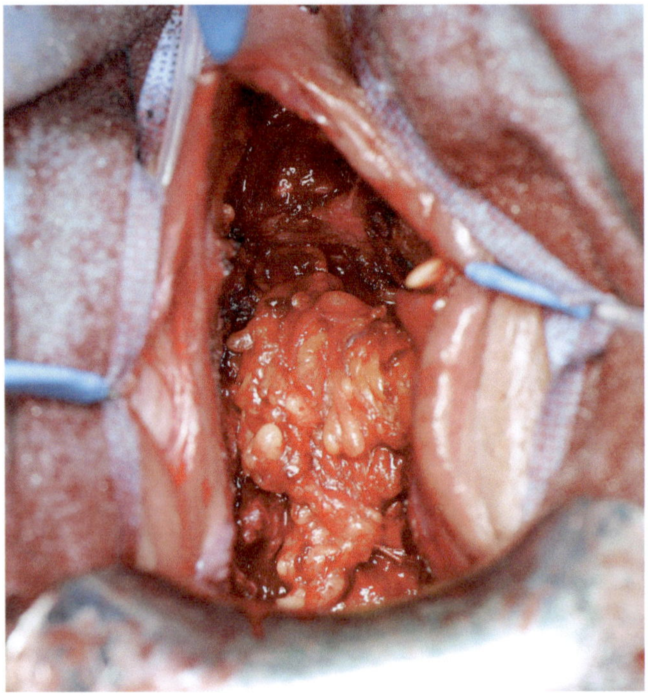

Fig. 6.39 The Martius flap has been transferred to the retropubic space. Multiple sutures are used to cover the bladder neck closure

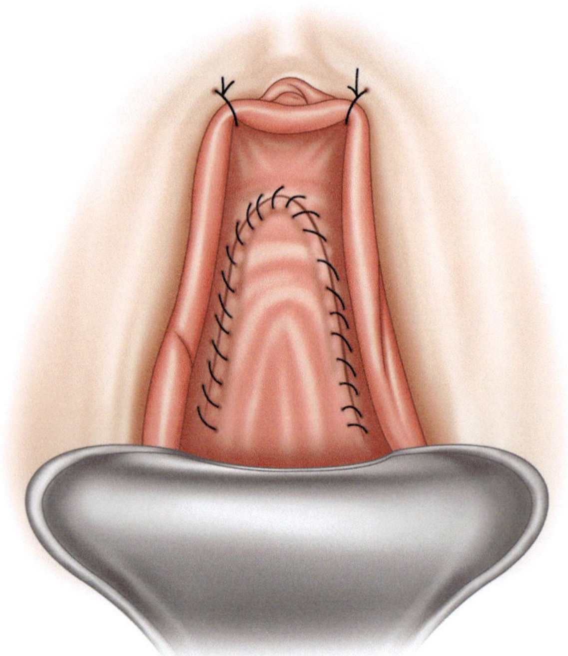

Fig. 6.40 Diagram showing the advancement of the vaginal wall distally to cover the area of the reconstruction

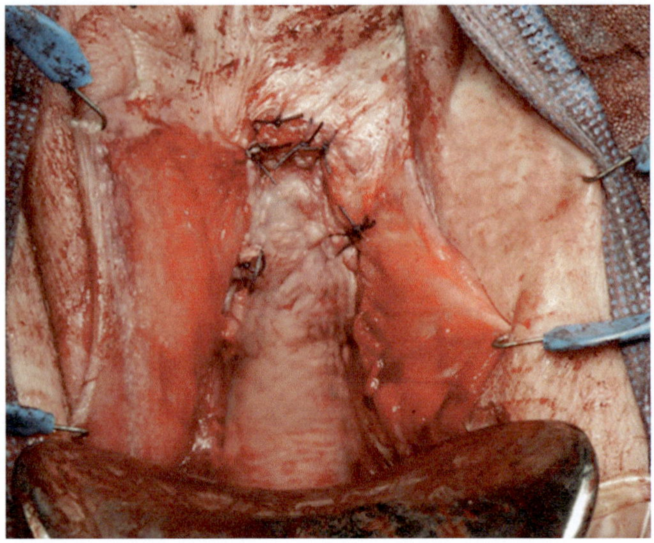

Fig. 6.41 The previously created anterior vaginal wall flap is advanced distally and anastomosed to the medial labial incisions. The closure should be tension-free. If required, distally interrupted sutures approximate the medial labial incisions, reducing the distance required for the flap advancement

6.2.4 Postoperative Care

Closure of the bladder neck only without bladder augmentation is usually done as outpatient surgery. Oral antibiotics are continued as indicated. In cases of additional continent or incontinent urinary diversion, patients are kept NPO until bowel activity resumes. In these patients, a suprapubic and stoma catheter will be inserted.

6.2.5 Intraoperative Complications

Bleeding in the form of profuse oozing is not uncommon, especially in patients with active infection. The lateral dissection of the bladder neck from the urethra and the detachment of the urethra from the inferior rami of the pubic bone can be the source of significant bleeding from the periurethral and perivesical vessels. Entering the retropubic space flush under the pubic bone to detach the pubourethral fascia will avoid the periurethral plexus. The lateral dissection to detach the urethropelvic fascia from the lateral levator should be performed with care, and the entrance to the retropubic space should be as far lateral as possible and parallel to the urethra, pointing the scissors superiorly. A vaginal packing and dedicated hemostasis with coagulation or interrupted sutures should control this oozing.

Difficulty in closing the bladder neck because of a large defect or radiation damage may require further mobilization of the bladder wall, with creation of an anterior flap. In this case, a Martius flap should be used to cover the defect.

Large proximal urethral diverticula may extend into the trigone and bladder, or ureteric injury may occur. Instillation of indigo carmine into the bladder will ensure bladder integrity. Cystoscopy after intravenous indigo carmine may be performed in selected cases to rule out ureteric injury.

6.2.6 Postoperative Complications

Perioperative antibiotic therapy is mandatory. The presence of chronic indwelling catheters or constant incontinence will increase the chances of wound infection and dehiscence. During surgery, copious irrigation with antibiotic solution is recommended.

The most important postoperative complication is a vesicovaginal fistula due to the disruption of the bladder neck closure. Obstructed or poor bladder drainage, infection, severe bladder spasms, or poor tissue quality contribute to this complication. Sometimes the fistula may close spontaneously, but many cases require re-exploration and reclosure of the bladder neck. Important factors in operative success and avoidance of fistula formation include a watertight closure, precise dissection, and anatomical closure of the urethral layers.

6.3 Construction of a Neourethra

6.3.1 Indications

Urethral reconstruction is required to rebuild a urethra lost by trauma, surgery, radiation, or anti-incontinence surgery. The surgery is aimed at constructing a full-length urethra that is fistula-free and continent. In patients with incontinence, sling procedures (fascial slings) can be used at the time of the reconstruction or in a second stage. Insertion of a concomitant fascial sling can lead to obstruction or fistula formation. Martius flaps are used all the time to cover the area of the reconstruction and prevent fistula formation.

To perform this type of reconstruction, a significant amount of anterior vaginal wall must be inverted and advanced; the anterior vaginal wall in the defective area should be mobile and well vascularized. Figures 6.42, 6.43, 6.44, 6.45, 6.46, 6.47, 6.48, 6.49, 6.50, 6.51, 6.52, 6.53, 6.54, 6.55, 6.56, 6.57, 6.58, 6.59, 6.60, 6.61, 6.62, and 6.63 show a few examples of the type of urethral reconstruction used in most cases.

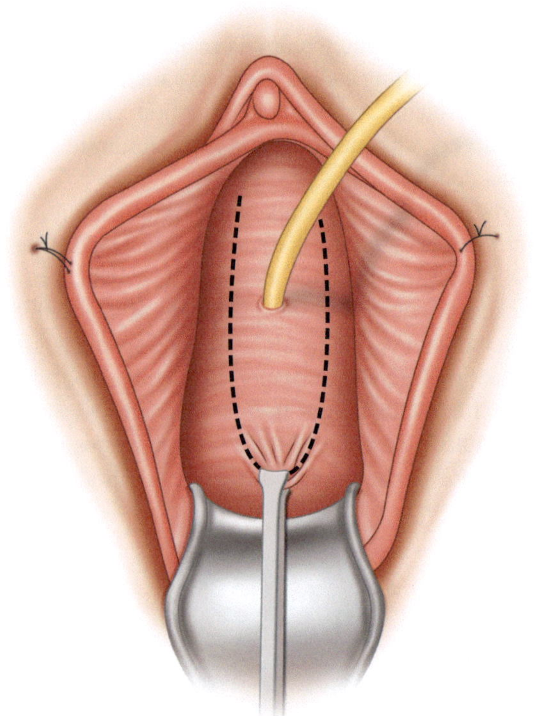

Fig. 6.42 Diagram of the incision used for urethral reconstruction. The area of the defect will be the posterior plate, and the anterior plate will be a flap of the anterior vaginal wall proximal to the defect. A U flap is created inferior to the displaced urethral meatus. The flap is dissected free. An incision lateral to the urethra is made on each side. The lateral margins of the incision are undermined and mobilized

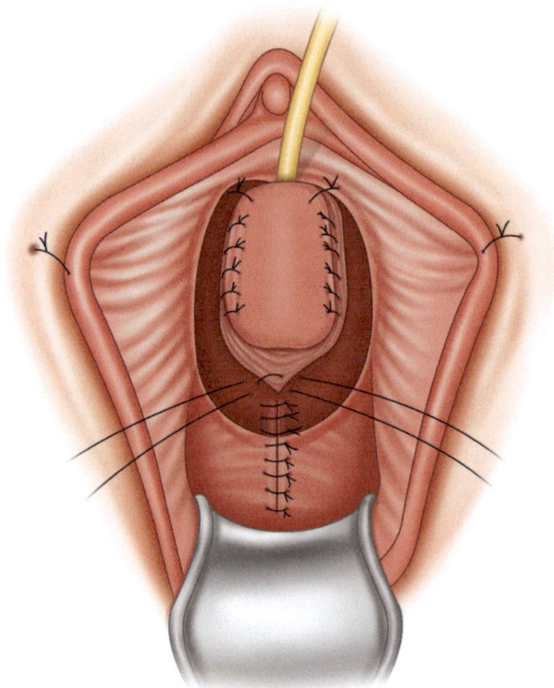

Fig. 6.43 The flap is advanced forward to cover the urethral defect. Interrupted sutures are used to anastomose the flap to the anterior vaginal wall incisions. The sutures should cover the catheter without tension. The undermined lateral incisions are sutured to cover the area of the reconstruction

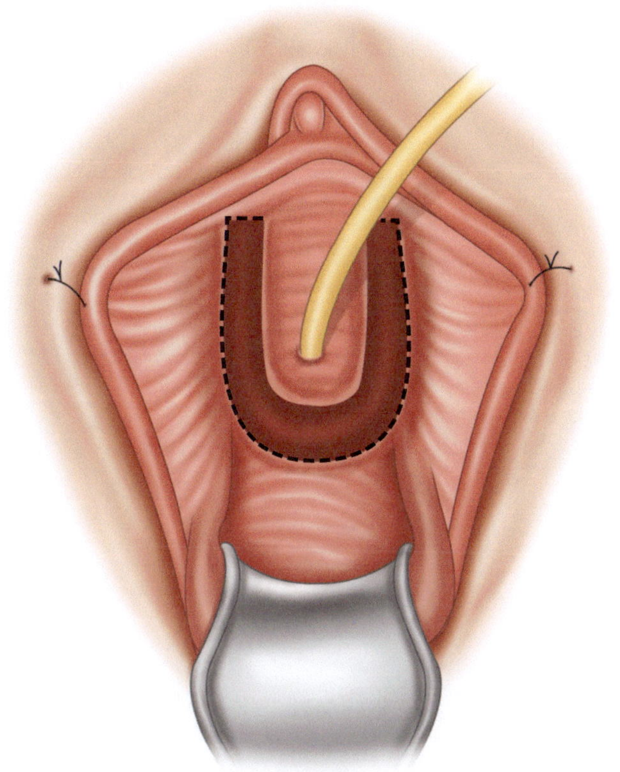

Fig. 6.44 Diagram of the urethral reconstruction using in situ vaginal wall as the tube. A U incision is made around the Foley catheter lateral enough to be able to cover the catheter tension-free. The lateral margins of the incision are dissected free and mobilized

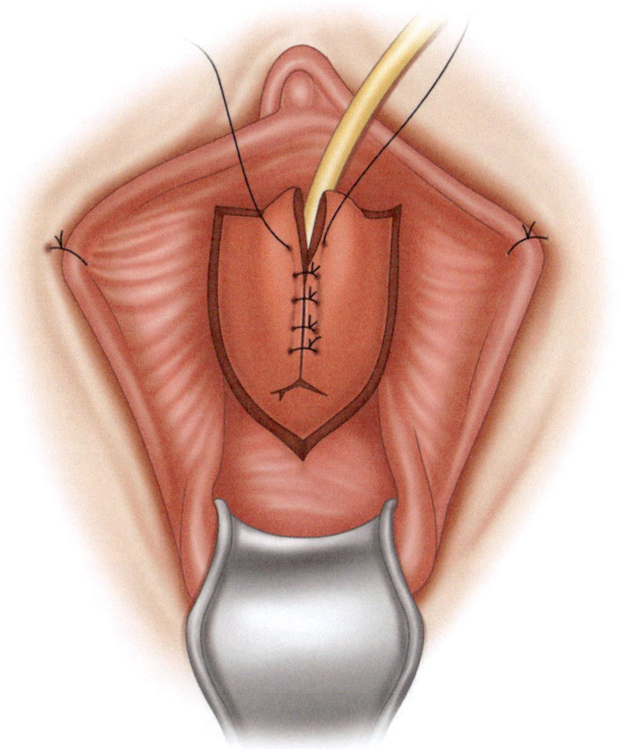

Fig. 6.45 Diagram of the next step of the reconstruction. The medial margins of the anterior plate are sutured around the catheter to form a tube. The lateral margins will be used to cover the defect

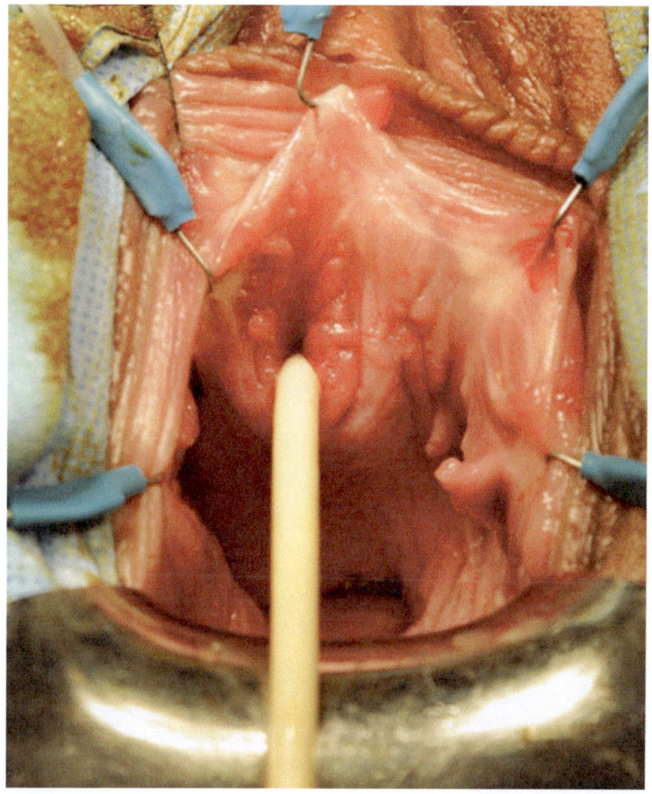

Fig. 6.46 Picture showing the urethral defect in a patient who lost half of the urethra through prior surgery. The Foley catheter is in place. The external meatus is located in a posterior location. The patient is continent and the main complaint is vaginal voiding and urethral discomfort

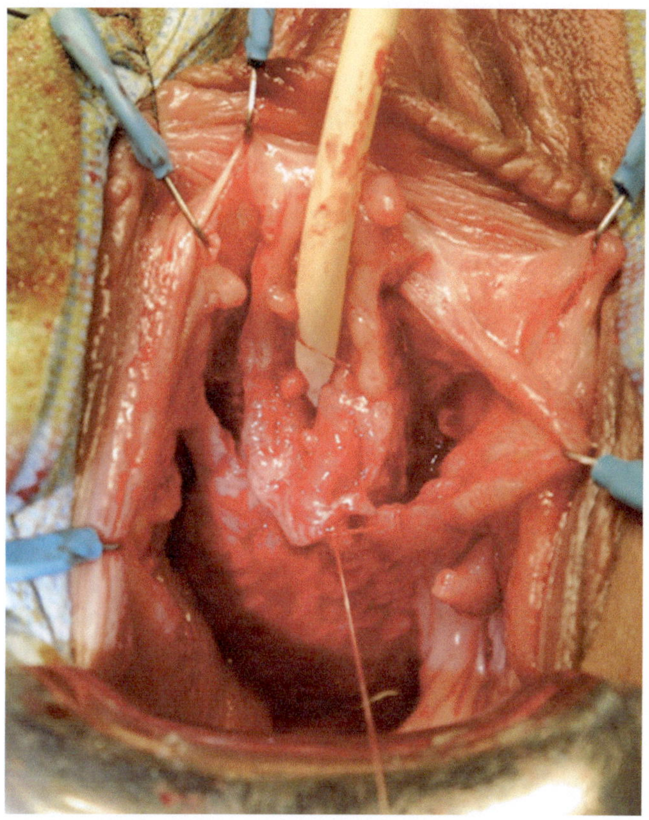

Fig. 6.47 Two incisions are made in the anterior vaginal wall, distal to the urethral meatus. The new location of the external meatus is selected

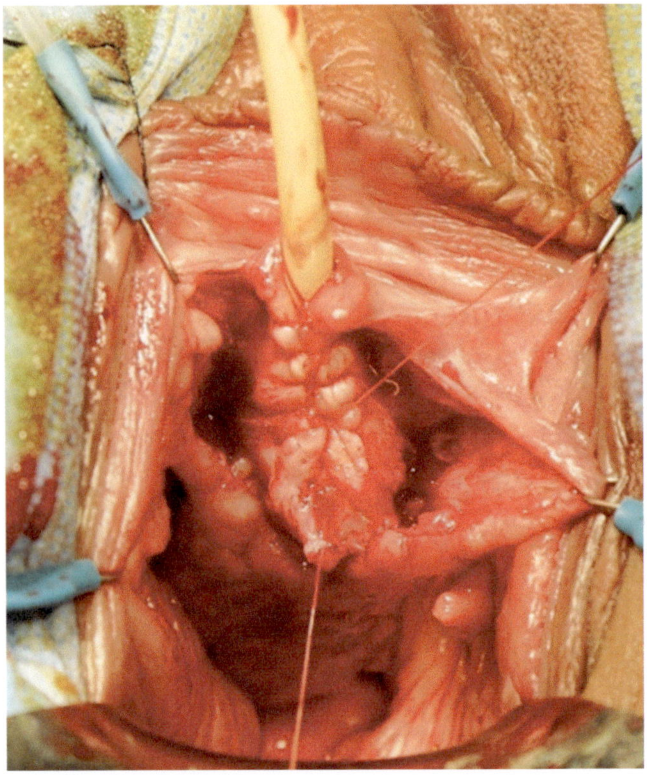

Fig. 6.48 The urethral margins are approximated and the distal half of the urethra is reconstructed with a two-layer closure using running and interrupted fine delayed absorbable sutures

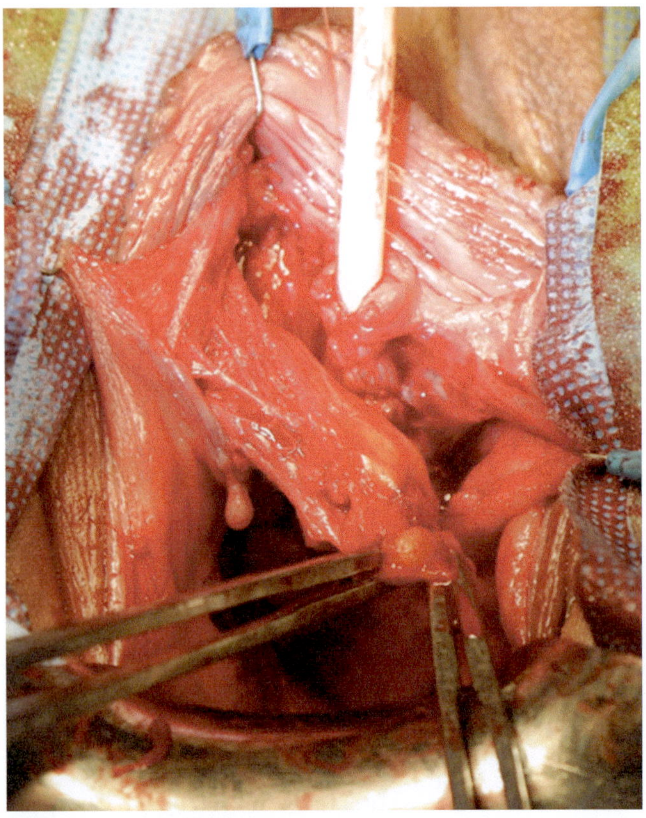

Fig. 6.49 An in situ Martius flap is prepared by dissection under the right labium, exposing the fibro-fatty tissue. The upper segment of the flap is transected and the base of the flap is rotated toward the vaginal canal

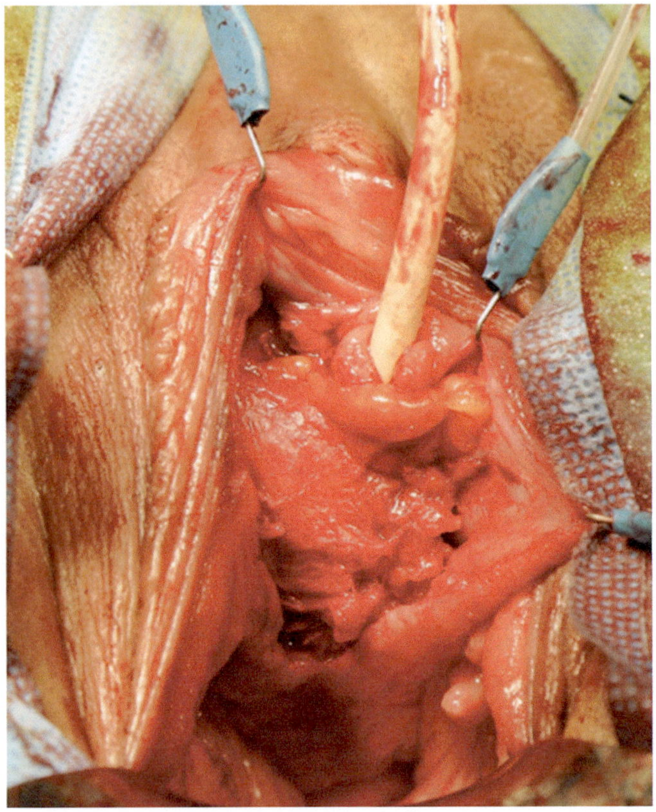

Fig. 6.50 The flap is transferred toward the left side and multiple sutures are applied to widely cover the area of the reconstructed urethra

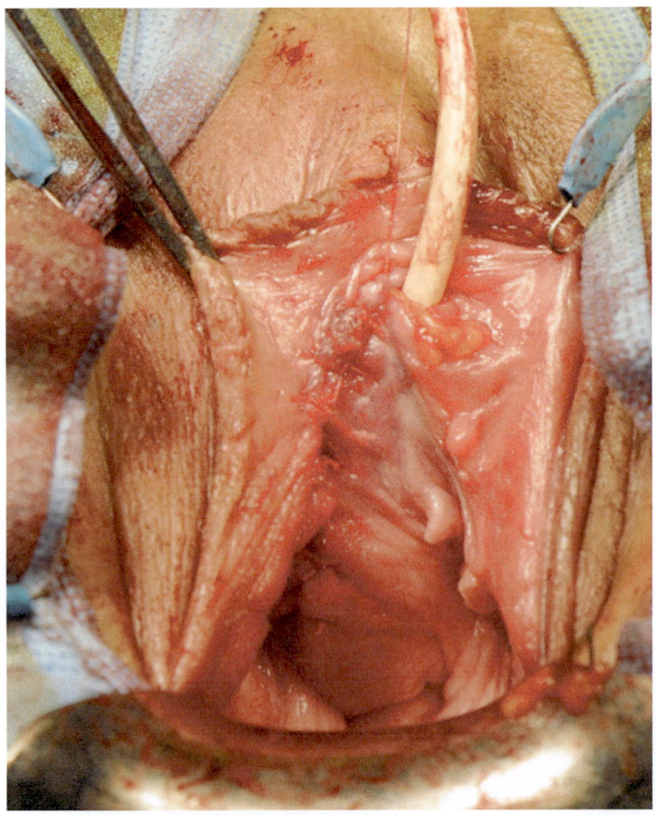

Fig. 6.51 Labial and distal vaginal tissue is used to cover the Martius flap and the area of the reconstruction

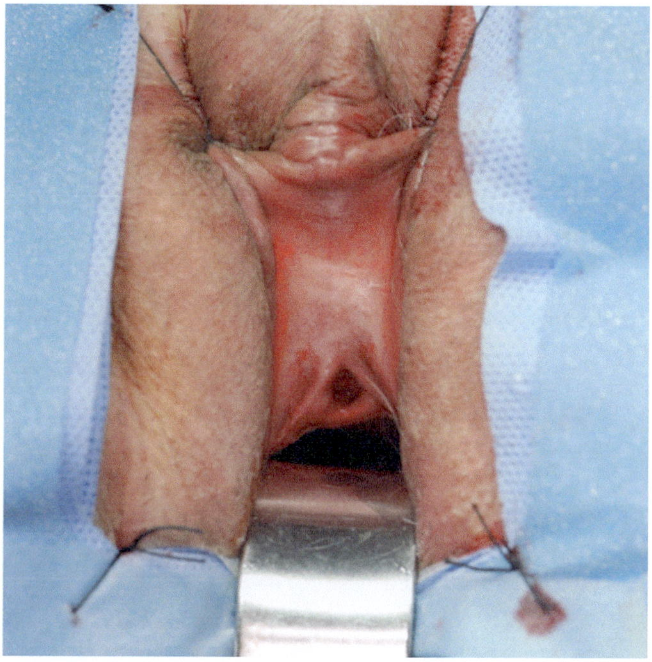

Fig. 6.52 View of the anterior vaginal wall in a patient with significant loss of the distal urethra after surgery. The urethra is hypospadiac and the patient complains of vaginal voiding

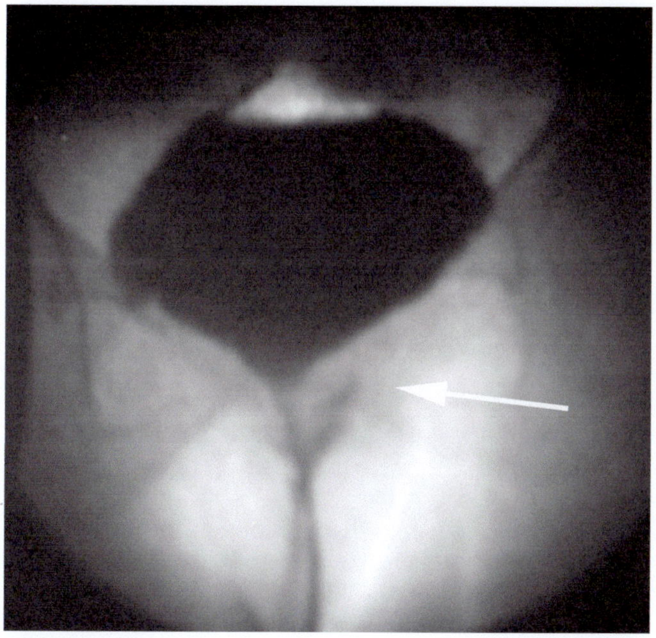

Fig. 6.53 Voiding cystogram showing the contrast filling the vaginal canal (*arrow*). No significant stress incontinence was present

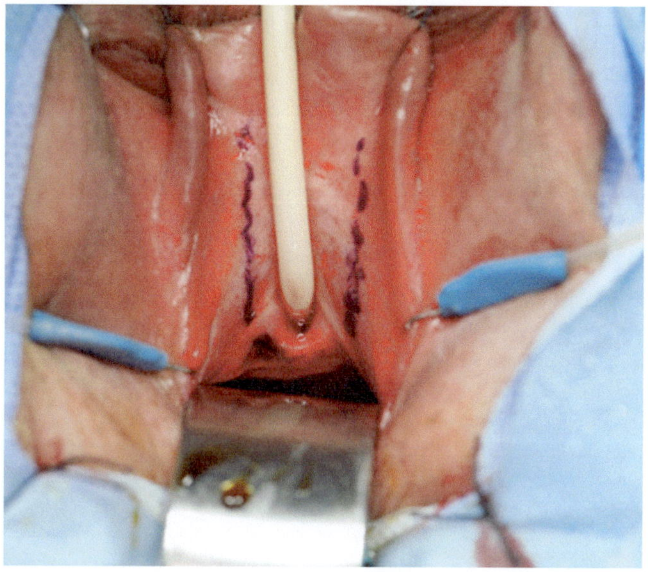

Fig. 6.54 Two longitudinal incisions will be made in the anterior vaginal wall in the area of the lost urethral wall

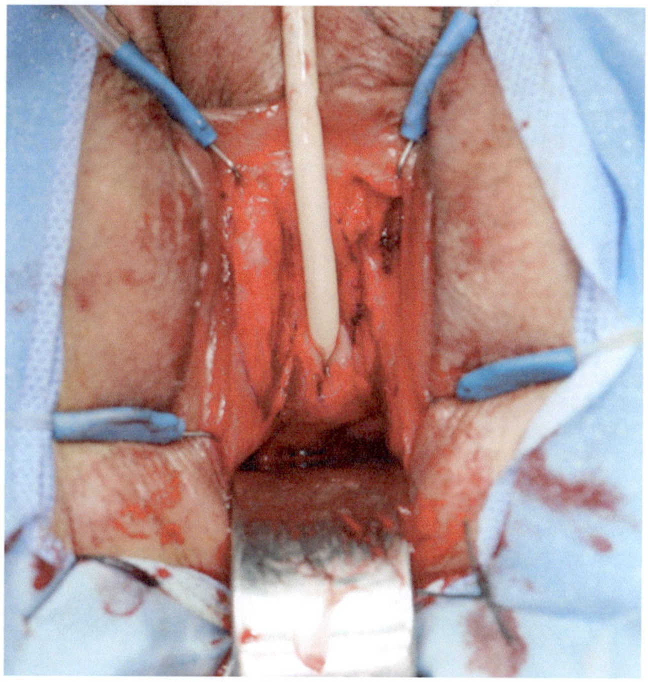

Fig. 6.55 Two incisions of the distal anterior vaginal wall are made that will be used to create the urethral tube. The incisions should be placed lateral enough to be able to rotate the margins and form a tension-free tube around the 12- or 14-Fr Foley catheter. The lateral margins of the incisions are undermined laterally and will be used to cover the urethral tube

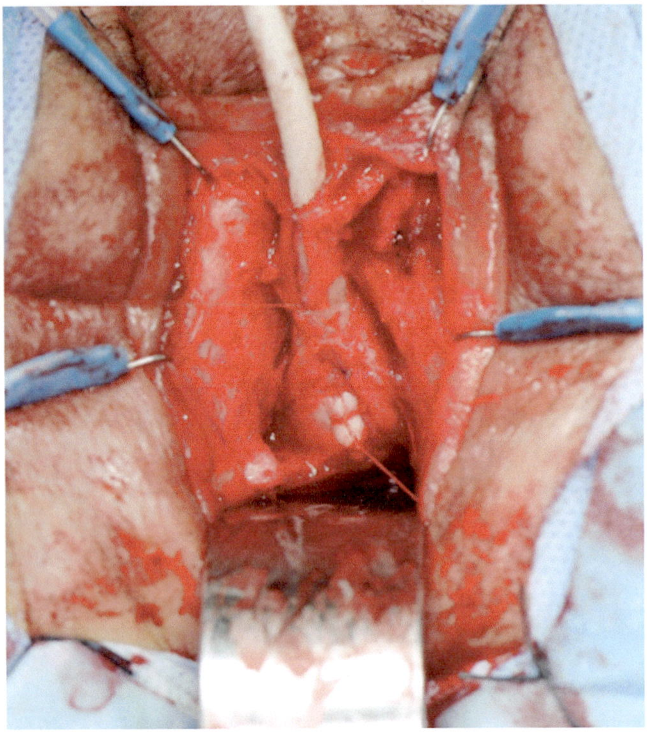

Fig. 6.56 The medial margins of the incision are sutured in a circular fashion around the Foley catheter. The reconstruction is done in two layers of running and interrupted fine delayed absorbable sutures. The catheter is moved back and forth to ensure tension-free closure

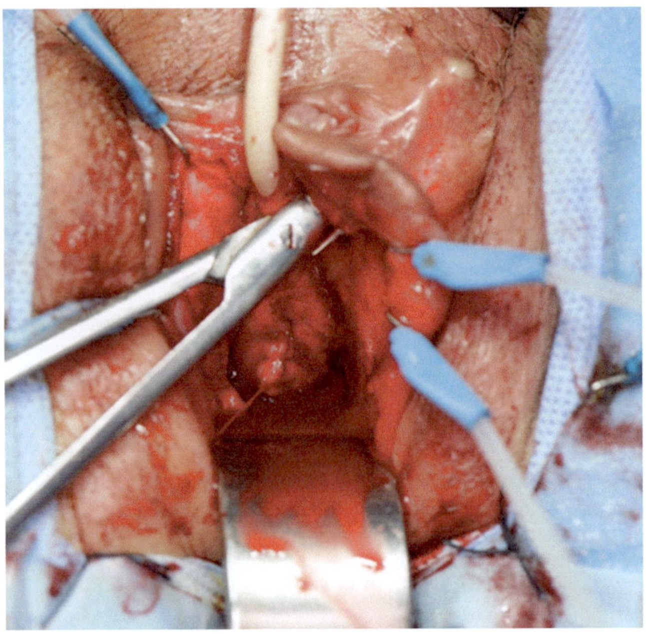

Fig. 6.57 An in situ Martius flap will be created from the left labial fibro-fatty tissue. Scissors are used to dissect under the left labial skin

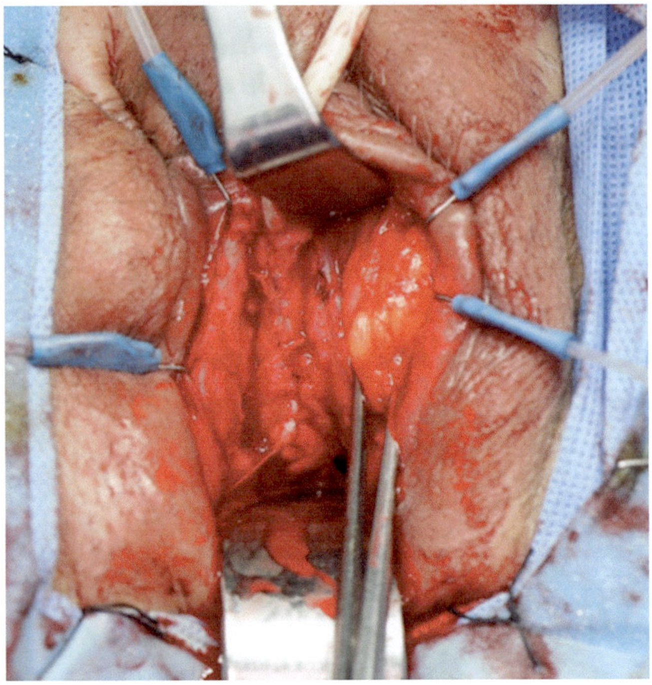

Fig. 6.58 The fatty tissue of the left labium is exposed and mobilized

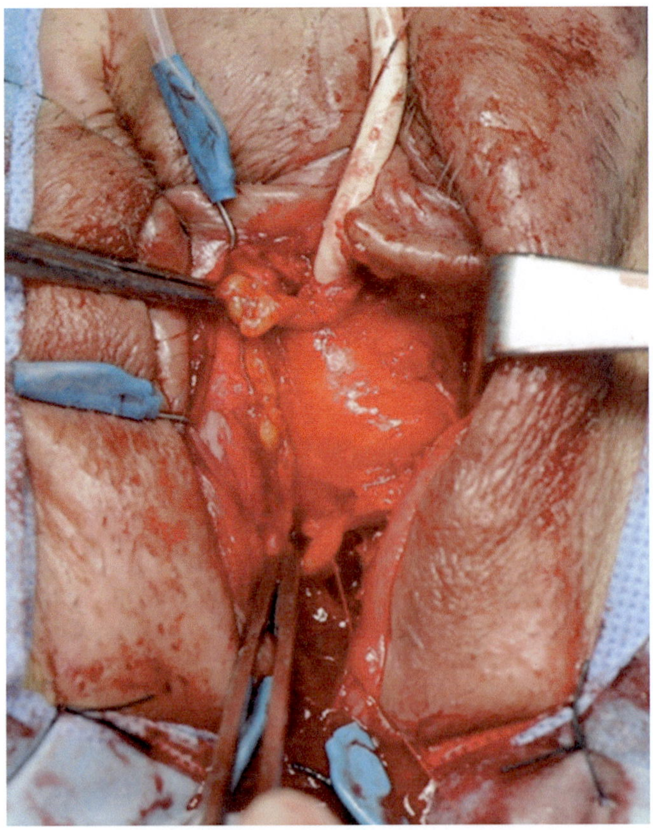

Fig. 6.59 The Martius flap has been mobilized and rotated toward the right to cover the area of reconstruction

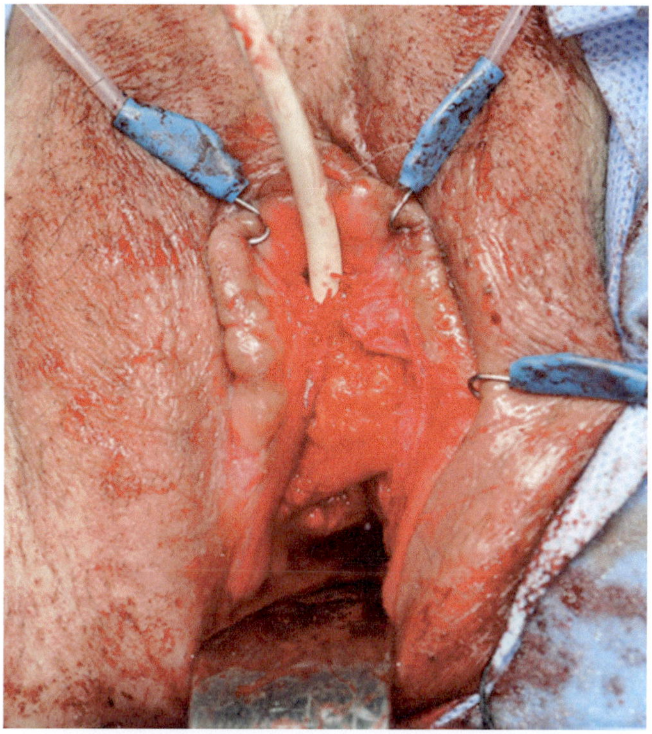

Fig. 6.60 Multiple sutures are used to fix and spread the Martius flap around the neourethra

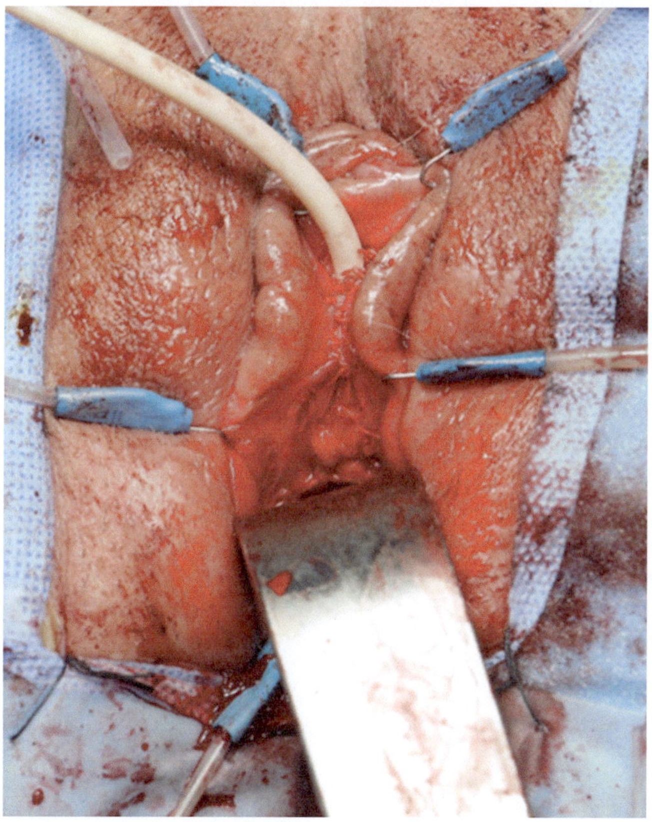

Fig. 6.61 The anterior vaginal wall and labial margins are used to cover the Martius flap. The anterior vaginal wall is seen at the end of the procedure with the new external meatus located in the normal distal position

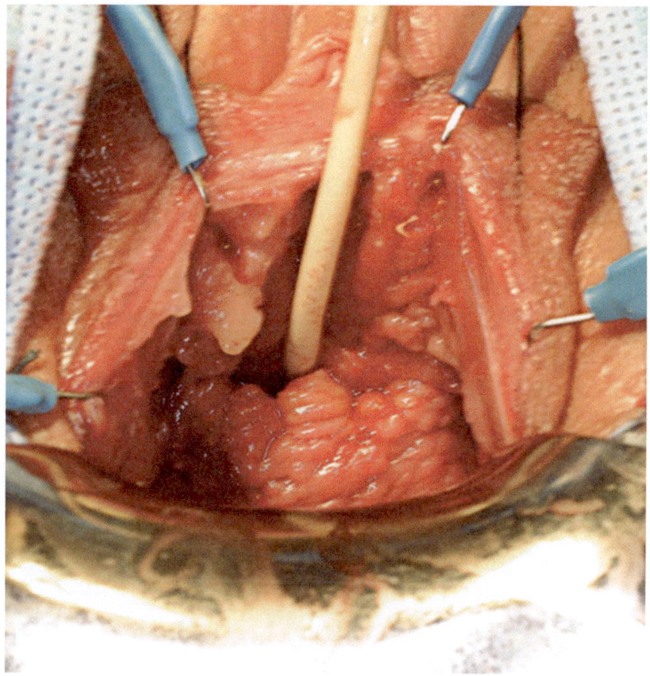

Fig. 6.62 Exposure of the anterior vaginal wall in a patient with an accidental surgical incision from the external meatus to the bladder neck resulting in total incontinence of urine and vaginal voiding

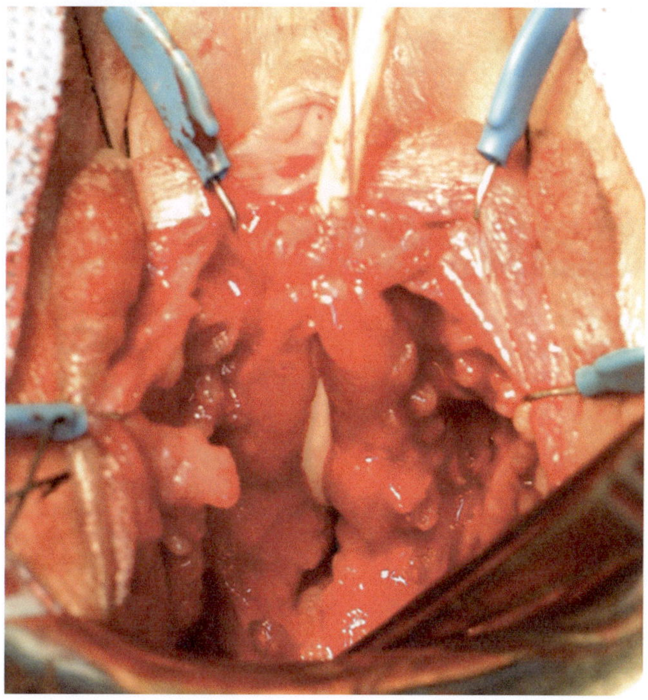

Fig. 6.63 Reconstruction of the urethra in this patient is described in detail in Chap. 5, on transvaginal repair of fistulas

6.4 Labioplasty for Excess Labia Majora

6.4.1 Indications

Though most of these surgeries are done for cosmetic reasons, some patients have clear medical indications. These include difficulties with spraying during urination, pain, discomfort, and dyspareunia.

On examination, other vaginal or urethral pathology should be ruled out. The excess labia are demonstrated by lateral traction of the upper margins of the labia.

6.4.2 Surgical Procedure

Figures 6.64, 6.65, 6.66, 6.67, 6.68, 6.69, 6.70, 6.71, 6.72, 6.73, 6.74, and 6.75 illustrate the technique for reduction labioplasty.

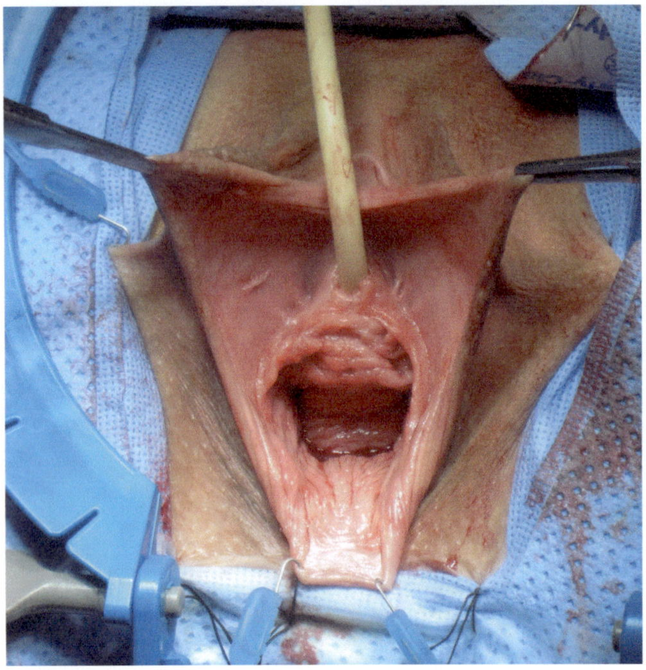

Fig. 6.64 The anterior vaginal wall is exposed after applying lateral traction to the labia

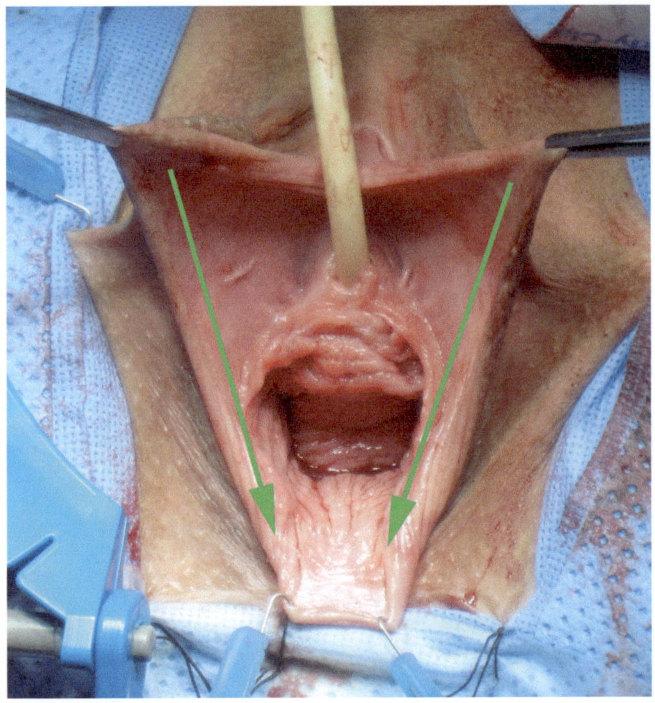

Fig. 6.65 The upper corner of the labium will be transferred to an inferior position after excision of the excess labial skin. The *arrows* indicate the extent of the line of incision of the inner labia majora

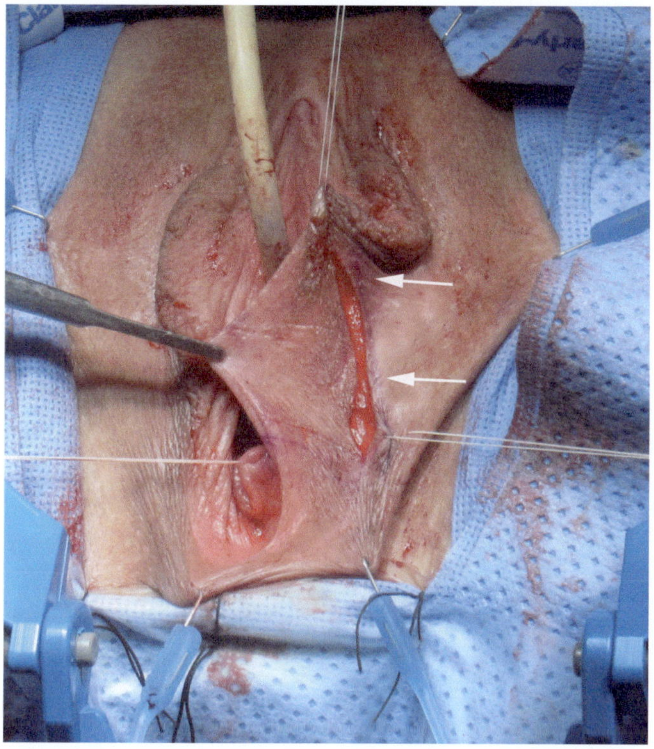

Fig. 6.66 A stay suture is applied to the upper margin of the labium. An oblique incision is made in the lateral aspect of the labium, extending to its base. The *arrows* indicate the lateral labial incision prior to excision

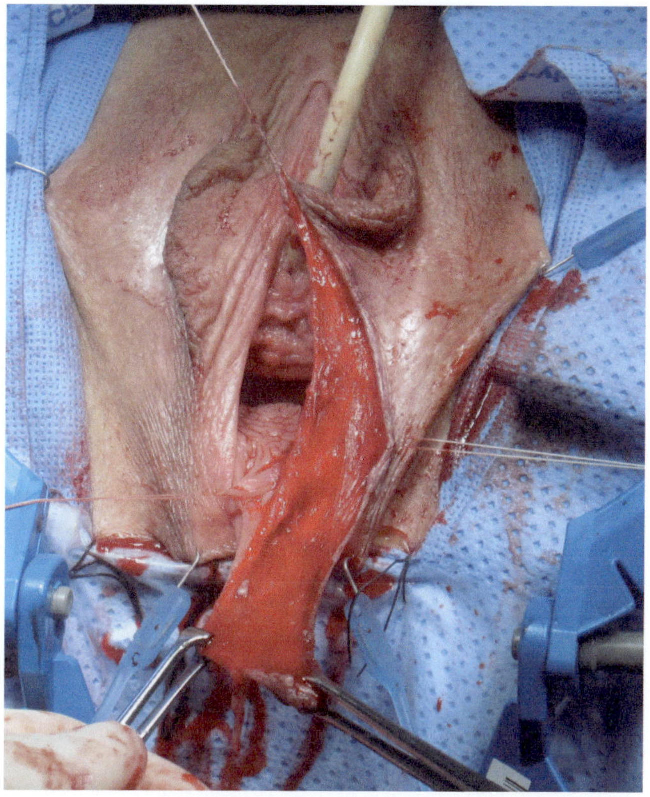

Fig. 6.68 The labial skin between the two incisions is excised, taking care to be very superficial and prevent any excision of the labial fibro-fatty tissue

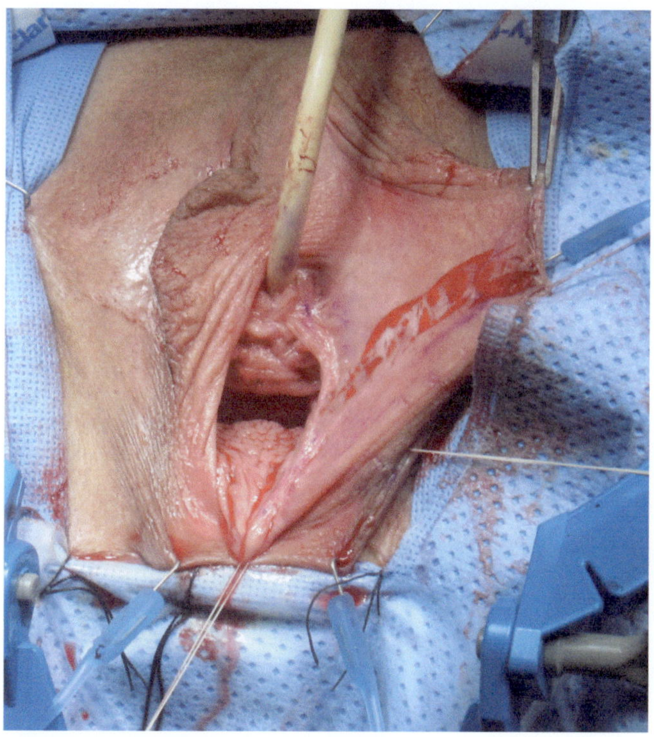

Fig. 6.67 Similarly to the lateral labial skin incision, an oblique incision is made in the medial aspect of the labial skin

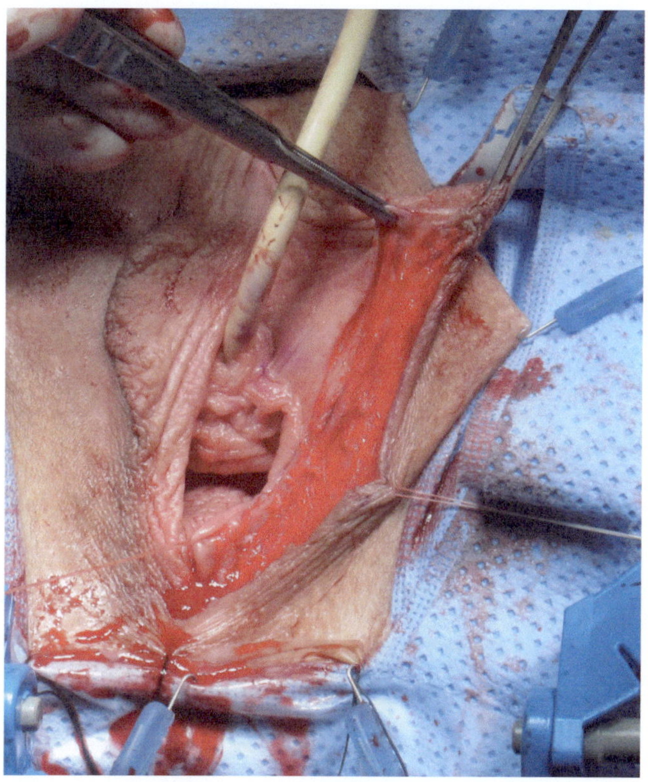

Fig. 6.69 The labium is retracted superiorly after the excision of the medial and lateral skin

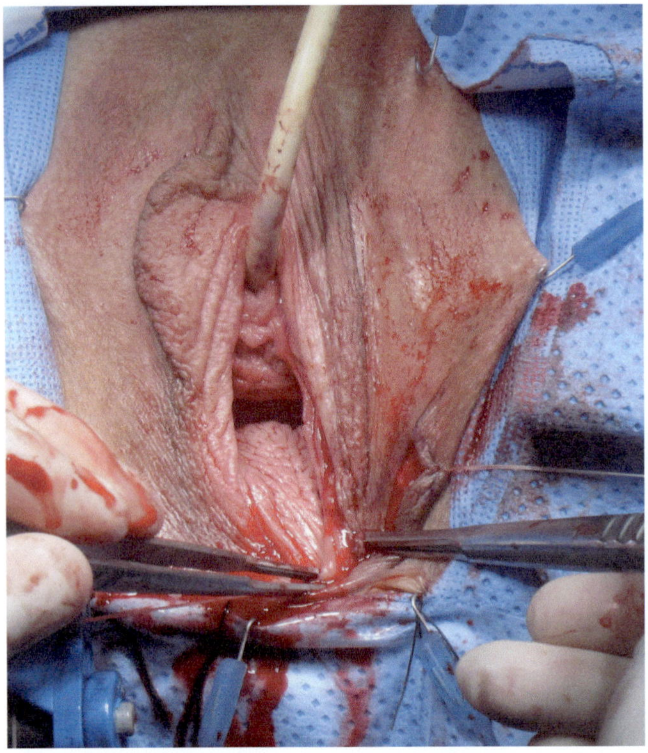

Fig. 6.70 The upper margin of the reduced labial skin is brought down to the inferior margin of the introitus

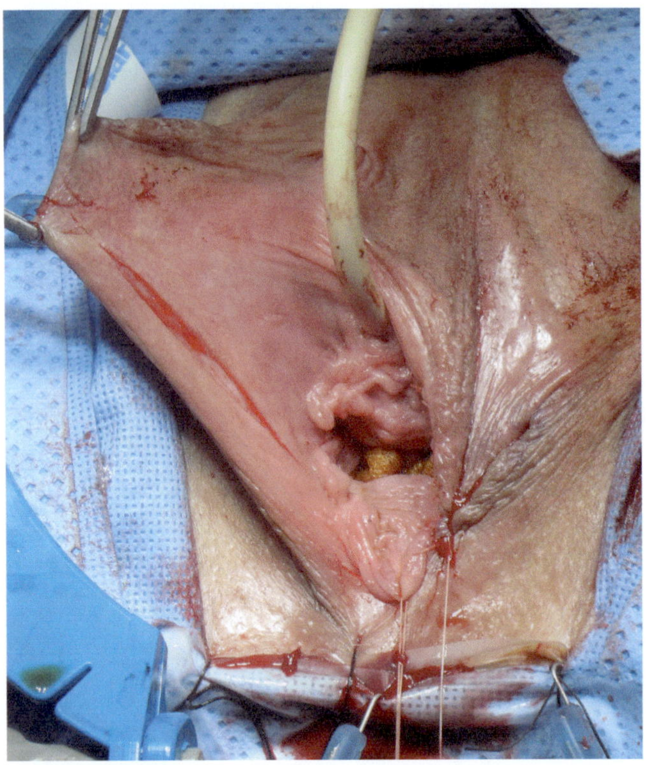

Fig. 6.71 Fine delay absorbable sutures are used to anastomose the reduced labium to the medial and lateral aspects of the initial incision

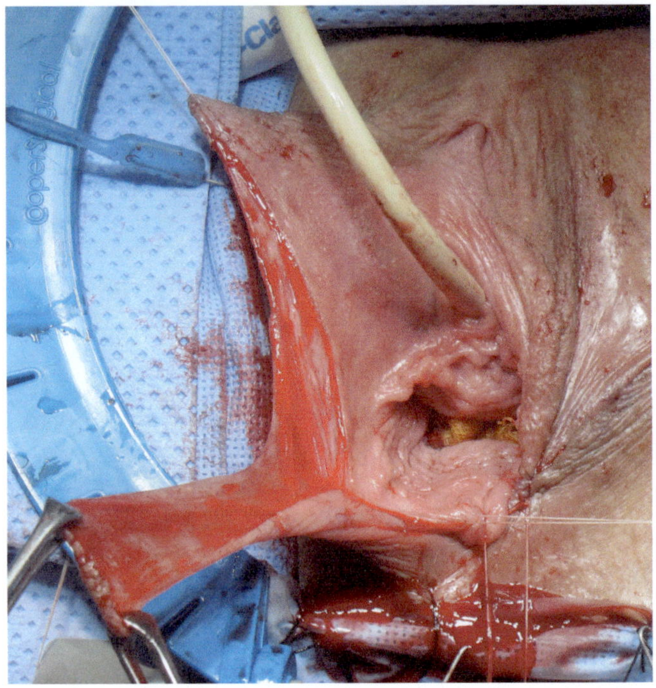

Fig. 6.72 A similar dissection is performed on the contralateral side. Medial and lateral incisions of the labium are performed and a triangular segment of skin is excised

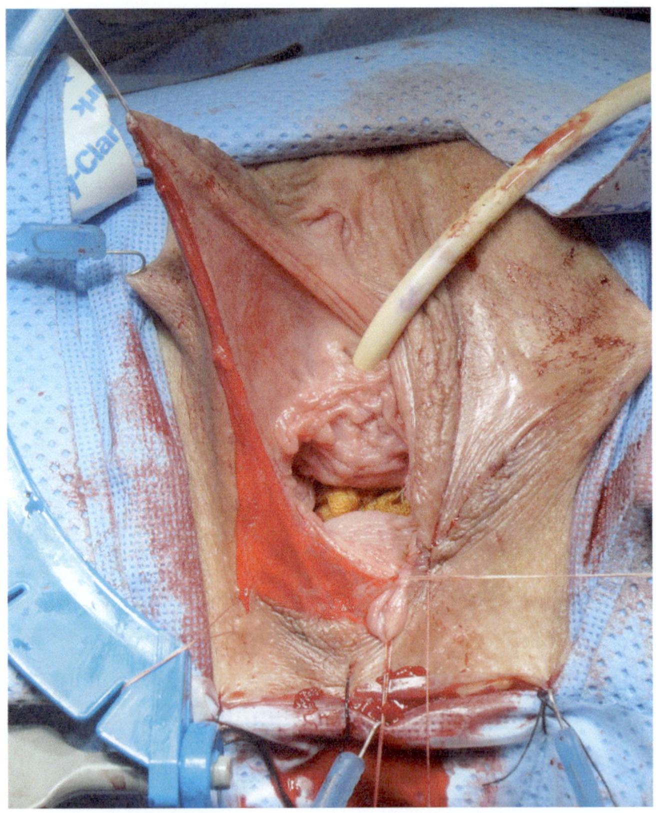

Fig. 6.73 The upper margin of the reduced labium is elevated superiorly

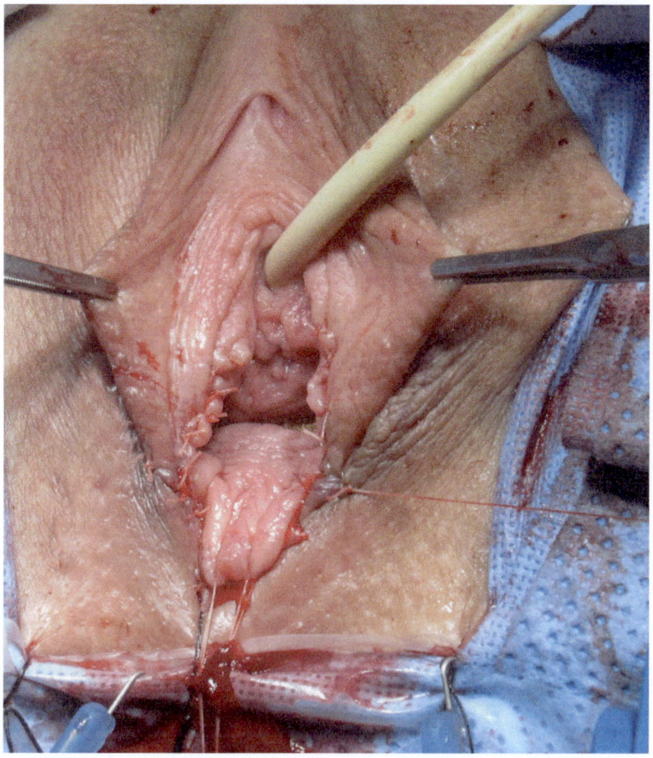

Fig. 6.74 The anastomosis of the reduced labium to the medial and lateral labial incisions is performed using fine delay absorbable sutures

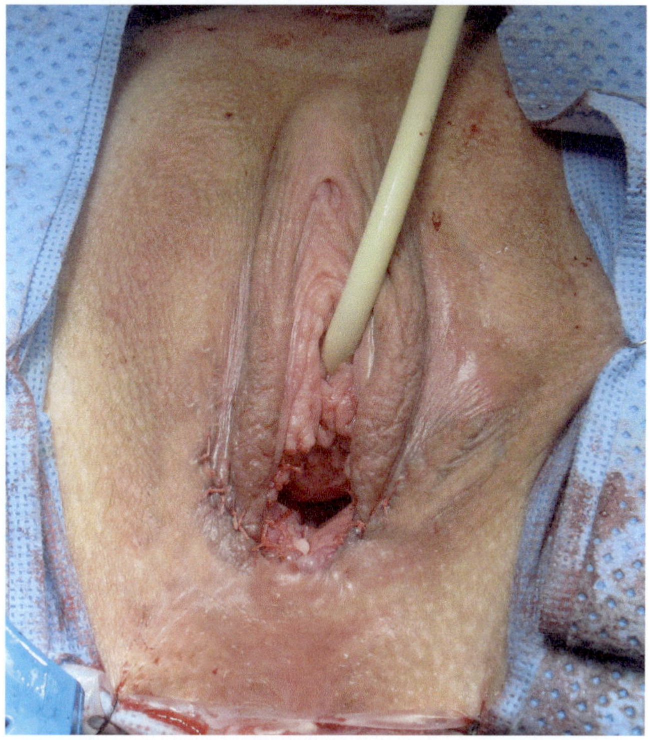

Fig. 6.75 Final result of the reduction labioplasty

6.4.3 Postoperative Care

A small dressing is applied for a few hours. The patient can resume normal activities but is prevented from sexual intercourse for 3–4 weeks.

6.4.4 Complications

Skin infection should resolve with antibiotics and drainage, if required. Bleeding or hematoma of the labia can occur and should resolve with conservative measures. Rarely, drainage is required. Dissatisfaction with the cosmetic result may require further intervention. Labial pain and numbness should resolve with time. Deep excision of the labial skin may result in long-term lack of labial sensations.

Suggested Reading

Abramov Y, Feiner B, Rosen T, Bardichev M, Gutterman E, Lissak A, et al. Primary repair of advanced obstetric anal sphincter tears: should it be performed by the overlapping sphincteroplasty technique? Int Urogynecol J Pelvic Floor Dysfunct. 2008;19(8):1071–4.

Blaivas JG, Flisser AJ, Bleustein CB, Panagopoulos G. Periurethral masses: etiology and diagnosis in a large series of women. Obstet Gynecol. 2004;103:842–7.

Blaschko SD, Yang JH, Baskin LS, Deng DY. Combined method of bladder neck closure and concomitant augmentation cystoplasty in the setting of refractory urinary incontinence. Urology. 2012;79(4):955–7.

Dmochowski RR, Ganabathi K, Zimmern PE, Leach GE. Benign female periurethral masses. J Urol. 1994;152:1943–51.

Dudding TC, Vaizey CJ, Kamm MA. Obstetric anal sphincter injury: incidence, risk factors, and management. Ann Surg. 2008;247(2):224–37.

Eilber KS, Raz S. Benign cystic lesions of the vagina: a literature review. J Urol. 2003;170(3):717–22.

Escribano Patiño G, Husillos Alonso A, Rodriguez Fernandez E, Cancho Gil MJ, Hernandez FC. Urethral stricture in women. (Article in Spanish.). Arch Esp Urol. 2014;67(1):129–37.

Fernando RJ, Sultan AH, Kettle C, Thakar R. Methods of repair for obstetric anal sphincter injury. Cochrane Database Syst Rev. 2013;12:CD002866. doi:10.1002/14651858.CD002866.pub3.

Hamori CA. Aesthetic surgery of the female genitalia: labiaplasty and beyond. Plast Reconstr Surg. 2014;134(4):661–73.

Kavanagh A, Afshar K, Scott H, MacNeily AE. Bladder neck closure in conjunction with enterocystoplasty and Mitrofanoff diversion for complex incontinence: closing the door for good. J Urol. 2012; 188(4 Suppl):1561–5.

Kowalik C, Stoffel JT, Zinman L, Vanni AJ, Buckley JC. Intermediate outcomes after female urethral reconstruction: graft vs flap. Urology. 2014;83(5):1181–5.

Norderval S, Røssaak K, Markskog A, Vonen B. Incontinence after primary repair of obstetric anal sphincter tears is related to relative length of reconstructed external sphincter: a case-control study. Ultrasound Obstet Gynecol. 2012;40(2):207–14.

Petrou SP, Rogers AE, Parker AS, Green KM, McRoberts JW. Dorsal vaginal graft urethroplasty for female urethral stricture disease. BJU Int. 2012;110(11 Pt C):E1090–5.

Radwan MH, Abou Farha MO, Soliman MG, El Refai M, Ragab MM, Shaaban AM, et al. Outcome of female urethral reconstruction: a 12-year experience. World J Urol. 2013;31(4):991–5.

Rovner ES, Goudelocke CM, Gilchrist A, Lebed B. Transvaginal bladder neck closure with posterior urethral flap for devastated urethra. Urology. 2011;78:208–12.

Soerensen MM, Pedersen BG, Santoro GA, Buntzen S, Bek K, Laurberg S. Long-term function and morphology of the anal sphincters and the pelvic floor after primary repair of obstetric anal sphincter injury. Colorectal Dis. 2014;16(10):O347–55.

Triana L, Robledo AM. Refreshing labioplasty techniques for plastic surgeons. Aesthetic Plast Surg. 2012;36:1078–86.

Willis H, Safiano NA, Lloyd LK. Comparison of transvaginal and retropubic bladder neck closure with suprapubic catheter in women. J Urol. 2015;193(1):196–202.

Wu JA, Braschi EJ, Gulminelli PL, Comiter CV. Labioplasty for hypertrophic labia minora contributing to recurrent urinary tract infections. Female Pelvic Med Reconstr Surg. 2013;19(2):121–3.

Zimmern PE, Hadley RH, Leach GE, Raz S. Transvaginal closure of bladder neck and placement of suprapubic catheter for destroyed urethra after long-term catheterization. J Urol. 1985;134:554–7.

Bladder Outlet Obstruction

7

Bladder outlet obstruction in the female is rare. The patient may complain of symptoms of obstruction such as the need to strain, difficulty in starting the stream, interrupted or prolonged stream, or the sensation of incomplete emptying. The patient's symptoms may not correlate with the residuals of urine, which can be low or high. Patients with chronic retention can present with minimal symptoms of obstruction but a significant residual of urine.

7.1 Etiology of Urethral Obstruction

Many factors can contribute to the etiology of urethral obstruction in women:

- Prior anti-incontinence surgery
- Urethral stricture
- Primary bladder neck obstruction
- Extrinsic compression
- Pelvic organ prolapse
- Neoplasm
- Infection
- Prolapsed urethral mucosa
- Urethral angulation (kinking)

After sling procedures, a number of factors can result in urinary retention and obstruction.

- Too much tension (tied too tight)
- Fixed, nonmobile urethra
- Sling that is into the urethral wall without entering mucosa
- Urethral fibrosis (post hematoma or infection)
- Sling material in the bladder or urethra
- Cystocele (secondary or primary)
- Bladder dysfunction (impaired contractility)

Electronic supplementary material The online version of this chapter (doi:10.1007/978-1-4939-2941-2_7) contains supplementary material, which is available to authorized users.

7.2 Diagnosis of Urethral Obstruction

The diagnosis of urethral obstruction in the female is not standard. Many patients present with clear lesions causing distal obstruction (thrombosis of distal urethra, Skene's gland diverticula). The inability to pass a catheter in the female requires further testing and may be diagnostic of the location of the stricture. In patients with bladder neck obstruction, the passage of a catheter through the urethra can be without difficulties. Urodynamic findings like high pressures and low flow often are not present. Since the present of a urethral catheter may distort the voiding pattern of the patient during the voiding phase. Also patients with a de-compensated large bladder will not develop high pressure voiding. Radiological findings of a stricture or narrowing of the urethra in the presence of a sustained bladder contraction appear to be the most reliable method of diagnosis. Cystoscopy is important to locate the stricture location and determine the size of the stricture.

The etiology of female outlet obstruction can involve various benign or malignant lesions, functional or anatomical, as listed above. The most common reason for urethral obstruction is urinary retention after an anti-incontinence procedure. Inability to void after surgery for stress incontinence is one of the most devastating complications for a patient who was voiding normally before surgery. Technical problems are the most common reason for the obstruction, but urethral obstruction can occur in spite of adherence to the most detailed surgical technique.

With abdominal surgery, the Marshall–Marchetti operation is most prone to create urethral obstruction because of the close proximity of the suspension sutures to the urethral wall, creating fixation and fibrosis of the urethra. In the Burch bladder neck suspension, sutures are placed laterally to the urethra, leaving the urethra free to contract, funnel, and open during voiding. But in the Burch suspension, close proximity of the suspending vaginal sutures to the urethra can entrap it, producing urinary obstruction.

S. Raz, *Atlas of Vaginal Reconstructive Surgery*, DOI 10.1007/978-1-4939-2941-2_7

In vaginal surgery, this complication is seen mainly in sling procedures and bladder neck suspension procedures, and very rarely with anterior colporrhaphy. Applying excessive tension on the suspension sutures, applying the sutures too close to the urethra, or bleeding or infection owing to fibrosis are all risk factors for postoperative urinary retention.

7.2.1 Diagnosis of Inability to Void After Surgery for Incontinence

Inability to void a few days or weeks after anti-incontinence surgery should initiate diagnostic maneuvers to rule out urethral obstruction. The patient should be taught intermittent self-catheterization to eliminate the Foley catheter as a factor in persistent retention. A history of urgency, frequency, and overactive bladder symptoms is a good predictor of bladder function. The physical examination should look for the presence of a large cystocele creating obstruction, urethral fixation, and elevation or scar tissue or granulating tissue present in the anterior vaginal wall. Cystoscopy will rule out any urethral or bladder injury from accidental suture penetration. The cystoscopy can be used to assess urethral fixation. One of the important features of organic obstruction is the loss of the normal elastic mobility of the urethra while moving the cystoscope sheath up and down. Urethral dilation and calibration can be performed, but organic urethral obstruction is rarely found. Urodynamic evaluation can be performed to study bladder contractility, sensations, compliance, level of continence, and pressure-flow studies. In urodynamics, we study sensations, compliance level or continence, and pressure-flow recording; they are important to show storage and voiding function. Urodynamic studies have been not predictable or correlated with the outcome of surgery to correct obstruction. If the patient is still unable to void after 3 or 4 months, surgical correction should be considered.

7.3 Preoperative Considerations

The surgical approach to urethrolysis (takedown) surgery can be transabdominal or transvaginal. The abdominal approach is rarely needed and reserved for very selected patients in whom abdominal anti-incontinence surgery is the reason for the retention. The use of omental flaps is recommended in this situation. The vaginal approach can be used for patients in whom either vaginal or abdominal surgery is the reason for the retention. Two types of transvaginal procedures are described in this chapter: anterior vaginal wall procedures and suprameatal urethrolysis. Urethrotomies and transurethral incisions of the bladder neck are to be discouraged in patients with obstruction after anti-incontinence surgery.

7.4 Surgical Techniques

The rest of this chapter presents a variety of cases of urethral obstruction and discusses their respective treatment strategies.

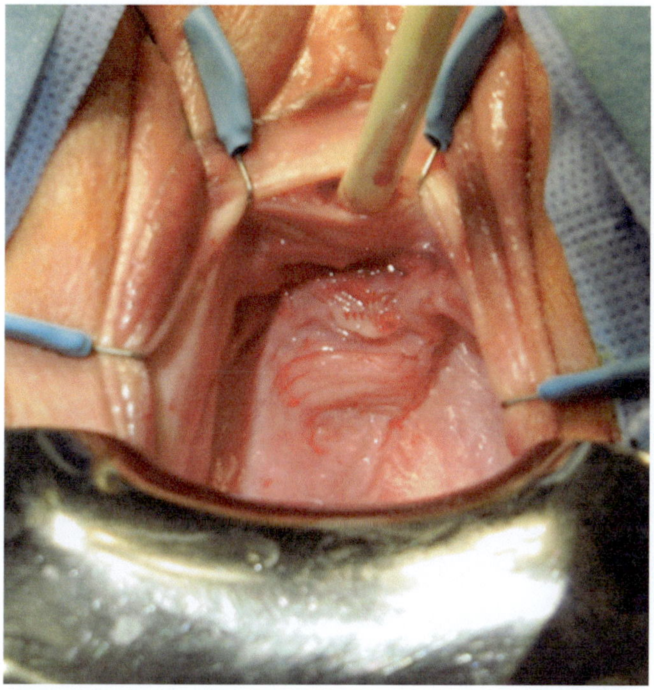

Fig. 7.1 Physical examination of a patient suffering from urinary retention after an obturator sling. On examination, the urethra is fixed (not mobile using Van Buren sounds), elevated, and angulated. Cystoscopy showed no erosion

7.4.1 Case 1: Urethral Obstruction After Sling

The patient is in urinary retention 2 months after the placement of an obturator sling. She is unable to void, performing self-catheterization (Figs. 7.1 and 7.2).

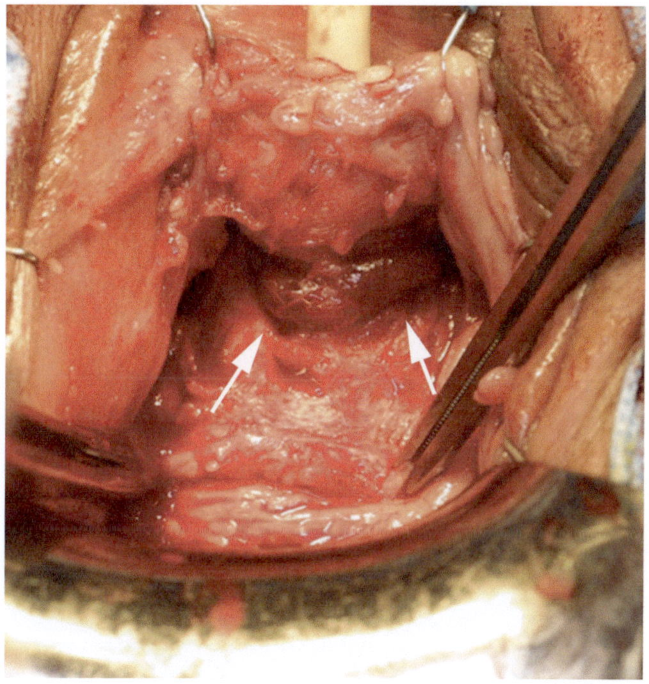

Fig. 7.2 On exploration, the mesh is found deep into the urethral wall (*arrows*) without penetration into the mucosa. Removal of the mesh corrected the retention

7.4.2 Case 2: Urethral Erosion After Sling

This patient had recurrent urinary tract infection, pain in urination, severe obstructive symptoms, and high residuals of urine after placement of a transobturator sling (Figs. 7.3 and 7.4).

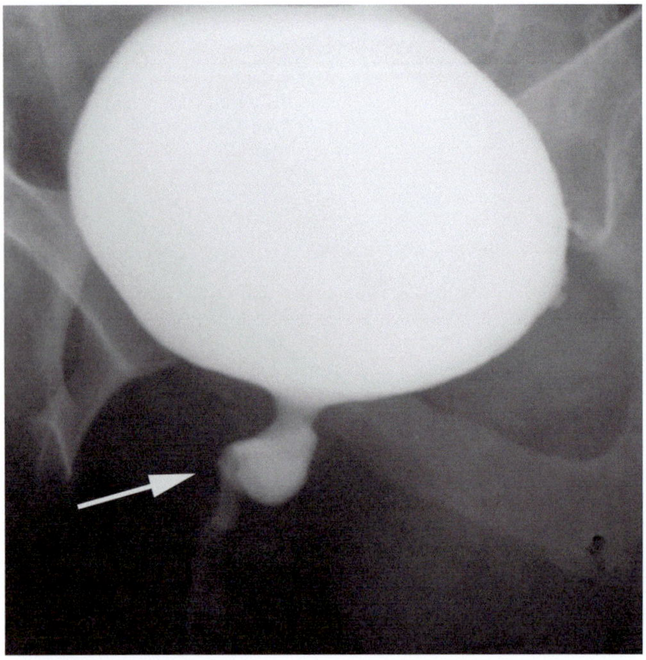

Fig. 7.3 Voiding cystogram showed an area of narrowing in the midurethra without extravasation. The *arrow* point the area of narrowing and deformity in the midurethra

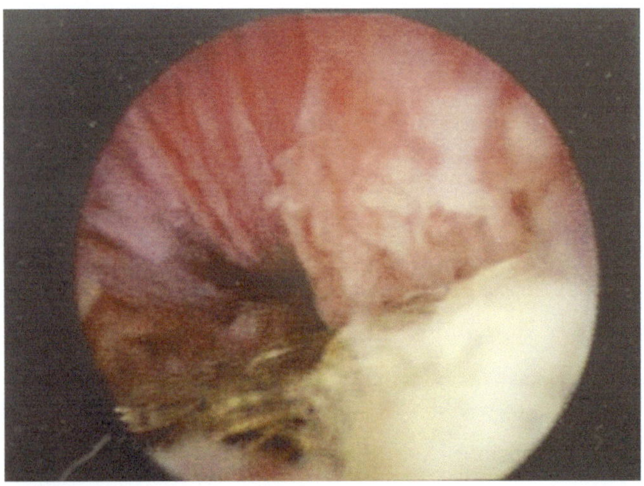

Fig. 7.4 Cystoscopy showed an erosion in the left side of the urethra that was not recognized at the time of surgery. Erosions of mesh into the urethra are unrecognized perforations during the surgery

7.4.3 Case 3: Secondary Cystocele After a Sling

The patient had a sling for stress incontinence. After voiding normally for 5 months, she started to suffer from symptoms of urinary obstruction. Postoperatively she noticed a progressive vaginal protrusion. The stream is poor and interrupted; manual reduction of the prolapse is required to void. The residual of urine is elevated (Figs. 7.5 and 7.6).

Because the patient was voiding fine after placement of the sling and the obstruction occurred many months later, the sling was left intact the cystocele was repaired correcting the problem; it was not the source of the obstruction.

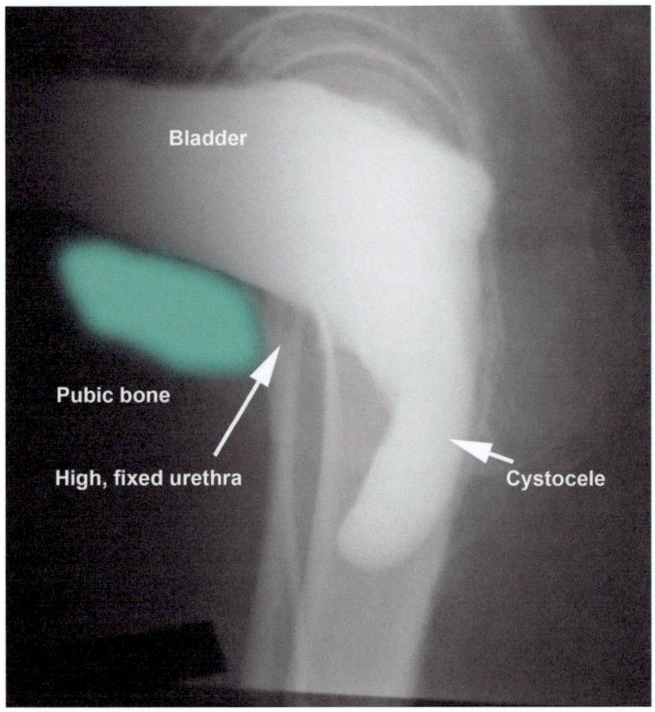

Fig. 7.5 A standing lateral cystogram shows a significant cystocele behind a highly supported urethra

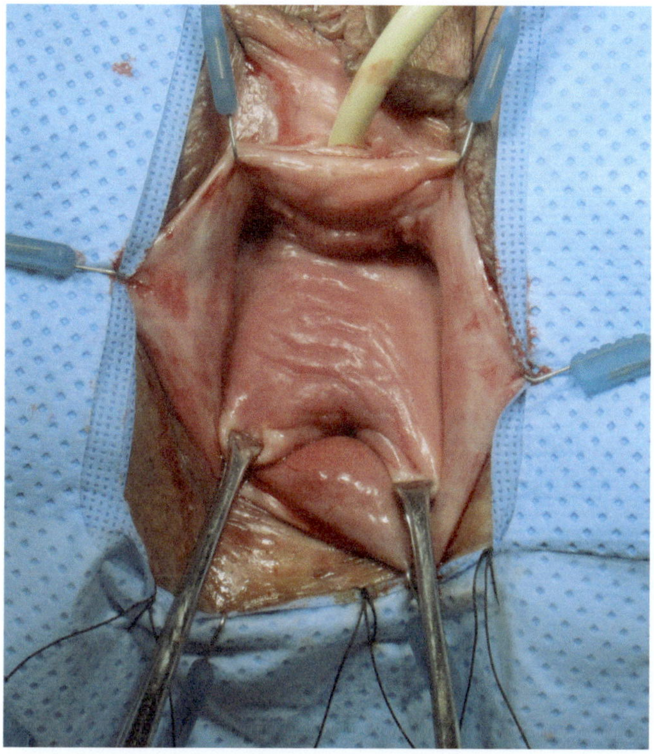

Fig. 7.6 Physical examination revealed a moderate cystocele coming out of the introitus with urethral elevation and fixation. Correction of the cystocele resulted in normal voiding, relief of the obstructive symptoms, and minimal residuals of urine

7.4.4 Case 4: Obstruction After a Burch Procedure

The patient suffered from urinary retention after a Burch procedure. She was using intermittent self-catheterization (Figs. 7.7, 7.8, and 7.9)

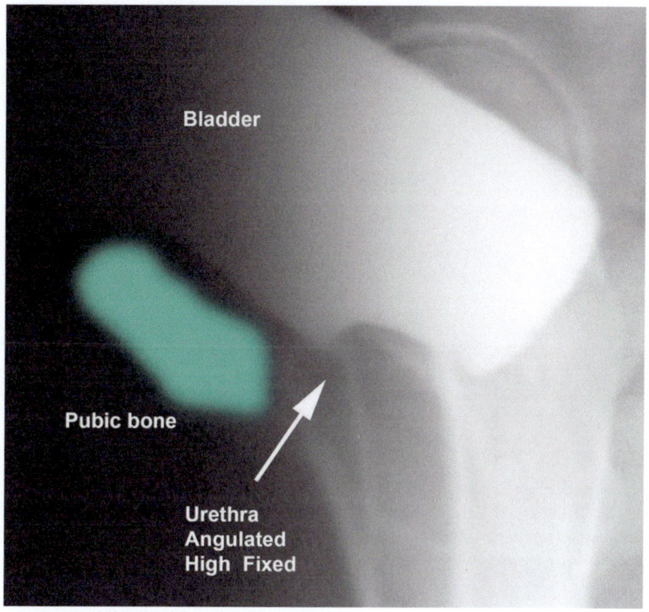

Fig. 7.7 A standing lateral cystogram shows a urethra in a high position, which is fixed and not mobile behind the pubic bone

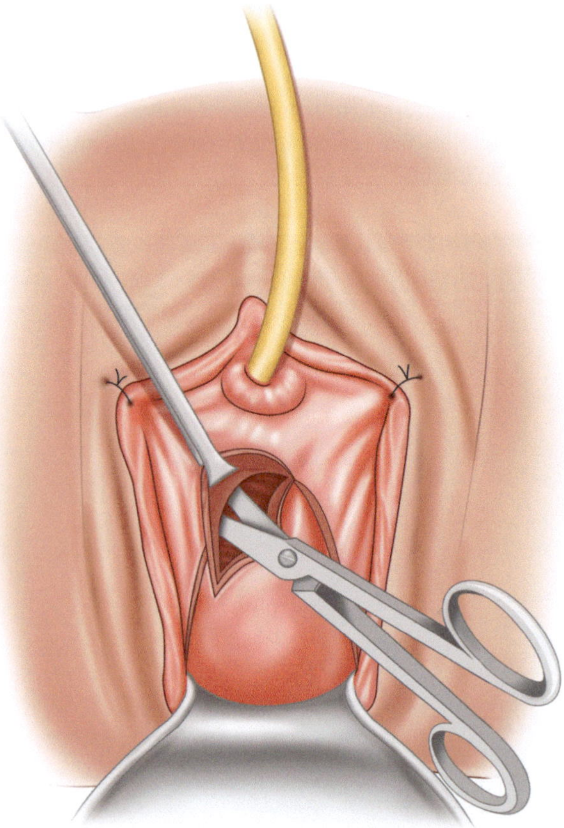

Fig. 7.8 Transvaginal retropubic urethrolysis is initiated by performing a lateral anterior vaginal wall incision and entering the retropubic space

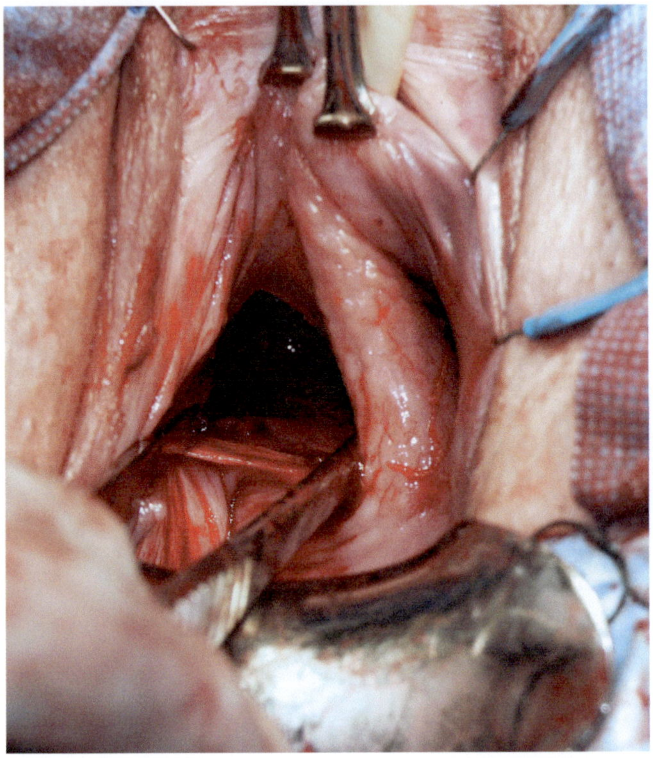

Fig. 7.9 The Burch sutures (Prolene sutures) are transected, and all adhesions of the bladder and urethra, from the posterior aspect of the pubic bone up to the Cooper ligaments, are freed. The patient was able to void on her own without retention

7.4.5 Case 5: Retention from Distal Urethral Diverticulum (Skene's Gland Cyst)

A young woman is in retention of urine owing to a large, tender, cystic lesion in the distal urethra (Figs. 7.10 and 7.11).

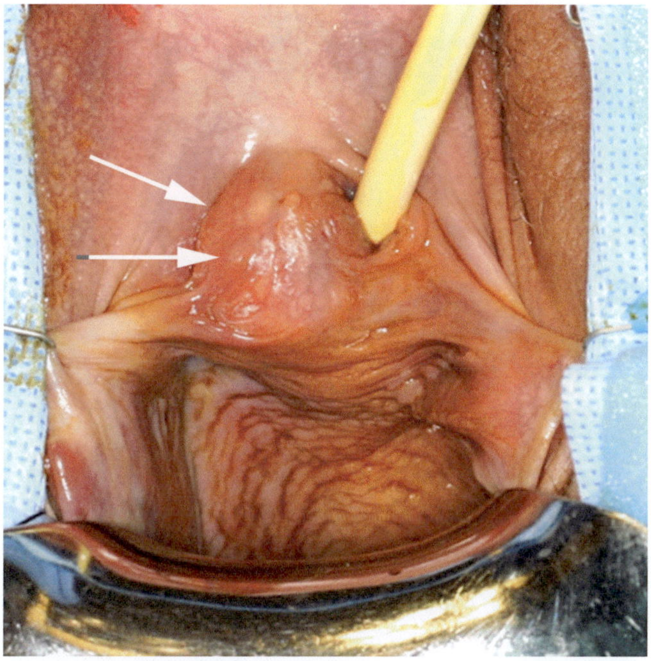

Fig. 7.10 A large, right distal cystic lesion (Skene's gland cyst) (*arrows*) displaces the urethra

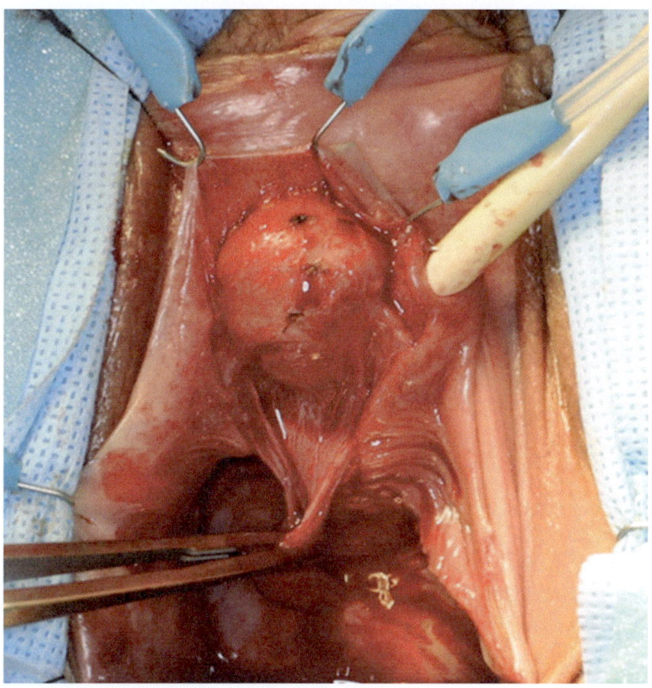

Fig. 7.11 A flap of the anterior distal vagina is performed to expose the cyst. The cyst will be excised, including the communication to the urethral meatus, leaving the urethra intact

7.4.6 Case 6: Obstruction from Distal Urethral Thrombosis

The patient developed acute urinary retention, urethral pain, and vaginal bleeding while receiving chemotherapy for advanced ovarian cancer (Figs. 7.12 and 7.13).

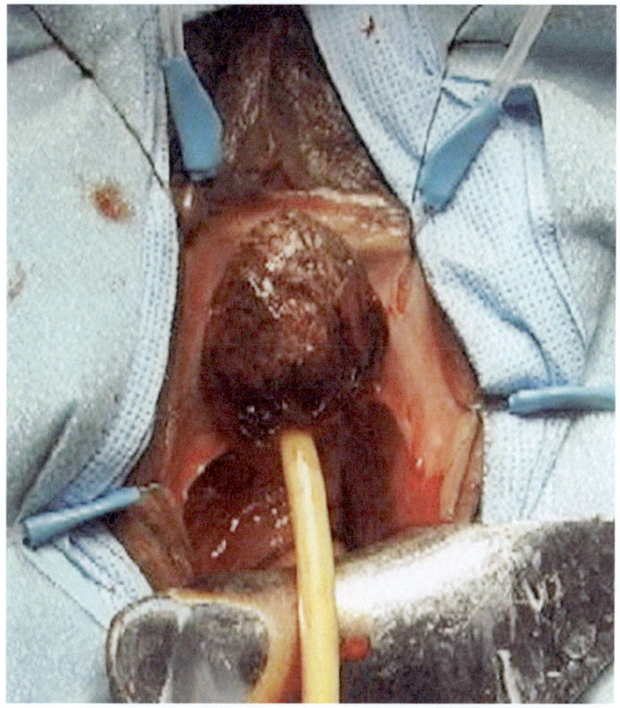

Fig. 7.12 A large, friable, tender mass is present in the distal urethra due to thrombosis and prolapse of the distal urethra, causing the urinary retention

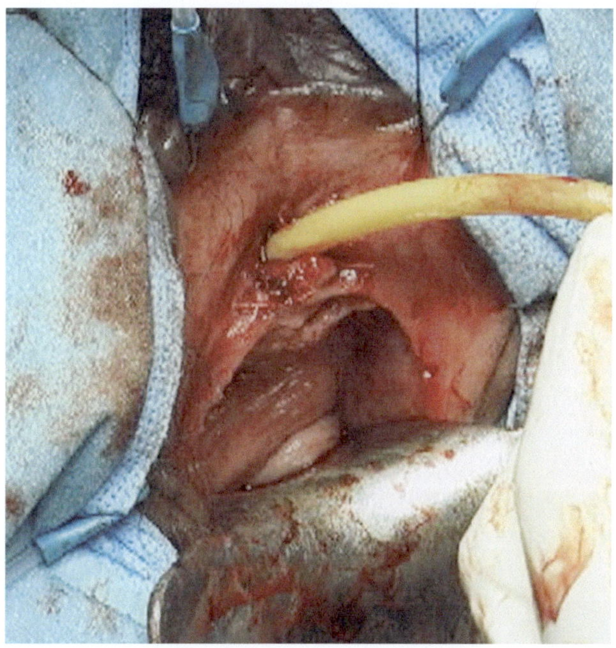

Fig. 7.13 After excision of the mass, a normal urethra is seen. The patient resumed normal voiding

7.4.7 Case 7: Urethrolysis and Retropubic Martius Flap for Recurrent Urinary Retention

The patient developed urinary retention after a retropubic and an obturator sling. She had three prior unsuccessful urethrolysis procedures for retention. The urethra is not mobile and is adherent to the pubic bone and the lateral pelvic wall (Figs. 7.14, 7.15, 7.16, 7.17, 7.18, 7.19, 7.20, and 7.21).

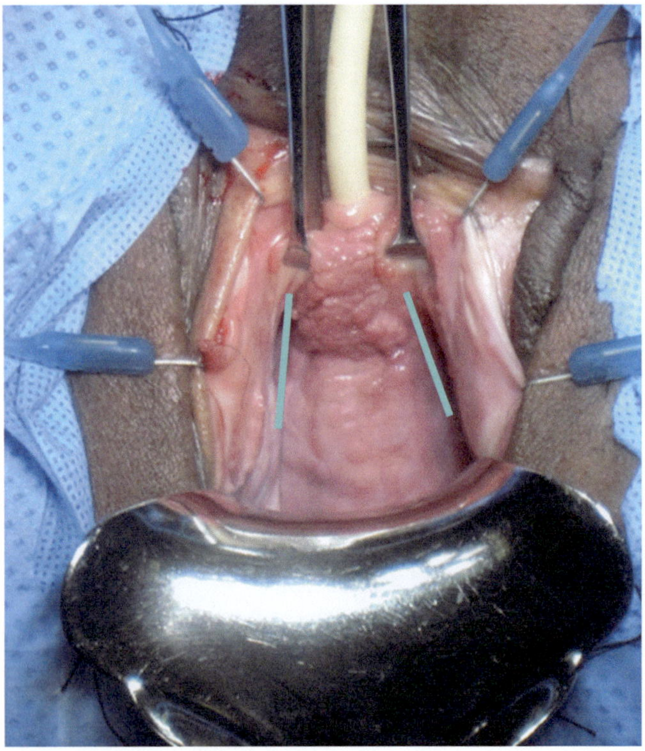

Fig. 7.14 Exposure of the anterior vaginal wall. Two oblique incisions will be made in the lateral distal vagina

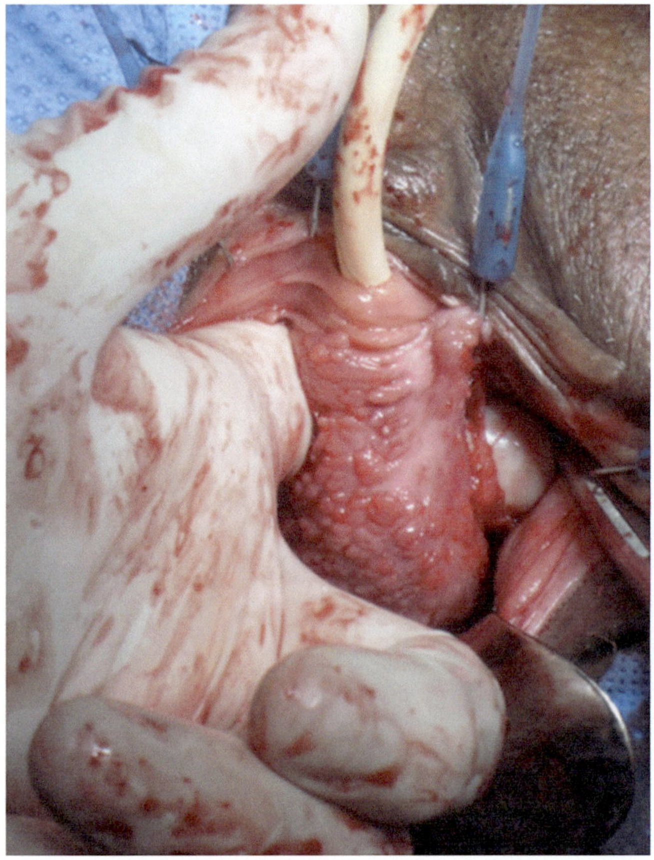

Fig. 7.15 A complete retropubic urethrolysis is performed, allowing the passage of a finger from the right to the left periurethral incisions

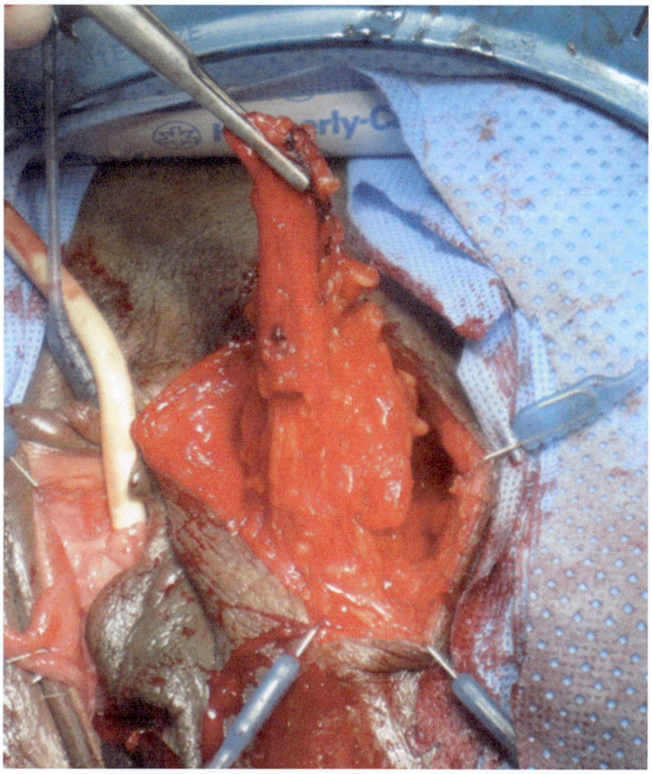

Fig. 7.16 A left Martius flap is prepared and the superior pedicle is incised, keeping intact the inferior pudendal blood supply

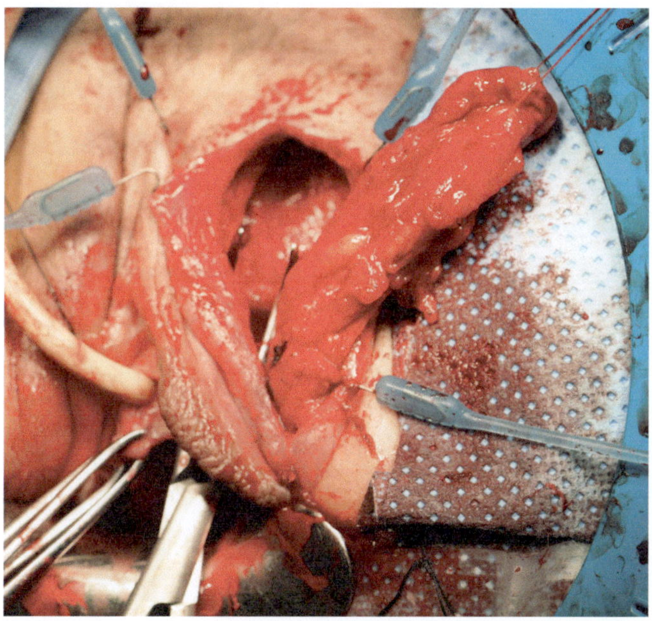

Fig. 7.17 A tunnel is made from the left vaginal incision to the labial incision and a large, curved clamp is inserted

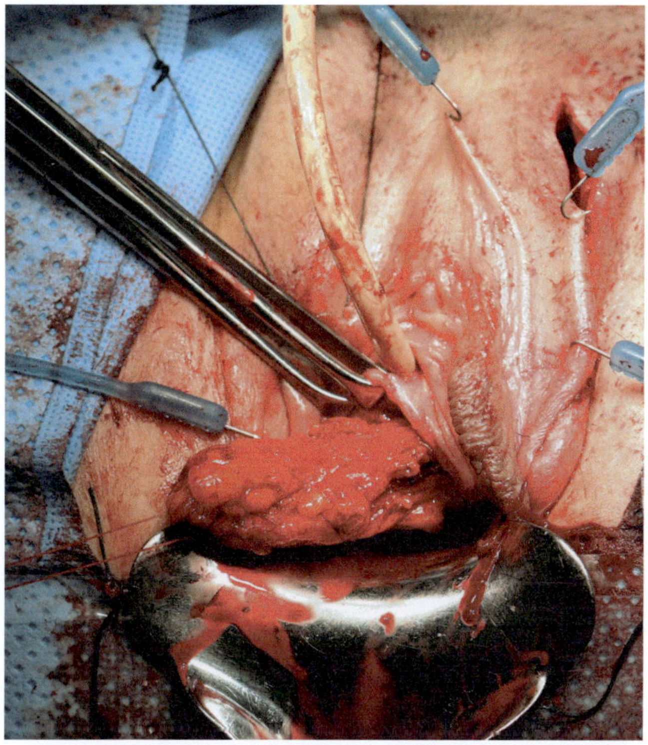

Fig. 7.18 The mobilized Martius flap is transferred from the labial incision to the left vaginal incision

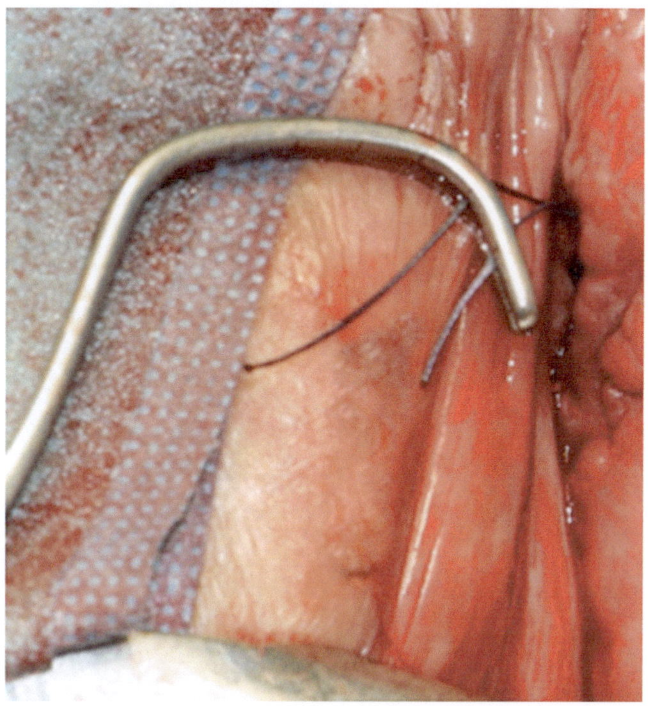

Fig. 7.19 An angulated curve clamp (Derra clamp) will be inserted in the right periurethral incision under finger control in the retropubic space and brought out at the left periurethral incision, where the end of the Martius flap will be anchored

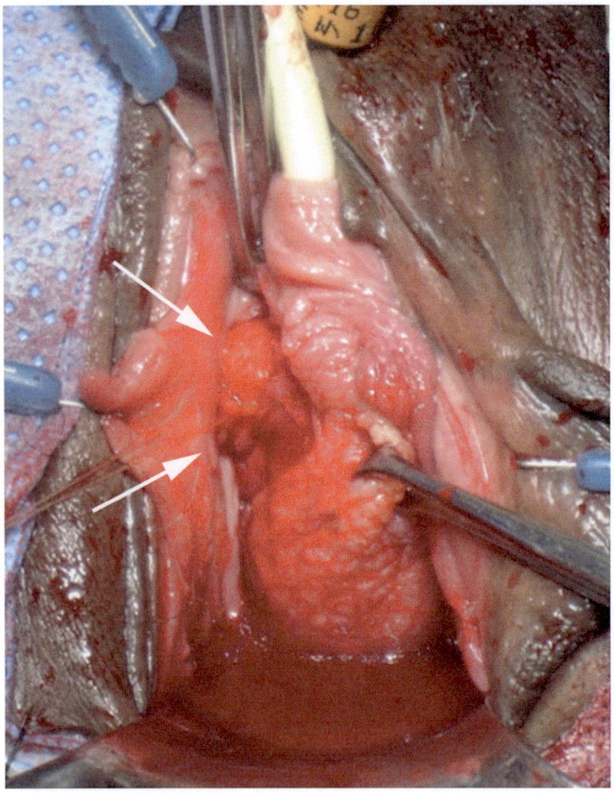

Fig. 7.20 The end of the Martius flap is transferred without tension from the left to the right periurethral incision. The end of the flap (*arrows*) is brought outside the incision

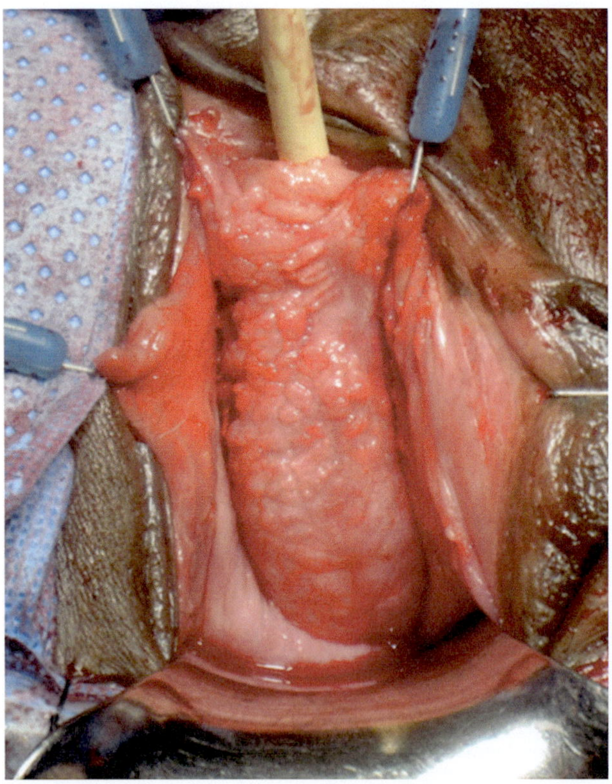

Fig. 7.21 The anterior vaginal incisions are closed with delayed absorbable sutures. On the right side, the end of the Martius flap is incorporated into the suture to prevent displacement. The urethra is now mobile

7.4.8 Case 8: Suprameatal Urethrolysis and Retropubic Martius Flap for Recurrent Retention

The patient presented with severe urethral obstruction after two retropubic slings complicated by infection and hematoma. Prior urethrolysis failed. The urethra is not mobile and is highly fixed to the posterior pubic bone (Figs. 7.22, 7.23, 7.24, 7.25, 7.26, 7.27, 7.28, and 7.29).

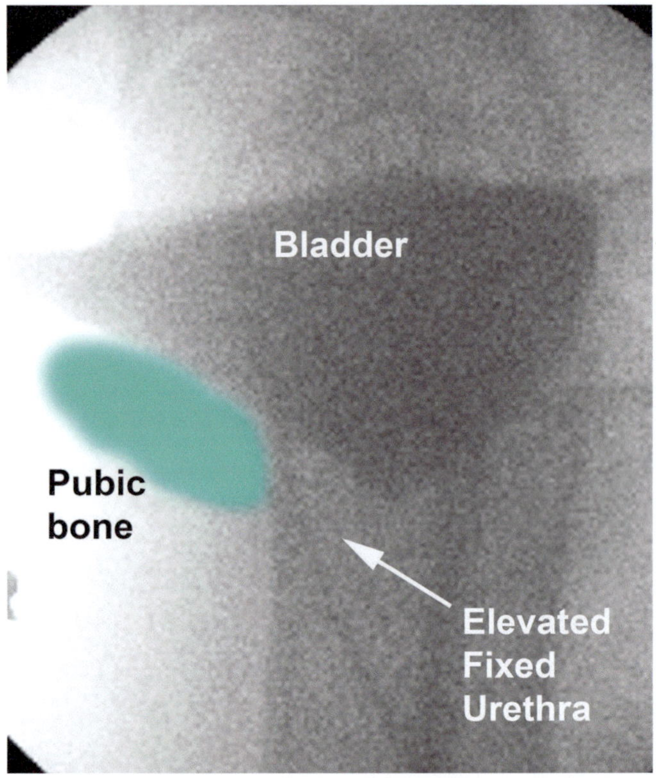

Fig. 7.22 Standing cystogram confirms urethral elevation and fixation without a cystocele

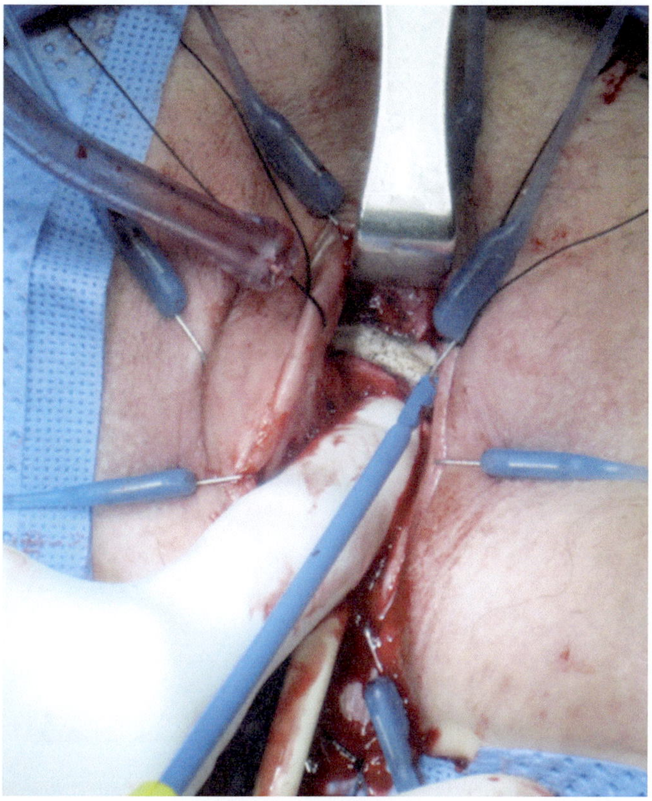

Fig. 7.23 A semicircular incision is made 1–2 cm anterior to the urethral meatus. The dissection is carried out toward the periosteum of the pubic bone. The urethra is dissected free from the inferior rami of the pubic bone by detaching the pubourethral fascia

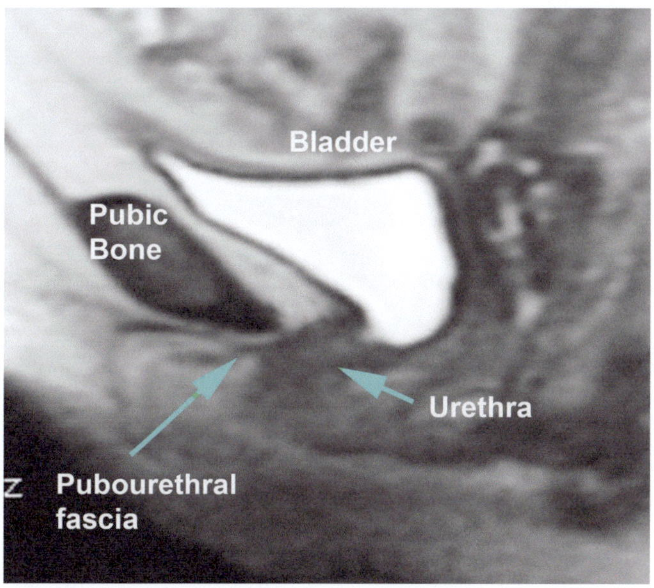

Fig. 7.24 Sagittal MRI of the urethra showing the attachment of the urethra to the inferior rami of the pubic bone by the pubourethral fascia. This fascia is the only direct connection of the urethra to the pubic bone

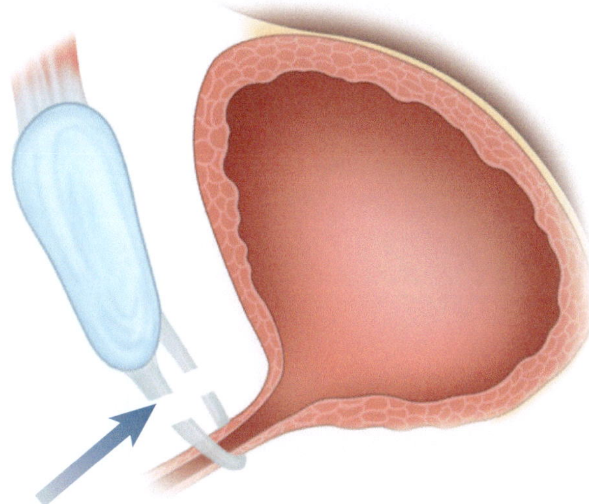

Fig. 7.25 Diagram of the surgical approach to suprameatal urethrolysis, with the dissection of the urethra from the inferior rami of the pubic bone

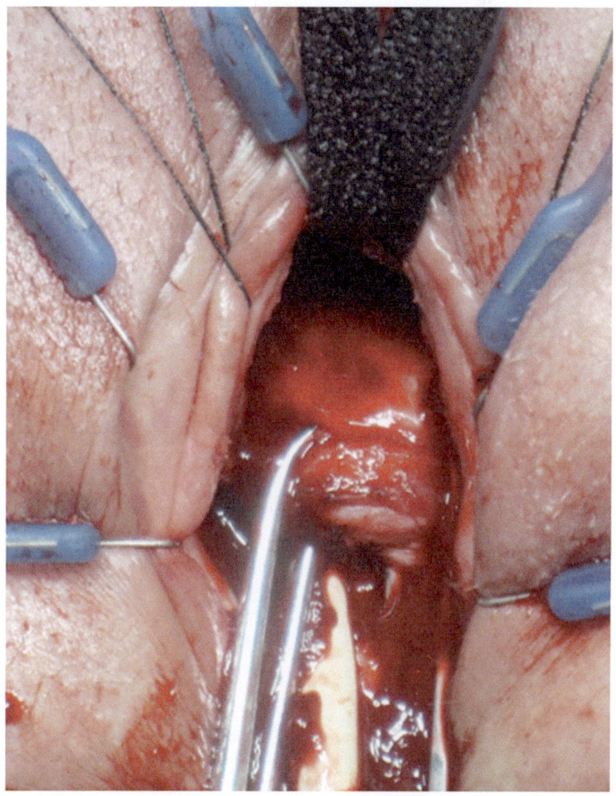

Fig. 7.26 Suprameatal exposure of the retropubic space. The urethropelvic fascia has been detached from the inferior rami of the pubic bone. Sharp dissection is carried out outside the periurethral fascia, in the direction of the anterior face of the pubic bone. With sharp dissection, the retropubic space is entered by detaching the pubourethral ligaments from the inferior margin of the pubic bone. The dissection must be kept superficial over the periurethral fascia because significant bleeding can occur if this fascia is penetrated. All adhesions in the retropubic space are freed using sharp and blunt dissection. The lateral attachments of the urethra to the lateral pelvic wall (urethropelvic ligaments) are left intact. Any sling material (fascia or synthetic) or suspending sutures are excised

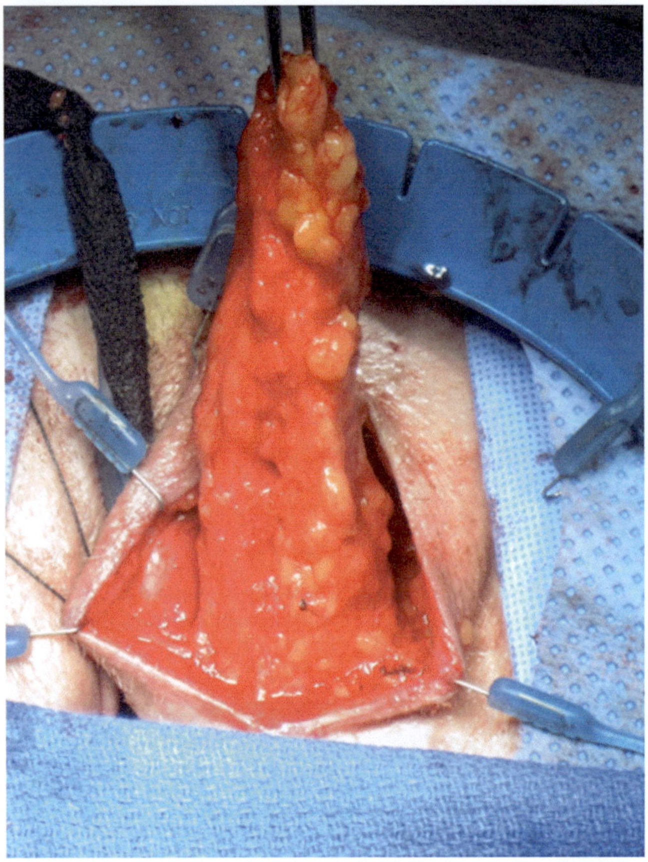

Fig. 7.27 A left Martius flap is isolated and mobilized to the base

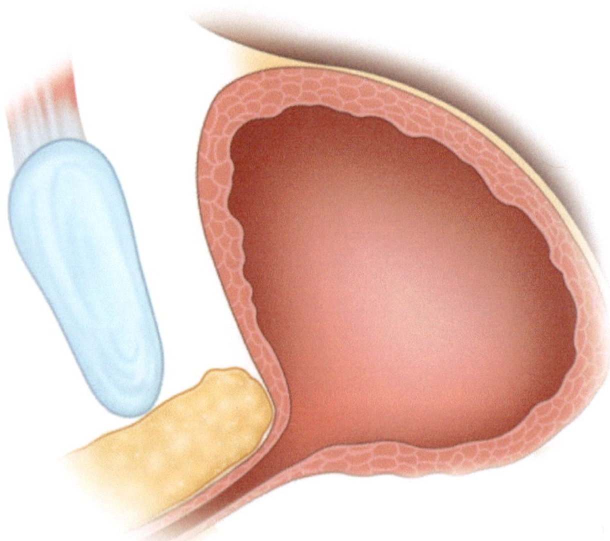

Fig. 7.28 Diagram of the transfer of the Martius flap under the pubic bone to the retropubic space

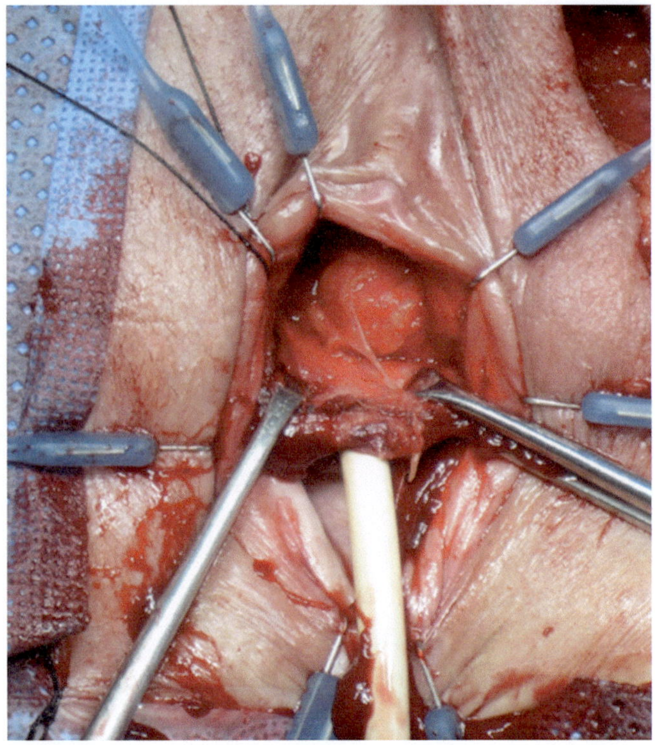

Fig. 7.29 A tunnel is made under the labia and the Martius flap is transferred to the retropubic space. The flap is anchored with absorbable suture to the anterior bladder wall and urethra to prevent recurrent adhesions. The patient resumed normal voiding after surgery

7.4.8.1 Intraoperative Complications

Bleeding of the retropubic space and periurethral area can be significant if the dissection is performed in the wrong cleavage of dissection. Bladder or urethral perforation should be repaired and a drain inserted in the retropubic space.

7.4.8.2 Postoperative Care

The operation can be performed in the outpatient setting. Ice packs and broad-spectrum antibiotics should be used in the perioperative period. Voiding trials should be postponed until the vaginal and urethral swellings subside, generally after 3–5 days. The patient may require self-catheterization for several weeks after surgery.

7.4.8.3 Postoperative Complications

Retropubic or labial incision infection or abscess may require drainage and proper antibiotic therapy. Secondary bleeding is very uncommon but can be significant. Continuation of the urinary retention may require further investigations after the healing period. Overactive bladder symptoms are common for several months after a successful urethrolysis; they will respond to cholinolytic therapy or other therapies if the obstruction is eliminated.

7.4.9 Case 9. Transurethral Incision of the Bladder Neck for Severe Bladder Neck Obstruction

A 70-year-old woman on self-catheterization for 3 years is experiencing urinary retention. She does not have urinary incontinence, has no neurological conditions, and has had no prior surgeries (Figs. 7.30, 7.31, and 7.32).

After the procedure, the patient does not require self-catheterization and residuals of urine are low. She remained minimally symptomatic. The diverticula were not treated.

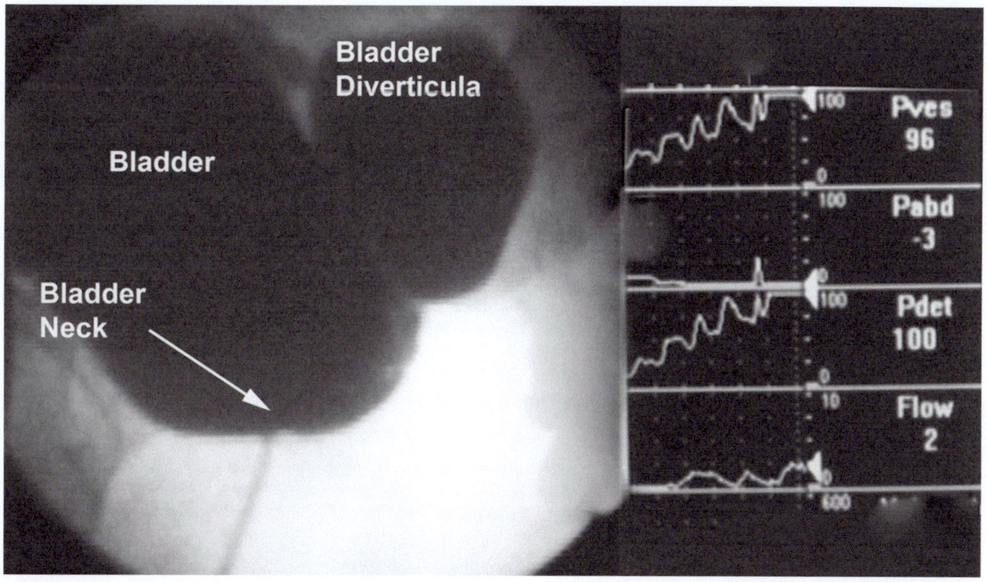

Fig. 7.30 Video urodynamics shows trabeculation of the bladder, multiple large diverticula, high-pressure voiding (detrusor pressures above 95 cm pressure), and flow of only 2 cc per second. At the time of voiding, the bladder neck is not funneling or opening

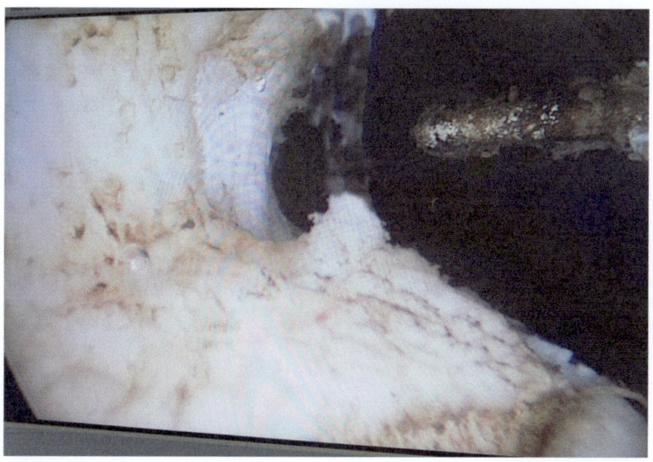

Fig. 7.31 After failing pharmacological treatment, a transurethral incision of the bladder neck was performed using the Collings knife. The incisions were done at the 3 o'clock and 9 o'clock positions

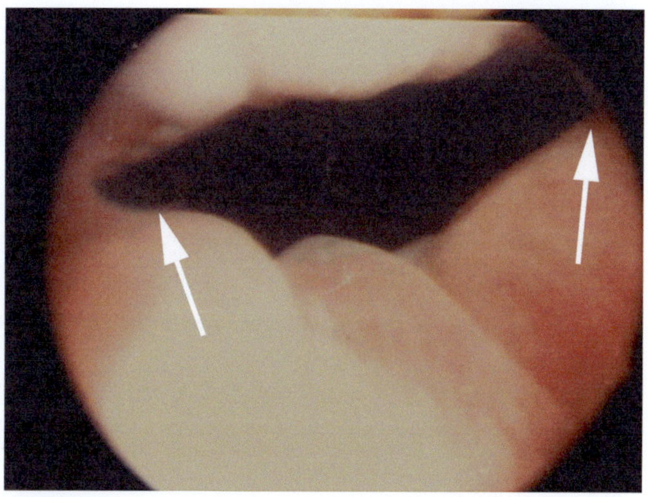

Fig. 7.32 Cystoscopy after surgery shows the bilateral incisions of the bladder neck (*arrows*) at the 3 o'clock and 9 o'clock locations

7.4.10 Case 10: Retention of Urine Due to Periurethral Abscess After Implant of Durasphere™

The patient presented with severe urethral pain, poor interrupted stream, recurrent urinary tract infections, and large residuals of urine. A few months before presentation, she had a transurethral implant of Durasphere™ (Coloplast, Minneapolis, MN) for stress incontinence (Figs. 7.33, 7.34, 7.35, 7.36, 7.37, and 7.38).

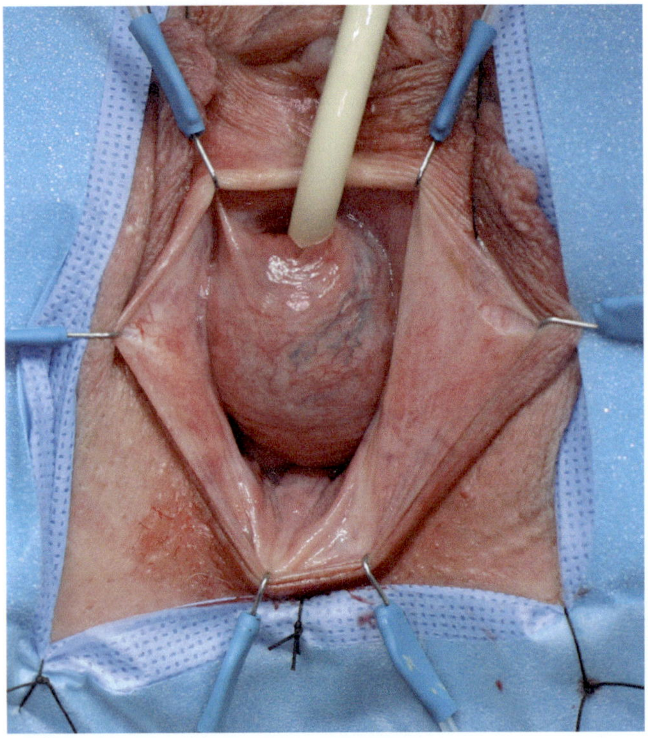

Fig. 7.33 Exposure of the anterior vaginal wall shows a cystic and tender mass. The vaginal skin is discolored by the Durasphere™ material

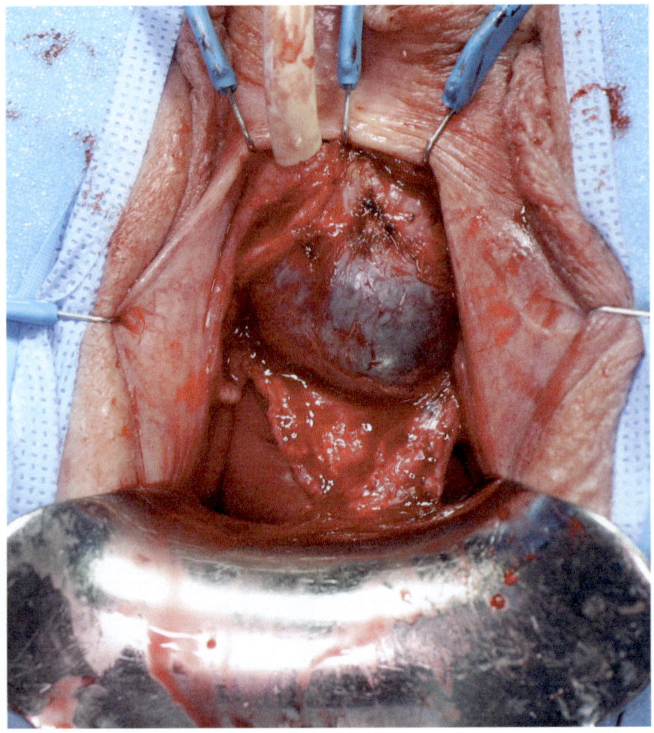

Fig. 7.34 A flap of the anterior vaginal wall is created to expose the periurethral fascia, which is very distended by the underlying collection

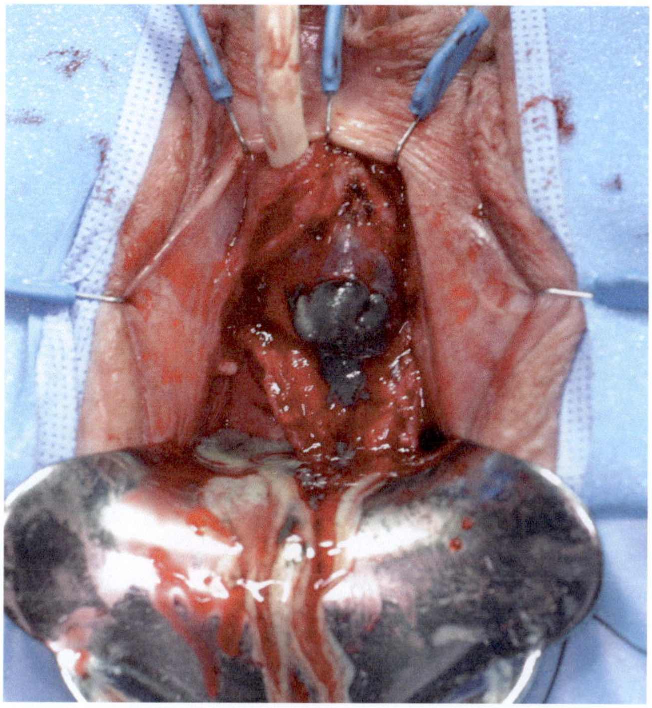

Fig. 7.35 Drainage of the collection shows a large amount of pus material and Durasphere™ adherent to the urethral mucosa

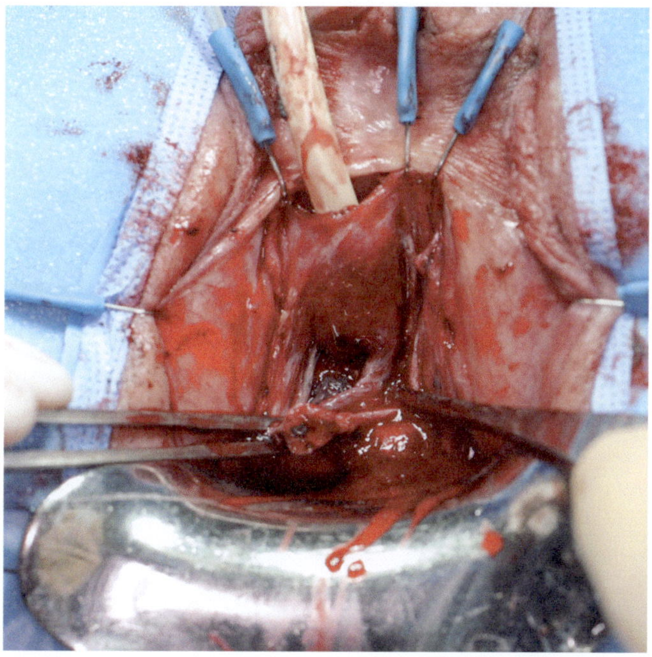

Fig. 7.36 After irrigation with antibiotic solution, a delicate dissection is required to excise the cystic cavity with the residual Durasphere™ material

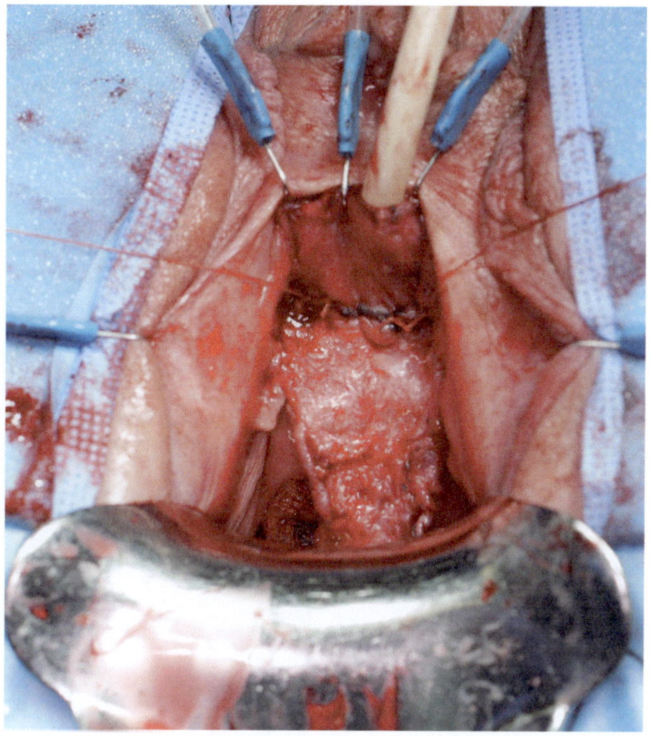

Fig. 7.37 The anterior vaginal wall is reconstructed by approximation of the periurethral fascia to cover the urethral mucosa

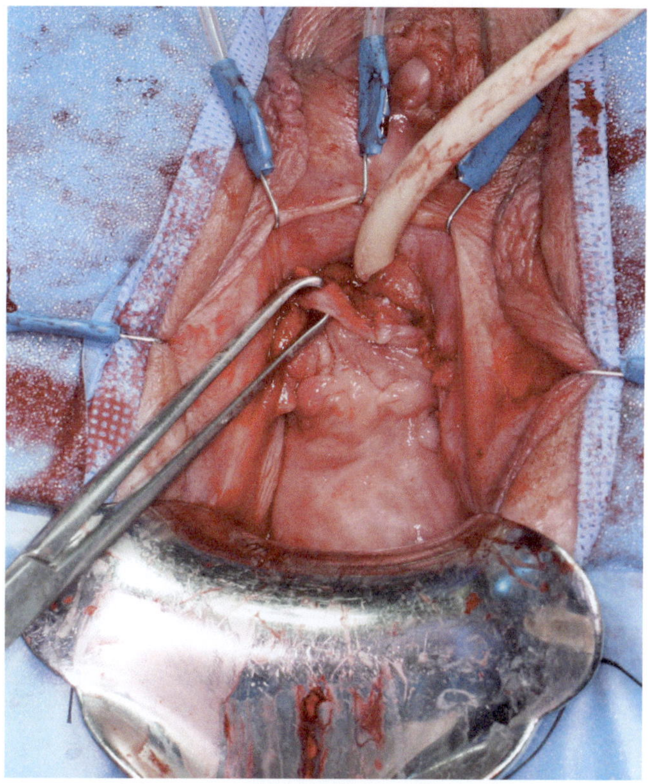

Fig. 7.38 A flap of the anterior vaginal wall is advanced distally to cover the area of the reconstructed urethral wall

7.4.11 Case 11: Distal Urethral Stricture

The patient presented with recurrent urethral stricture, poor stream, elevated residuals of urine, and inability to perform cystoscopy. Urethral catheterization was possible only after urethral dilation over a guidewire (Figs. 7.39, 7.40, 7.41, and 7.42).

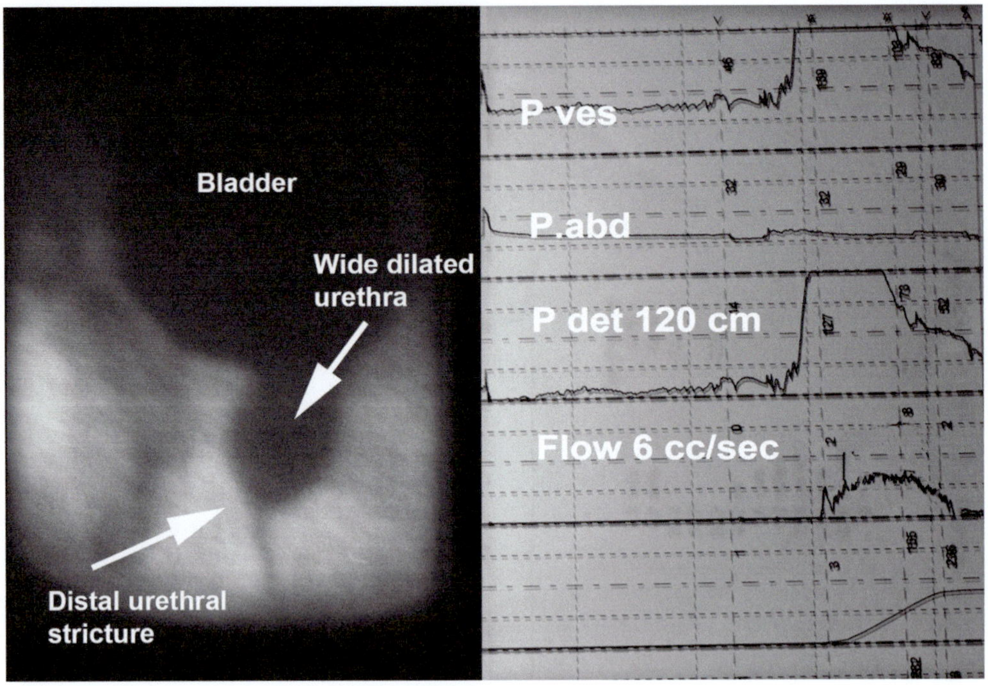

Fig. 7.39 Video urodynamics of the patient during voiding shows a pattern of very high pressures (true detrusor pressures of 120 cm H_2O) and a flow of 6 cc per second

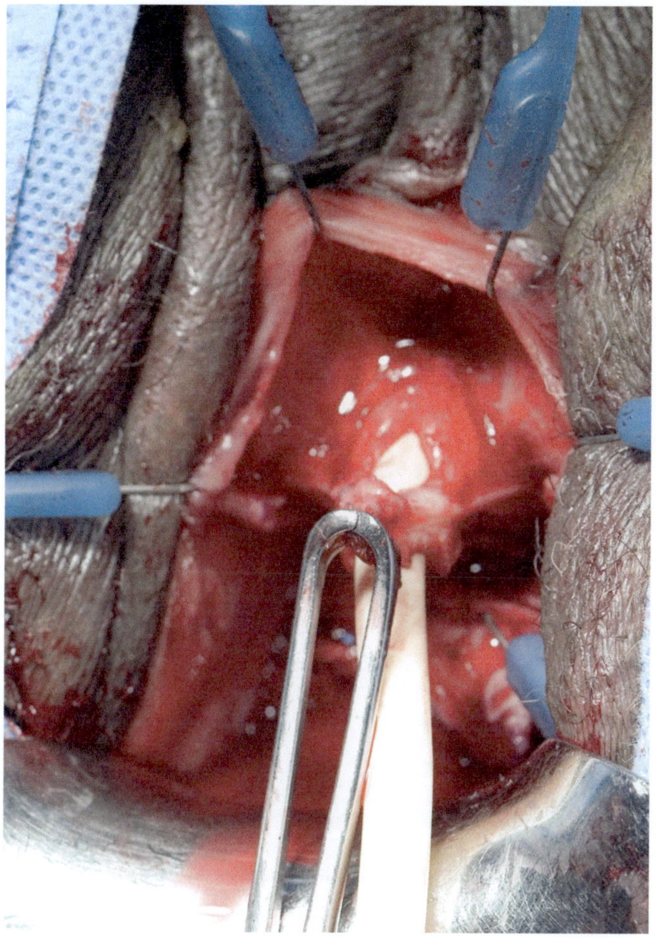

Fig. 7.40 A circular incision around the urethra was performed. A flap of the anterior distal vaginal wall was created. Exposure and incision of the distal anterior urethra were performed

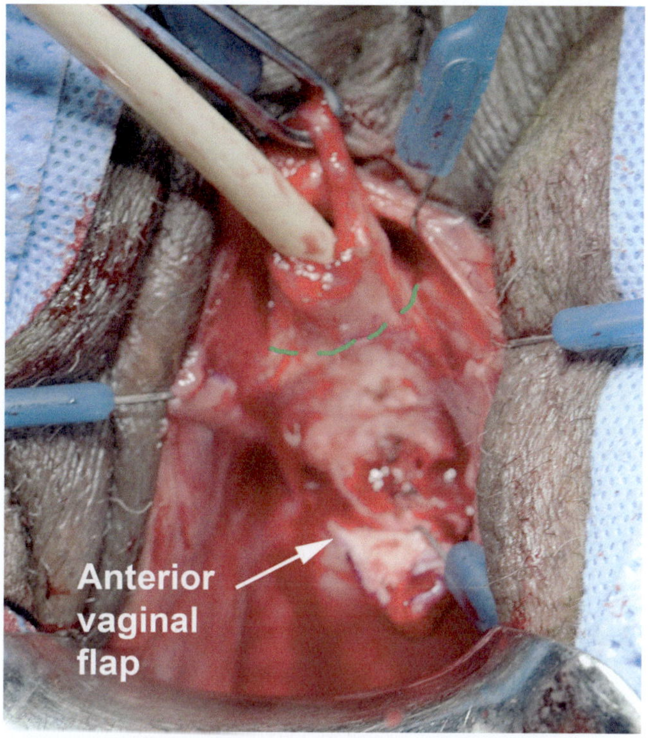

Fig. 7.41 Exposure of the distal posterior urethral wall is obtained, and a circular incision will be performed to complete the excision of the distal urethra with the stricture

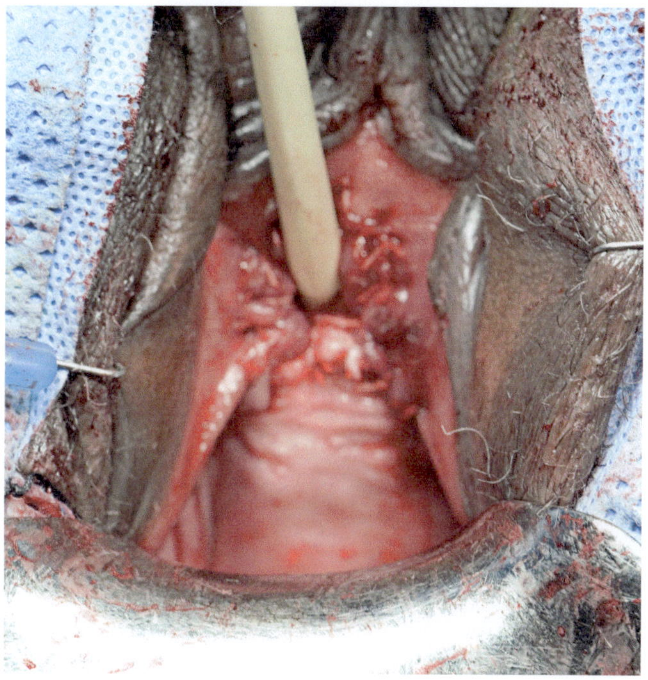

Fig. 7.42 The end of the excised urethra is anastomosed to the distal vagina in a circular line of delayed absorbable sutures

7.4.12 Case 12: Repair of Midurethral Stricture using the Heineke–Mikulicz Technique

A 62-year-old patient presented with symptoms of obstruction, large post-void residuals, and difficulty in passing a catheter. She was diagnosed with a recurrent midurethral stricture. Multiple urethrotomies failed, and she required frequent dilation of the urethra to prevent complete retention (Figs. 7.43, 7.44, 7.45, 7.46, 7.47, 7.48, 7.49, and 7.50).

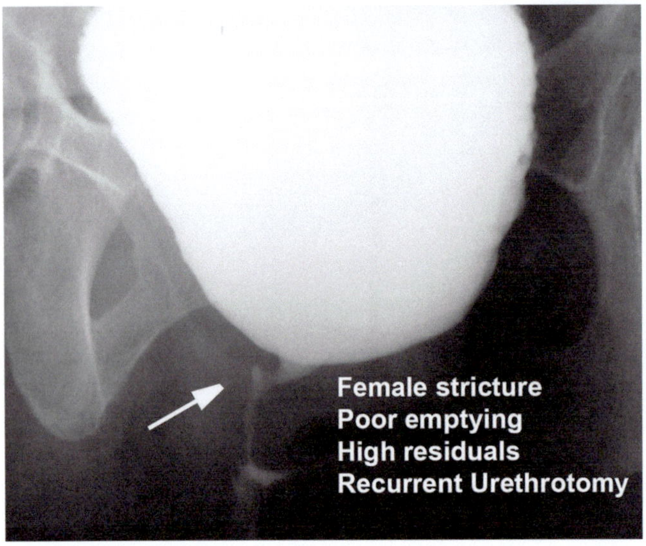

Fig. 7.43 Voiding cystogram demonstrating the narrowing of the midurethral area. Cystoscopy confirms the finding of a urethral stricture

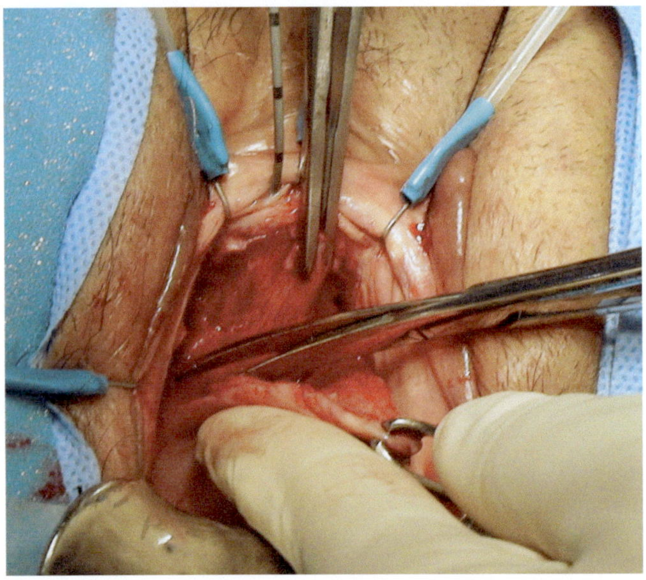

Fig. 7.44 An inverted U flap of the anterior vaginal wall is created to expose the urethra. The top of the flap reaches the distal urethra

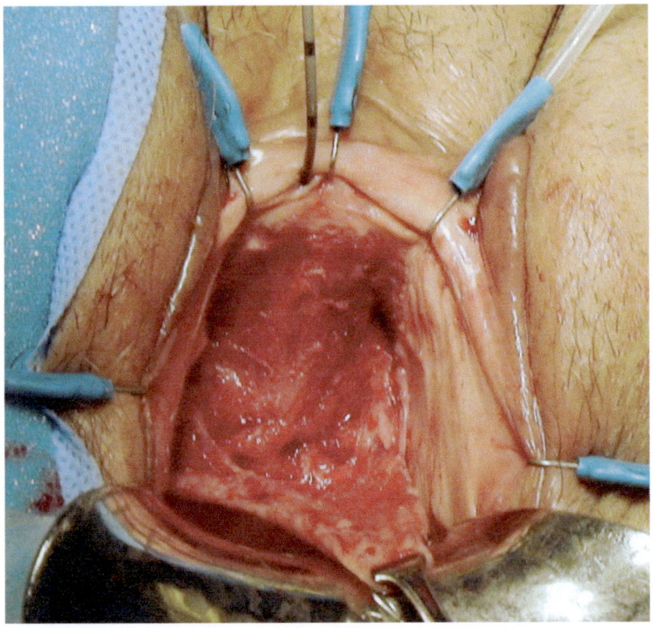

Fig. 7.45 The length of the urethra and the periurethral fascia are exposed just proximal to the bladder neck

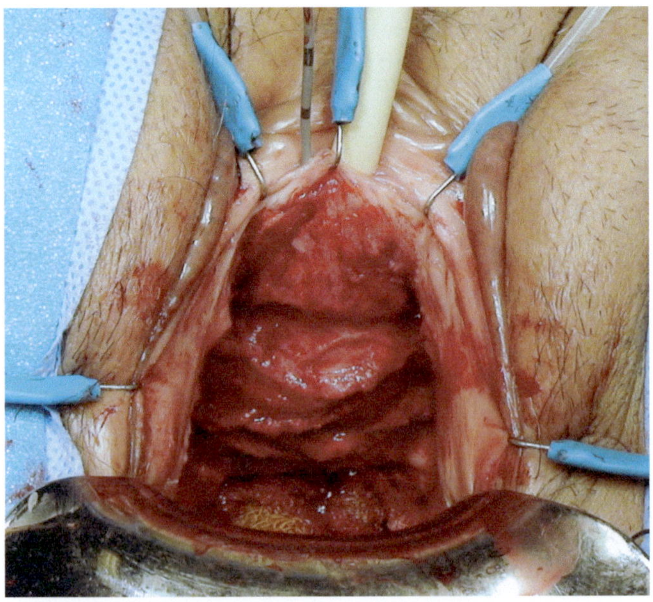

Fig. 7.46 A transverse incision is made over the periurethral fascia, and two flaps (superior and inferior) are created to expose the urethral wall

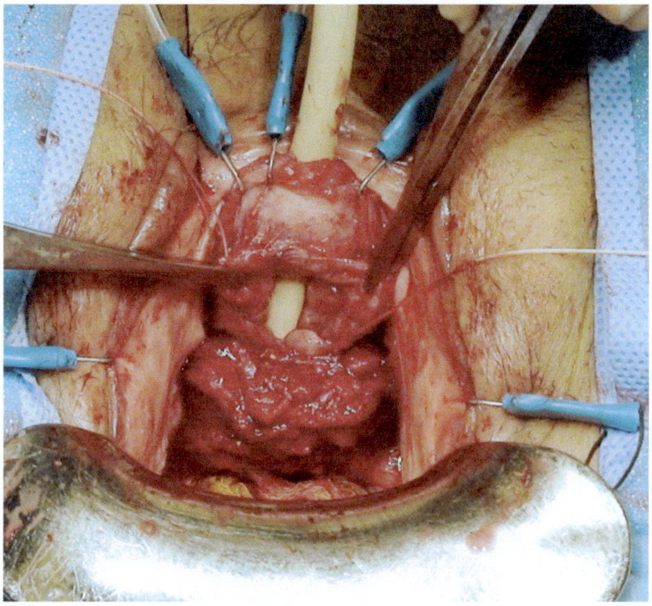

Fig. 7.47 A longitudinal incision of the whole urethral wall is made. The urethral wall is dissected proximally and distally for a distance of at least 1 cm in each direction

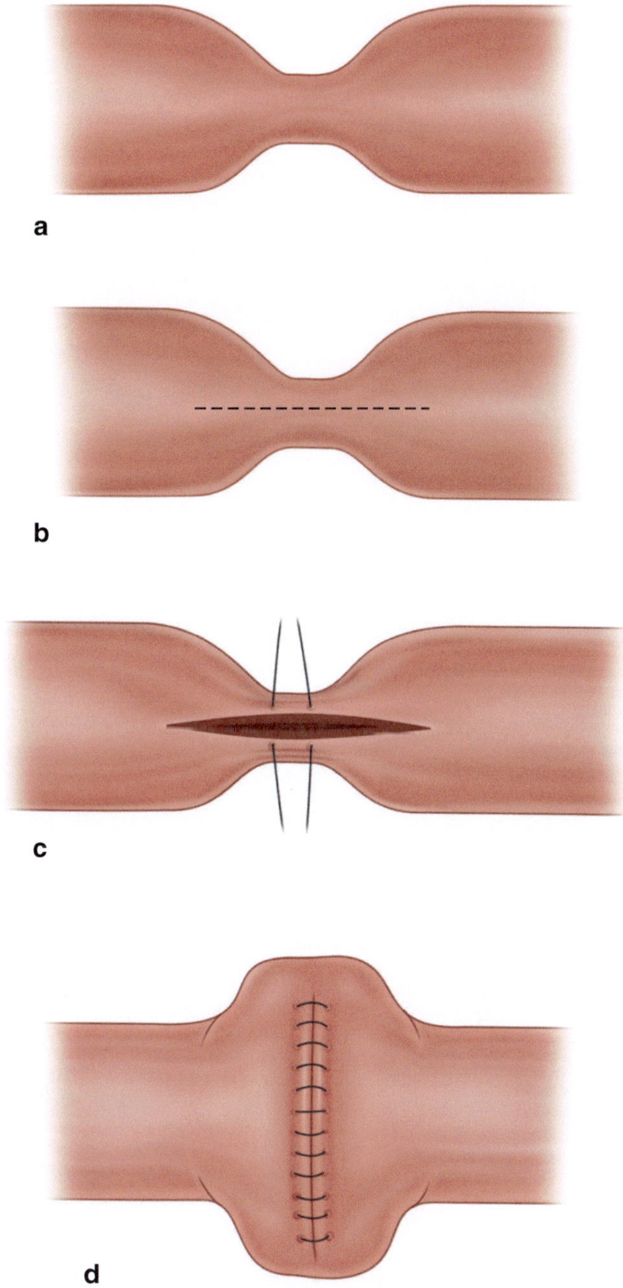

Fig. 7.48 Diagram of the Heineke–Mikulicz technique to widen a midurethral stricture (**a**). A longitudinal incision (**b**, **c**) is made proximal and distal to the stricture. The closure is done in a horizontal fashion (**d**), widening the stricture area

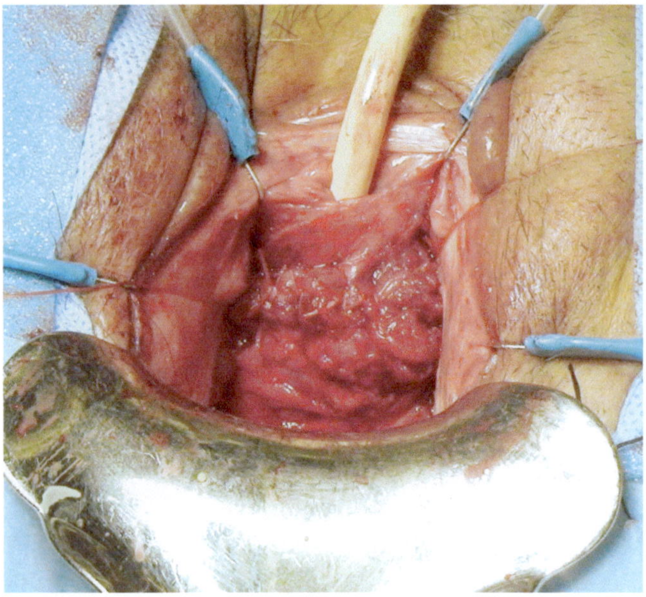

Fig. 7.49 The margins of the open urethra are approximated in a horizontal fashion using delayed absorbable sutures, providing a wide caliber to the urethra

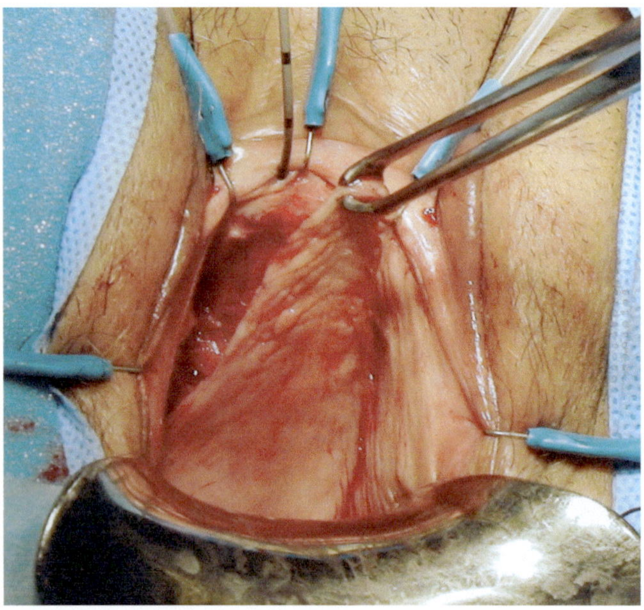

Fig. 7.50 The flaps of periurethral fascia are closed in a transverse fashion, covering the urethral closure. The vaginal wall flap is advanced distally to cover the area of reconstruction

7.4.13 Case 13: Suprameatal Anterior Urethral Pediculated Rotational Labial Flap to Correct Urethral Stricture

A 67-year-old patient presented with progressive obstructive symptoms after prior vaginal surgery. The stream is poor and interrupted, and there is a high residual of urine. The patient has required numerous urethral dilations and visits to the emergency room for complete retention. Cystoscopy revealed a tight midurethral and distal urethral stricture with a length of 1.5 cm (Figs. 7.51, 7.52, 7.53, 7.54, 7.55, 7.56, 7.57, 7.58, 7.59, and 7.60). We will use a rotational vascularized labial flap to correct the stricture. Alternatively a buccal graft can be used.

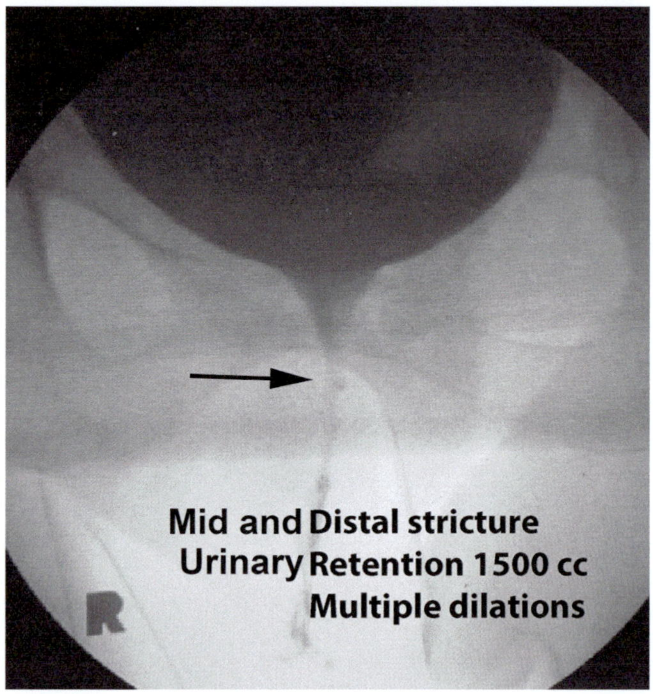

Fig. 7.51 Voiding cystogram showing the area of urethral narrowing persistent throughout the study. The post-void residuals of urine were 1500 cc

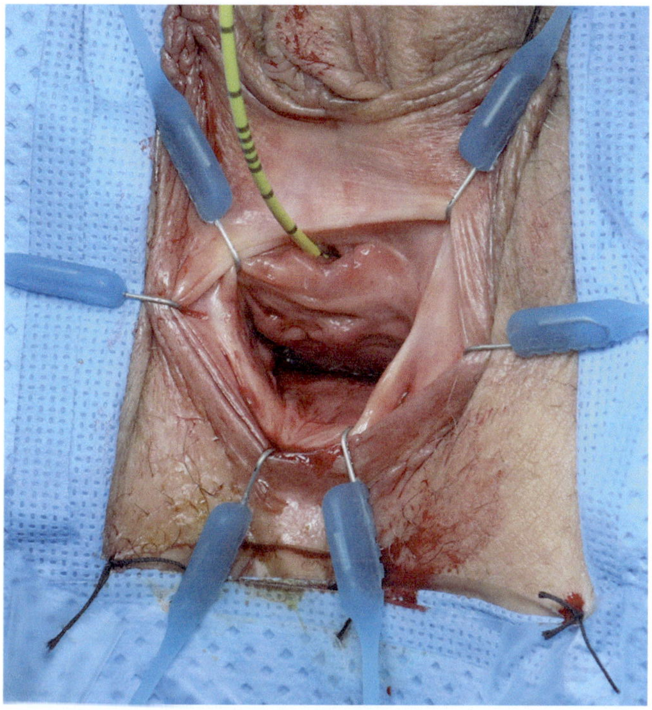

Fig. 7.52 Under cystoscopy, a guidewire and an open-ended 5-Fr ureteric catheter is inserted into the urethra. No dilation of the urethra is performed

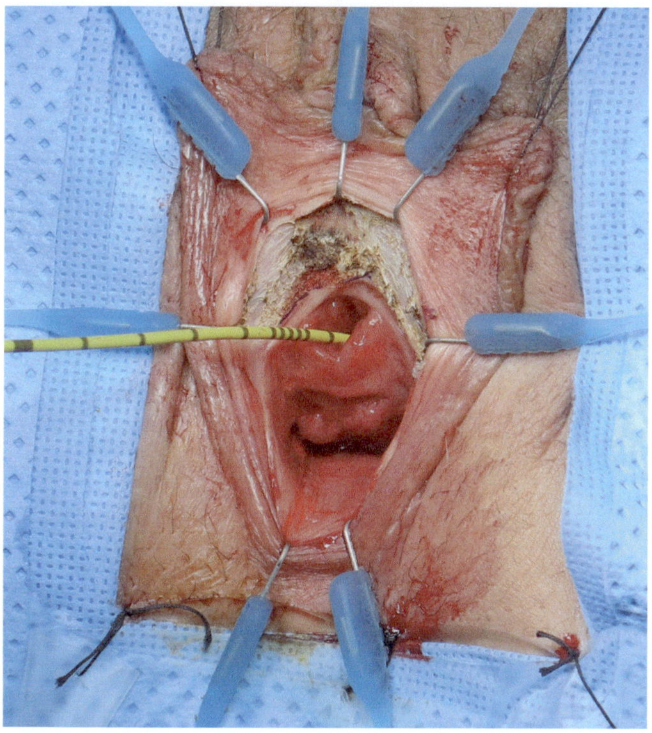

Fig. 7.53 A suprameatal semicircular incision is made anterior to the urethra, 1 cm or more from the external meatus

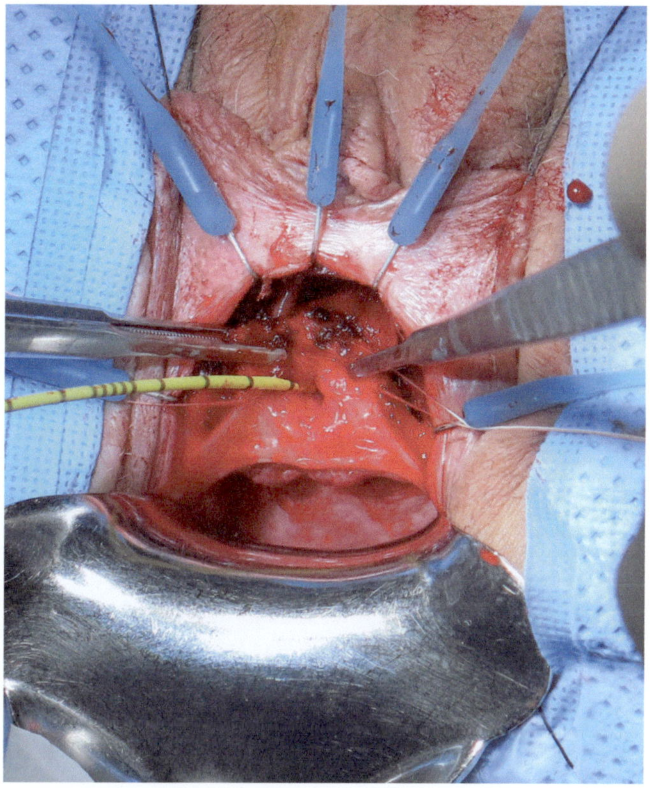

Fig. 7.54 Dissection is carried out anterior to the urethra toward the pubic symphysis and the inferior margin of the pubic bone. The anterior distal urethra is mobilized

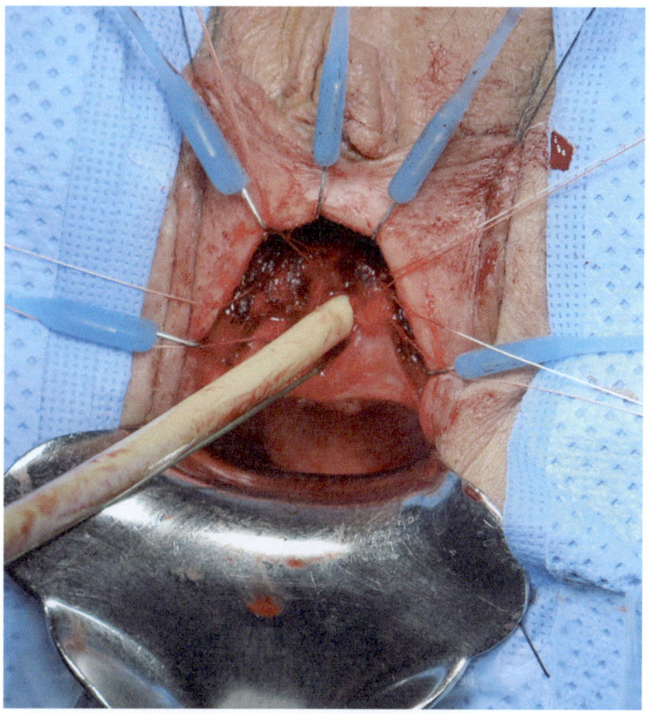

Fig. 7.55 The anterior urethra is incised from the meatus to the midurethra, until a normal wide urethral lumen is seen. The urethra is calibrated to show patency, and a Foley catheter is inserted without difficulty. A series of #3-0 delayed absorbable sutures are applied to the margins of the incision, keeping the needle for later use

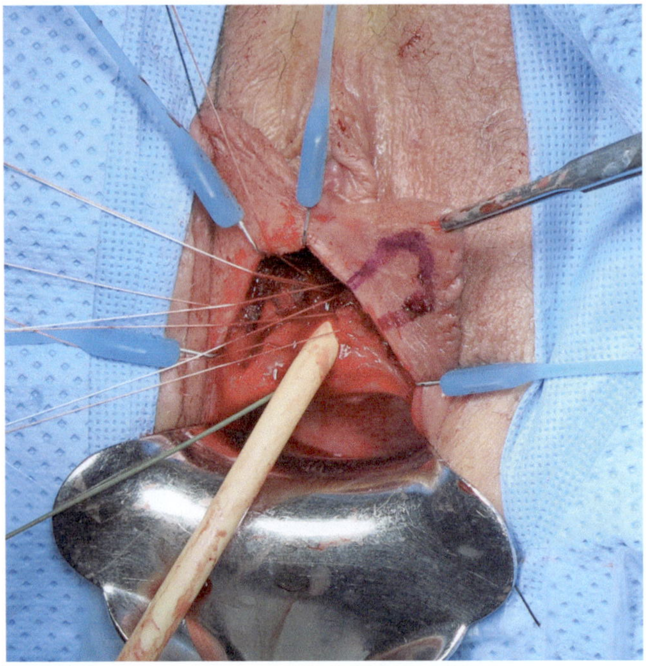

Fig. 7.56 The inner aspect of the labia minora will be the donor site. An inverted U incision will be made to create the pediculated flap of the labial skin

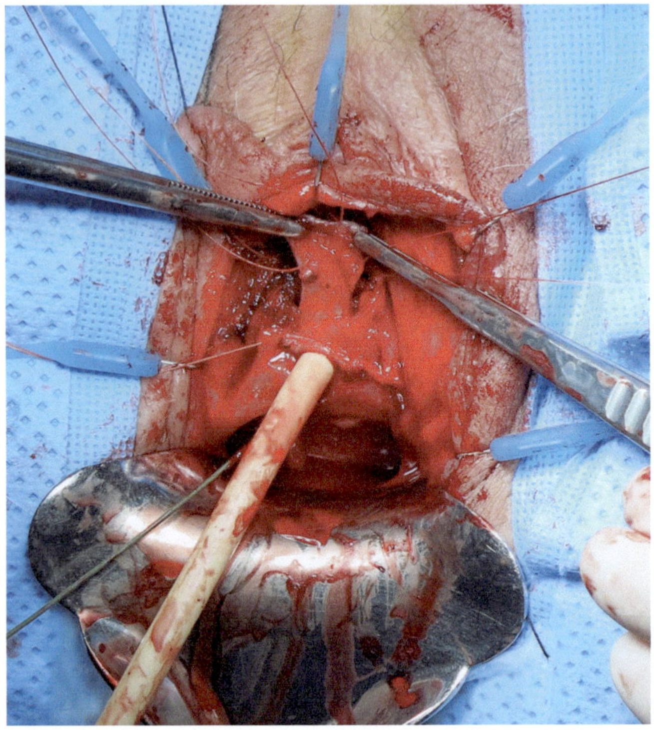

Fig. 7.58 The flap is rotated and anastomosed to the urethra, using the preplaced urethral sutures

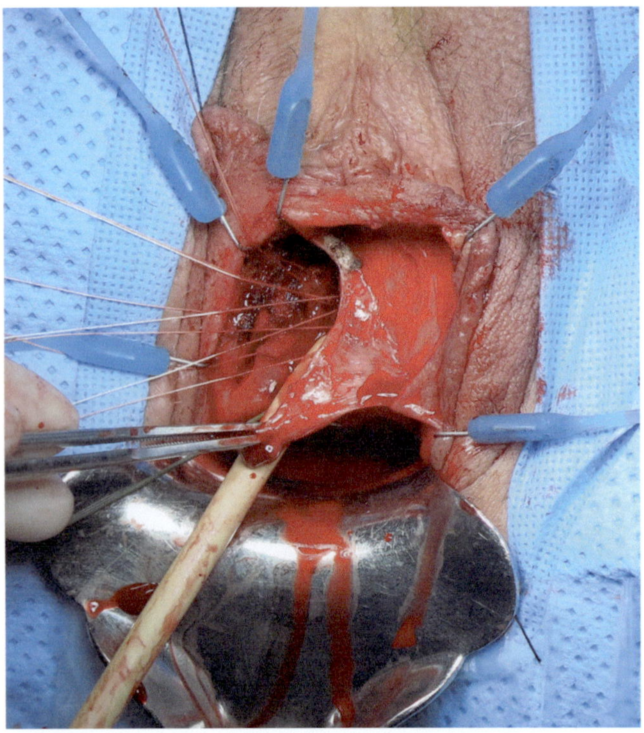

Fig. 7.57 A flap of the inner labium is mobilized, keeping the inferiorly based vascular supply intact

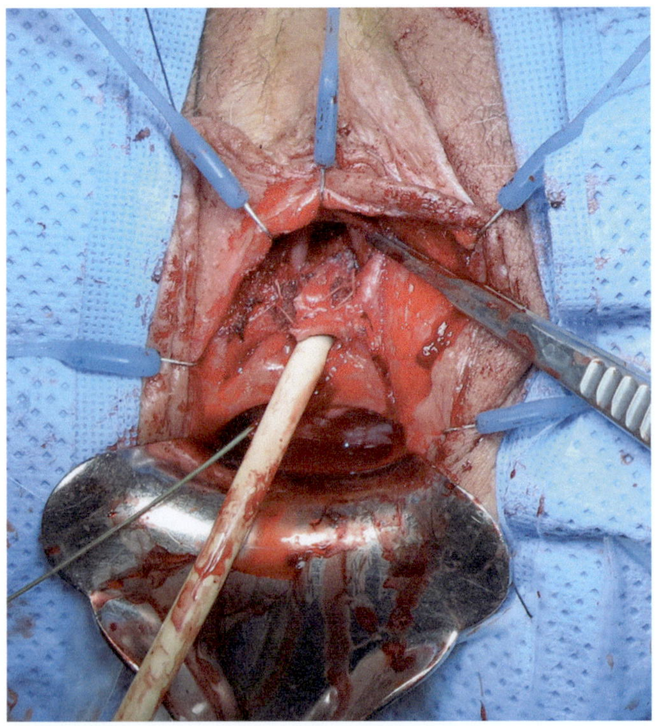

Fig. 7.59 The anastomosis is completed and the fatty tissue of the inner labium is used to cover the anastomosis

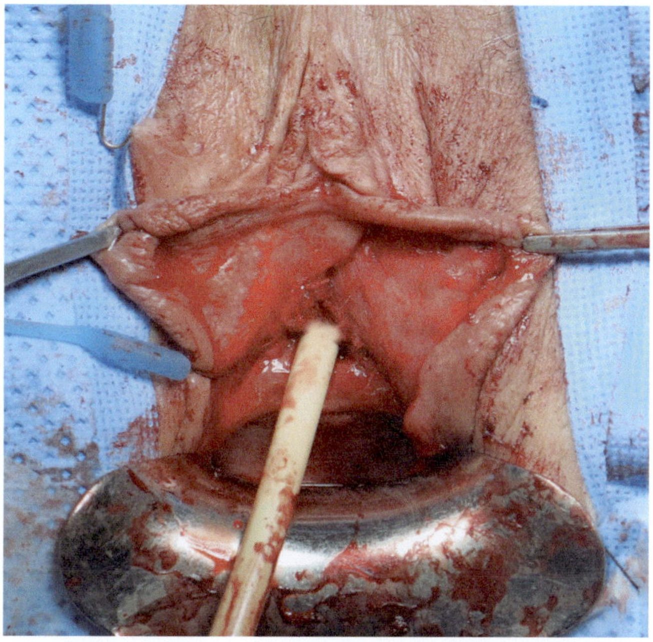

Fig. 7.60 The incision of the inner labium is closed toward the superior aspect of the urethra, using running intradermal delayed absorbable sutures

Suggested Reading

Klutke C, Siegel S, Carlin B, et al. Urinary retention after tension-free vaginal tape procedure: incidence and treatment. Urology. 2001;58:697–701.

Laurikainen E, Killholma P. A nationwide analysis of transvaginal tape release for urinary retention after tension-free vaginal tape procedure. Int Urogynecol J Pelvic Floor Dysfunct. 2006;17:111–9.

Sokol A, Jelovsek J, Walters M, et al. Incidence and predictors of prolonged urinary retention after TVT with and without concurrent prolapse surgery. Am J Obstet Gynecol. 2005;192:1537–43.

8 Vaginal Cysts and Masses

This chapter discusses a variety of conditions presenting as a vaginal mass unrelated to prolapse. The patient can be asymptomatic or may have bowel or urinary symptoms related to the mass. Masses can be found by the patient herself, but many times they are seen on a routine pelvic examination. The patient can complain of vaginal discomfort, dyspareunia, incontinence of urine, or vaginal bleeding.

Many types of cysts are found in the vagina:

- Cysts of embryonic origin
  - Müllerian (paramesonephric) cysts
  - Mesonephric–Wolffian (Gartner's duct) cysts
  - Skene's (paraurethral) duct cysts
  - Bartholin's gland cysts
  - Vaginal adenosis
  - Cysts of the canal of Nuck (hydrocele)
- Cysts of urethral origin
  - Diverticula
  - Iatrogenic cyst
  - Skene's gland cyst (secondary)
- Epidermal inclusion cysts
- Endometriosis
- Ectopic ureterocele

S. Raz, *Atlas of Vaginal Reconstructive Surgery*, DOI 10.1007/978-1-4939-2941-2_8

8.1 Bartholin's Gland Cyst

Bartholin's gland cysts have their embryological origin in the urogenital sinus. These glands are the homologues of the bulbourethral gland (Cowper glands) in the male. These cysts are present lateral to the introitus and medial to the labia minora. They are covered with transitional or stratified squamous epithelium. Their size and rapidity of growth are influenced by sexual stimulation. The treatment for these cysts is marsupialization of the cyst in the inner aspect of the labia (Figs. 8.1, 8.2, 8.3, and 8.4). Surgery is indicated only in symptomatic patients with pain, discomfort, or abscess formation.

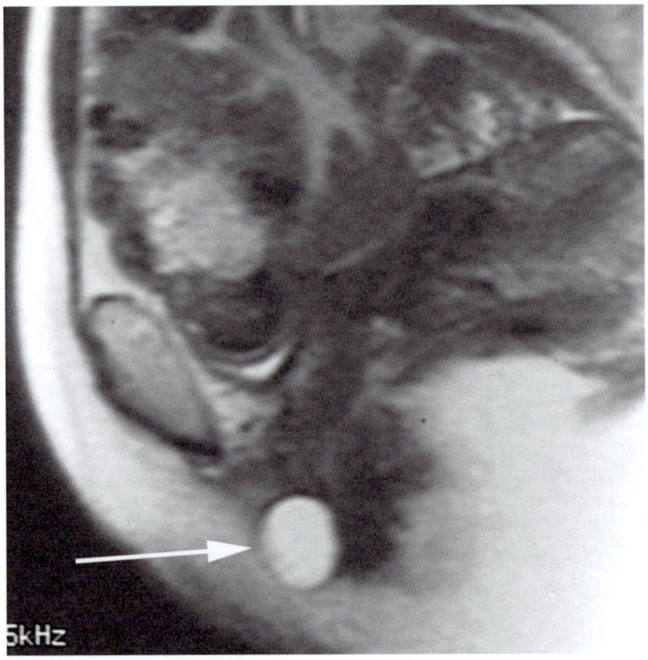

Fig. 8.1 Sagittal midpelvis MRI of a patient suffering from right labial pain and swelling, with pain during intercourse. A cystic lesion is seen in the distal vagina (*arrow*)

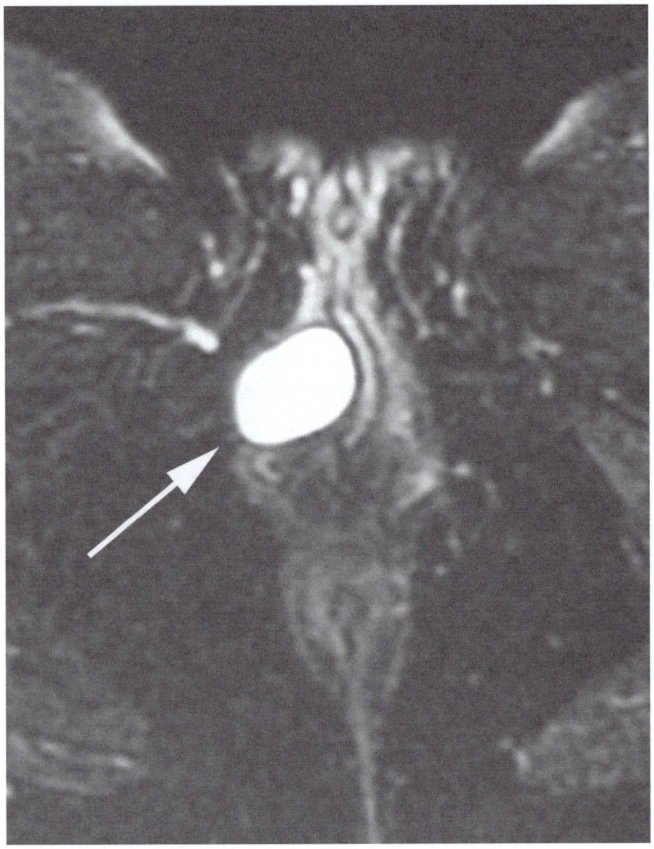

Fig. 8.2 Axial MRI showing a cystic lesion in the right labia. The cyst contains clear fluid (*arrow*)

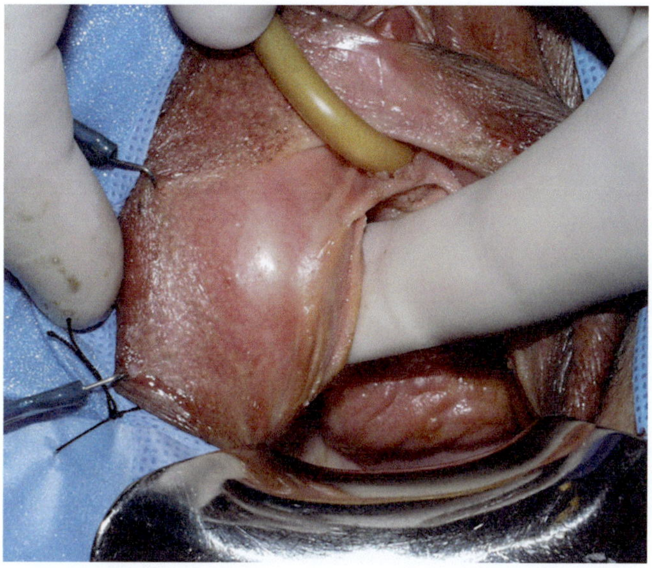

Fig. 8.3 Vaginal examination of the patient with a finger in the vagina under the right labia minora shows the cystic lesion in the inner aspect of the labia

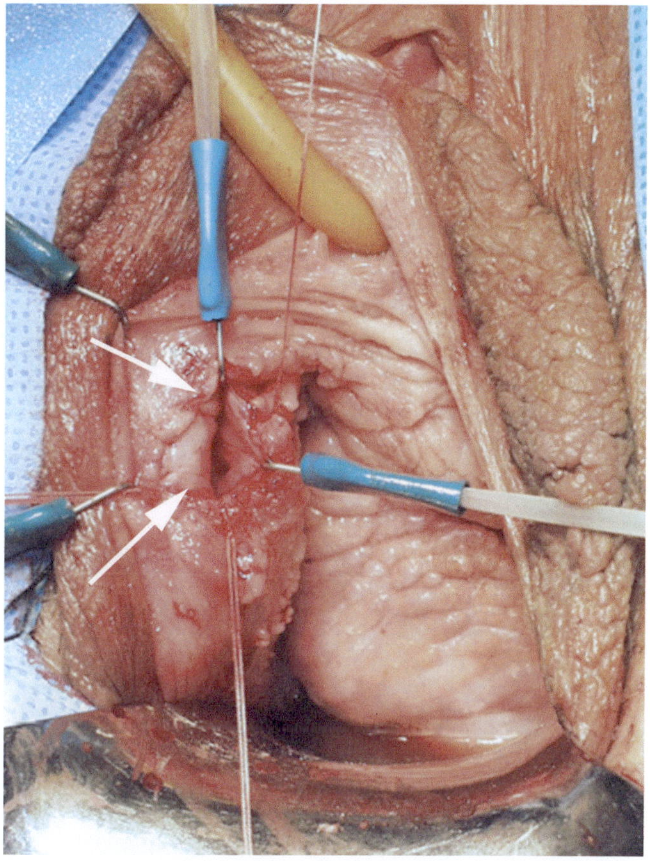

Fig. 8.4 Marsupialization of the cyst was performed. An incision was made in the inner aspect of the vagina medial to the labial minora, the cyst was opened, and the margins of the cyst were anastomosed to the vaginal wall. *Arrow* shows the line of anastomosis between the cystic wall and the inner aspect of the labia majora

8.2 Skene's Gland Cyst

The Skene's glands are the prostatic homologue in the female, with ducts covered by transitional or stratified columnar epithelium. They are located on each side of the urethra at the 5 and 7 o'clock positions. Skene's duct cysts (paraurethral) originate from the distal urethral gland. Cysts can be congenital (urogenital sinus origin) or can be acquired owing to inflammation or trauma of the drainage tract of the gland.

Obstruction of the distal urethral glands can lead to infection, abscess, and symptoms of severe urethral pain and voiding dysfunction. The abscess can drain into the vagina, creating a small fistulous tract, or less commonly reenter the urethra, forming a diverticulum (Figs. 8.5 and 8.6). Symptoms of these cysts include urethral pain, voiding symptoms, and urethral discharge. On physical examination, the area of the distal urethra may be reddish or inflamed, and pus can be drained by pressing the periurethral area. In some cases, a small or large, tender distal mass can be found. Endoscopy is not very useful. Ultrasound or MRI can be performed in selected cases.

Usually these cysts are asymptomatic, but when they are larger, they can produce pain, obstruction, and dyspareunia. Surgery, consisting of excision of the cyst and occlusion of the urethral communication, is indicated for patients with significant symptoms not responding to antibiotic therapy (Figs. 8.7, 8.8, 8.9, and 8.10).

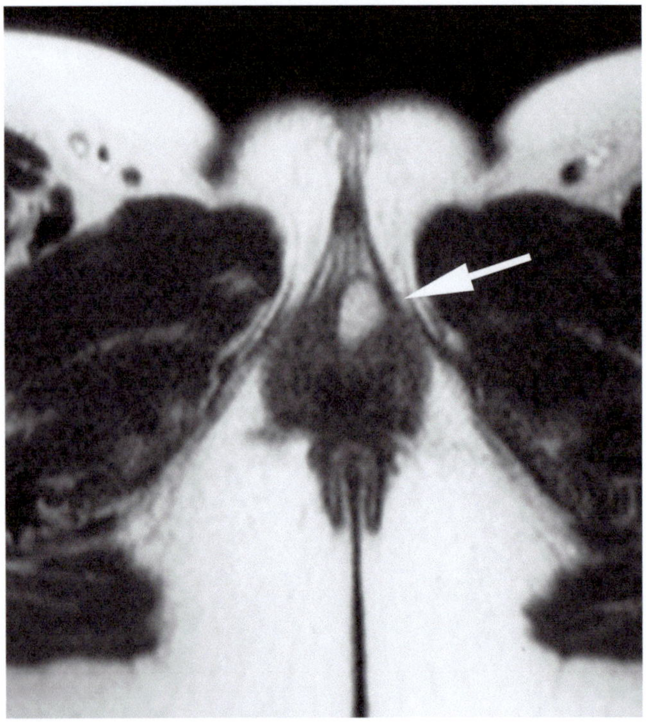

Fig. 8.5 Axial MRI of the distal vagina showing a cystic lesion in the distal urethra (*arrow*). The patient presented with pain during intercourse, difficulty in emptying the bladder, and urethral burning

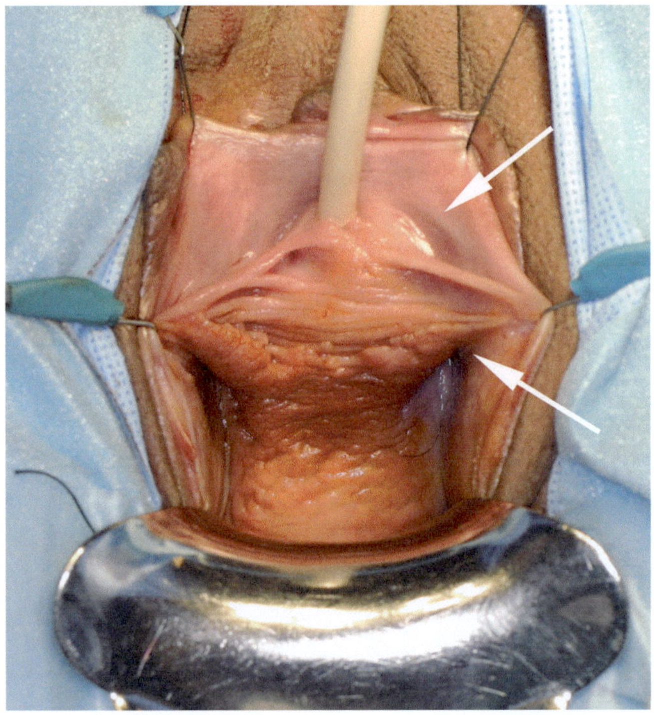

Fig. 8.6 Exposure of the vaginal wall shows a tender, cystic lesion in the left distal periurethral area. The *arrows* point toward the cystic area around the urethral meatus

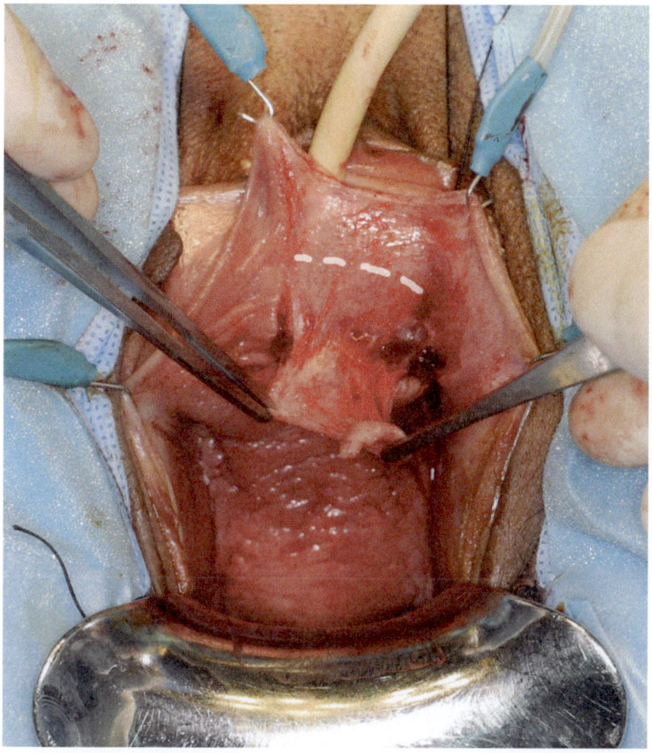

Fig. 8.7 An inverted U flap is created in the left distal vagina to expose the periurethral fascia. The *line marks* the line where the periurethral fascia will be incised

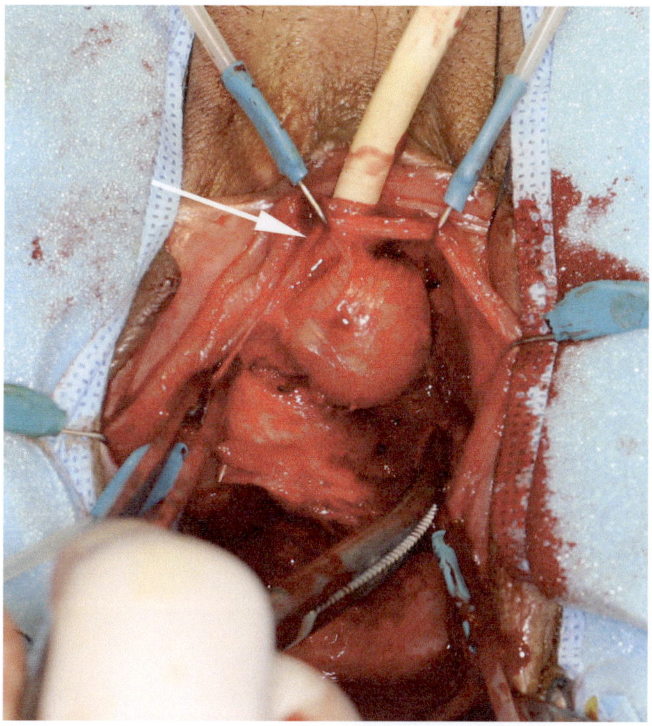

Fig. 8.8 The periurethral fascia is opened in a transverse fashion; superior and inferior flaps are created. The entrance of the cyst at the distal urethra is seen. The *arrow* point to the attachment of the cyst to the distal urethral wall

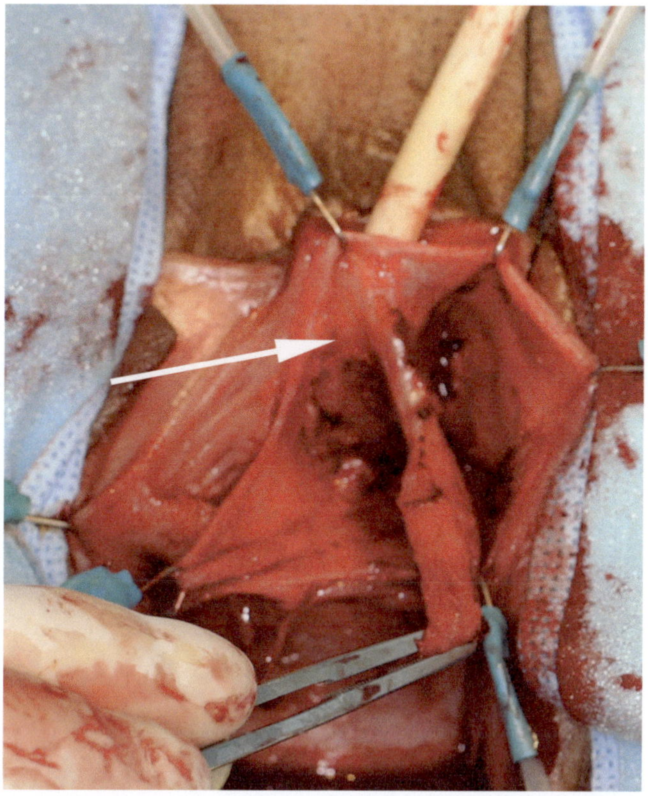

Fig. 8.9 The cyst is drained and the duct of the Skene's gland is dissected free toward the distal urethra and excised. The connection to the urethra is sutured and tied. The duct communicating to the urethra is seen (*arrow*)

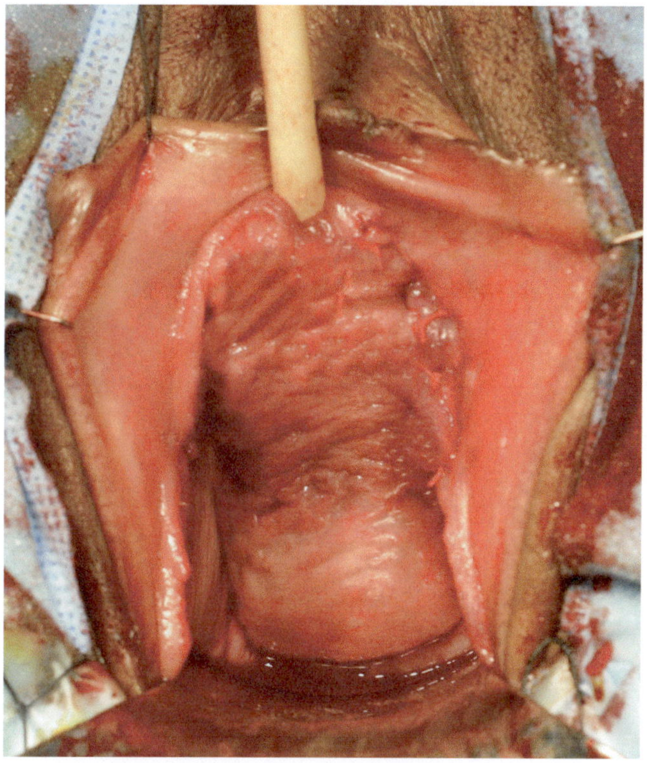

Fig. 8.10 The periurethral fascia is closed in a transverse fashion, and the vaginal flap is advanced distally to cover the area of the reconstruction. The Foley catheter is left in place for 24 h

8.3 Ectopic Ureterocele Presenting as a Vaginal Cyst

The patient, 23 years old, presented with difficulty in emptying the bladder, recurrent urinary infection, and distal urethral pain. Figures 8.11, 8.12, 8.13, and 8.14 illustrate the finding of an ectopic ureterocele. The patient had a side-to-side anastomosis of the ureters, with ligature of the affected ureter. The urethral cyst and her voiding dysfunction were corrected and she remained asymptomatic.

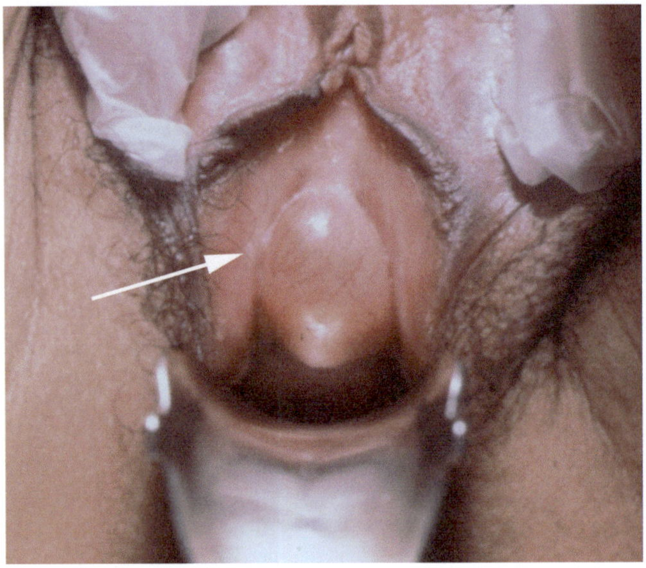

Fig. 8.11 Physical examination reveals a large, cystic mass emerging from the urethra (*arrow*)

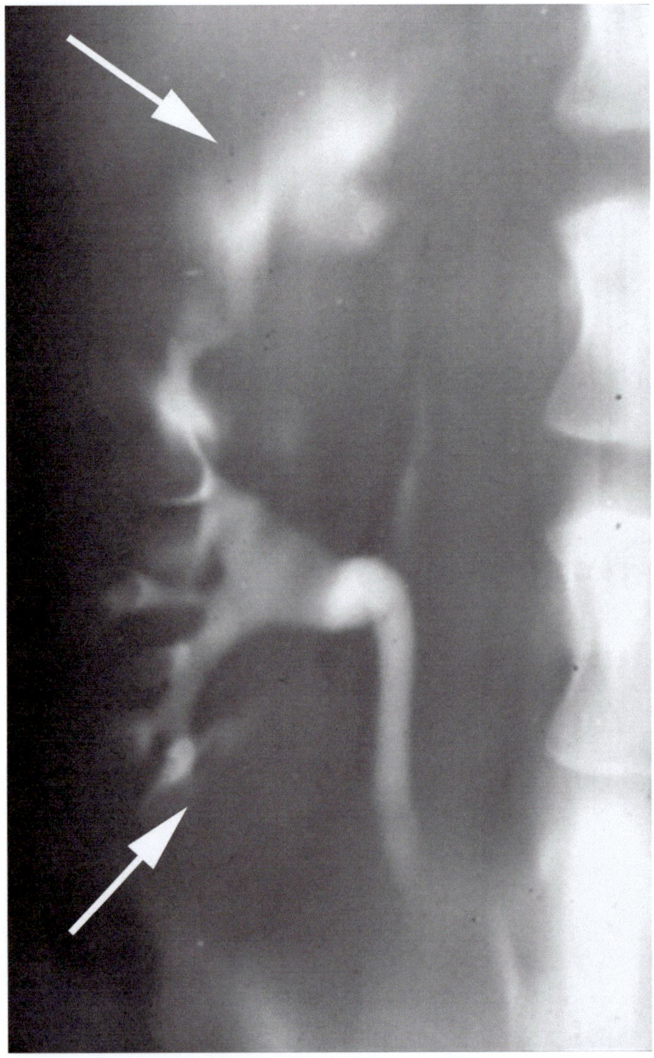

Fig. 8.12 A CT urogram reveals a double collecting system with the upper segment having mild dilatation with good function. *Arrow* pointing toward right duplicated system

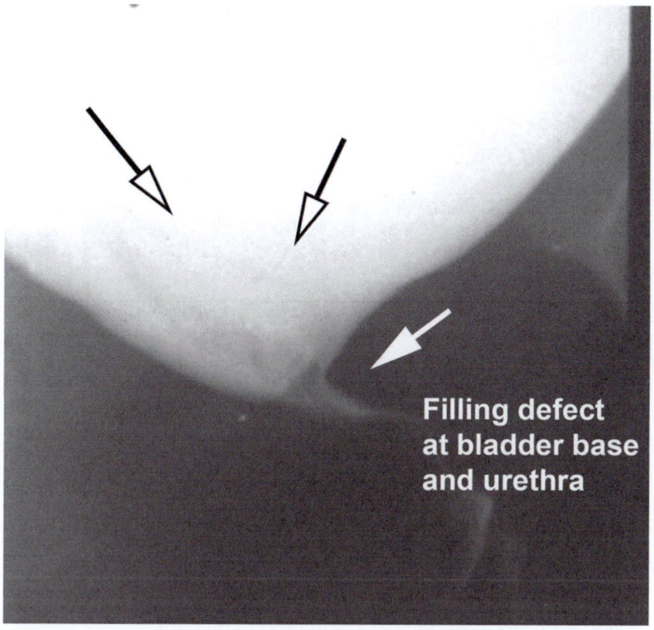

Fig. 8.13 A voiding cystogram showing a filling defect of the bladder base extending toward the urethra. The *arrows* delineated the cystic defect

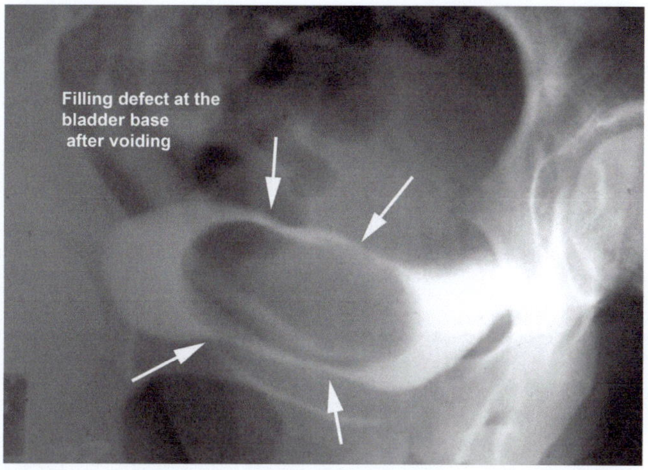

Fig. 8.14 A post-void film shows a large cystic filling defect of the bladder base, typical of an ectopic ureterocele. The *arrows* outline the cyst

8.4 Inclusion Cyst of the Anterior Vaginal Wall

Inclusion cysts are secondary to buried epithelial fragments following surgical procedures in the vagina. The location varies with the prior surgery. The cyst has a stratified squamous epithelial lining and cheese-like contents. If symptomatic, the cyst should be treated by excision.

The patient in Figs. 8.15, 8.16, 8.17, and 8.18 presented with a cystic mass of the anterior vaginal wall. The patient previously had a vaginal hysterectomy and several vaginal procedures for cystocele repair. The patient did not have urinary symptoms and the mass was not tender.

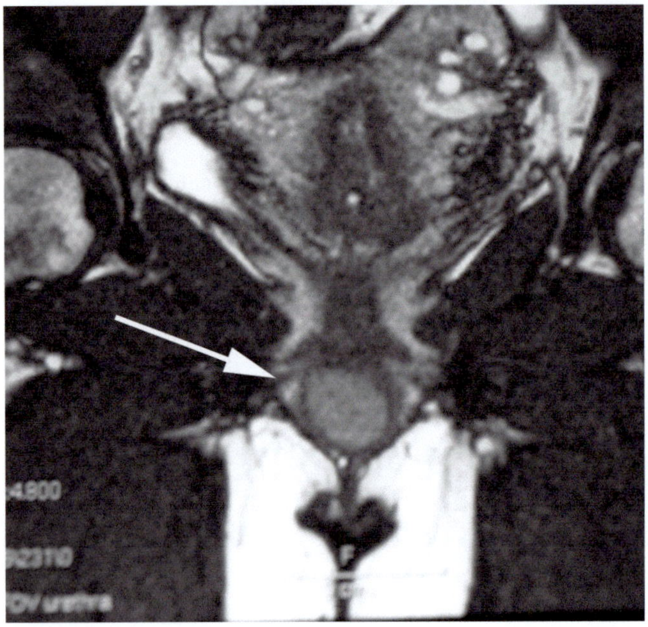

Fig. 8.15 Coronal T2 MRI image of the pelvis showing a gray filled cystic mass of the vagina (*arrow*)

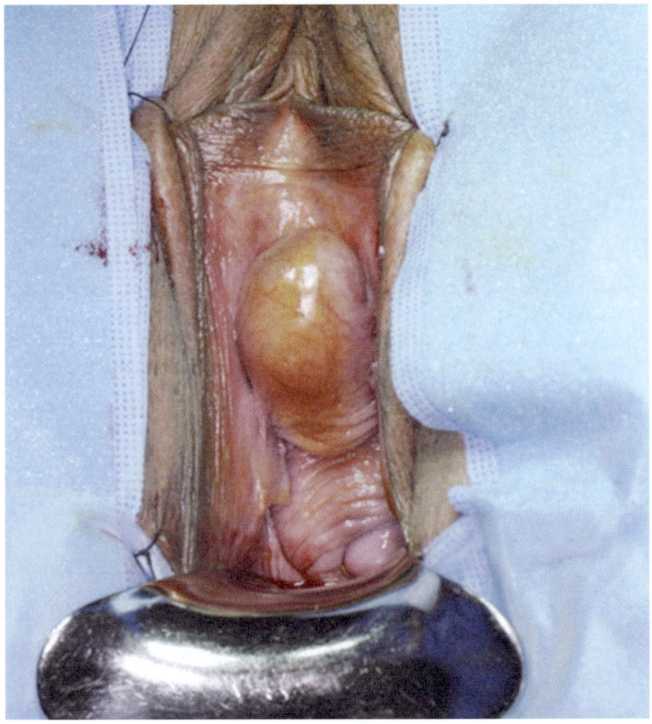

Fig. 8.16 Exposure of the anterior vaginal wall shows a large cystic mass, which is not tender

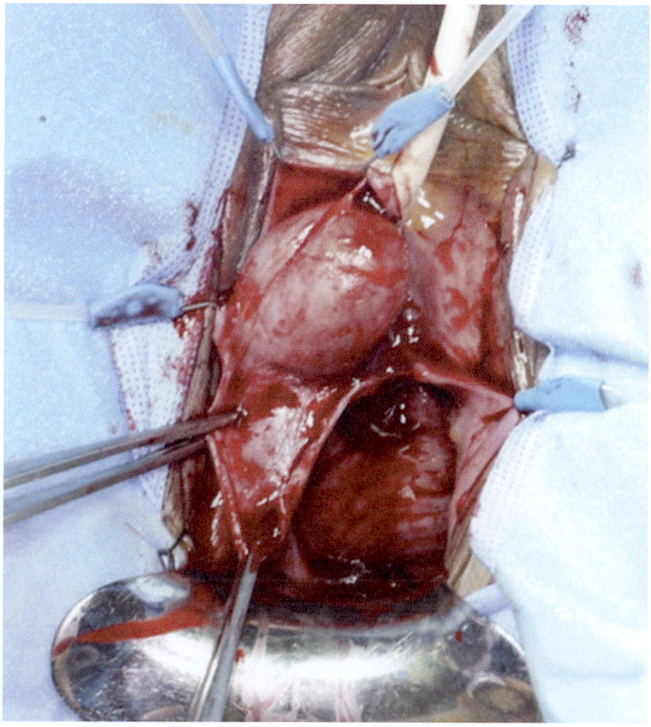

Fig. 8.17 An inverted U flap of the anterior vaginal wall is created to expose the wall of the cyst

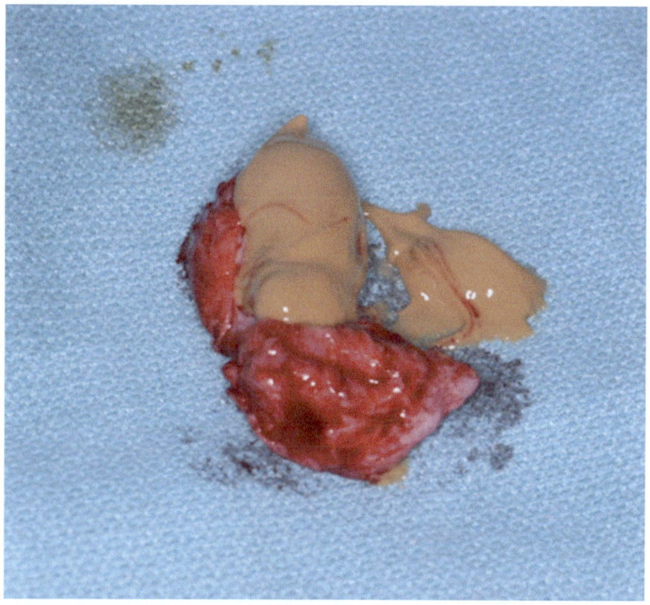

Fig. 8.18 After the excision, the cyst is opened, revealing the typical yellow-gray, cheese-like material

8.5 Endometrioma

A patient known to have pelvic endometriosis presented with a tender, cystic small mass of the anterior vaginal wall (Fig. 8.19). The symptoms did not improve with medical therapy, so excision of the cyst, an endometrioma, was performed (Fig. 8.20).

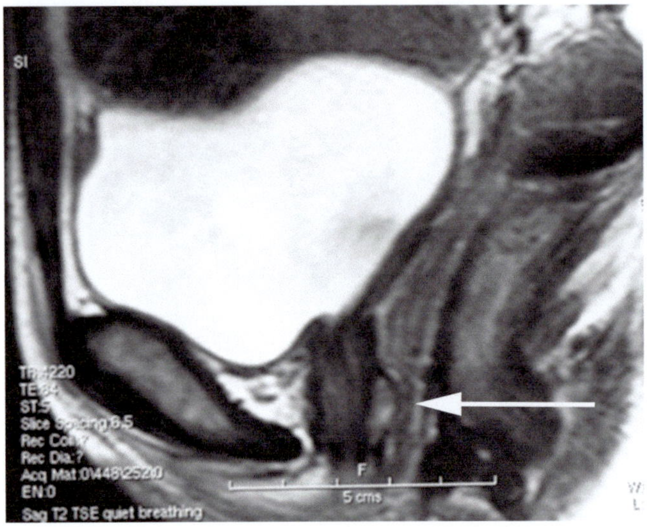

Fig. 8.19 A sagittal MRI image shows a small lesion of the anterior vaginal wall that is not clear fluid (*arrow*)

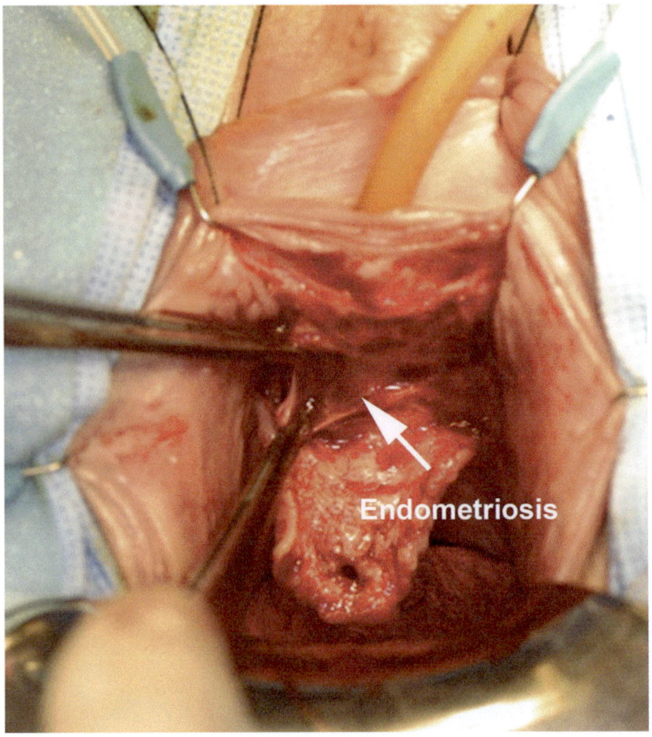

Fig. 8.20 The anterior vaginal wall is exposed and the cyst is opened, draining a small amount of chocolate-colored fluid. The cyst was excised and pathology confirmed the findings of an endometrioma

8.6 Leiomyoma (Fibroid) of the Vaginal Wall

A patient complained of pain during intercourse and feeling a mass in her vagina. Examination detected a hard, non-tender, mobile mass in the right mid-vaginal area (Fig. 8.21). The mass was excised and confirmed to be a benign leiomyoma (Figs. 8.22 and 8.23).

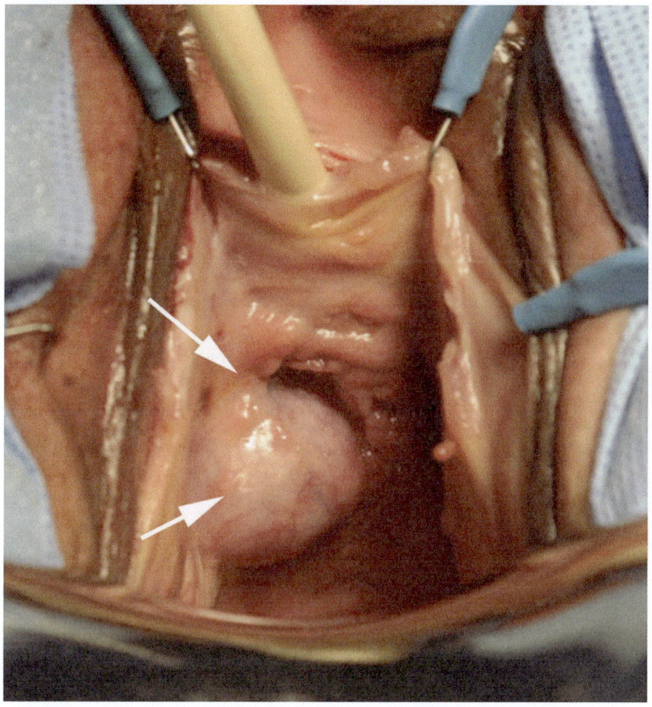

Fig. 8.21 Exposure of the anterior vaginal wall was obtained, showing the mass on the right (*arrow*)

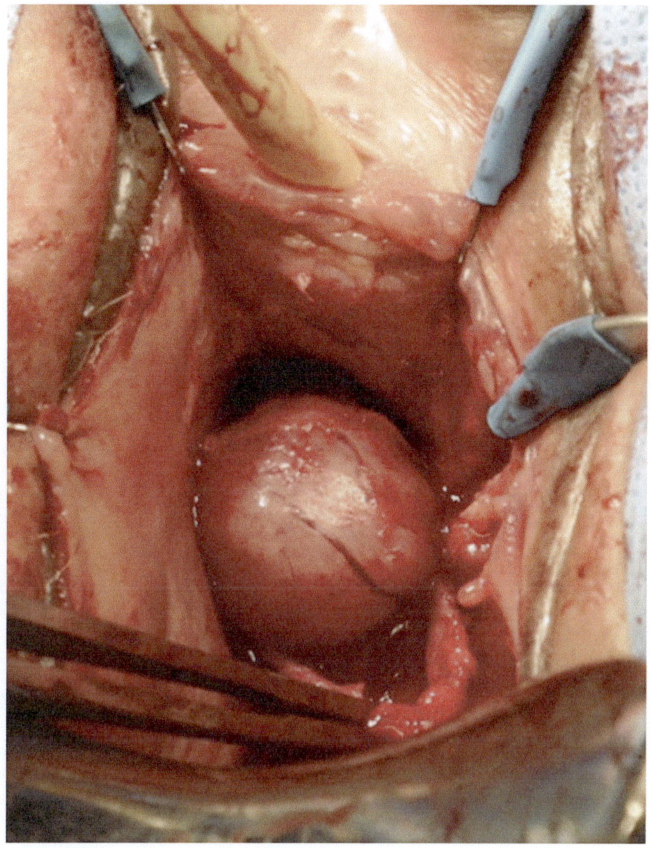

Fig. 8.22 An incision is made over the lesion, and superior and inferior flaps are created to expose the mass

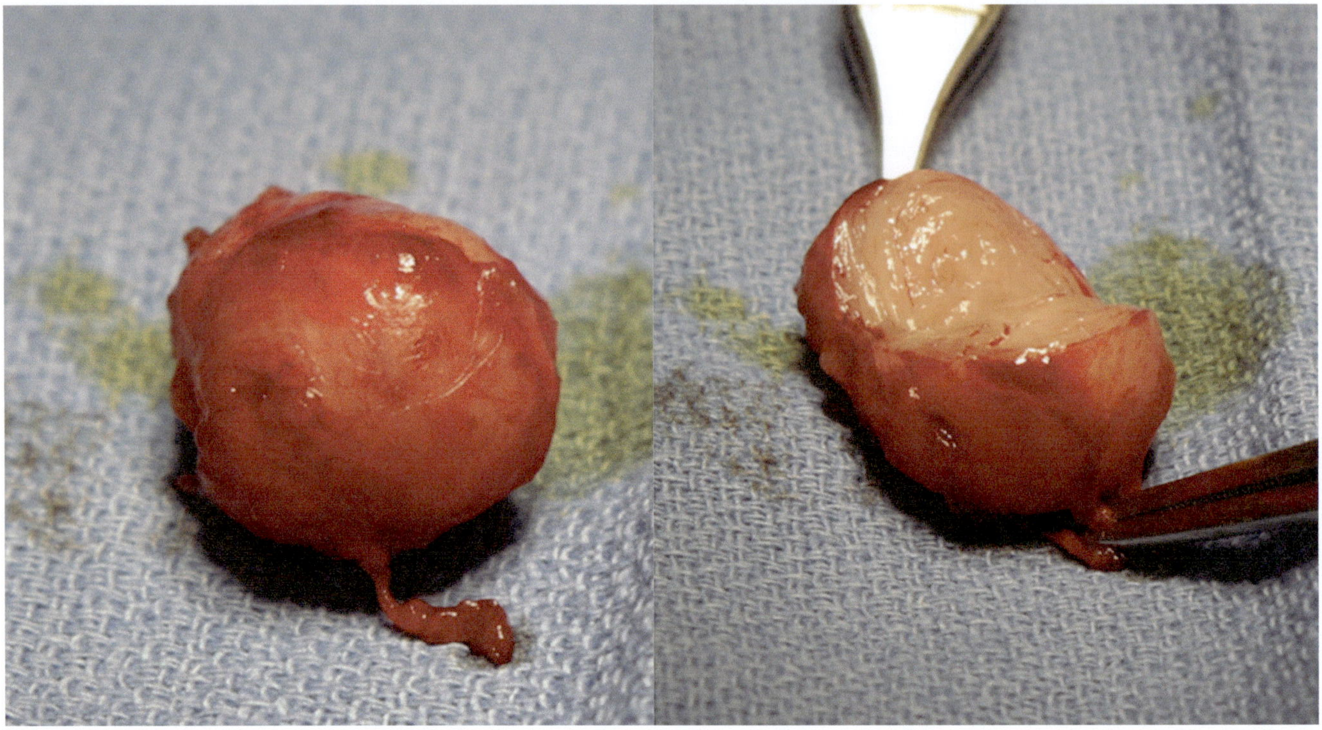

Fig. 8.23 After excision (*left*), the mass is incised (*right*), showing a uniform, hard, fibrous structure. The final pathology confirms the diagnosis of a benign leiomyoma

8.7 Fibroadenoma of the Urethra

An 82-year-old patient presented with difficulty in emptying her bladder and tenderness in the distal vagina. The lesion seen in Fig. 8.24 was excised and shown to be a fibroadenoma of the urethra.

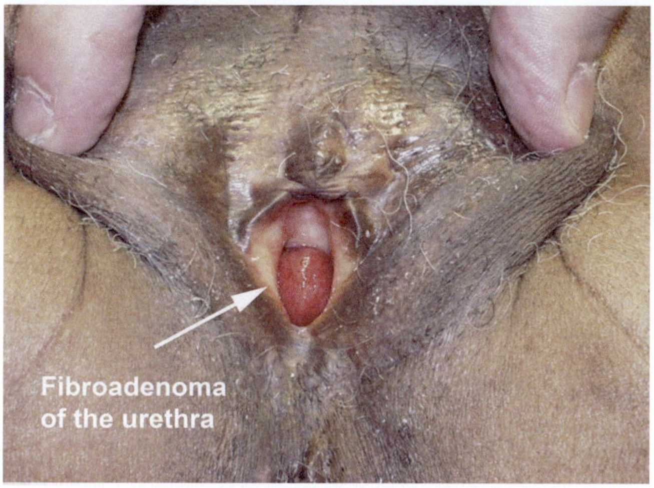

Fig. 8.24 After excision, the pathology showed this lesion to be a fibroadenoma of the urethra originating from the periurethral glands (*arrow*)

8.8 Gartner's Cyst of the Anterior Vaginal Wall

Mesonephric–Wolffian Gartner's duct cysts usually present in the anterolateral vaginal wall. The Wolffian duct will develop into the ureter and trigone. The epithelial cyst is cuboidal and nonciliated, with nonmucinous fluid. These cysts are generally small, averaging 2 cm in diameter.

The patient in Figs. 8.25 and 8.26 was found on routine examination to have a small cystic area of the anterior vaginal wall. After excision, pathology confirmed that it was a Gartner's cyst.

Another patient (Figs. 8.27, 8.28, 8.29, and 8.30) presented with a much larger Gartner's cyst, which had grown for 7 years prior to presentation.

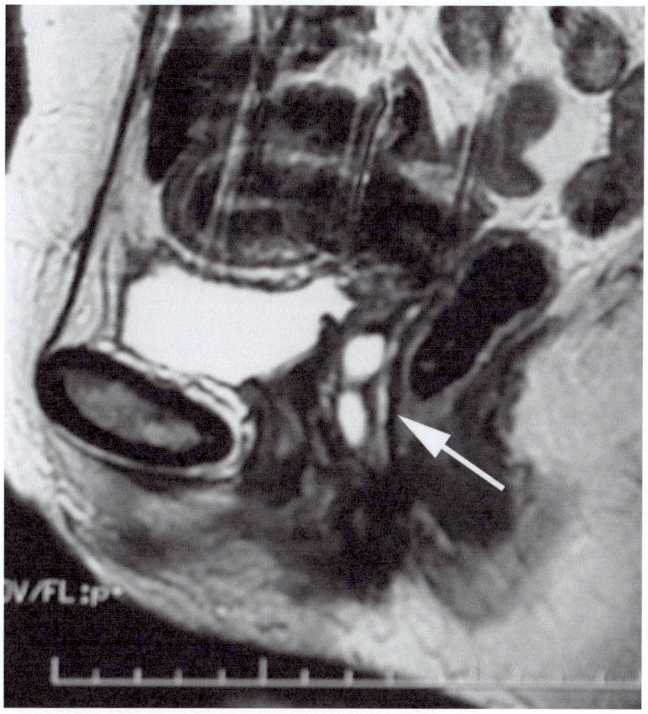

Fig. 8.25 Sagittal MRI confirms the presence of a clear-fluid cystic mass. No solid areas or blood features were seen. The *arrow* point toward the cystic areas in the anterior vaginal wall

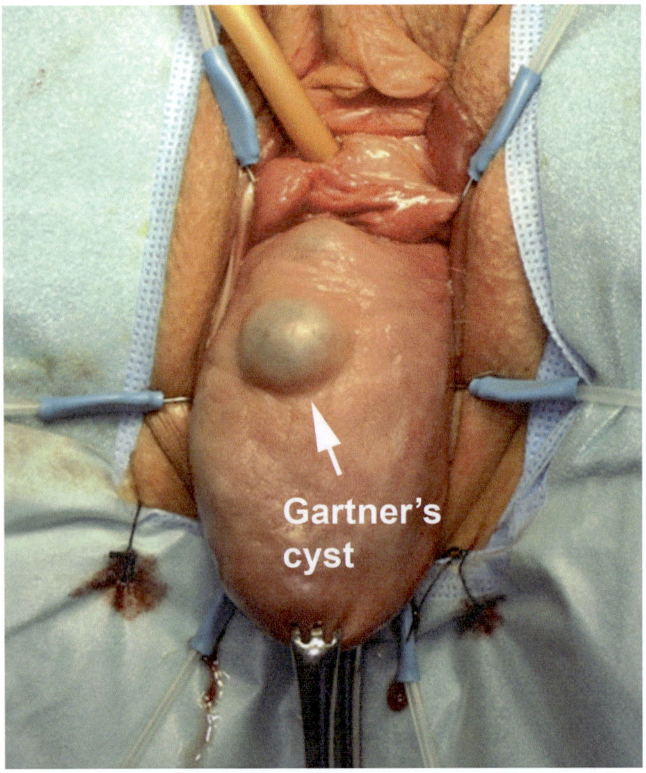

Fig. 8.26 Exposure of the anterior vaginal wall was obtained and the cystic area was excised. It was filled with clear, nonmucinous fluid. Pathology confirmed the diagnosis of Gartner's cyst

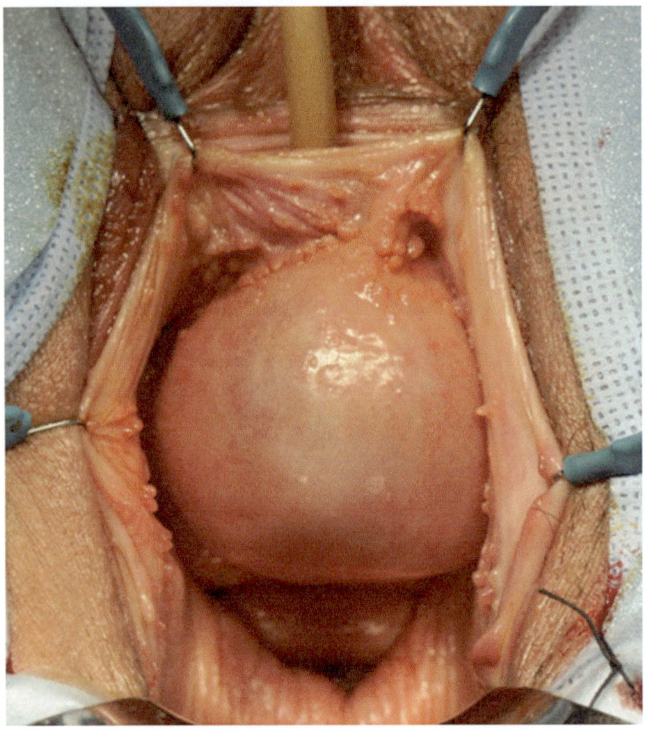

Fig. 8.27 This patient presented with a large, nontender mass of the anterior vaginal wall. The mass had progressively grown for 7 years prior to presentation

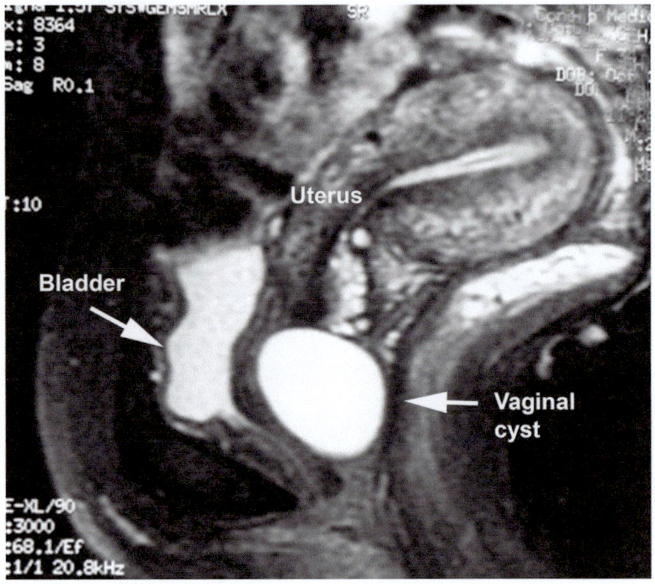

Fig. 8.28 A sagittal T2 MRI image showed a clear-fluid cystic mass of the anterior vaginal wall

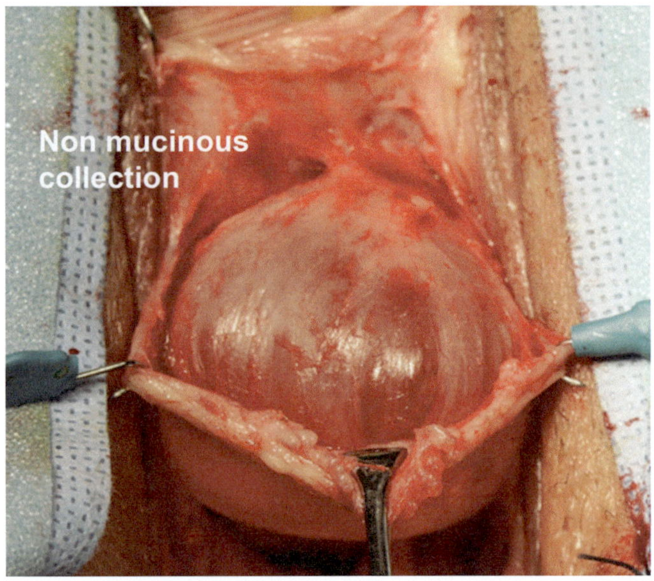

Fig. 8.29 A superior and inferior flap of the anterior vaginal wall was created to expose the cystic area. The mass was excised superficially to the perivesical fascia

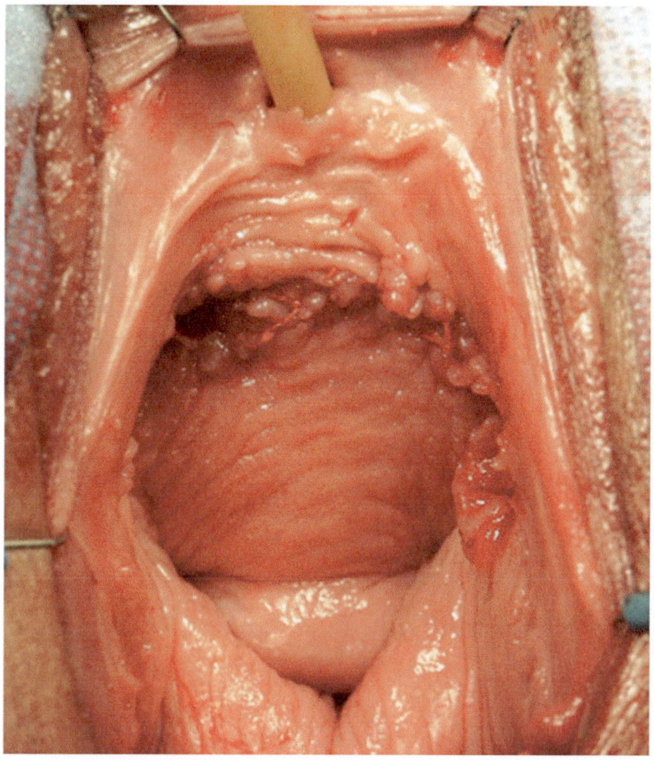

Fig. 8.30 The excess of vaginal wall was excised and the anterior vaginal wall was reconstructed. The final pathology confirmed the diagnosis of Gartner's cyst

8.9 Müllerian Cyst

Müllerian or paramesonephric vaginal cysts may be present in the anterior vaginal wall (generally anterolateral). The Müllerian ducts normally develop into the uterus and upper vagina. The epithelium is pseudostratified columnar cells and is mucin producing. These cysts are usually small (1–7 cm) and asymptomatic. Treatment is required only if the cyst is symptomatic.

Figures 8.31 and 8.32 depict a patient who was found on routine examination to have a small, cystic, nontender mass of the anterior vaginal wall.

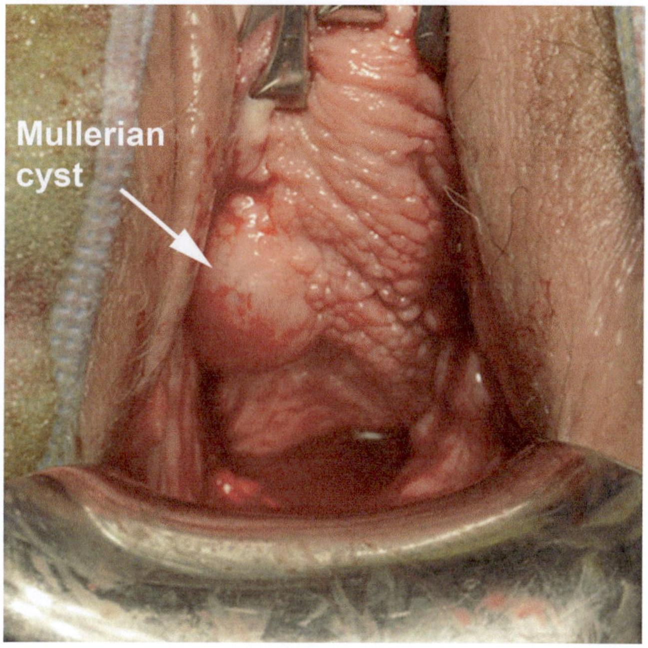

Fig. 8.31 Exposure of the anterior vaginal wall, showing the location of the small cystic mass

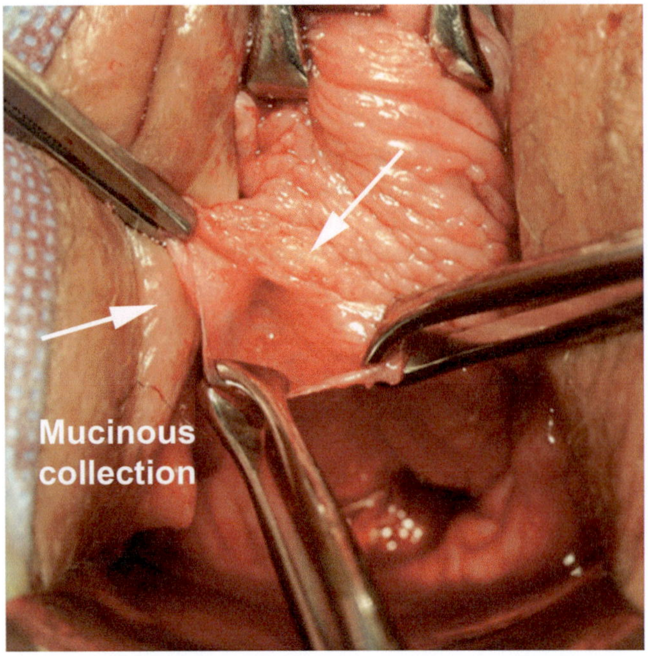

Fig. 8.32 Excision of the cyst was performed and a mucous type of fluid was drained. The final pathology confirmed the diagnosis of Müllerian cyst. The *arrows* outline the margins of the cyst

8.10 Distal Thrombosis of Urethral Mucosa

The patient in Figs. 8.33 and 8.34 developed acute urinary retention, urethral pain, and vaginal bleeding while receiving chemotherapy for advanced ovarian cancer.

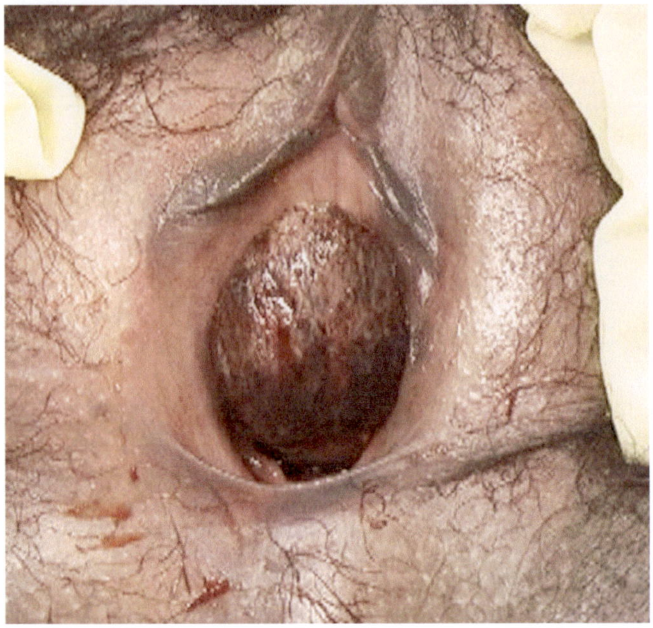

Fig. 8.33 Vaginal examination revealed a large, necrotic, hemorrhagic mass occluding the urethra

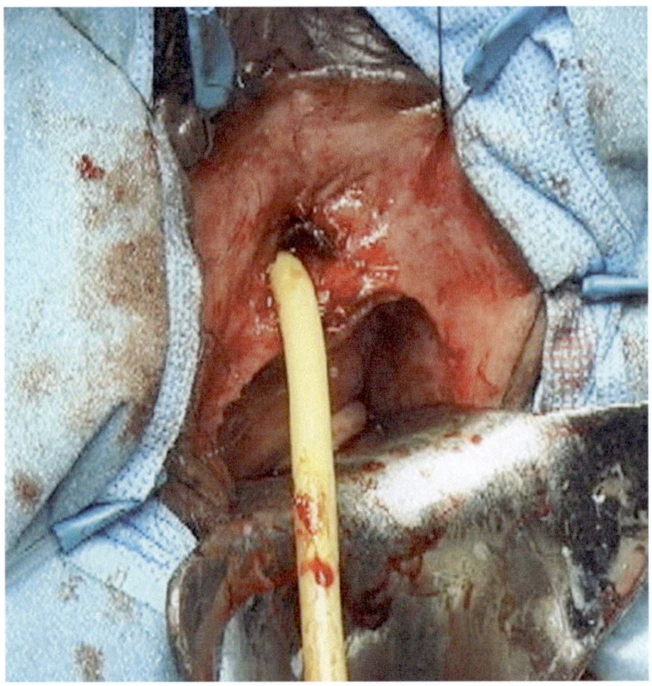

Fig. 8.34 The mass was excised and the urethral mucosa anastomosed to the vaginal wall over a Foley catheter

8.11 Posterior Vaginal Wall and Perineal Leiomyoma (Fibroid)

The patient in Figs. 8.35, 8.36, 8.37, 8.38, and 8.39 presented with vaginal discomfort, defecatory dysfunction, and a large, nontender mass of the posterior vaginal wall extending to the perineum.

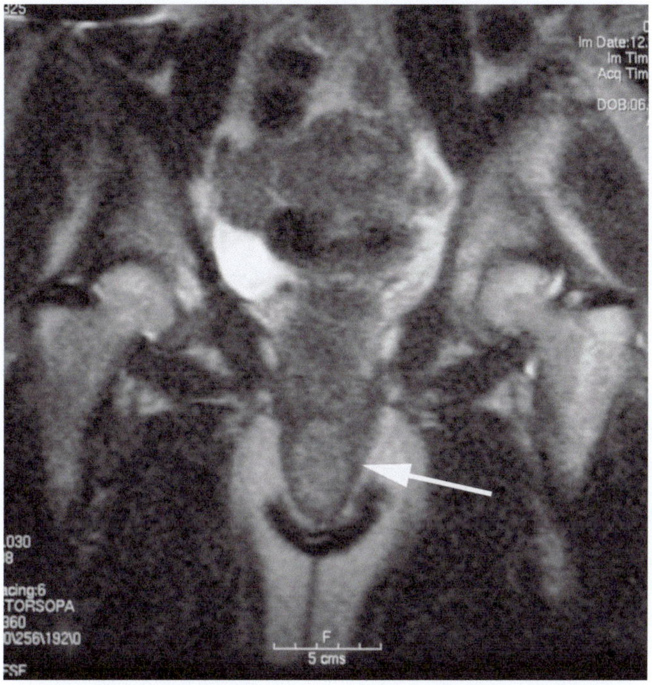

Fig. 8.35 A coronal MRI shows the presence of a solid, well-circumscribed mass of the perineum (*arrow*)

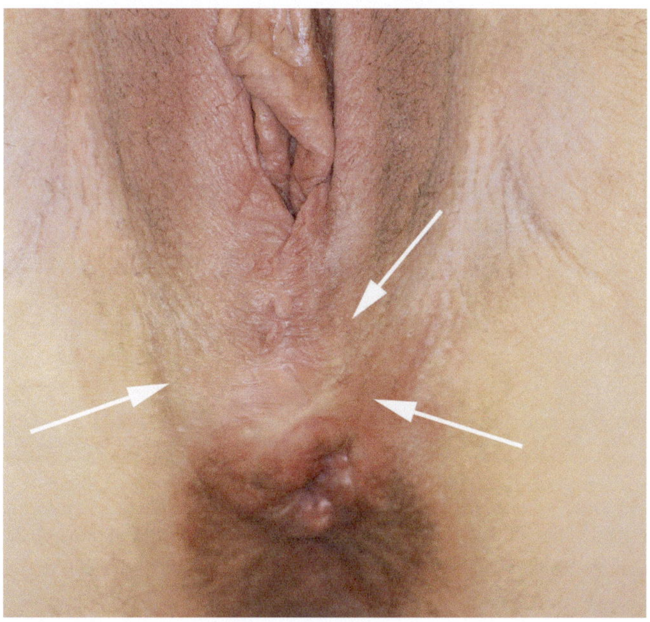

Fig. 8.36 Exposure of the posterior vaginal wall and perineum shows a hard mass that extends from the posterior vaginal wall to the perineum. A perineal approach to remove the mass was performed. The *arrows* outline the lesion in the perineum

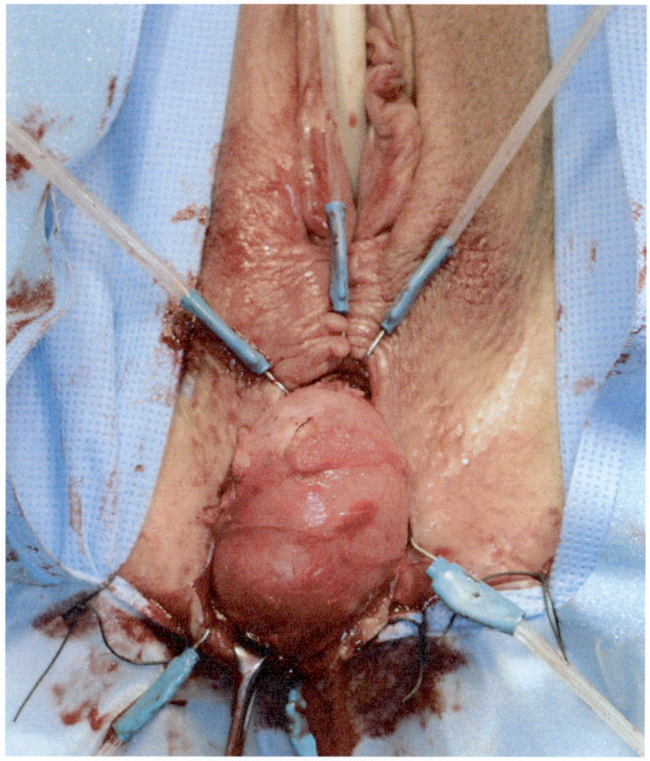

Fig. 8.37 A superior and inferior flap of the perineal skin was created to expose the mass. The mass is dissected free, without difficulty, from the posterior vaginal wall and prerectal area

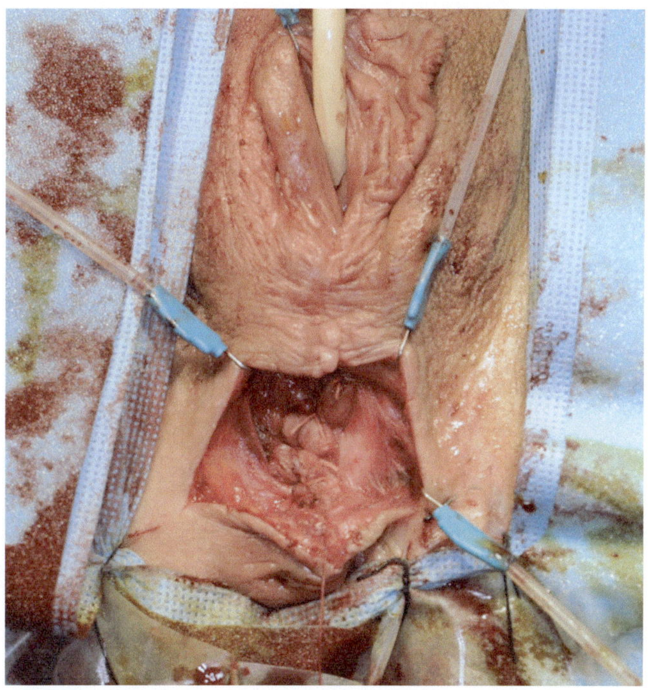

Fig. 8.38 After removal of the mass, the prerectal area, the perineum, and the posterior vaginal wall were reconstructed

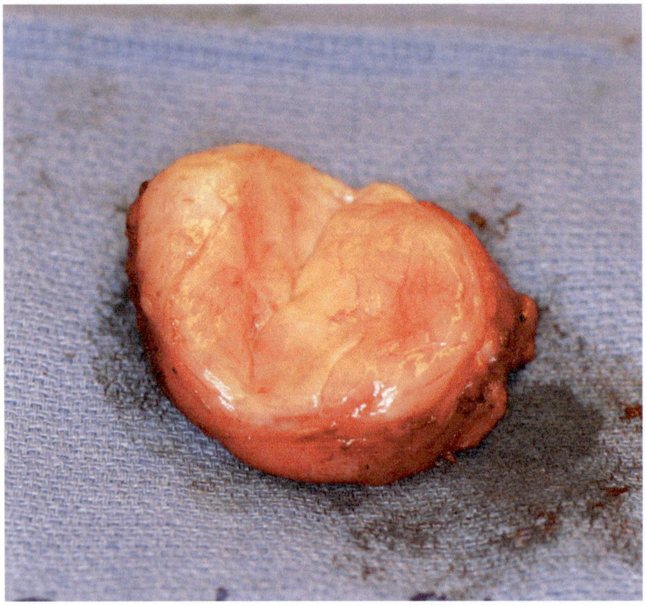

Fig. 8.39 The mass was removed and transected. The final pathology confirmed the diagnosis of benign leiomyoma (fibroid)

8.12 Chondroma of the Inferior Pubic Rami

The patient in Figs. 8.40, 8.41, and 8.42 presented with difficulty in voiding and a feeling of a hard mass growing in the anterior vaginal wall.

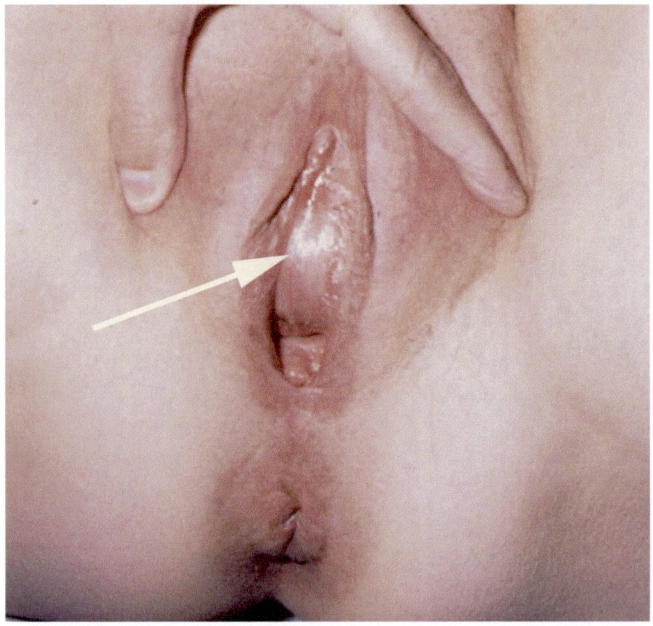

Fig. 8.40 Physical examination revealed a very hard, fixed mass anterior to the urethra, under the pubic bone (*arrow*). The mass was not mobile or tender

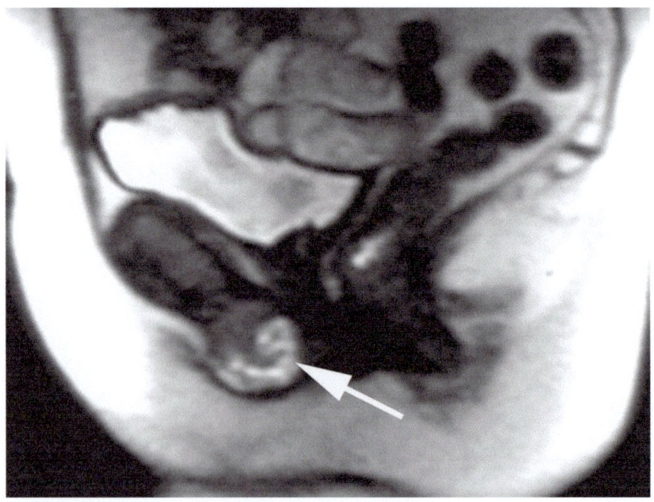

Fig. 8.41 A sagittal MRI shows a mass emerging from the inferior ramus of the pubic bone (*arrow*), displacing the urethra posteriorly. The mass is well circumscribed and is not invading surrounding tissues

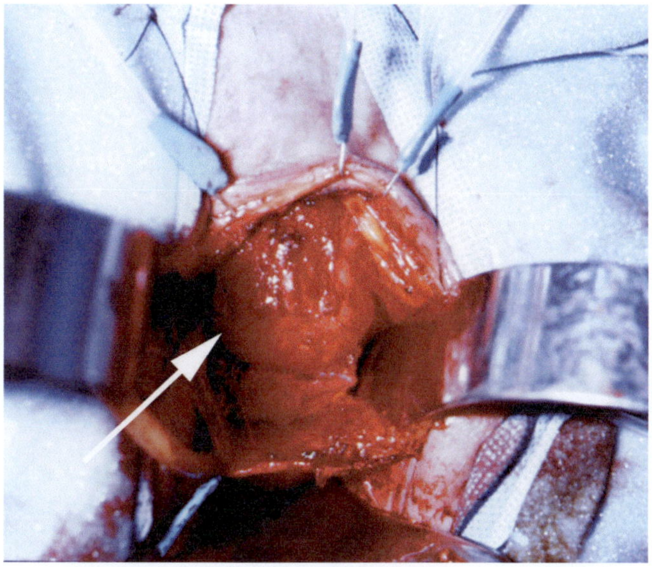

Fig. 8.42 A suprameatal incision was made to separate the urethra from the inferior ramus of the pubic bone (*arrow*). The mass was removed entirely, and the final pathology confirmed the diagnosis of a benign chondroma

8.13 Large Urethral Leiomyoma Causing Urethral Obstruction

During her second pregnancy, the young patient in Figs. 8.43, 8.44, 8.45, 8.46, 8.47, 8.48, 8.49, 8.50, 8.51, 8.52, 8.53, 8.54, 8.55, 8.56, 8.57, and 8.58 presented with difficulty in voiding, tenderness in the anterior vaginal wall, and the feeling of a mass. Physical examination revealed a large, nontender, elastic, nonmobile mass inferior to the pubic bone. The mass displaced the urethra inferiorly.

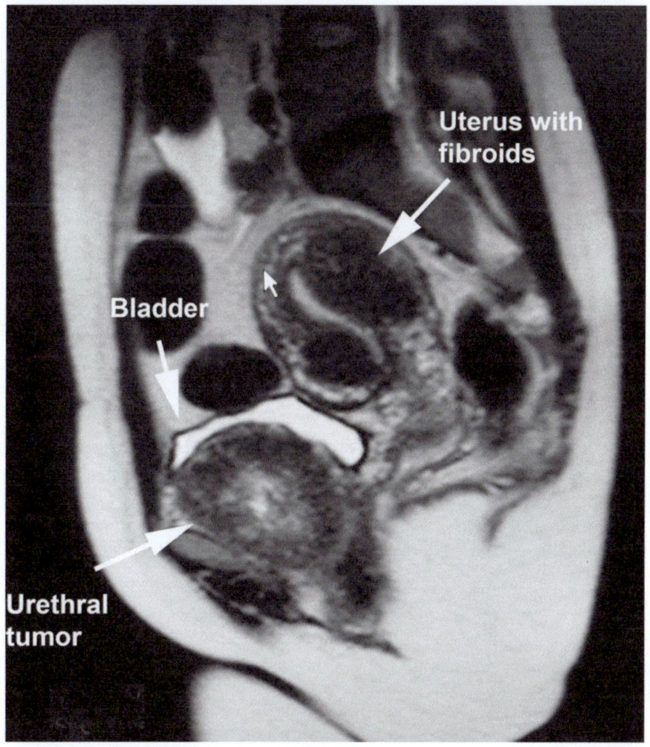

Fig. 8.43 Sagittal T2 MRI of the midpelvis reveals a large mass, mostly solid, with areas of necrosis and fluid displacing the anterior vagina and urethra inferiorly. The uterus is normal except for several small fibroids, and the adnexa are normal

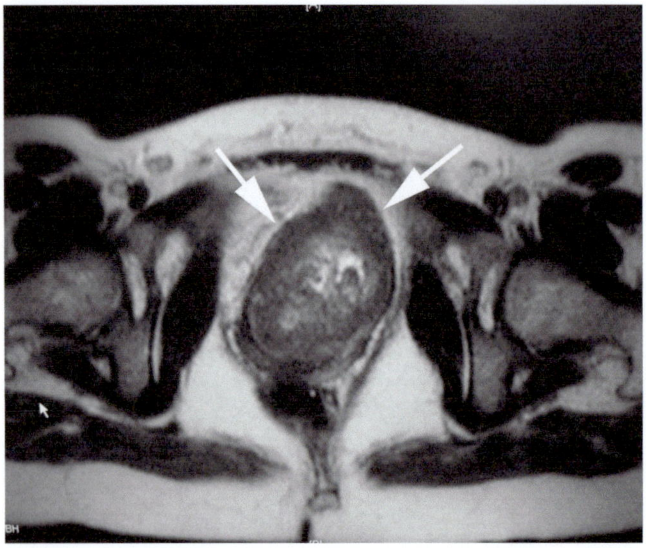

Fig. 8.44 An axial MRI shows the replacement and displacement of the urethra by the large mass. Multiple areas of necrosis are seen. The *arrows* outline the tumor

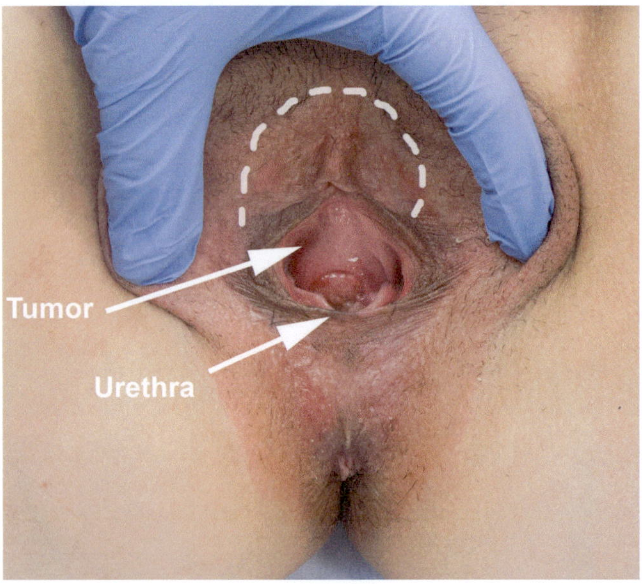

Fig. 8.45 On examination, a large mass is displacing the urethra inferiorly. The mass extends below the inferior ramus of the pubic bone toward the retropubic space. The rest of the anterior and posterior vaginal wall was normal. The *arrows* point toward the extension of the tumor inferior to the pubic bone

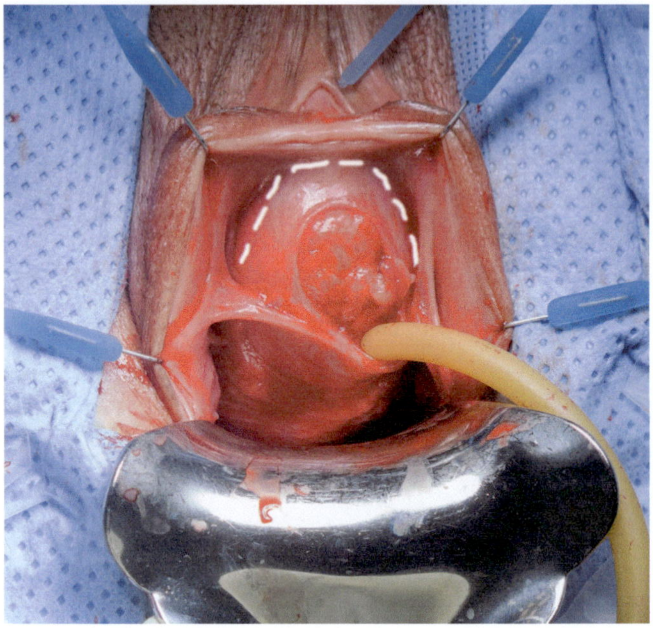

Fig. 8.46 An inverted U flap of the anterior vaginal wall was created over the lesion. The *line* outlines the incision of the anterior vaginal wall

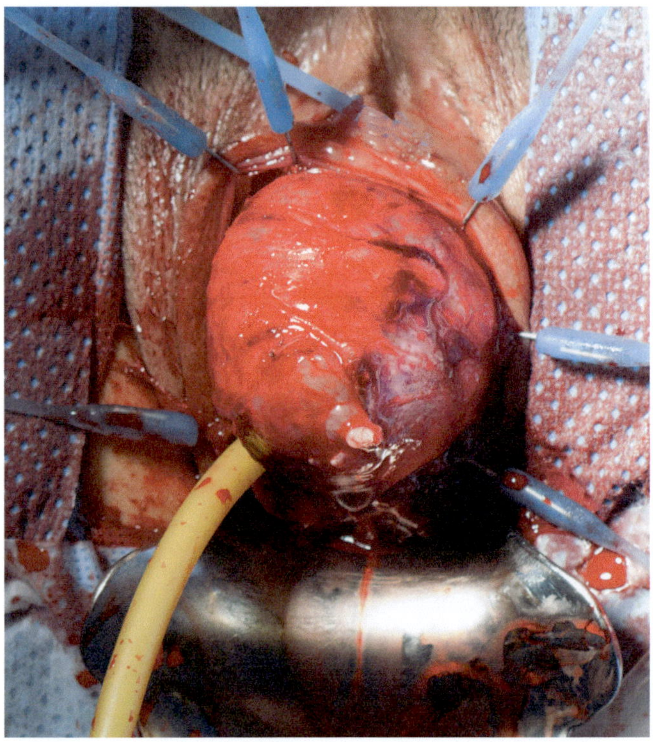

Fig. 8.47 Dissection of the mass required extensive mobilization of the anterior vaginal wall and urethral area. The retropubic space was entered by detaching the pubourethral ligaments from the inferior margin of the pubic bone. The lateral attachments of the mass to the levator muscles also required extensive dissection

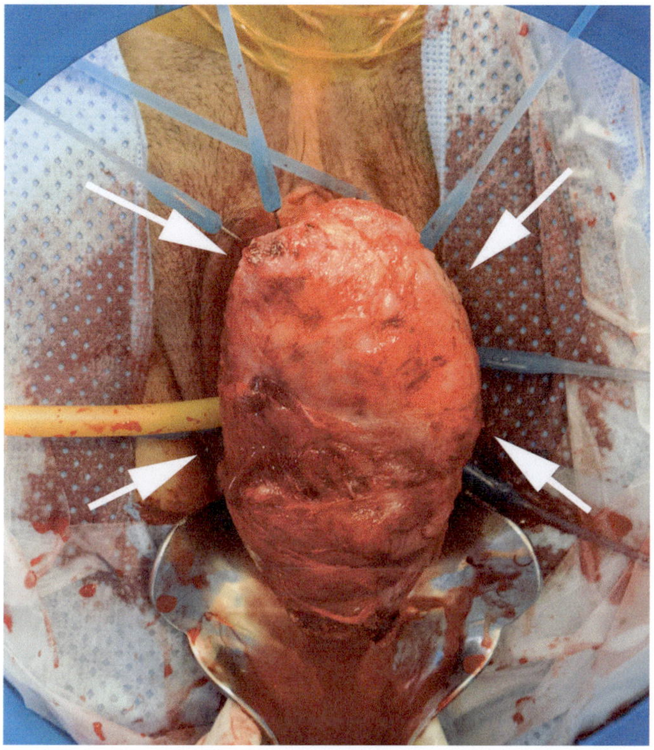

Fig. 8.48 The mass is mobilized and freed from the surrounding structures. The *arrows* outline the tumor before removal

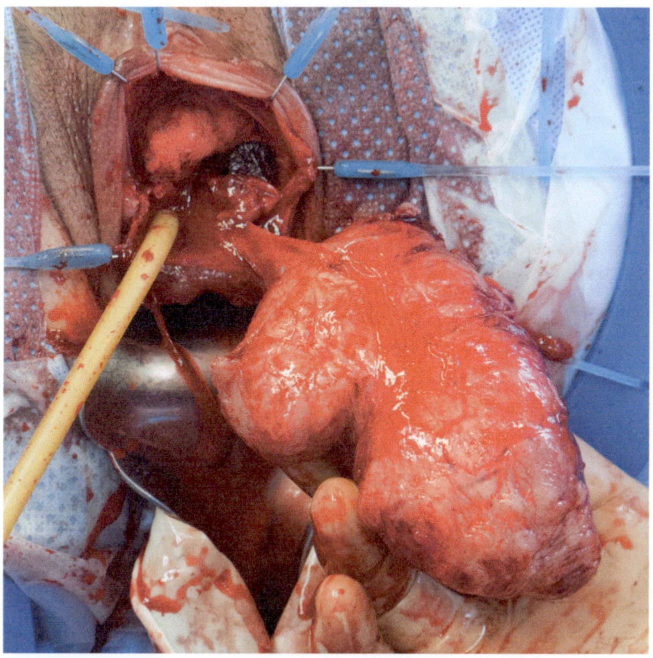

Fig. 8.49 The mass has been removed, and the remaining adhesions have been transected

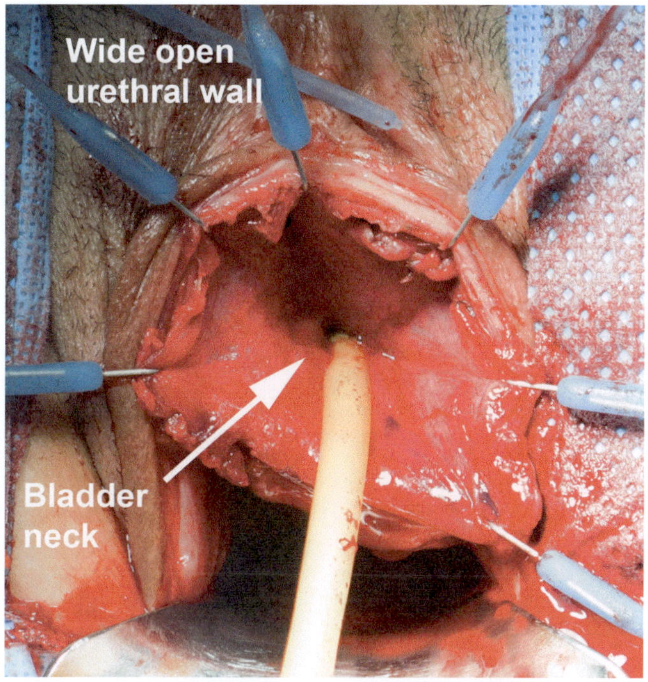

Fig. 8.50 The distal and proximal urethras are wide open (like a cone with the tip representing the bladder neck). The bladder neck is the only area intact and competent. Construction of a neourethra will be performed

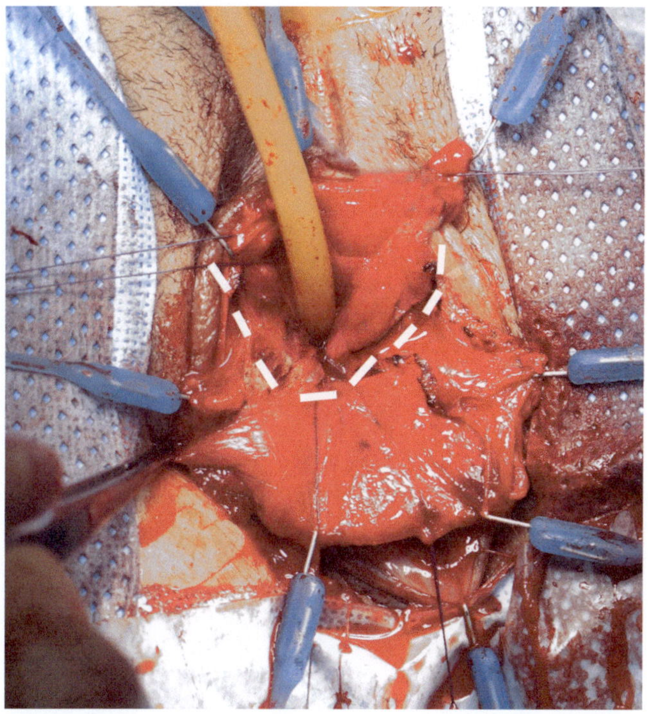

Fig. 8.51 Two parallel incisions (*broken white line*) are made in the anterior, widely dilated defect of the urethral wall, lateral to the Foley catheter, starting at the bladder neck

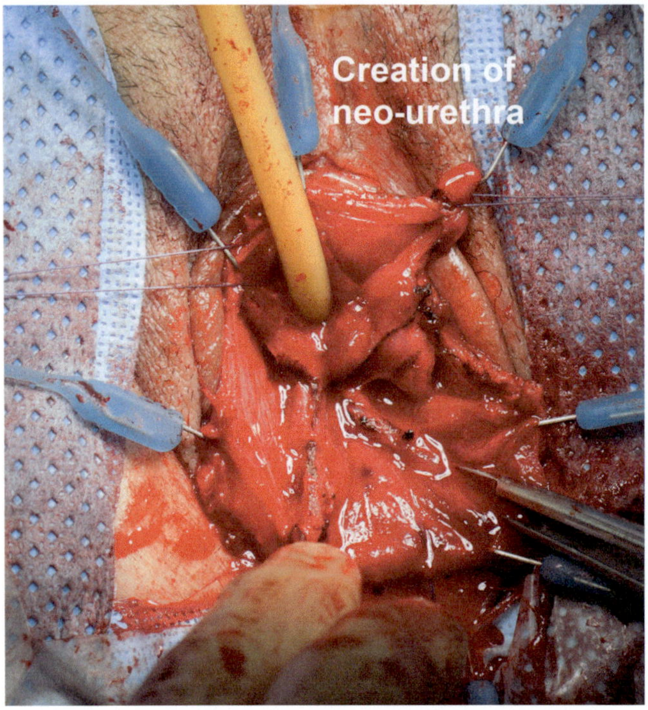

Fig. 8.52 The margins of the anterior incisions are approximated over the Foley catheter to construct a tube of the anterior defect. Two layers of running and interrupted sutures are applied

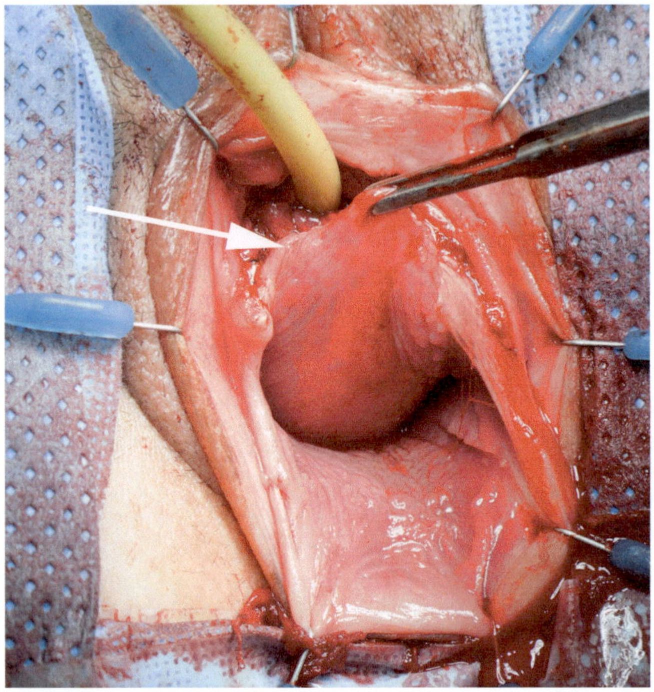

Fig. 8.54 The neourethra was reconstructed. Bladder irrigations are done to rule out any extravasation. The excess of periurethral fascia was excised. An anterior vaginal wall flap (*arrow*) is advanced distally to cover the area of the reconstructed urethra

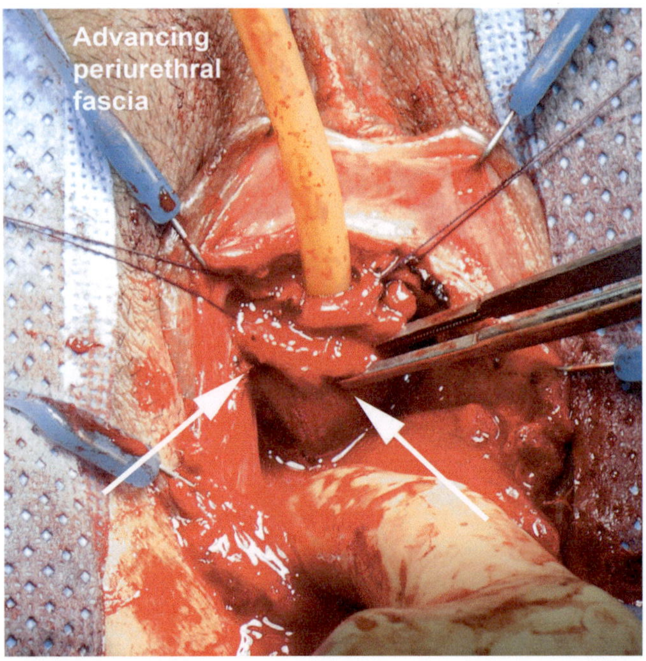

Fig. 8.53 The mucosa of the lateral and posterior defect was excised and trimmed. The periurethral fascia was advanced distally to cover the area of the reconstructed urethra. The *arrows* indicate the margin of the advanced periurethral fascia

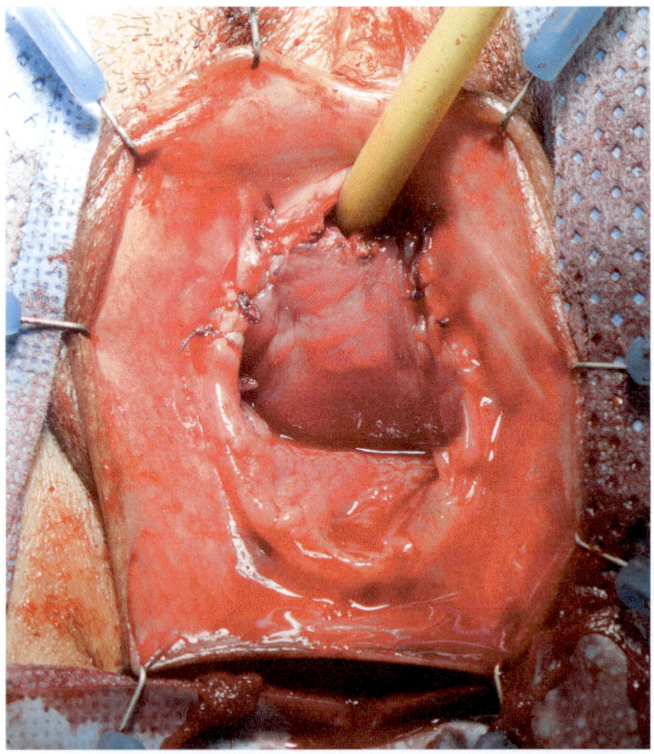

Fig. 8.55 The anterior vaginal wall reconstruction is completed. The flap of the anterior vaginal wall is anastomosed distally to the new urethral meatus and laterally to the vaginal wall

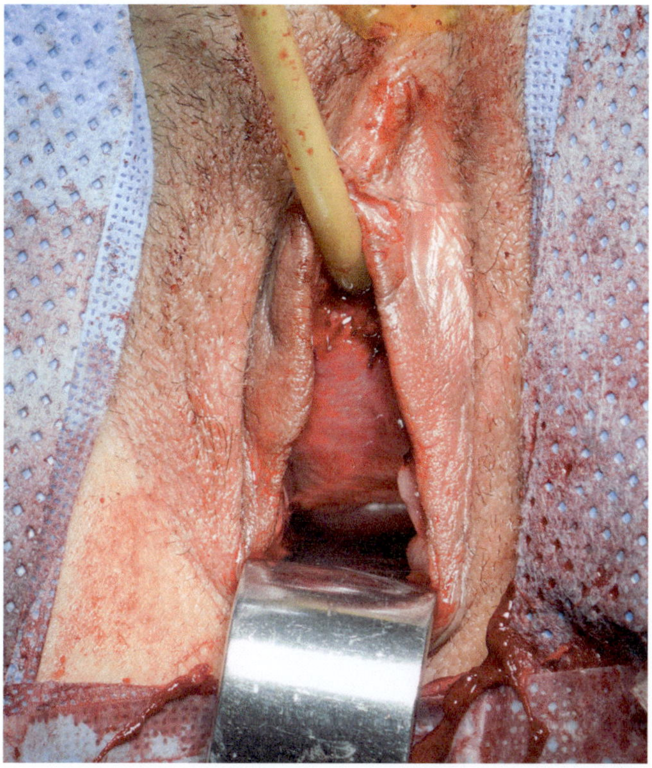

Fig. 8.56 Postoperative view of the anterior vaginal wall after the surgery was completed

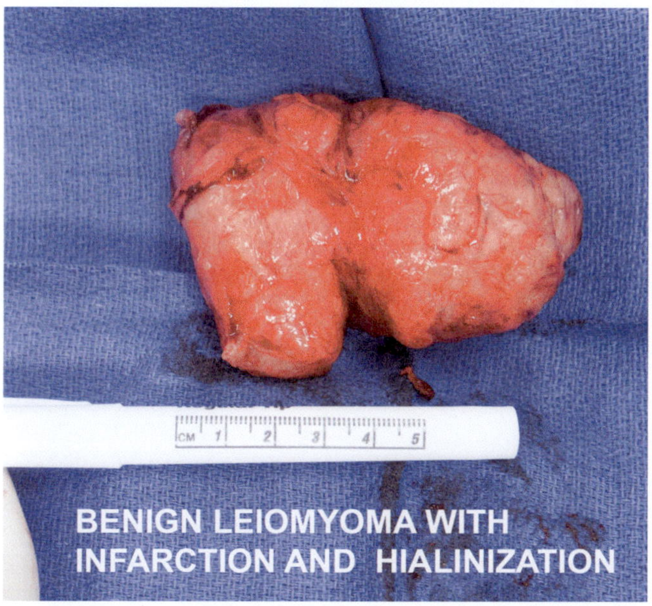

Fig. 8.57 The specimen after removal. The final pathology showed a benign leiomyoma with areas of infarction and hyalinization

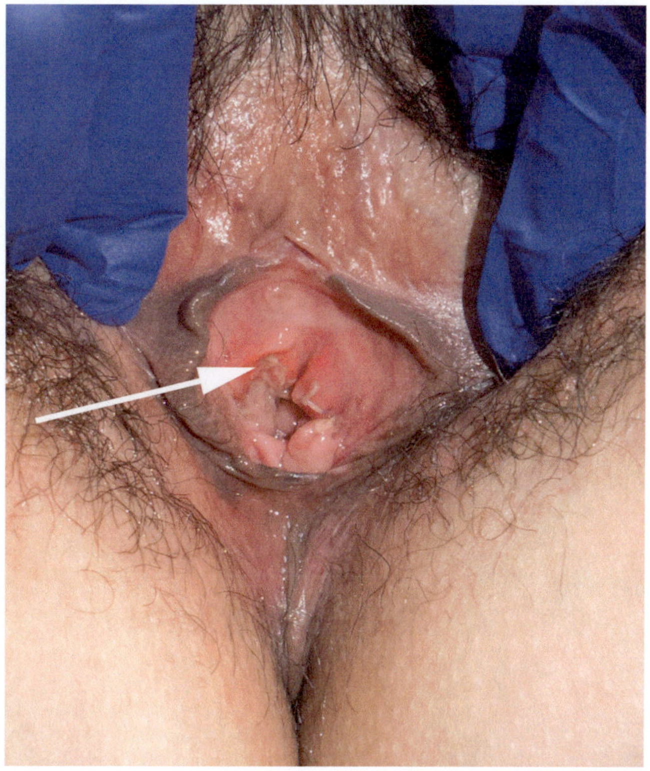

Fig. 8.58 Picture of the anterior vaginal wall 5 months after surgery. The patient is voiding normally and without any incontinence. The anterior vaginal wall is well supported. The *arrows* point toward the external reconstructed urethral meatus

Suggested Reading

Blaivas JG, Flisser AJ, Bleustein CB, Panagopoulos G. Periurethral masses: etiology and diagnosis in a large series of women. Obstet Gynecol. 2004;103:842–7.

Dmochowski RR, Ganabathi K, Zimmern PE, Leach GE. Benign female periurethral masses. J Urol. 1994;152:1943–51.

Eilber KS, Raz S. Benign cystic lesions of the vagina: a literature review. J Urol. 2003;170(3):717–22.

9 Complications of Vaginal Surgery

Vaginal surgery complications can at times be difficult to manage. Clearly the best management scheme entails steps to prevent complications. These steps require judicious preoperative planning with detailed knowledge of the patient's case, operative anatomy, surgical indications, and expectations, as well as prudent use of preoperative diagnostic testing. This kind of preparation facilitates better recognition of intraoperative complications and consequent expeditious treatment.

Proper identification of the intraoperative complication, with thorough knowledge of the surgical principles of repair, will help to prevent late complications or adverse outcomes. Delay in operative management will only prolong the problem and may result in longer hospitalization and greater patient discomfort, cost, and inconvenience.

A thorough preoperative evaluation will assist in outlining the best surgical approach and properly identifying optimal surgical candidates. Depending on the pathology to be treated, one can tailor the preoperative approach accordingly.

The identification and management of many important complications of vaginal surgery are discussed in this chapter:

- Bleeding
- Infection
- Bladder injury (perforation)
- Urethral injury
- Ureteric injury
- Bowel/rectal injury
- Neurologic injury
- Pelvic pain, mesh exposure or extrusion
- Recurrent prolapse
- De novo urgency incontinence
- Urinary outlet obstruction
- Vaginal narrowing/stenosis
- Recurrent stress incontinence
- Pelvic pain, dyspareunia

Electronic supplementary material The online version of this chapter (doi:10.1007/978-1-4939-2941-2_9) contains supplementary material, which is available to authorized users.

S. Raz, *Atlas of Vaginal Reconstructive Surgery*, DOI 10.1007/978-1-4939-2941-2_9

9.1 Bleeding

Most cases of bleeding during transvaginal surgery are self-corrected. Clearly, patients at risk for bleeding complications (such as those using aspirin, NSAIDs, or warfarin and those who have a history of a bleeding diathesis) should be screened and the risk possibly corrected prior to surgery. Nonetheless, significant bleeding can be encountered intraoperatively, especially if one dissects into the wrong tissue planes or structures. Bleeding encountered intraoperatively can be controlled with judicious use of electrocoagulation, suture ligatures, or both. These techniques should be performed cautiously if done in the anterior vaginal wall or retropubic space, in order to avoid ureteric injury. Most cases of mild bleeding subside with packing or placement of a tampon. Alternatively, intravaginal inflation of a Foley catheter with 50–60 mL of water can help tamponade bleeding (Fig. 9.1). If bleeding becomes severe or the patient becomes unstable, the source of bleeding may be extraperitoneal or retroperitoneal (Fig. 9.2). Appropriate resuscitative measures should be taken in these cases. Persistent or postoperative bleeding may require re-exploration or even a laparotomy. If the bleeding area cannot be identified, one may consider selective angioembolization or, if necessary, bilateral hypogastric artery ligation.

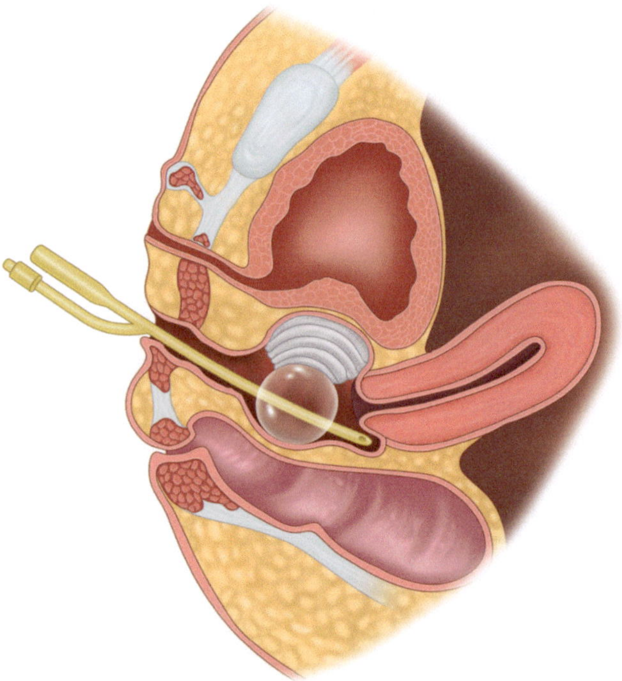

Fig. 9.1 In cases of persistent vaginal bleeding after surgery, the insertion of the Foley catheter behind a vaginal packing can provide further control of the bleeding

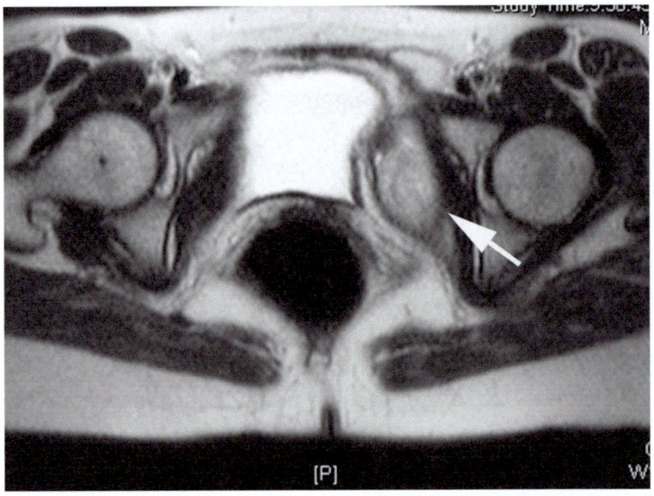

Fig. 9.2 MRI was done for pain occurring immediately after insertion of an obturator sling. The image shows a hematoma (*arrow*) in the left obturator fossa. The hematoma expanded, requiring surgical drainage

9.2 Infection

As bacteria potentially contaminate the vagina, it is a frequent site of infections in the postoperative period. These infections can be avoided with judicious use of broad-spectrum antibiotics administered perioperatively, along with a careful and thorough vaginal preparation and scrub prior to incision, along with proper draping of the surgical field so that the rectum/anus is out of the area of the operation. Additionally, preoperative urine culture and sensitivity testing may be indicated in patients at risk for recurrent urinary tract infections (UTIs) or those with abnormal urinalyses (e.g., presence of leukocytes, nitrites, or blood). Prevention again is key to helping avoid complications in the postoperative period.

Infections may affect the vaginal incision areas, suprapubic incisions, retropubic spaces, or urinary tract. Incisional infections or vaginal cuff infections occur more commonly after hysterectomy and may result from retained secretions or inadequate cleansing of the vaginal apex. Nonetheless, these infections may drain spontaneously or require antibiotics and daily gentle digital examination of the vagina. Prevention of this complication requires thorough cleansing of the entire vagina prior to surgery and during closure of the cuff and avoidance of dead space, where fluid and bacteria may collect. Retropubic infections may occur from similar mechanisms and may require drainage by interventional radiology or rarely open drainage and antibiotic irrigation and insertion of a Penrose of other drains type to ensure that the collection resolves. Suprapubic infections and infected sutures may occur if bacteria become entrapped and are transferred to the suprapubic incision. Again, copious antiseptic irrigation helps to avoid this problem, as do preoperative antibiotics. If this area becomes infected, one must judge whether the infection requires open drainage or simply antibiotics. Additionally, if the sutures are painful, they may be infected and can be removed suprapubically. Often, there may be sufficient scar formation inferiorly to provide adequate bladder neck support despite removal of the suspending sutures. Erosion from suture or synthetic material in the vagina leads to vaginal drainage, bleeding, and pain, and these materials usually must be removed (Figs. 9.3 and 9.4).

UTIs may cause an exacerbation of incontinence symptoms after the catheters are removed, so one must always realize that an infection may be present in the setting of postoperative incontinence or urge symptoms. Postoperative antibiotics are not required but the avoidance of long-term urethral Foley catheters help to reduce the incidence of UTIs. We try to use suprapubic catheters in the postoperative period, as they lessen the likelihood of bacterial contamination of the urinary tract. Rarely, the cystitis may result in a pyelonephritis, requiring hospitalization and intravenous antibiotics.

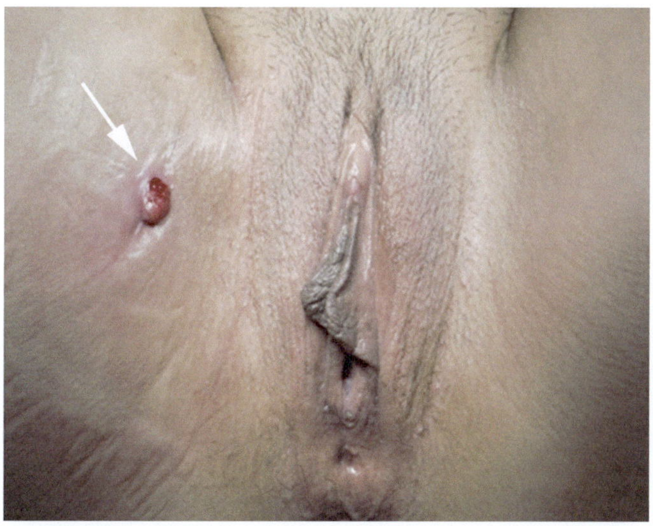

Fig. 9.3 Chronic sinus tract and recurrent abscess of the inner thigh after an obturator sling. The sling was removed by a combined groin and vaginal approach, correcting the problem

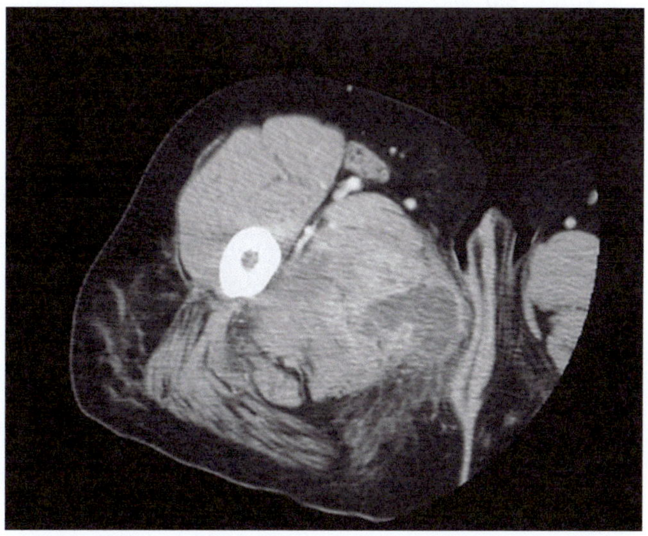

Fig. 9.4 CT scan of a patient admitted with high fever, pain, and inability to walk after an obturator sling. The scan showed diffuse inflammatory changes and a pelvic abscess. The collection was drained and the mesh was removed after resolution of the infection

9.3 Bladder Injury (Perforation)

Injuries to the bladder may occur during dissection of the vaginal wall off of the underlying perivesical fascia or during suture or trocar passage in patients with slings or cystocele repairs. The urethral Foley allows palpation of the urethra and bladder neck. The catheters are plugged during surgery, so if bladder entry occurs, one may notice urine extravasating into the operative field. Any blood in the urine should be considered suspicious of bladder or urethral injury. In the course of dissecting tissue flaps of vaginal wall off of the perivesical fascia, one must stay very superficial in the dissection on the side of the wall in order to prevent bladder entry. Another area in which bladder injury may occur is during entry into the retropubic space. If the retropubic space is entered, using curved Mayo scissors and keeping them pointed directly superior and parallel to the urethra at the level of the distal urethra should prevent bladder injury.

Bladder perforations are not rare when blind passage of trocars is used. They may occur when using trocars to transfer mesh from the suprapubic area to the vagina (SPARC procedure) or from the vagina to the suprapubic area (TVT procedure). Cystoscopy is mandatory in these cases. Unless a large perforation occurred, the trocar can be reinserted lateral to the area of the perforation. When bladder entry is suspected, instillation of indigo carmine dye into the Foley catheter can be helpful in identifying the entry site and subsequently confirming the repair. Lack of recognition of an intraoperative bladder injury can lead to a vesicovaginal fistula (Figs. 9.5 and 9.6) or the presence of mesh in the bladder.

Suture perforation of the bladder may occur in the course of transvaginal surgery and incontinence procedures (Fig. 9.7). It may be easily identified with the use of intraoperative cystoscopy and should rarely be problematic. If one discovers a bladder entry, the sutures are simply removed. Other important steps in the prevention of bladder entry at this time include emptying the bladder of accumulated urine prior to retropubic space dissection and proper entry in the lateral fornix and not through the levator fascia laterally or too medially into the bladder.

If a bladder entry is encountered, a multilayer repair using absorbable sutures is recommended. The initial layer reapproximates the mucosal surface with fine absorbable sutures, and the outer layer (perivesical fascia) is closed with interrupted absorbable sutures. Cystoscopy is performed, and indigo carmine may be instilled through the catheter to ensure a watertight closure. If ureteric injury is contemplated, intravenous indigo carmine dye is administered and visualized cystoscopically from each ureteric orifice. Extensive bladder injury may require the use of a fibro-fatty labial flap (Martius flap) as an added layer of protection from future fistula formation. Finally, the vaginal epithelium is advanced over the repair in such a way that none of the suture lines are overlapping. Long-term catheter drainage is required for at least 1 week, and a voiding cystourethrogram should be performed to confirm healing and absence of extravasation.

Perforations unrecognized at the time of surgery can result in erosion of mesh into the bladder (Figs. 9.8, 9.9, and 9.10). Mesh is not migrating into the bladder. Mesh in the bladder is due to an unrecognized perforation at the time of surgery.

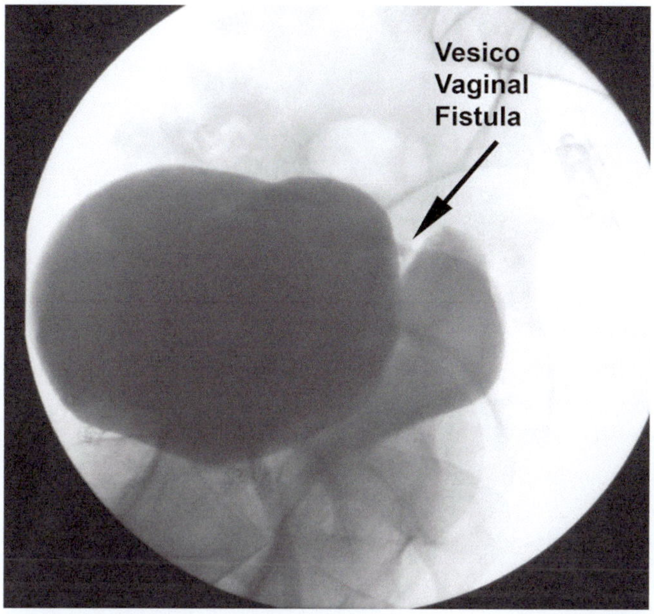

Fig. 9.5 Cystogram of a patient 1 month after cystocele repair with mesh. The study shows extravasation of contrast into the vagina through a vesicovaginal fistula

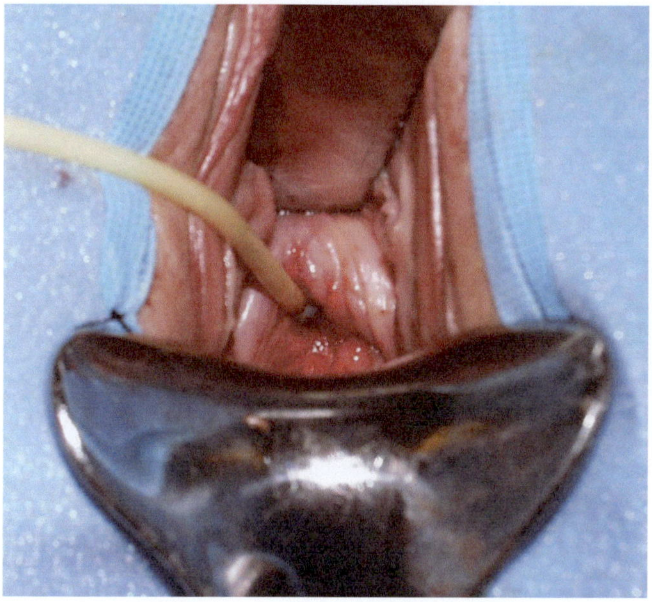

Fig. 9.6 Examination of the vaginal wall shows localized inflammatory changes, eroded mesh and the fistula of the anterior vaginal wall. A catheter was inserted in the fistula prior to surgery

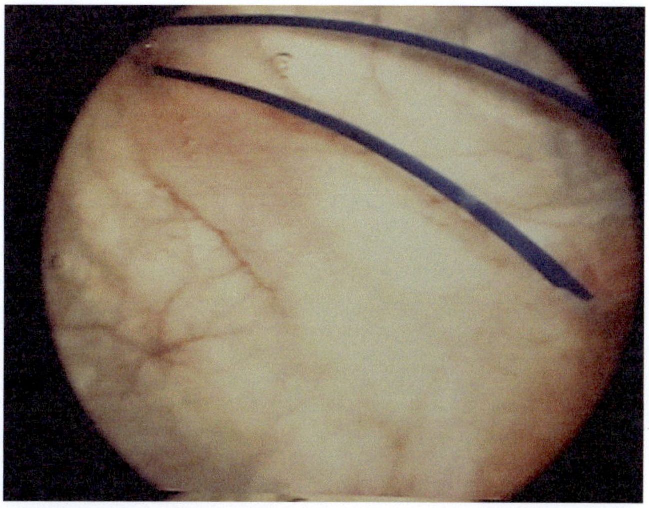

Fig. 9.7 Cystoscopy of a patient suffering from frequency, urgency, and urinary infections after placement of an autologous fascial sling supported by nonabsorbable sutures. The sutures have perforated the bladder. Endoscopic incision and excision of the sutures was performed

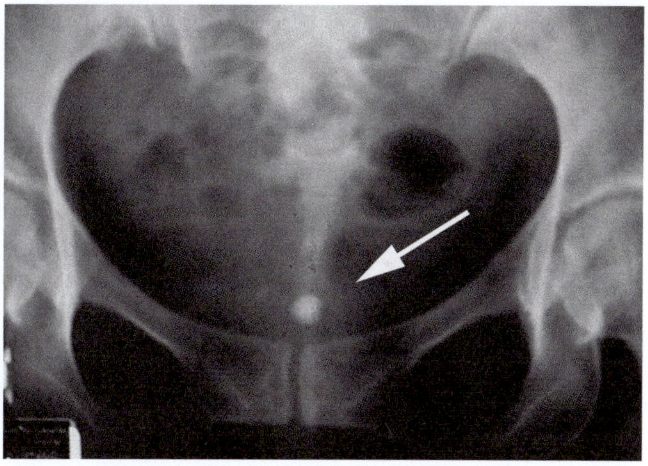

Fig. 9.8 This plain pelvic X-ray of a patient after a retropubic sling procedure shows a bladder calcification (*arrow*). Endoscopy confirms the presence of a fixed bladder stone. The mesh and the stone in the bladder were removed

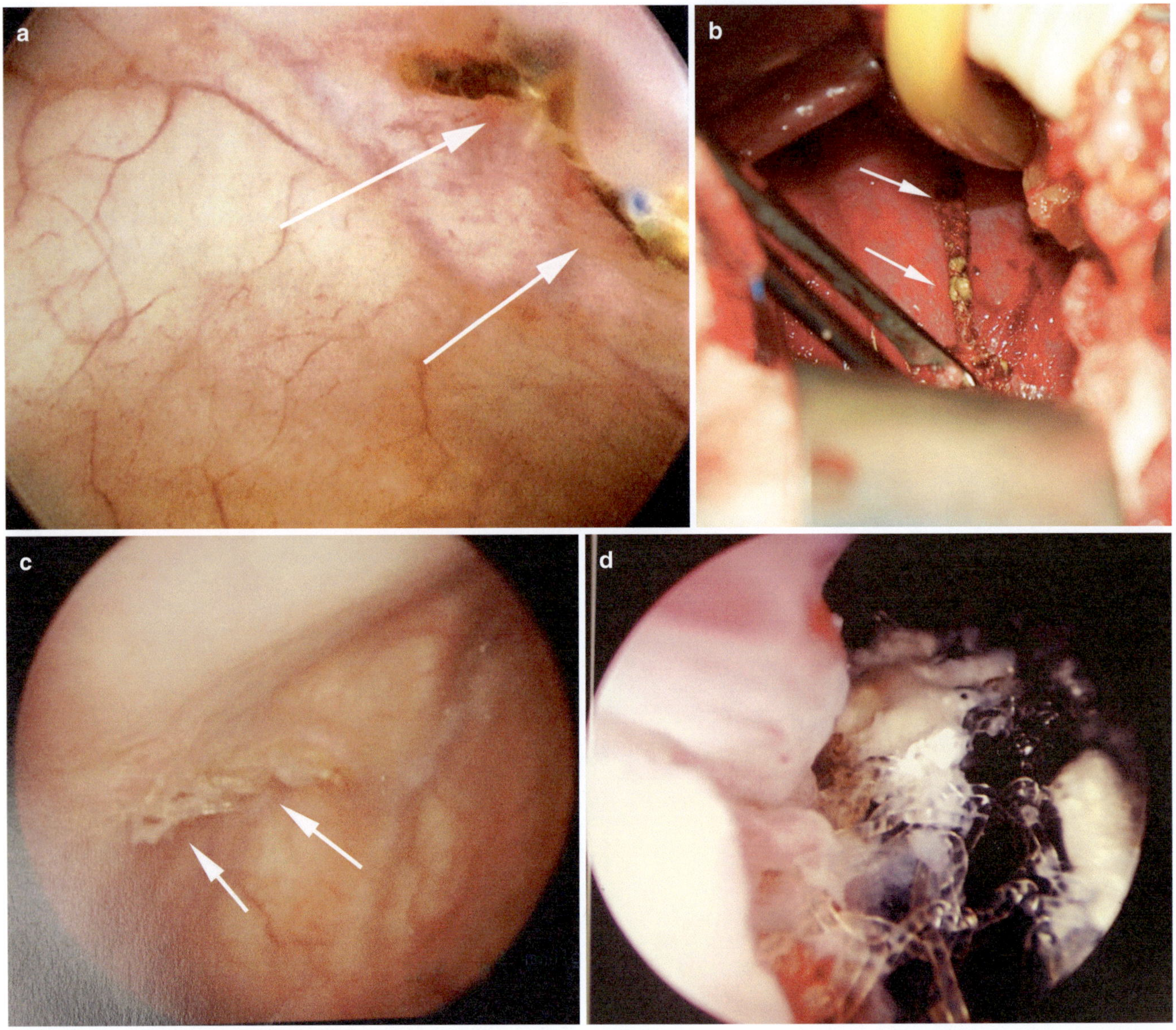

Fig. 9.9 (**a**) Cystoscopy of a patient with recurrent urinary infection and pelvic pain after placement of retropubic mesh. The mesh has eroded the urethra (*arrows*). It was totally removed transvaginally (including a partial cystectomy), and a Martius flap was used to cover the defect. (**b**) Open bladder at the time of exploration showing a segment of mesh eroded into the bladder wall. There are multiple stones on the mesh (*arrows*). All the mesh was removed by a transvaginal and open bladder removal. (**c**) Cystoscopy finding of mesh (*arrow*) on the left lateral bladder wall 3 months after a retropubic mesh insertion for urinary incontinence. (**d**) Cystoscopy of a patient with complications of a retropubic mesh insertion. The mesh has eroded the bladder wall, requiring open removal

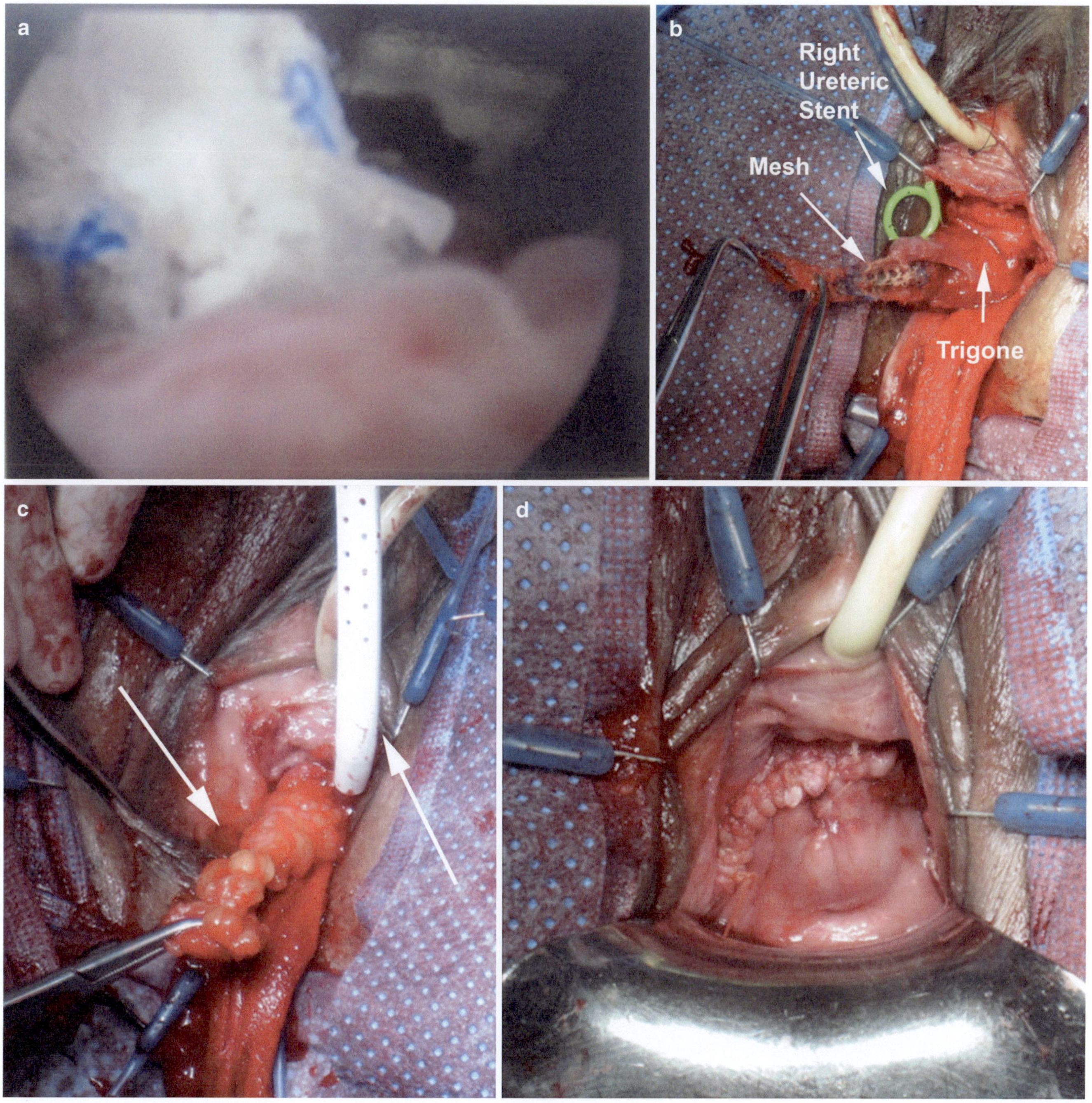

Fig. 9.10 (**a**) Cystoscopy of a patient with frequency, urgency, pain, hematuria, and recurrent urinary infection after insertion of an anterior vaginal wall mesh. The mesh traversed the bladder from the trigone to the right lateral bladder wall. (**b**) Exposure of the anterior vaginal wall is obtained and the mesh is dissected from the trigone. A ureteric stent was inserted in the right ureter. The bladder was opened and the mesh was excised from the bladder wall. (**c**) The bladder is closed in layers. An in situ Martius (*arrow*), a flap is created and rotated to cover the area of surgery. A retropubic flat drain is inseted (*arrow*). (**d**) A flap of the anterior vaginal wall is advanced to cover the area of the reconstruction. (**e**) Translabial ultrasound in a patient complaining of pelvic pain, urinary infections, and hematuria after insertion of a retropubic mesh. The *arrows* outline the periurethral mesh. (**f**) Cystoscopy revealed that the mesh has eroded the left half of the bladder wall. Transvaginal exploration of the left perivesical space is performed, the bladder is opened, and the eroded mesh is exposed (*arrow*). (**g**) Suprapubic exploration is performed, and the mesh is transferred through the retropubic space from the abdominal to the vaginal incision (*arrow*). A transvaginal partial cystectomy is performed because of the extent of the inflammatory changes and stones. The bladder is irrigated with diluted indigo carmine to ensure integrity of the closure. (**h**) The bladder wall is closed in two layers, and a Martius flap from the left labium is rotated to the left retropubic space

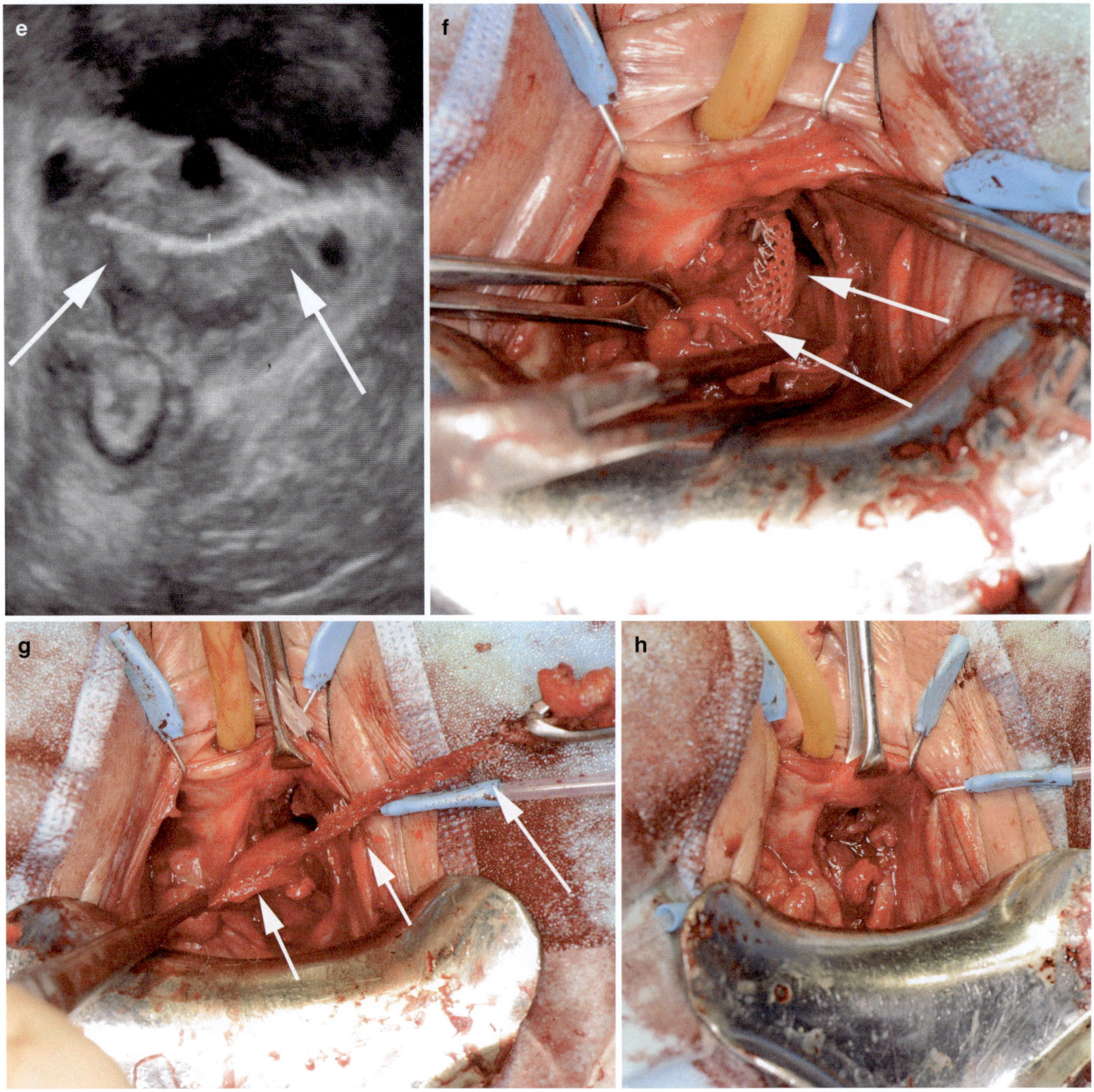

Fig. 9.10 (continued)

9.4 Urethral Injury

Intraoperative injuries to the urethra should be an infrequent occurrence because it is easily identifiable with a Foley catheter in place. One must stay lateral and superficial to the periurethral fascia in all dissections. Similar to avoiding bladder injury, if entry into the retropubic space is necessary, it should be done lateral to these structures. Too medial an entry can risk urethral injury, but this injury should still be infrequent. If injury does occur in the course of dissection, immediate repair should be undertaken in order to properly orient the anatomic layers and prevent postoperative fistula, stricture, or diverticula. Interrupted or running sutures of fine absorbable material should be used to close the mucosal defect. A separate, interrupted layer of absorbable suture should be placed to reapproximate the periurethral fascia in such a way as to avoid overlapping suture lines. The vaginal wall should be advanced over the repair, again avoiding overlapping suture lines. Large entries can also be closed with the assistance of a fibro-fatty Martius flap graft prior to epithelial closure.

Injury to the urethra may be discovered in the postoperative period. When a patient presents with persistent loss of urine despite restoration of normal anatomy and no objective demonstration of urethral incontinence, the surgeon should also consider the possibility of an iatrogenic ureterovaginal, vesicovaginal, or urethrovaginal fistula. This may occur as a result of an unrecognized intraoperative complication, postoperative infection, or ischemic necrosis of the pelvic tissues, especially in patients with poorly estrogenized tissues or previous radiotherapy. Voiding cystourethrogram is helpful in confirming this diagnosis.

Sling erosions are occurring with greater frequency with the increasing use of synthetic substances in vaginal sling surgery. One must be cognizant of the issues related to synthetics: the body may reject the tissue, the sling may become infected, or both. The symptoms, which may vary from patient to patient, are often pain with voiding, frequency, vaginal discharge, and dyspareunia.

We have abandoned the use of synthetic mesh in vaginal surgery. Although they provide a better immediate outcome than other procedures, long-term complications (even 5–10 years later) are a concern, as 5–10 % of patients will develop erosions, pelvic pain, and dyspareunia. Proper management once sling erosion is identified entails careful transvaginal excision of the sling, which may be infected. The sling may have eroded into the urethral wall, so optimal repair may require urethral reconstruction with or without interposition of flaps (Figs. 9.11, 9.12, 9.13, and 9.14).

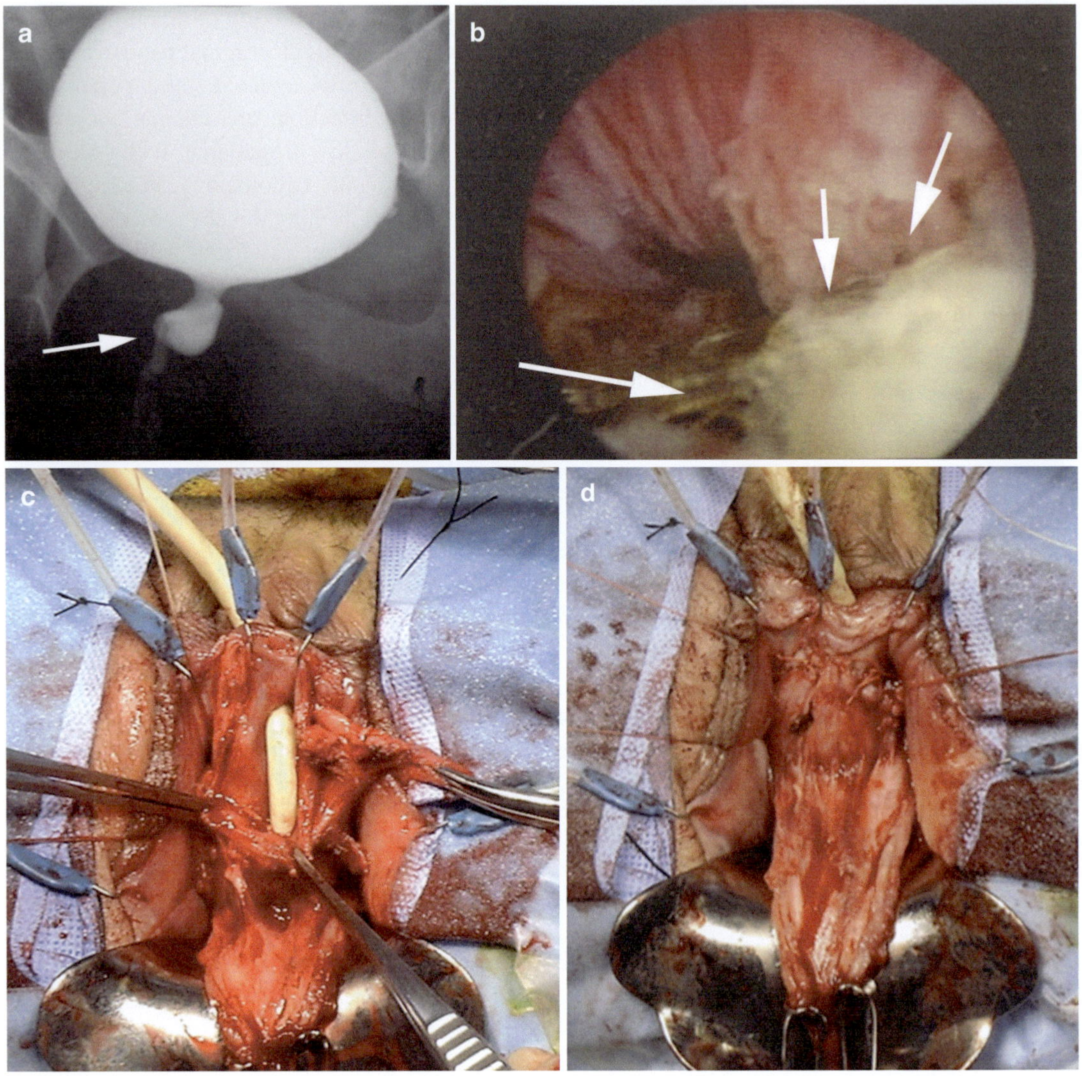

Fig. 9.11 (**a**) Voiding cystogram of a patient after an obturator mesh insertion. The patient complains of obstructive symptoms, pain, and urinary infections. The study shows deformity and narrowing of the midurethra (*arrow*). (**b**) Cystoscopy of the patient, showing urethral erosion due to mesh (*arrows*). (**c**) An anterior vaginal wall flap was created. The periurethral fascia is opened horizontally and the urethral wall is opened. (**d**) The mesh is isolated and totally excised. The urethral wall was reconstructed, and the periurethral fascia was approximated horizontally. A Martius flap was rotated to cover the defect and the vaginal wall advanced to cover the area of reconstruction

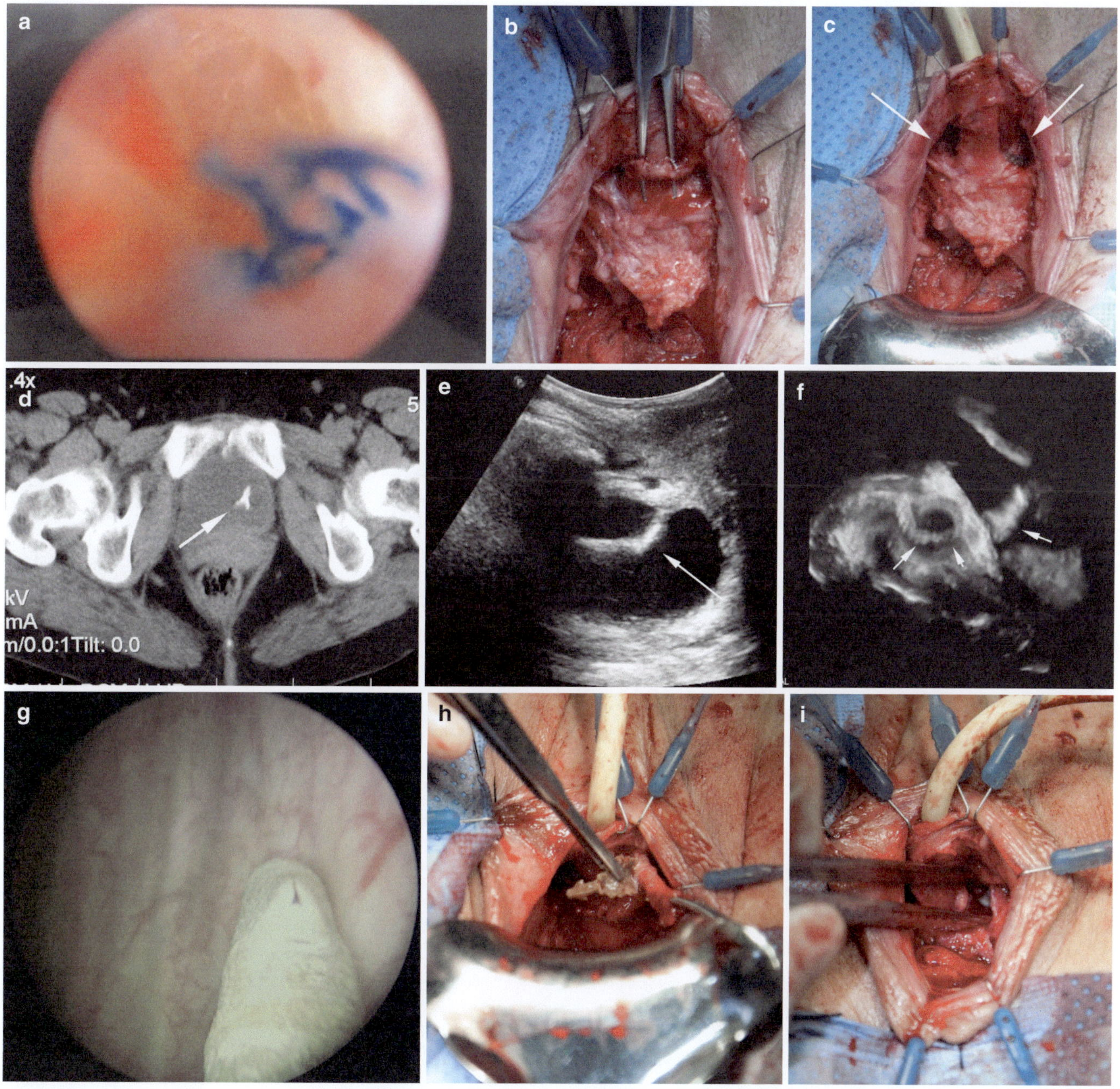

Fig. 9.12 (**a**) Cystoscopy of a patient with pain, infection, and dyspareunia after a retropubic sling. The mesh is seen to be eroded at the bladder neck. (**b**) The anterior vaginal wall was exposed. The mesh is dissected from the periurethral fascia. (**c**) The retropubic space was entered and the mesh removed from the urethral wall. All the mesh was removed by vaginal and suprapubic exploration. The two areas of erosion are closed in layers, and a Martius flap was used to cover the area of reconstruction. Arrows indicate the area of urethral erosion at each side of the urethra. (**d**) Plain pelvic X-ray of a patient with recurrent urinary tract infection 1 year after the insertion of a MiniArcTM Single-Incision Sling (AMS, Minnetonka, MN). A triangular calcification (*arrow*) represents the mesh anchor in the bladder. (**e**) Sagittal cuts of translabial ultrasound show mesh (*arrow*) in the bladder. (**f**) Tridimensional reconstruction of the translabial ultrasound shows the penetration of the mesh in the bladder neck area (*arrow*). (**g**) Cystoscopy showing the end segment of the mesh sling in the bladder lumen. The mesh did not migrate; rather, it was not recognized at the time of surgery. (**h**) The sling is removed from the bladder neck after removal of the right side of the mesh from the obturator fossa on the right. The mesh anchor removed from the bladder is held by a forceps. (**i**) After the removal of the mesh, the fistula at the bladder neck is seen. (**j**) The fistula is closed in layers. Irrigation of the bladder with diluted indigo carmine shows no extravasations. (**k**) A Martius flap from the left labium is prepared and will be rotated and transferred to the vaginal area. (**l**) The Martius flap has been transferred and covers the area of reconstruction. (**m**) The flap of the anterior vaginal wall created at the time of the initial incision is advanced distally to cover the area of the Martius flap

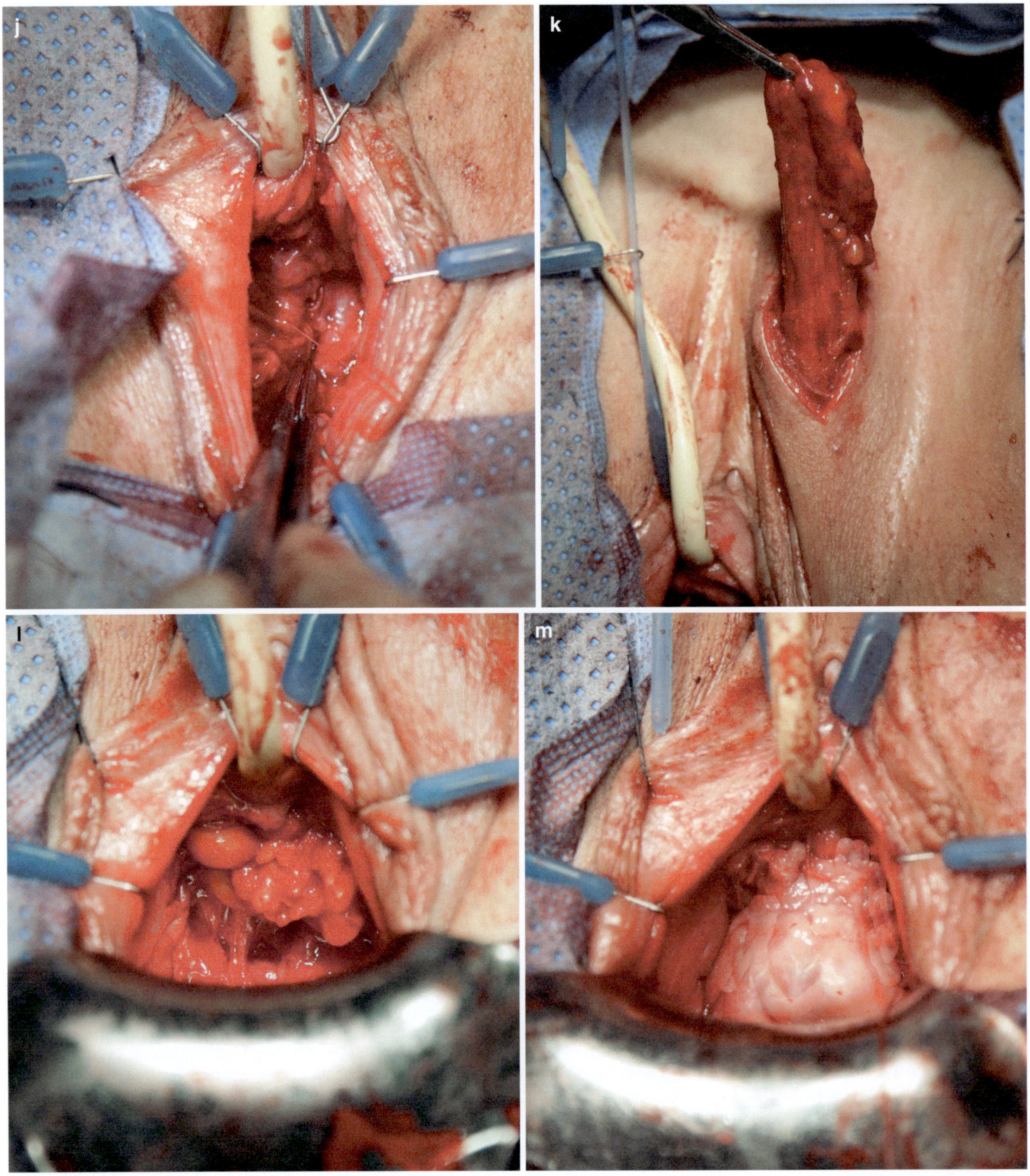

Fig. 9.12 (continued)

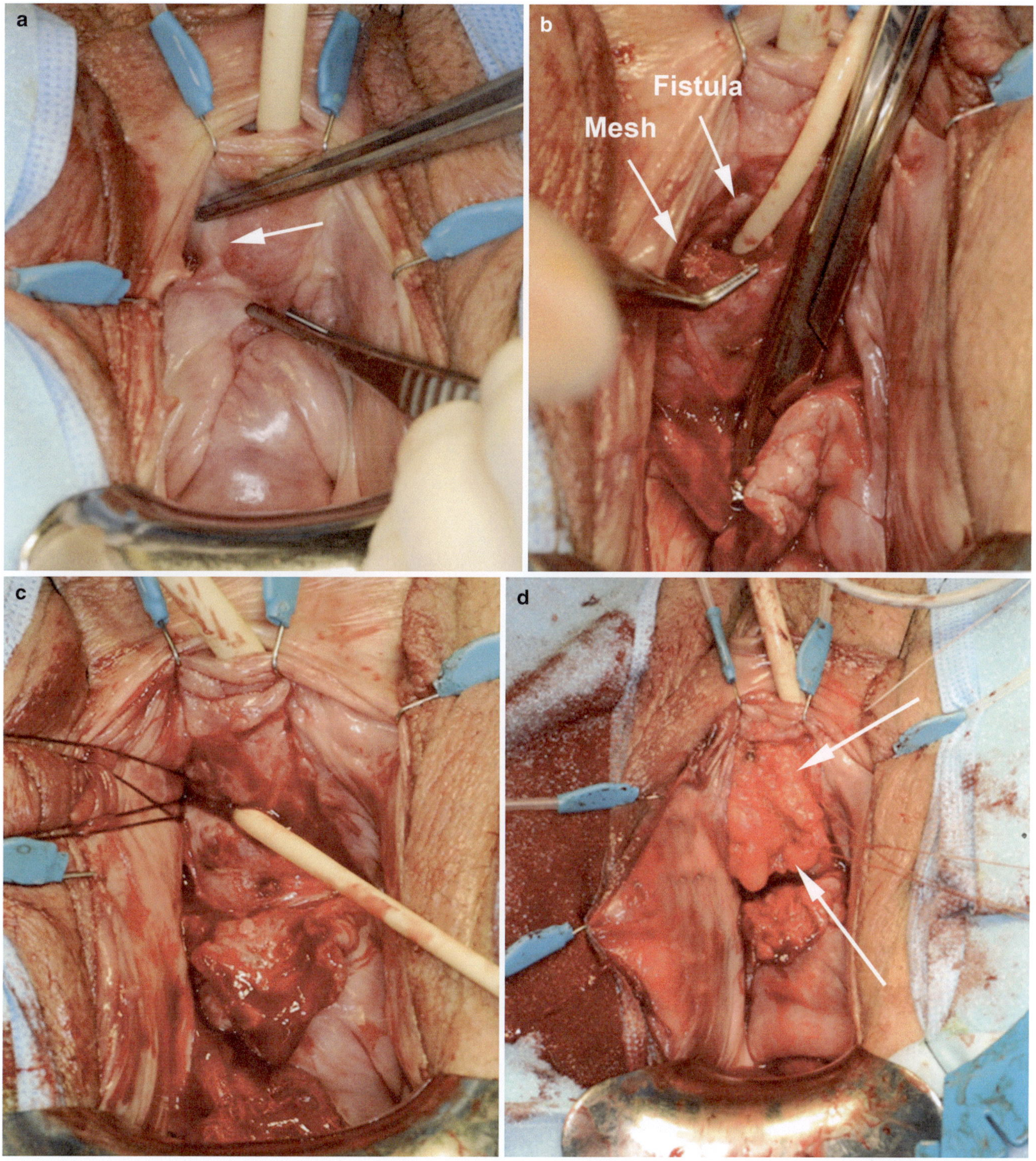

Fig. 9.13 (**a**) In a patient with constant and stress leakage of urine after a retropubic sling, a bladder neck fistula is seen, with mesh exposure on the margin of the fistula (*arrow*). (**b**) A superior and inferior flap of the vaginal wall was developed to isolate the fistula. A Foley catheter is inserted into the tract to facilitate the dissection. All the mesh is removed. (**c**) The fistulous tract is closed in two layers. The first layer includes the whole fistulous tract, and the second layer includes the periurethral fascia to cover the area of the closure. The bladder is irrigated with diluted indigo carmine solution to confirm closure of the fistula. (**d**) An in situ Martius flap (*arrow*) is brought from the right labium to cover the area of reconstruction. The anterior vaginal flap will be advanced distally, providing new vaginal tissue covering the repair. *Arrow* indicates the Martius flap covering the area of the reconstruction

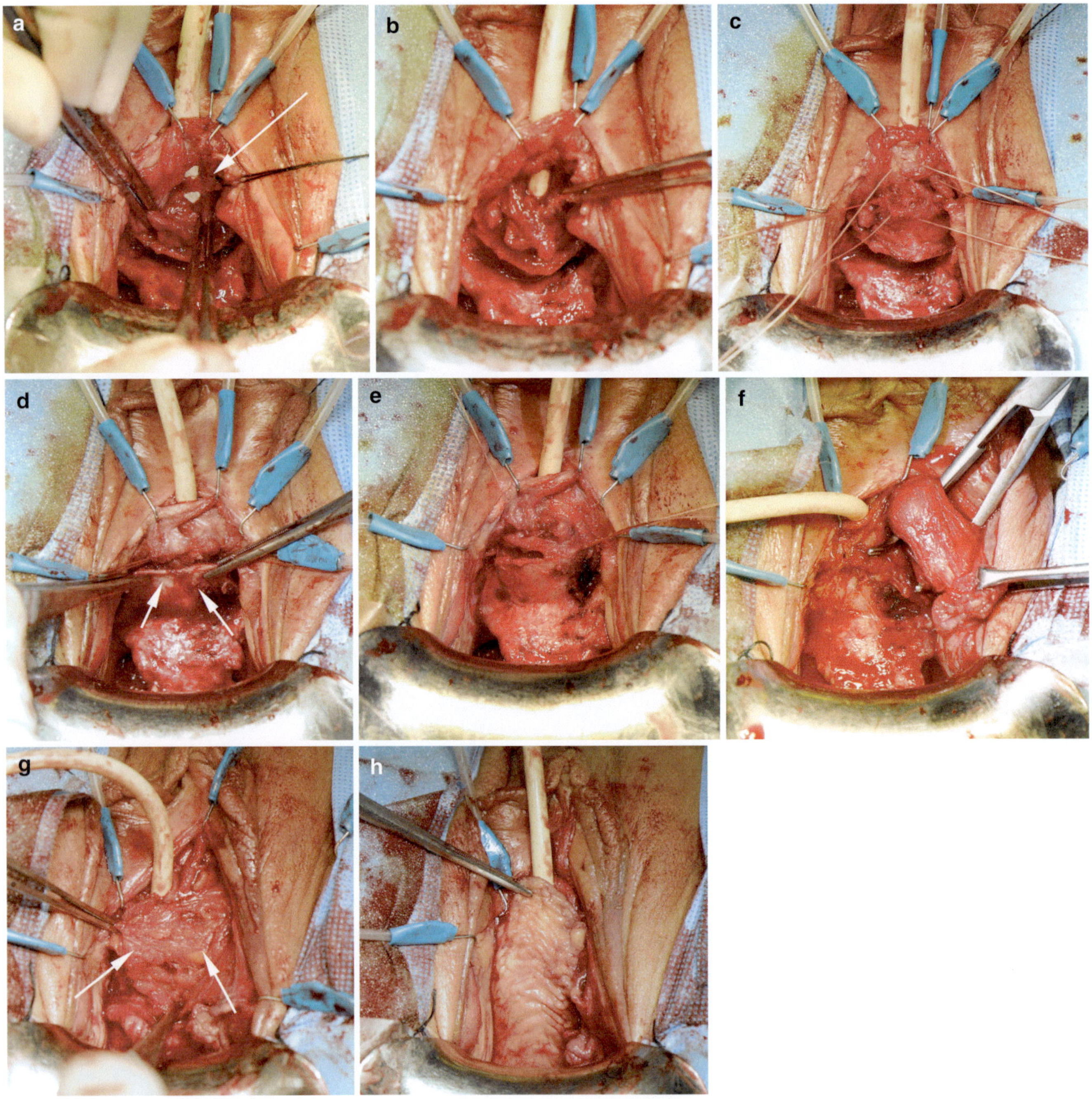

Fig. 9.14 (**a**) Surgical findings in a patient with urinary retention after a retropubic sling. Exploration of the anterior vaginal wall was performed. An inverted U flap was developed. A transverse incision of the periurethral fascia was performed and superior and inferior flaps are developed. The mesh has perforated the urethra (*arrow*). (**b**) The mesh has been removed after a vaginal and suprapubic exploration. A large urethral defect is seen. (**c**) An end-to-end anastomosis of the urethra is performed after mobilization of the margins of the urethra. (**d**) The periurethral fascia (*arrows*) is advanced distally to cover the area of the reconstruction. (**e**) Interrupted figure-of-eight sutures are applied to the periurethral fascia from the inferior to the distal margins, covering the urethral repair. (**f**) An in situ Martius flap of the left labium is developed. (**g**) The Martius flap (*arrows*) has been mobilized and rotated to cover the urethra. (**h**) The anterior vaginal flap is advanced distally to cover the Martius flap, providing new vaginal tissue to cover the area of reconstruction

9.5 Ureteric Injury

Ureteric injuries occur in 0.3–3 % of patients undergoing gynecologic surgery. Over two thirds of these injuries occur during the course of transabdominal surgery, however, so ureteric complications of transvaginal surgery are fortunately rare. The chances of ureteric injury increase if the patient has had previous pelvic surgery or a history of fibrosis and adhesions after transabdominal surgery. Proper preoperative planning may allow the placement of a stent if there is a concern about possible injury.

Ureteric injuries in the course of transvaginal surgery can be prevented in several ways. During sling surgery and entry into the retropubic space, as previously outlined, ensuring that entry is distal to the level of the bladder neck and not more proximal on the bladder reduces the chances of ureteric injury. More commonly, injury occurs during the placement of sutures or mesh over the perivesical fascia during cystocele repairs. One can avoid the ureters by careful and superficial placement of the sutures after reducing the trigone and elevating the base of the bladder with gentle retraction. Deep dissection of the vaginal wall during placement of anterior mesh may perforate the bladder but affect the ureters. Placement of mesh over a very thin perivesical fascia may lead to late erosions and ureteric obstruction. Intravenous administration of indigo carmine dye ensures patency of the ureters if dye is seen effluxing from the orifice; seeing blood or a lack of dye efflux should alert one to the possibility of ureteric injury.

The usual management is repositioning of the sutures and repeated cystoscopic examination. If the injury is detected late (i.e., postoperatively), proper drainage is achieved via placement of an endoscopic stent or percutaneous nephrostomy tube. If the ureter fails to resume patency with these measures, operative correction with a ureteric reimplant is undertaken after a prudent period of observation (Figs. 9.15 and 9.16).

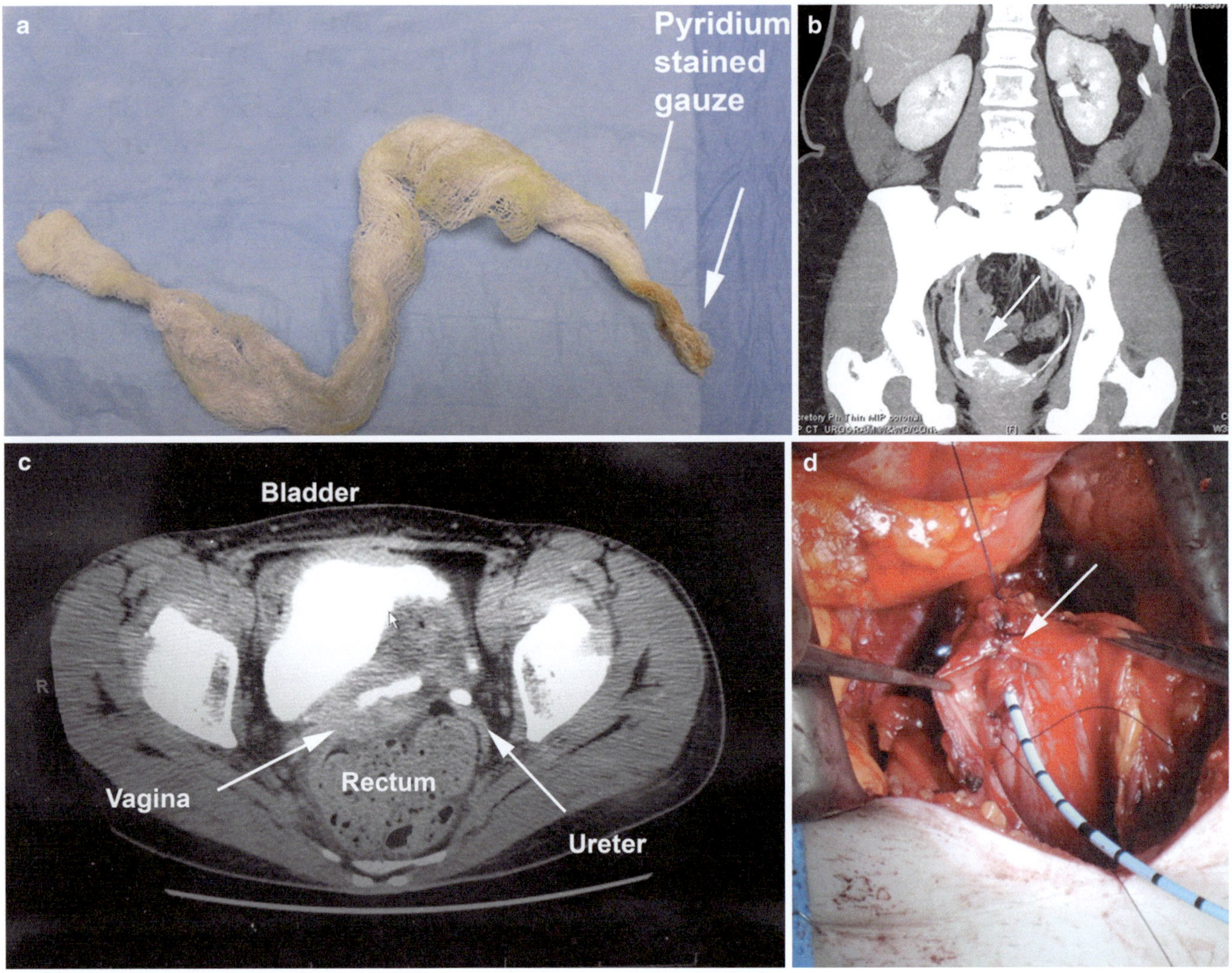

Fig. 9.15 (**a**) A patient presents with low-grade constant leakage of urine from the vagina after a vaginal hysterectomy and cystocele repair. There is no stress incontinence on examination. The patient was given phenazopyridine (Pyridium) for 24 h prior to the examination. When the bladder was filled with diluted indigo carmine, no blue dye was seen on a pad test, but the gauze was stained with orange dye at the proximal part (*arrow*). The cystoscopy was normal. (**b**) A CT urogram reveals normal, bilateral functioning kidneys without hydronephrosis. In patients with ureteric fistula without obstruction, the ureter involved is not hydronephrotic. *Arrow* indicates the area of the extravasation of contrast into the vaginal cuff. (**c**) Extravasation of contrast is seen in the vaginal cuff area, confirming the presence of a ureterovaginal fistula. (**d**) A Boari flap and a 4-cm tunnel were created to reimplant the ureter (*arrow*)

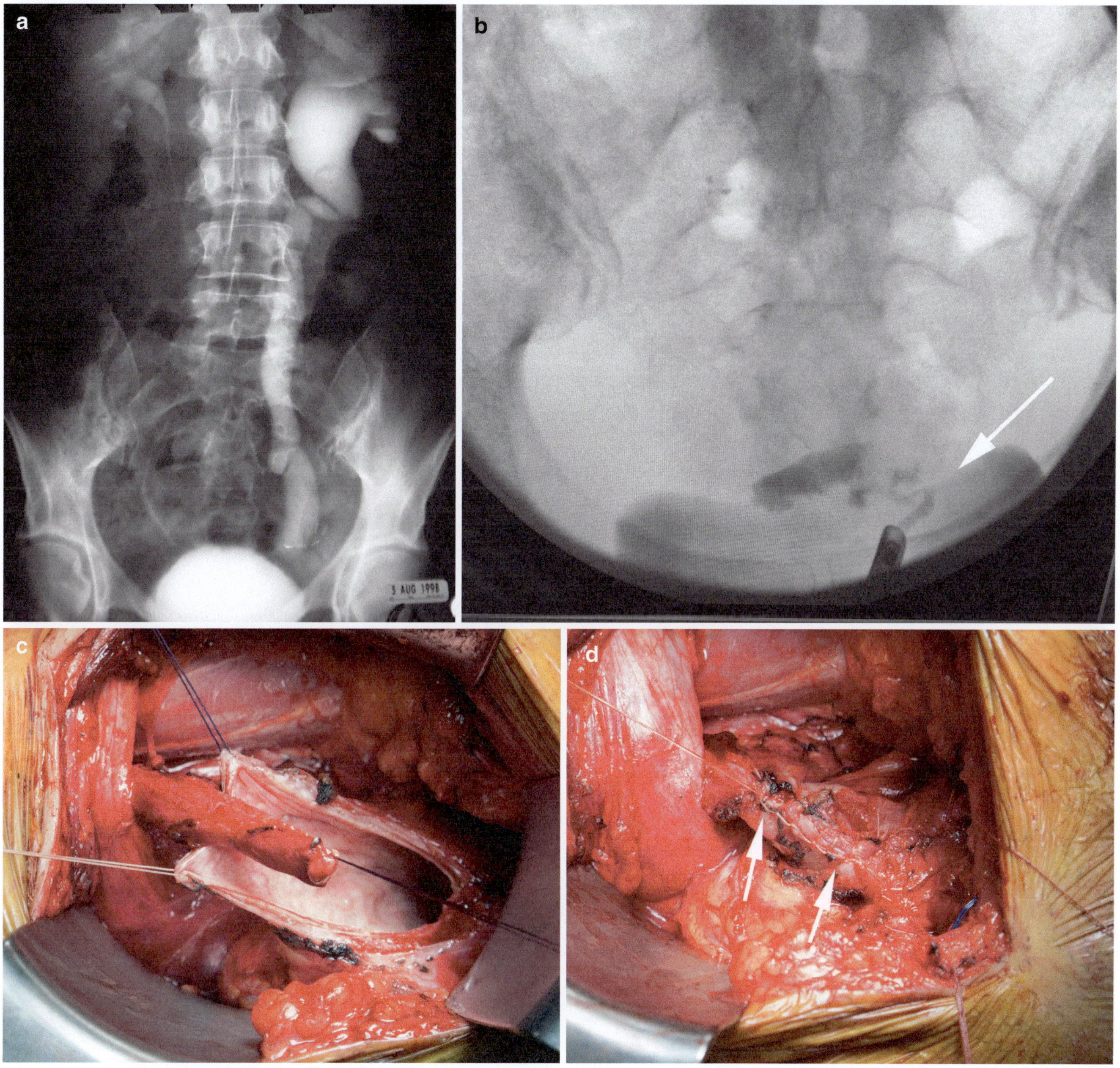

Fig. 9.16 (**a**) CT urogram of a patient complaining of left flank pain and urinary leakage per vagina after a vaginal hysterectomy and cystocele repair. There is severe hydronephrosis of the left kidney. The cystoscopy and the cystogram were normal. (**b**) Retrograde ureteric imaging was attempted. The left ureter was totally obstructed. Multiple attempts to pass a stent or guide wire were not successful. The diagnosis was made of left ureteric obstruction (*arrow*) and ureteric fistula. (**c**) A Boari flap and a stented left ureteric reimplantation were performed. (**d**) The Boari flap is made into a tube (*arrow*) and the bladder is closed. A suprapubic and urethral catheter will drain the bladder for 3 weeks

9.6 Bowel and Rectal Injury

Rectal and bowel injury should be an uncommon complication, but when injury does occur, it must be approached seriously (Figs. 9.17 and 9.18). Steps to avoid intraoperative bowel complications include good preoperative bowel preparation and proper intraoperative identification of the bowel to prevent its injury. In the course of rectocele repairs, one should stay very superficial in the dissection of the vaginal wall off of the prerectal fascia. Enterocele repairs also may be complicated by bowel injury, but careful packing of the intra-abdominal contents with a laparotomy pack will reduce the incidence of injury.

When bowel injury occurs, one must decide on the nature of the injury prior to deciding on therapy. In the event of a clean, small opening in the bowel, transvaginal closure may be performed in a multilayer, watertight fashion. Interposition of fatty tissue or other local tissue adjacent to the closure is wise, as it may help to prevent postoperative fistula formation. Large, extensive lacerations or those contaminated with stool may require colostomy fecal diversion after termination of the vaginal procedure. Rarely, the placement of suprapubic catheters may lead to a bowel fistula.

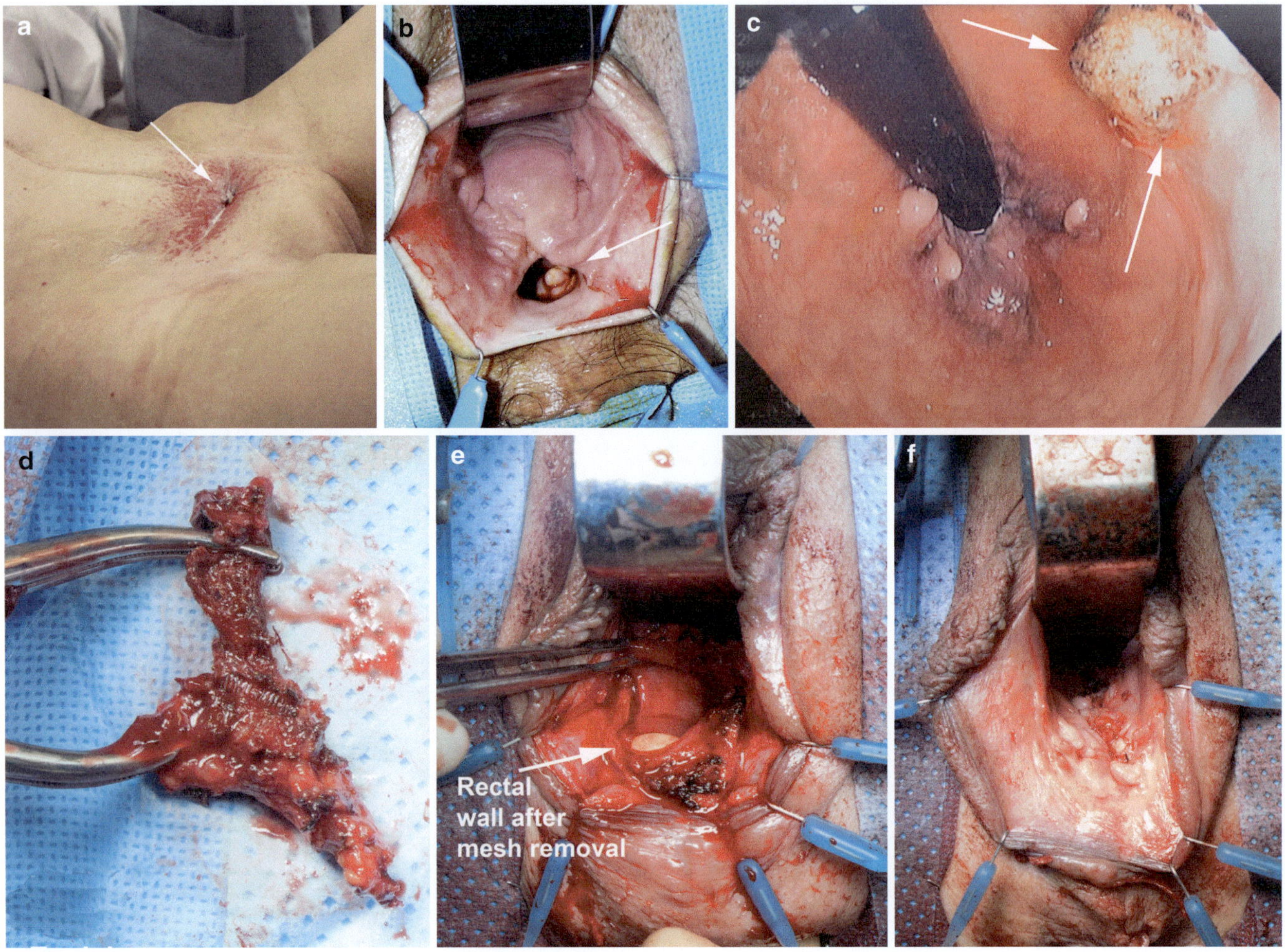

Fig. 9.17 (**a**) View of the lower abdomen of a patient suffering from an enterocutaneous fistula after placement of a retropubic sling (*arrow*). She had had prior abdominal surgeries, including hysterectomy. Abdominal exploration revealed that the mesh was placed in the middle of a small bowel segment. The mesh was removed and a small bowel resection was performed. (**b**) View of the posterior vaginal wall in a patient with a rectovaginal fistula (*arrow*) after posterior repair with mesh. The fistula was repaired by removing the mesh and repairing the rectal defect in layers, including a Martius flap. More details on the surgical technique to repair a rectovaginal fistula are described in Chap. 5. (**c**) Colonoscopy was performed on this patient suffering from pelvic pain and vaginal and rectal bleeding after the insertion of a posterior mesh. The mesh has traversed the left lateral wall and the lumen of the rectum (*arrow*), causing severe inflammatory changes (*arrows*) in the left posterior perirectal and vaginal areas. *Arrows* indicate the finding at the time of colonoscopy showing the eroded mesh. (**d**) Exploration of the posterior vaginal wall was performed, and the whole posterior mesh (including the rectal mesh) was removed. Shown is a segment of the mesh removed from the rectum. (**e**) The defect in the left lateral rectal wall is seen (*arrow*). A finger in the rectum demonstrates the defect. (**f**) The rectal wall and the posterior vaginal wall were repaired in layers. A loop colostomy was performed, owing to the extent of the defect and the inflammatory changes in the lateral posterior pelvis

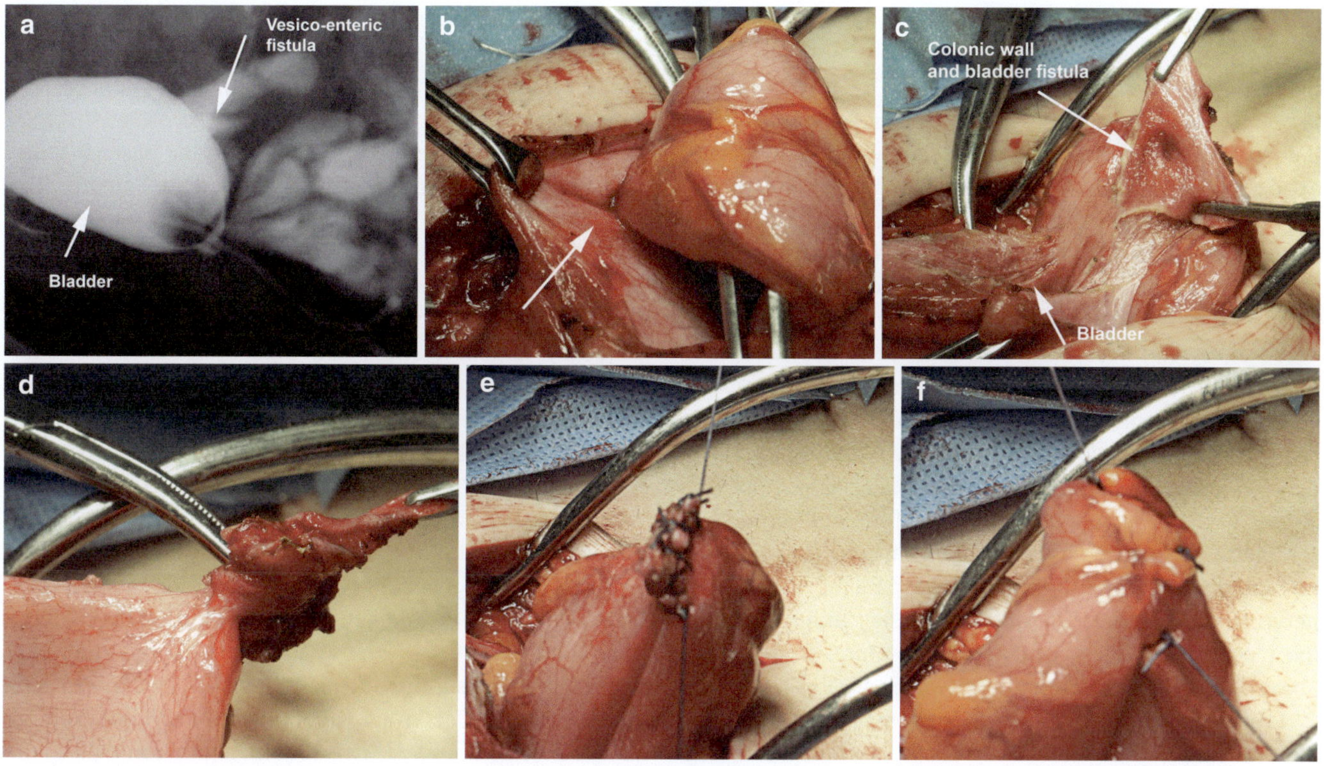

Fig. 9.18 (**a**) Lateral cystogram of a patient after a retropubic sling, with recurrent infection and stool matter in the urine. The patient had multiple prior abdominal surgeries. The cystogram shows a vesicoenteric fistula (*arrow*) with dye entering the colon. (**b**) Exploration of the abdomen shows the communication of the bowel to the bladder, where the mesh was found traversing the area (*arrow*). The mesh was removed entirely. (**c**) The bladder was opened and a circular segment of the bladder with the fistulous tract was excised and left on the colonic wall. (**d**) The bladder was closed in layers. The fistulous tract is seen over the colonic wall. No bowel resection was performed. (**e**) The fistulous tract is partially excised and was sutured in layers, without opening the colonic wall. (**f**) The serosa of the colon and the fatty tissue of the mesocolon are used to cover the area of reconstruction

9.7 Neurologic Injury

Sacrospinous fixation can be complicated by nerve injury, as the pudendal and sciatic nerve branches lies in proximity to the sacrospinous ligament. Clearly, one must maximize exposure with the use of Breisky–Navratil retractors and must palpate the ligament prior to suture placement. Additionally, the suture should be placed through the ligament without incorporating lateral tissue, to decrease the chance of nerve injury. Rarely, sciatic nerve or obturator nerve injury can occur with lateral or extensive retropubic dissection or placement of an obturator mesh.

More commonly, one sees entrapment of the ilioinguinal nerve branches that course immediately lateral to the pubic bone on either side. This entrapment can cause quite disabling, constant suprapubic pain. Therefore, in the course of retropubic procedures, if the transfer of the mesh is done too far laterally over the ilioinguinal nerve, pain may result from nerve entrapment. Ideally, one should stay more medial in the placement of mesh or suspension sutures immediately above the pubic bone, as opposed to laterally.

Proper patient positioning can help avoid complications of peroneal palsy or femoral neuropathy. Gentle positioning with the use of padded lithotomy props and the avoidance of excessive pressure or tension on the lower extremities can prevent problems. Recovery from these injuries is usually spontaneous but may take several weeks to months.

9.8 Pelvic Pain, Mesh Exposure or Extrusion

Pain after a pelvic surgical procedure is a normal occurrence, but pain that continues beyond the normal healing period requires full evaluation. Obstruction, infection, pelvic collection, or bleeding can be all sources of persistent pain. Mesh exposure or extrusion can be present. A physical examination and adequate imaging should diagnose the problem, and steps to correct it should be undertaken (Fig. 9.19).

With the extensive the use of mesh in the past 15 years, the incidence of vaginal exposure has increased greatly. The exposure can appear early after surgery or as late as 5–10 years afterward. The mesh exposure can be asymptomatic, but many times it is accompanied by pelvic pain, groin and suprapubic pain, hip pain, and dyspareunia. Urinary frequency, urgency, stress and urgency incontinence, and defecatory dysfunction can be present. The etiology of mesh exposure is unclear. Factors involved can be suture separation, chronic mesh infection, vaginal atrophy, and superficial placement of the mesh on the vaginal wall. As with other implants, it is possible that a biofilm is formed on the mesh, explaining the delayed appearance of symptoms.

Simple mesh exposure without urinary or bowel symptoms can be excised and new vaginal wall used to cover the area. When mesh exposure is accompanied by significant pelvic, groin, or suprapubic pain, however, it is our experience that a segmental removal of the mesh will not improve the symptoms. These patients require a total removal of the mesh. Retropubic mesh removal requires a vaginal exploration, division of the mesh into two segments, separation of the mesh from the periurethral tissues, and entrance into the retropubic space and dissection of the mesh free from the bladder, levator, and obturator muscles and the posterior aspect of the pubic bone. A combined suprapubic exploration is done to entirely remove the mesh. In patients with complications of obturator mesh, the mesh is dissected from the obturator fossa (the obturator internus, membrane, and externus). If the mesh is not a single incision mesh exploration of the mesh should be removed from the adductor fossa as well (gracilis, adductor longus, and brevis).

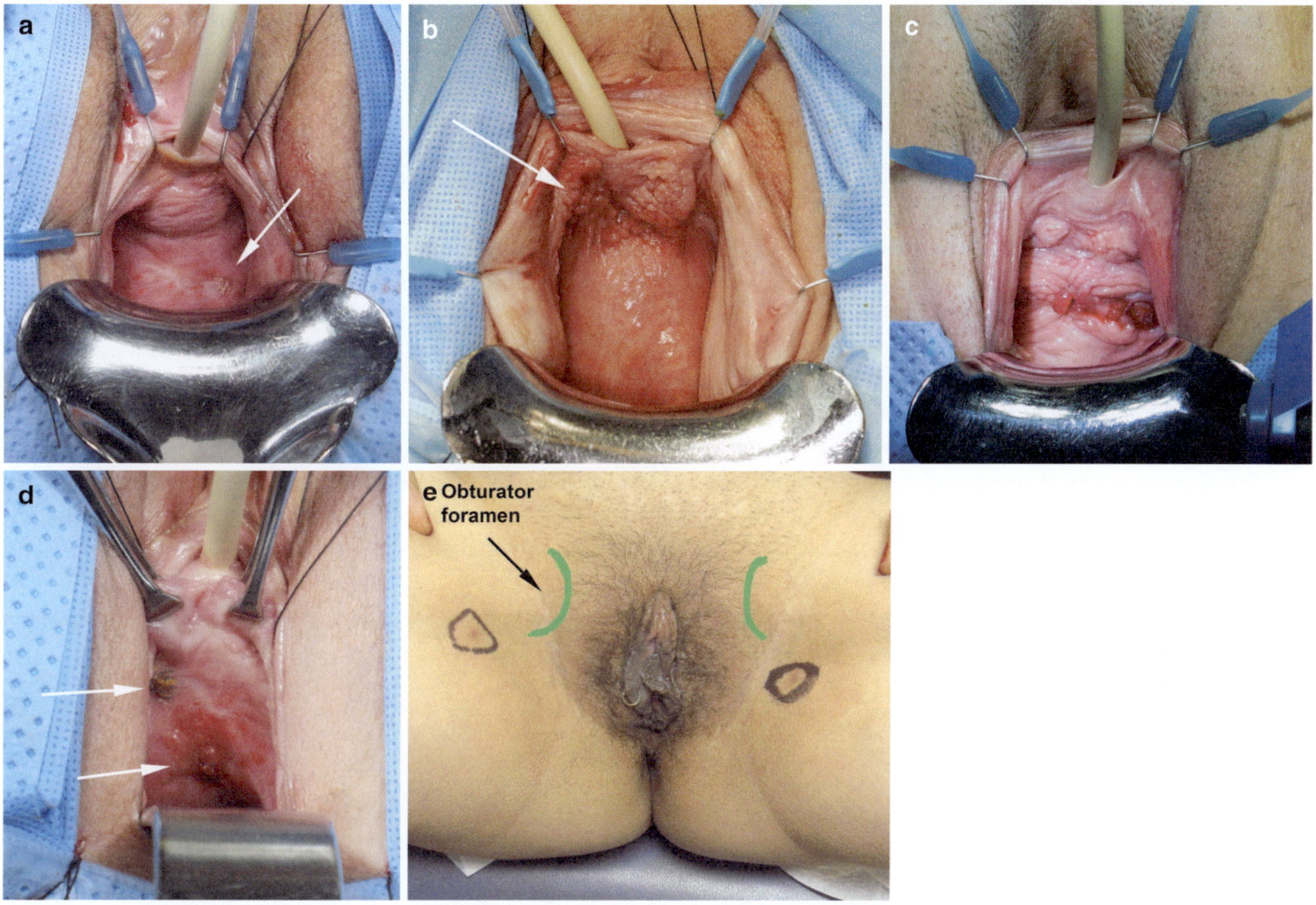

Fig. 9.19 (**a**) Anterior mesh exposure (*arrow*) after anterior mesh insertion for cystocele. The patient complained of dyspareunia but not pelvic pain, leg or groin pain, or urinary symptoms. A localized excision of the mesh was performed, with good outcome over 2 years. Estrogen cream was added to the treatment. (**b**) Anterior vaginal wall exposure of a patient complaining of pelvic pain, dyspareunia, hispareunia, groin and leg pain, and vaginal discharge after an obturator sling insertion. There is an erosion in the right distal vagina (*arrow*). The mesh was totally removed by exploration of the obturator and adductor fossa. (**c**) Erosion of the anterior vaginal wall after anterior mesh placement with arms extending to the sacrospinous ligament and paravesical space. The patient complained of back pain, tail bone pain, dyspareunia, vaginal bleeding, and leg pain. An extensive operation was required to remove the whole anterior mesh, with removal of the attachments to the obturator musculature and sacrospinous ligament area. (**d**) Extensive anterior vaginal wall erosion after anterior mesh placement for cystocele and vault prolapse. There is extensive infiltration and erosion of the anterior vaginal wall toward the cuff. The vaginal wall is atrophic and thin from prior explorations and attempted mesh removal. The whole anterior mesh, including the arms, was removed. A rotational flap of the vaginal cuff and posterior vaginal wall was required in order to cover the large anterior vaginal defect after the mesh removal. *Arrows* indicate areas of mesh erosion into the anterior vaginal wall. (**e**) This patient complained of significant groin, hip, and leg pain after obturator sling surgery for stress incontinence. The point of entrance of the trocars was found to be far lateral and inferior from the normal location next to the inner descending pubic rami. Removal of the mesh resulted in a cure of the pelvic pain

9.8.1 Removal of Pelvic Mesh: Indications and Preoperative Evaluation

Removal of mesh is indicated after insertion of a sling and anterior or posterior mesh if the patient complains of significant pelvic pain, suprapubic and groin pain, leg pain, obstructed urination or defecation, dyspareunia, vaginal drainage, or extensive vaginal wall erosion. Some patients also present with systemic effects.

The preoperative evaluation consists of a good medical history and a review (if available) of the prior operative report and any prior partial mesh removal. The anterior vaginal wall can be indurated by mesh (intra-epithelial infiltration), or an obvious exposure can be seen and palpated. A rectal examination will detect rectal involvement, found in patients with arms of mesh extending to the sacrospinous ligament. Urine examination and a check of post-void residuals are mandatory. In patients with obstructive symptoms, video urodynamics will help to assess the degree and location of the obstruction and its impact on bladder function. In patient with erosions of the urethra, a filling defect may be present. Cystoscopy is also mandatory to rule out urethral or bladder erosion, as the mesh can be found eroding the urethral wall or the lateral and anterior bladder wall. Stones are not uncommon around mesh.

Translabial ultrasound is the only means to visualize the mesh location, integrity, and proximity to the urethral wall in cases of prior partial removal (Fig. 9.20). Erosion of the mesh in the bladder will also be visualized. The test is done with sagittal, axial, and coronal cuts, as well as in the relax and strain maneuvers. The mesh can be found mobile or fixed. The anterior and posterior meshes are commonly found folded. Tridimensional reconstruction of the urethra and vaginal canal also can be performed.

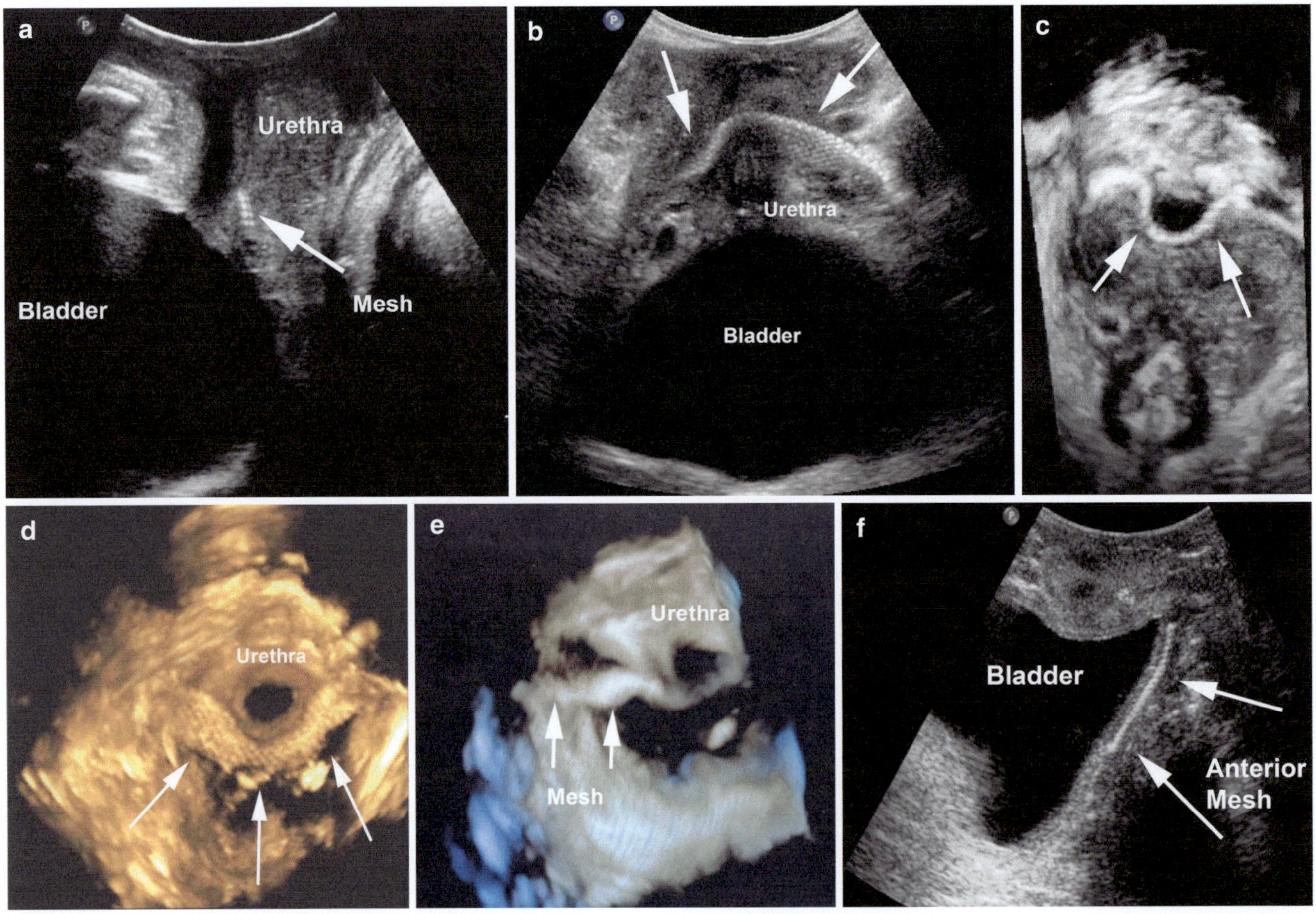

Fig. 9.20 (**a**) Sagittal ultrasound view at the midurethral area showing the bladder, the urethra, and the location of a retropubic mesh (*arrow*) located at the bladder neck. In more than 600 ultrasound studies, fewer than 50 % of midurethral slings have been found in the midurethral area. (**b**) Coronal cut through the urethra showing the mesh (*arrow*) at the midurethral area. (**c**) Axial image in a patient with urethral obstruction and burning after an obturator sling procedure. The mesh (*arrows*) is deep in the urethral wall but has not eroded into the lumen. (**d**) Tridimensional reconstruction of a sling (*arrows*) and its relation to the urethral wall. (**e**) Axial image of the anterior vaginal wall in a patient with complications of a urethral sling procedure. The patient had a partial mesh removal previously. The image reveals the residual mesh (*arrow*) in the right periurethral area. (**f**) Sagittal cuts showing a flat segment of mesh (*arrow*) covering the anterior bladder wall in a patient with vaginal wall erosion after anterior mesh insertion. (**g**) Sagittal image of a patient with vaginal wall erosion, pain, and urinary urgency after placement of anterior vaginal wall mesh. The mesh (*arrow*) is folded and shortened. (**h**) Sagittal cut of a patient with complications of posterior vaginal mesh. The extent of the mesh is seen anterior to the rectum (*arrow*)

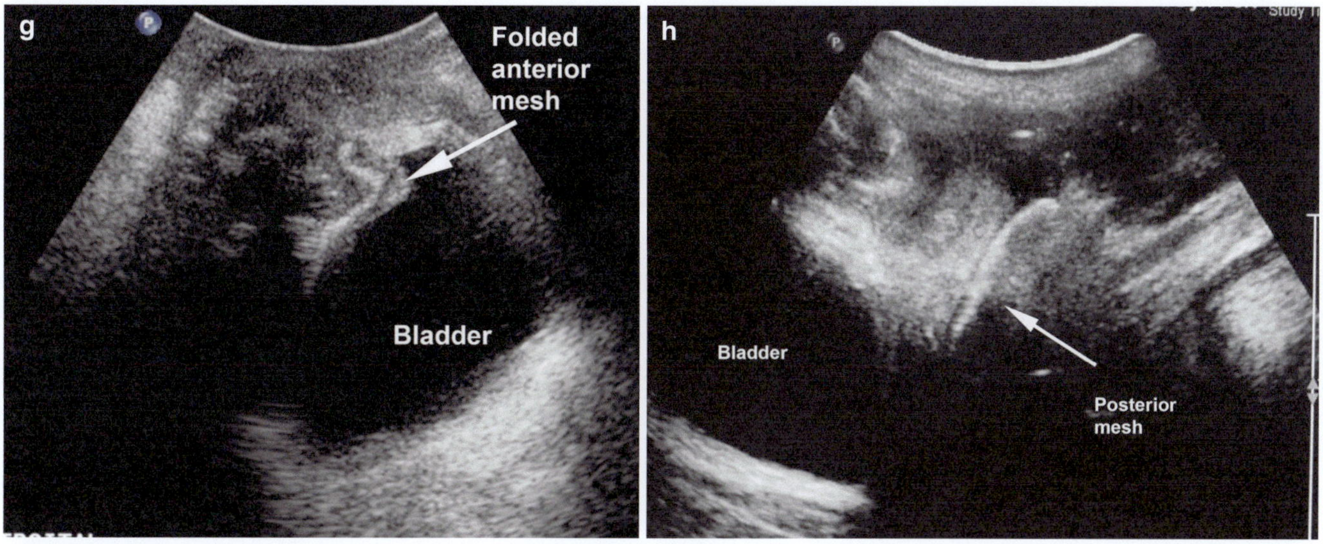

Fig. 9.20 (continued)

9.8.2 Removal of Suburethral Segment of Mesh

The patient shown in Fig. 9.21 presented with vaginal wall exposure, vaginal drainage, and dyspareunia after a retropubic sling. There was no pelvic, suprapubic, or leg pain and no incontinence. The patient decided to have only the suburethral segment of the mesh removed in order to preserve continence.

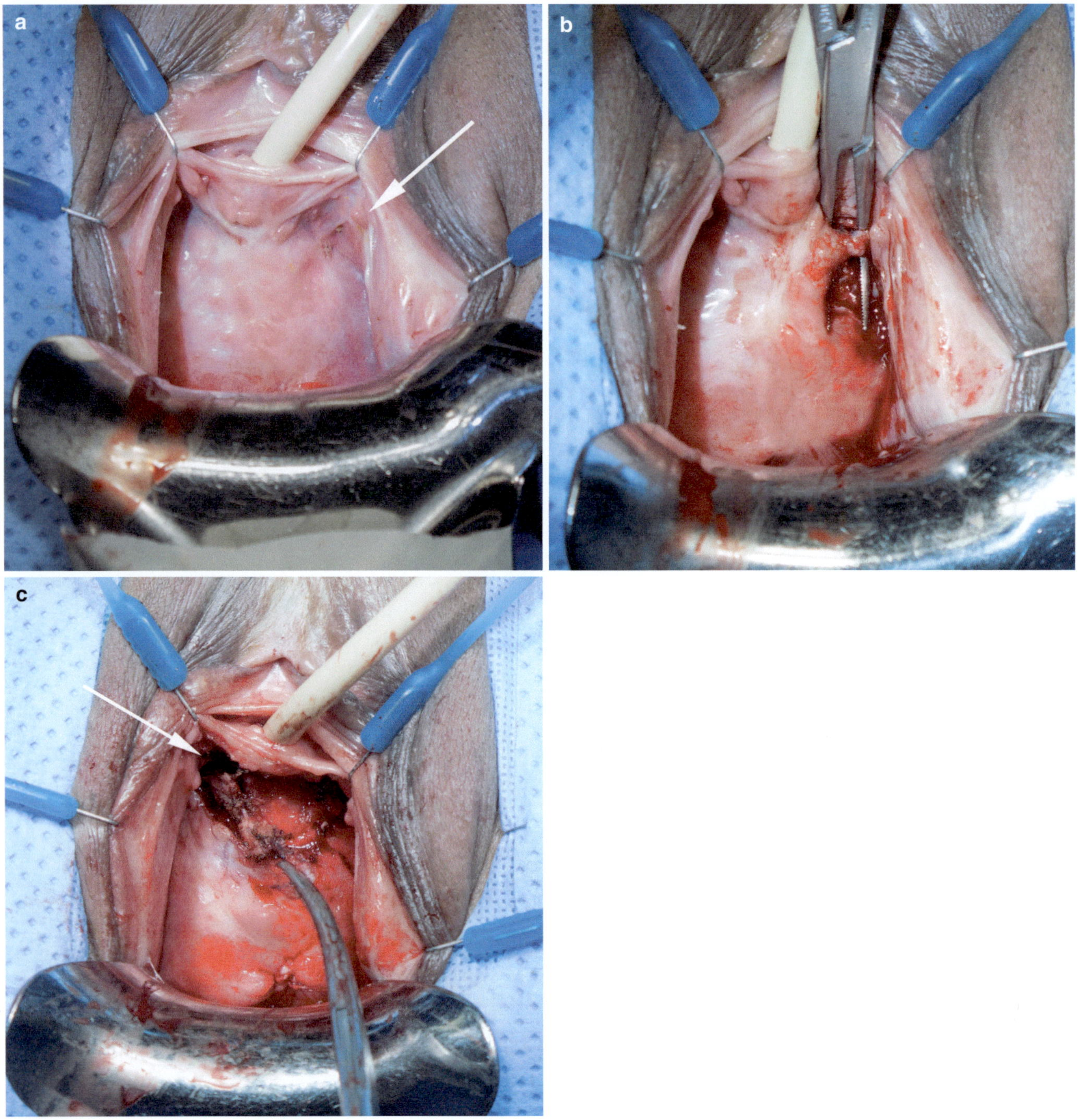

Fig. 9.21 (**a**) With exposure of the anterior vaginal wall, erosion is seen in the left distal vagina (*arrow*). (**b**) An oblique incision is made in the distal left vaginal wall and the mesh is isolated using a fine right-angle clamp. The mesh is transected as it enters the retropubic space. (**c**) A similar oblique incision has been made in the right side and a transverse incision of the anterior vaginal wall is performed, creating superior and inferior flaps. The mesh is dissected free from the urethra and is transected at the entrance to the retropubic space, in the lateral periurethral area

9.8.3 Removal of Retropubic Mesh

The patient in Fig. 9.22 suffers from suprapubic and groin pain, difficulty in emptying the bladder, and dyspareunia 2 years after a TVT mesh insertion. She was found to have a small exposure on the left distal vagina. She had prior revision of the mesh. The patient is placed in lithotomy position. The vagina and lower abdomen are prepared. A Foley catheter is inserted in the bladder.

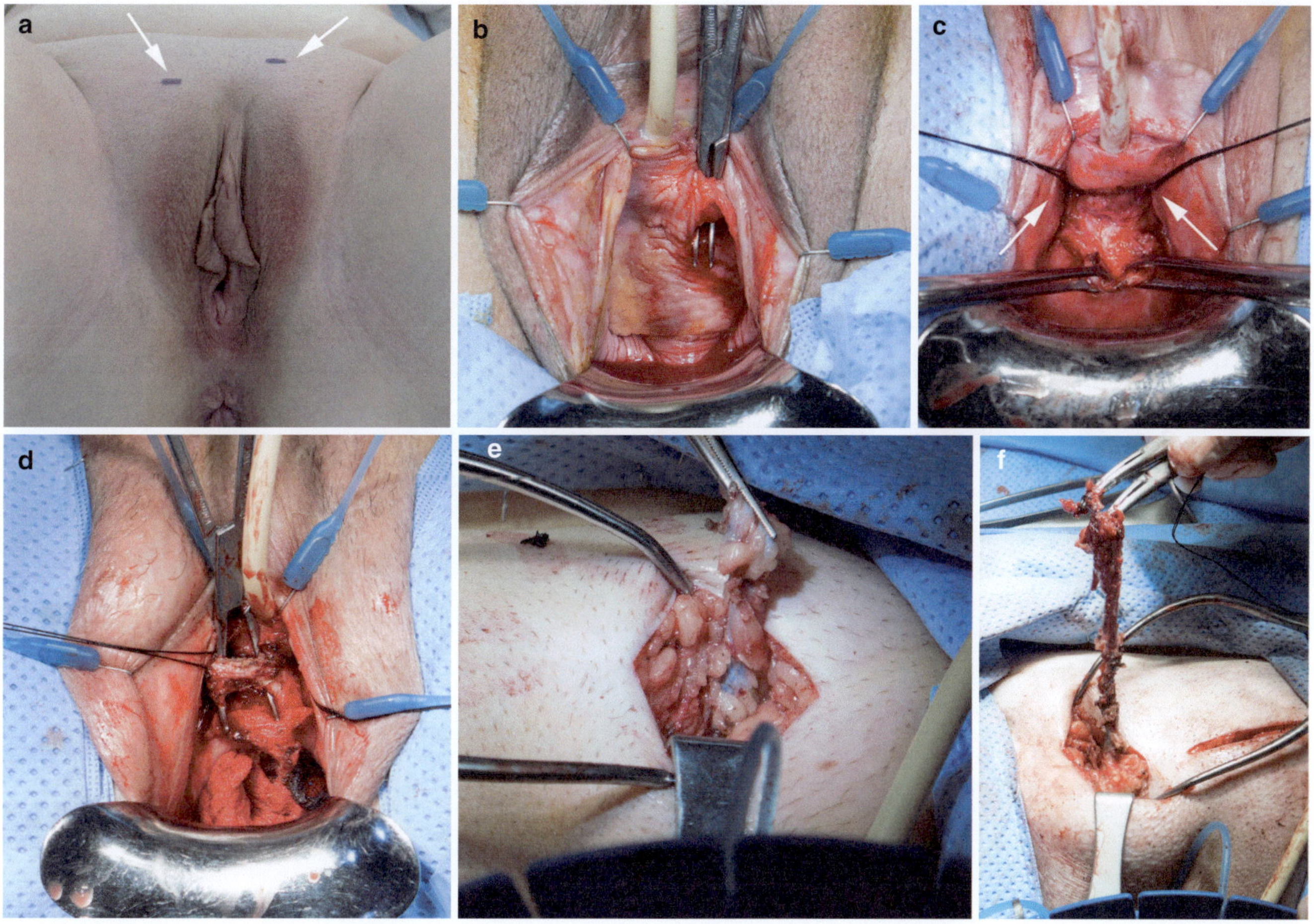

Fig. 9.22 (**a**) Prior to surgery the suprapubic area is examined and the exit points of the trocars are marked (*arrows*). More commonly, these points are not seen. The patient is placed in lithotomy position and the vagina and lower abdomen are prepared. A Foley catheter is inserted in the bladder. (**b**) Two oblique incisions are made in the distal vagina. The mesh is isolated over a silk suture. (**c**) A transverse incision is made in the anterior vaginal wall between the sutures, and a superior and an inferior flap are created to expose the mesh (*arrows*). The area of mesh erosion is excised with the creation of the flaps. (**d**) The mesh is dissected free from the periurethral tissues and will be divided in two. The silk tie at the end of the mesh is used to facilitate its dissection and removal. (**e**) The retropubic space is entered. The mesh is dissected free from the urethral wall, from the posterior aspect of the pubic bone, and from the bladder wall. Often the mesh is inserted more laterally, incorporating the levator musculature. The mesh may have been inserted flush over the posterior pubic bone, penetrating the obturator fascia. Under finger control in the vagina, the dissection is carried out up to the suprapubic area. The skin is incised under finger guidance and dissection is carried out down to the insertion of the fascia to the pubic bone. The fascia is open under finger guidance in the retropubic space for a distance of several centimeters. The end of the mesh is grasped with a clamp. Further dissection of the mesh from the surrounding subcutaneous tissue and fascia is performed. The mesh is also separated from the periosteum of the pubic bone. All dissection of the mesh is performed using a coagulation knife, because sharp dissection can easily transect the mesh. The mesh in the retropubic space must be totally free, so that a finger can be inserted through the anterior fascial incision into the retropubic space. (**f**) A finger is inserted through the fascial incision in the retropubic space. A large pedicle clamp is inserted from the vaginal incision, grasping the end of the mesh. Under finger control in the retropubic space, the mesh is transferred from the vagina to the suprapubic area. (**g**) Sometimes the mesh is firmly attached to the bladder wall and levator muscle next to the vaginal incision, making it difficult to transfer the mesh from the vagina to the suprapubic incision. In these cases, we use a large clamp to transfer the mesh from the suprapubic to the vaginal incision. Under direct vision, the attachments of the mesh to the levator and bladder wall are separated to free up the mesh. *Arrows* indicate the mesh segment as it is removed from the retropubic space; mesh is attached to the perivesical fascia and levator musculature. (**h**) The removed mesh is seen. The specimen must contain all the mesh; leaving fragments of mesh may result in continuation of the patient's symptoms and uncertainty about the outcome of the procedure

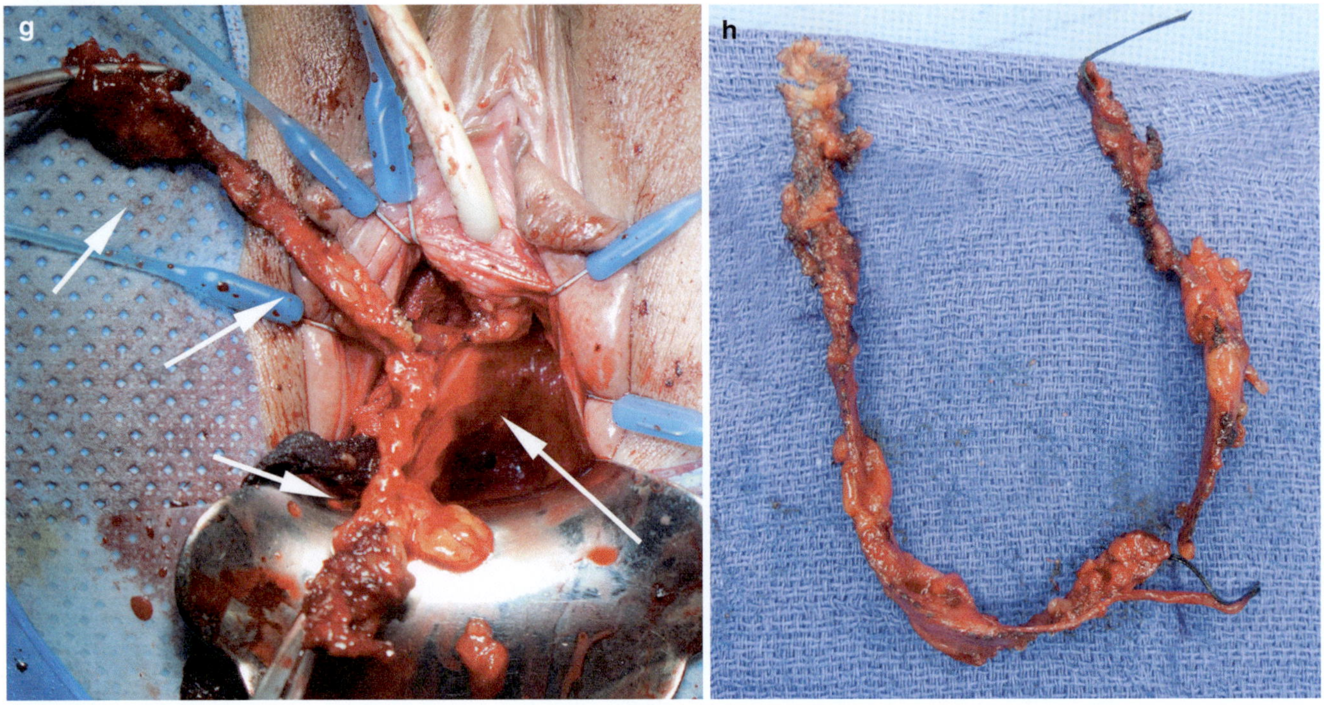

Fig. 9.22 (continued)

9.8.4 Removal of Obturator Sling

The patient in Fig. 9.23 had an obturator sling for stress incontinence. She presented with symptoms of urinary obstruction, vaginal and groin pain, and dyspareunia.

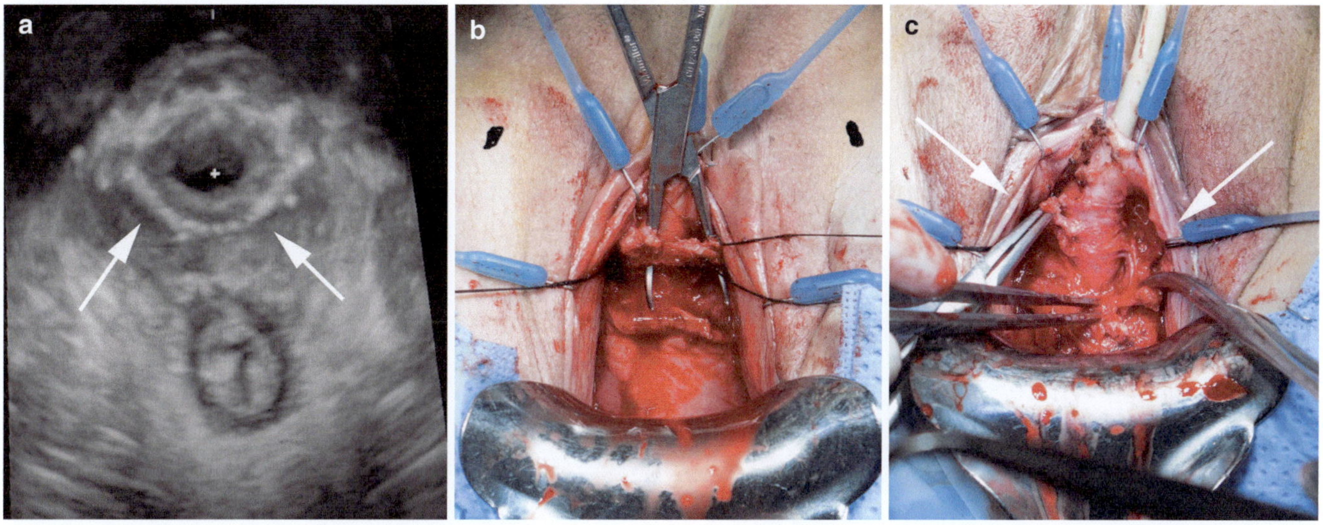

Fig. 9.23 (**a**) Translabial ultrasound showing the mesh as a strip of hyperechoic areas around the urethra (*arrow*). (**b**) The mesh was isolated laterally over a silk suture. A transverse incision was made in the anterior vaginal wall between the sutures, creating a superior and an inferior flap of vaginal wall. (**c**) The mesh is divided in two in the midline. At the end of each segment, a silk suture is applied to facilitate the transfer and dissection of the mesh. Each half of the mesh is dissected free from the periurethral tissues and directed toward the obturator fascia. The obturator fascia is open. The mesh is dissected free from the descending inner rami of the pubic bone, from the obturator internus, the obturator membrane, and the obturator externus. The mesh is sometimes surrounded by dense adhesions and fixed to the pubic bone, in which case we use a periosteum elevator to separate the mesh from the periosteum of the pubic bone. The dissection is very delicate, and excess traction must be avoided to prevent transection of the mesh. *Arrows* indicate the mesh after transaction in the midline, showing two segments of mesh, right and left. (**d**) Guided by the puncture side of the trocar (or more often by the finger in the obturator fossa), an oblique incision is made 1 cm lateral to the descending pubic bone. The skin and subcutaneous dissection allows for exposure of the adductor fascia that covers the adductor longus and gracilis muscles. Occasionally, a small segment of mesh is found, but more often no mesh is found over the fascia. The adductor fascia is open. Under blunt dissection the adductor musculature is split, allowing the passage of a finger to the already dissected obturator fossa. (**e**) In the vagina, the end of the mesh with the silk suture is grasped with an angulated pedicle clamp. Under finger control in the obturator fossa, the mesh and the clamp are transferred toward the adductor fossa. The mesh and the clamp are seen emerging from the adductor fossa (*arrow*). (**f**) The silk suture is transferred to the adductor fossa. The mesh (*arrow*) is dissected free from the lateral periosteum of the descending rami of the pubic bone and from the adductor musculature (adductor longus, brevis, and gracilis), using a coagulation knife to prevent transection of the mesh. The more difficult part is the removal of the mesh attachment to the periosteum. Care should be taken to remove all the mesh, which may extend laterally and deeper into the adductor fossa. (**g**) The mesh in the left obturator fossa has been removed entirely. A small laparotomy pad soaked with antibiotics is inserted in the adductor fossa. (**h**) A similar maneuver was performed on the right side. The mesh is removed from the right adductor fossa. (**i**) The two lateral labial incisions are seen after the mesh removal. A vaginal packing soaked with antibiotics is inserted in the vagina for 24 h. The Foley catheter is left in place for 5 days

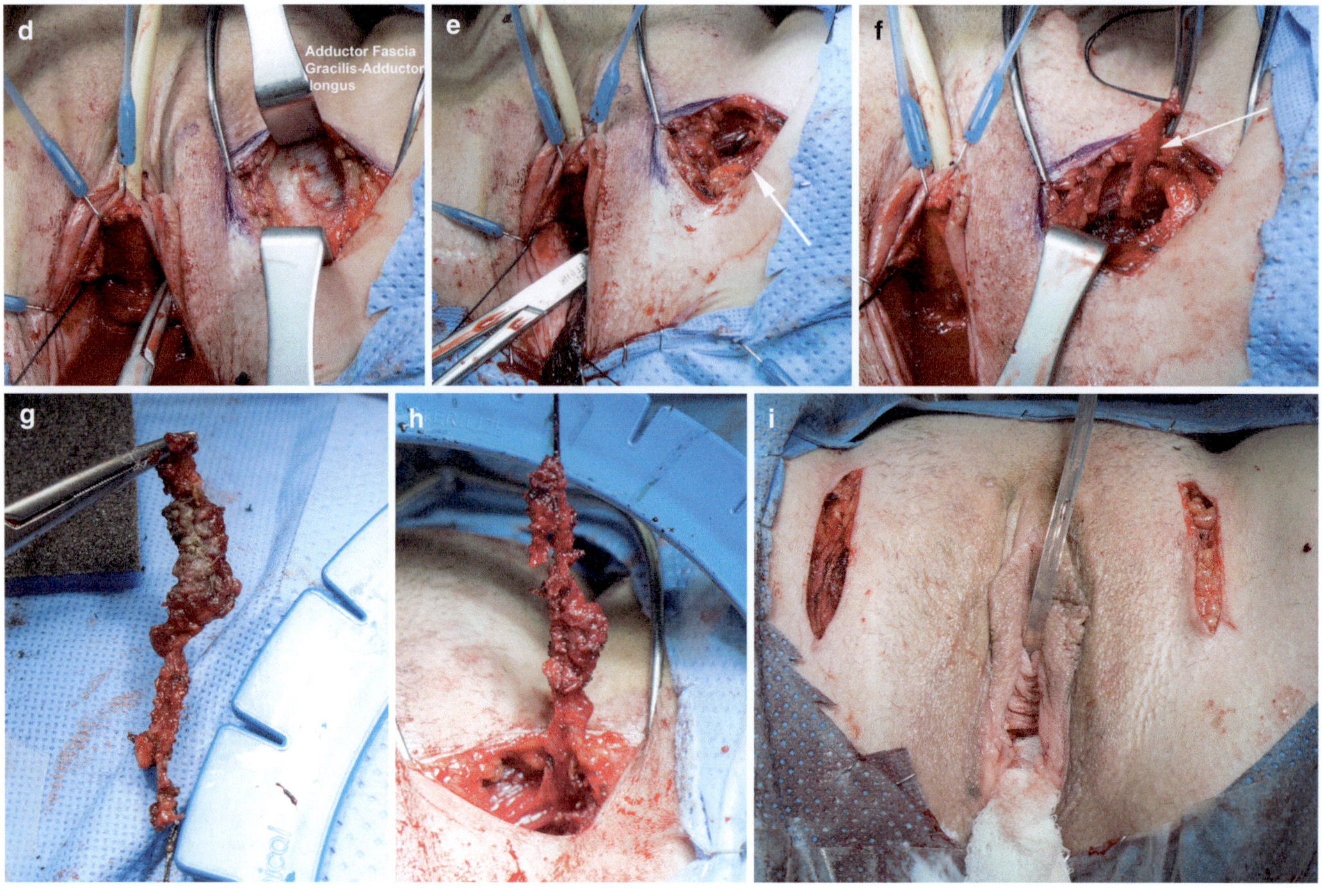

Fig. 9.23 (continued)

9.8.5 Removal of Anterior Mesh for Cystocele Repair Without Arms

When pelvic pain, dyspareunia, vaginal drainage, urgency incontinence are present in a patient with anterior mesh insertion for prolapse, the whole mesh should be removed.

Anterior mesh can be inserted as a free segment into the paravesical space and anterior vaginal wall without arms (Prosima) (Fig. 9.24), with an arm toward the sacrospinous ligament and paravesical space, crossing the obturator fossa (Avaulta, Perigee, Prolift), or with a single incision in which the fixation is toward the sacrospinous ligament and obturator muscle without trocars through the obturators (Elevate). Removal of each of these types of mesh requires an extensive and difficult dissection of the mesh from the bladder, paravesical space, and sacrospinous ligament area, where nerves (sacral plexus, pudendal nerve, and sciatic nerve) and the uterine and gluteal arteries are present. The mesh may cause only vaginal wall changes (exposure, extrusion), but often extensive infiltration of the anterior vaginal wall requires excision of large areas of affected vagina. Occasionally, rotational flaps of the labia, vaginal wall, or inner thigh may be required.

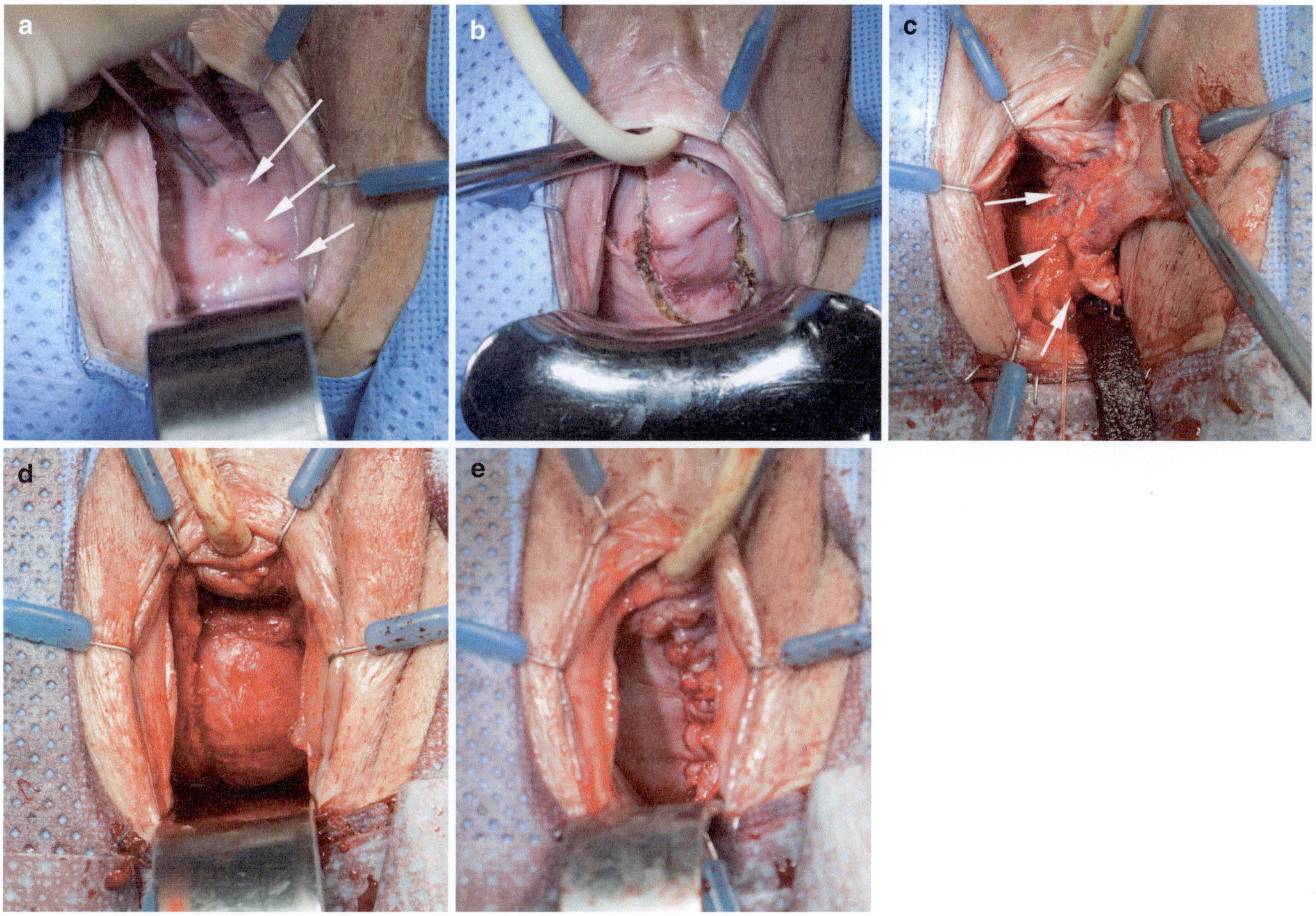

Fig. 9.24 (**a**) Extensive anterior vaginal wall exposure and infiltration of mesh (*arrows*) after an anterior vaginal wall mesh repair (Prosima). (**b**) A large elliptical incision is made in the anterior vaginal wall to include the affected area. (**c**) The anterior vaginal wall and the mesh are dissected free laterally to enter the paravesical space, where the mesh (*arrows*) is detached from the obturator musculature. (**d**) The entire mesh has been removed, exposing the perivesical fascia from the bladder neck to the vaginal cuff. (**e**) Figure-of-eight delayed absorbable sutures are used to approximate the margins of the intact anterior vaginal wall. This patient had enough anterior vaginal wall leftover to do a primary closure

9.8.6 Removal of Anterior Mesh for Cystocele Repair with Four Arms

The patient in Fig. 9.25 presents with vaginal pain, drainage, and pelvic pain after a cystocele repair with four arms: two to the obturator musculature and two to the sacrospinous ligament.

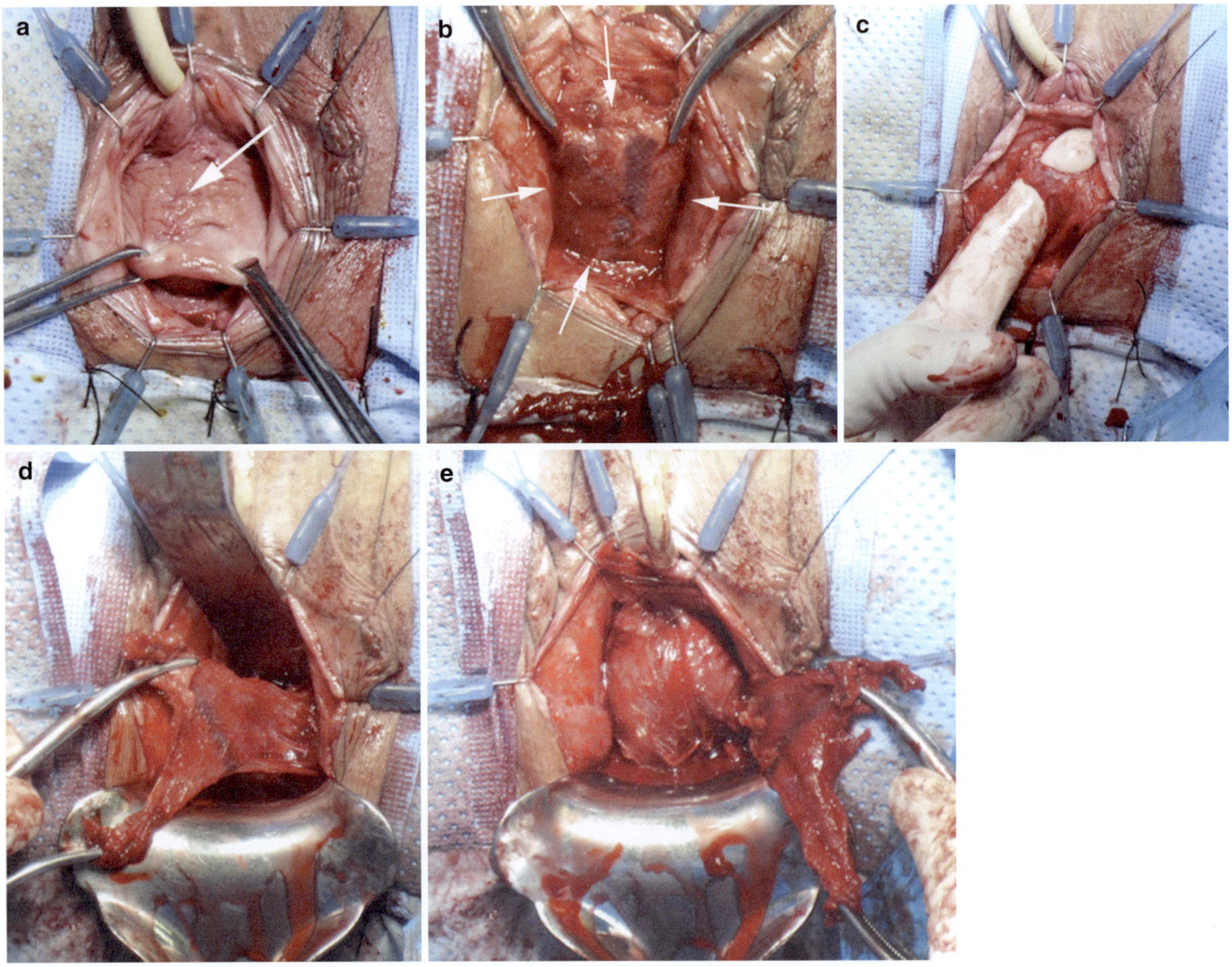

Fig. 9.25 (**a**) The anterior vaginal wall is retracted. An area of vaginal exposure and erosion is seen (*arrow*) with multiple areas of infiltration of the vaginal wall by the mesh. (**b**) A vertical incision is made in the anterior vaginal wall. The vaginal wall is dissected free from the mesh. The dissection is extended toward the vaginal cuff and distal to the bladder neck. *Arrows* indicate the anterior mesh after separation from the anterior vaginal wall; it will be dissected free from the bladder wall. (**c**) The right arm of the mesh is dissected free from the perivesical tissues. The arm is followed toward the obturator muscle and detached. The lower arm is detached from the sacrospinous ligament in the right side, providing mobility to the mesh. The finger holds one of the arms of the mesh. (**d**) The mesh is dissected free from the perivesical fascia. Care is taken during this dissection not to penetrate the bladder wall. Diluted indigo carmine can be inserted in the bladder through the Foley catheter to ensure its integrity. (**e**) The upper arm of the mesh has been dissected from the obturator muscle. The inferior arm is followed toward the paravesical and pararectal space and dissected free from the attachment to the sacrospinous ligament

9.8.7 Removal of Posterior Mesh

The patient in Fig. 9.26 presents with severe defecatory dysfunction, posterior vaginal pain, and anal pain after insertion of a posterior mesh.

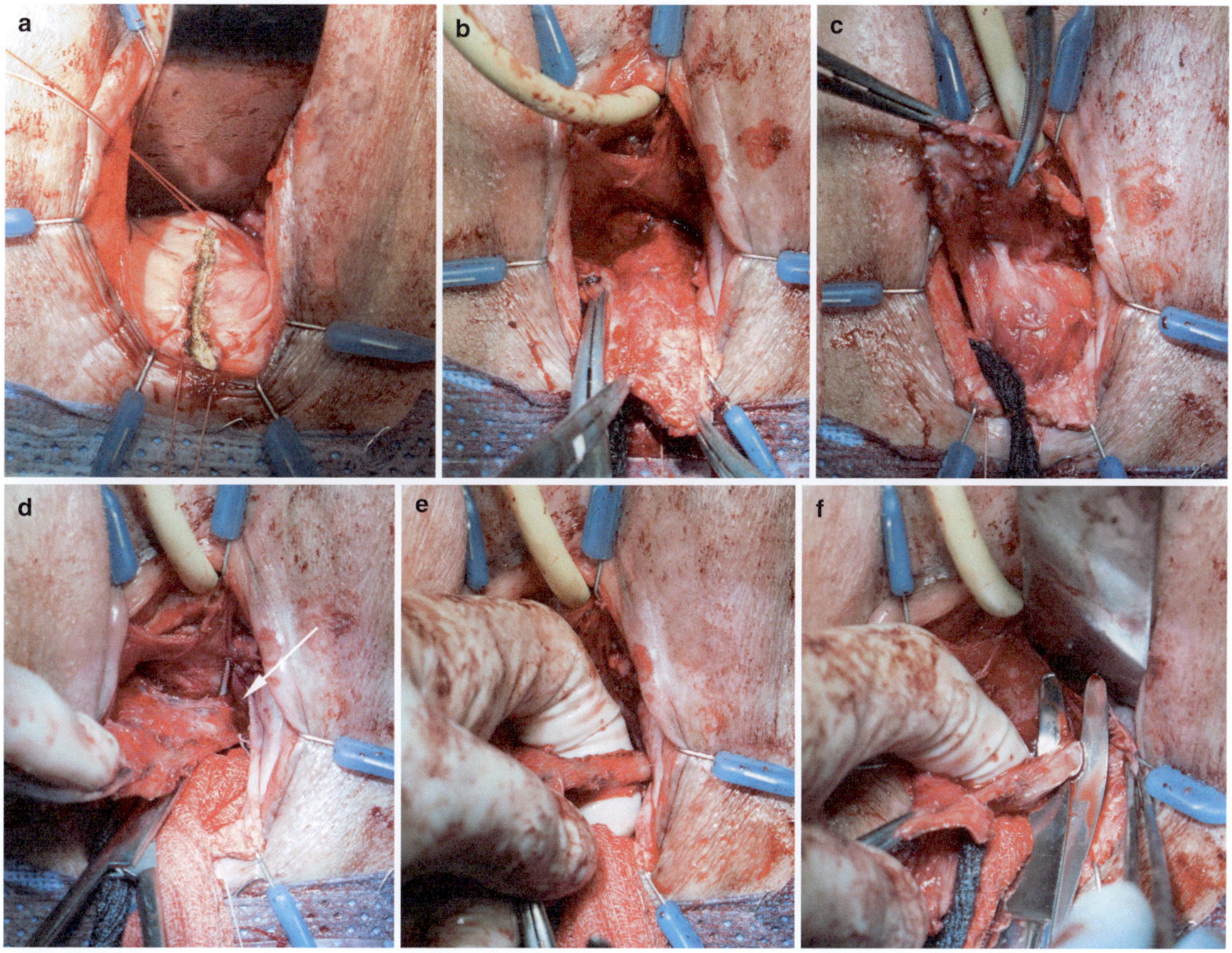

Fig. 9.26 (**a**) A vertical incision is made in the posterior vaginal wall from the cuff to the distal vagina. (**b**) Dissection is carried out under the vaginal wall on each side of the incision to expose the pararectal fascia and the lateral margins of the mesh. The dissection is carried out superficial to the mesh, proximal toward the vaginal cuff. (**c**) The distal segment of the mesh is detached from the posterior distal vagina and elevated, in order to dissect the rectal wall from the mesh. (**d**) The mesh is dissected toward the pararectal space, where the arms of the mesh are isolated over a right-angle clamp (*arrow*). (**e**) The left proximal arm of the mesh is dissected free toward the sacrospinous ligament area. (**f**) Using a right-angle scissors, the mesh is transected flush over the sacrospinous ligament. Branches of the uterine artery require coagulation or suture ligature. (**g**) The posterior bladder mesh was dissected free from the rectal wall. This is a very delicate dissection and care should be taken to avoid rectal injury. (**h**) Posterior vaginal mesh after excision

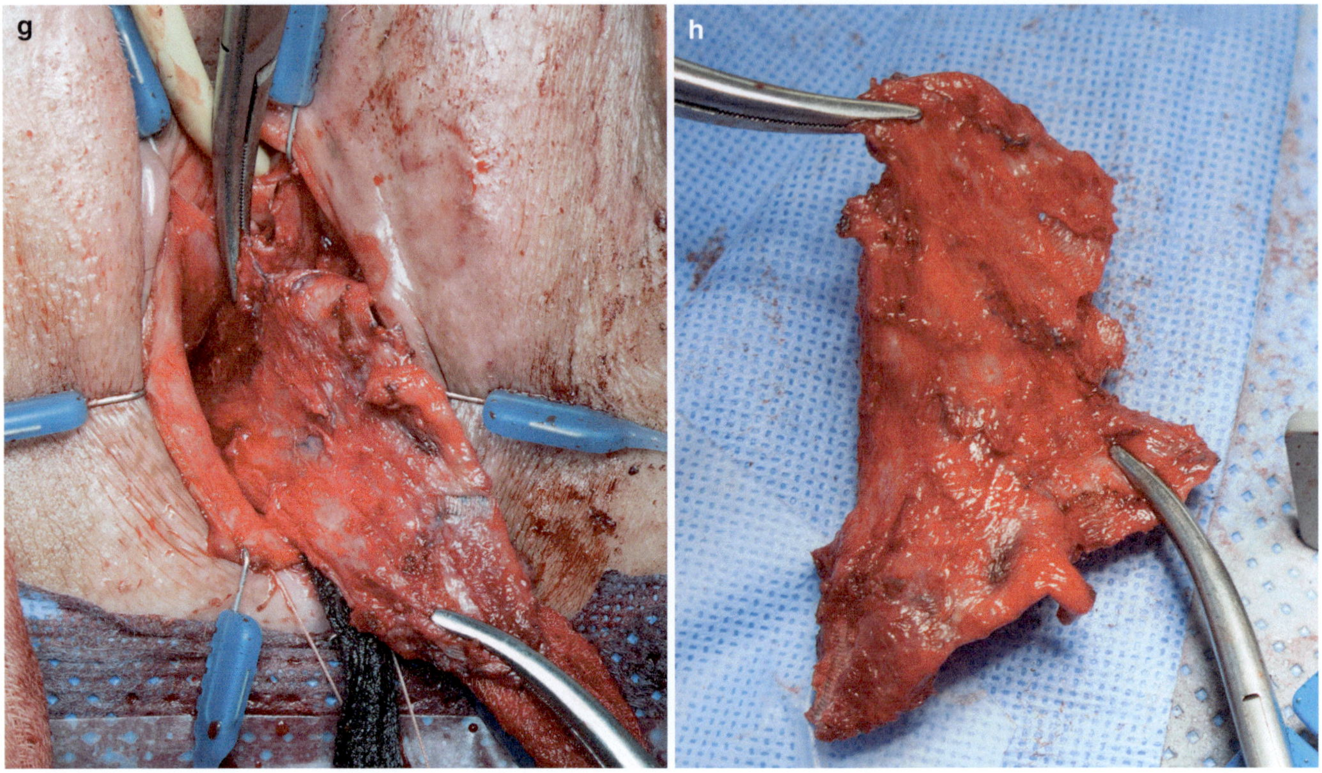

Fig. 9.26 (continued)

9.9 Recurrent Prolapse

Recurrent prolapse may occur in the setting of almost any vaginal repair where the anatomic axis of the vagina is changed. Such repairs may change the dynamic forces of where the intra-abdominal pressure is transmitted and may cause exacerbation of preexistent prolapse. Therefore, one must aggressively seek to identify any moderate to severe degrees of prolapse that may potentially worsen with time. We perform dynamic MRI evaluation of the pelvic floor in patients with high-grade prolapse and have found unrecognized pelvic floor pathology in approximately 20 % of these patients. We then approach these patients with the intent to identify and correct the pathology in order to prevent recurrent prolapse in the future. If recurrent prolapse occurs, one must decide if it is severe or symptomatic enough to require operative management (Fig. 9.27).

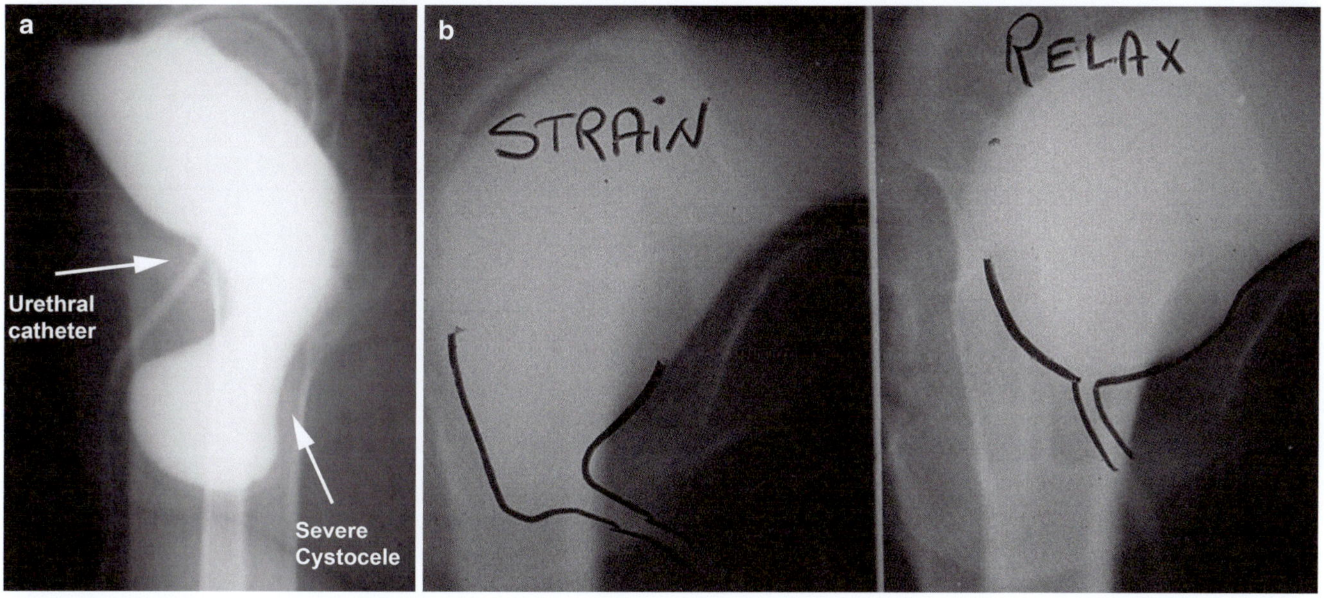

Fig. 9.27 (**a**) Lateral cystogram of a patient after a cystocele repair. The patient complains of a vaginal bulge and difficulties in emptying the bladder. The study confirms a well-supported urethra and a significant recurrent cystocele. (**b**) Lateral cystogram in a patient with recurrent stress incontinence after a sling procedure for stress incontinence. The relax and strain pictures show significant urethral hypermobility and a mild cystocele. The sling procedure failed to support the urethra and prevent mobility. (**c**) Lateral straining MRI of the midpelvis showing a large enterocele (*arrows*). The patient underwent a sling procedure and a cystocele repair. The vault was not repaired, and 6 months after surgery, the patient presents with significant vault prolapse. *Arrows* indicate the enterocele sac. (**d**) The patient presented to the emergency room 2 months after an uneventful vaginal hysterectomy. She was found to have evisceration of the small bowel through a small defect of the cuff closure. (**e**) The same patient was taken to the operating room immediately, where the bowel was reduced to the abdominal cavity without any bowel resection. The defect of the cuff after reduction of the bowel is seen. (**f**) The cuff of the vagina was closed, the vault resuspended, and the vaginal wall reconstructed

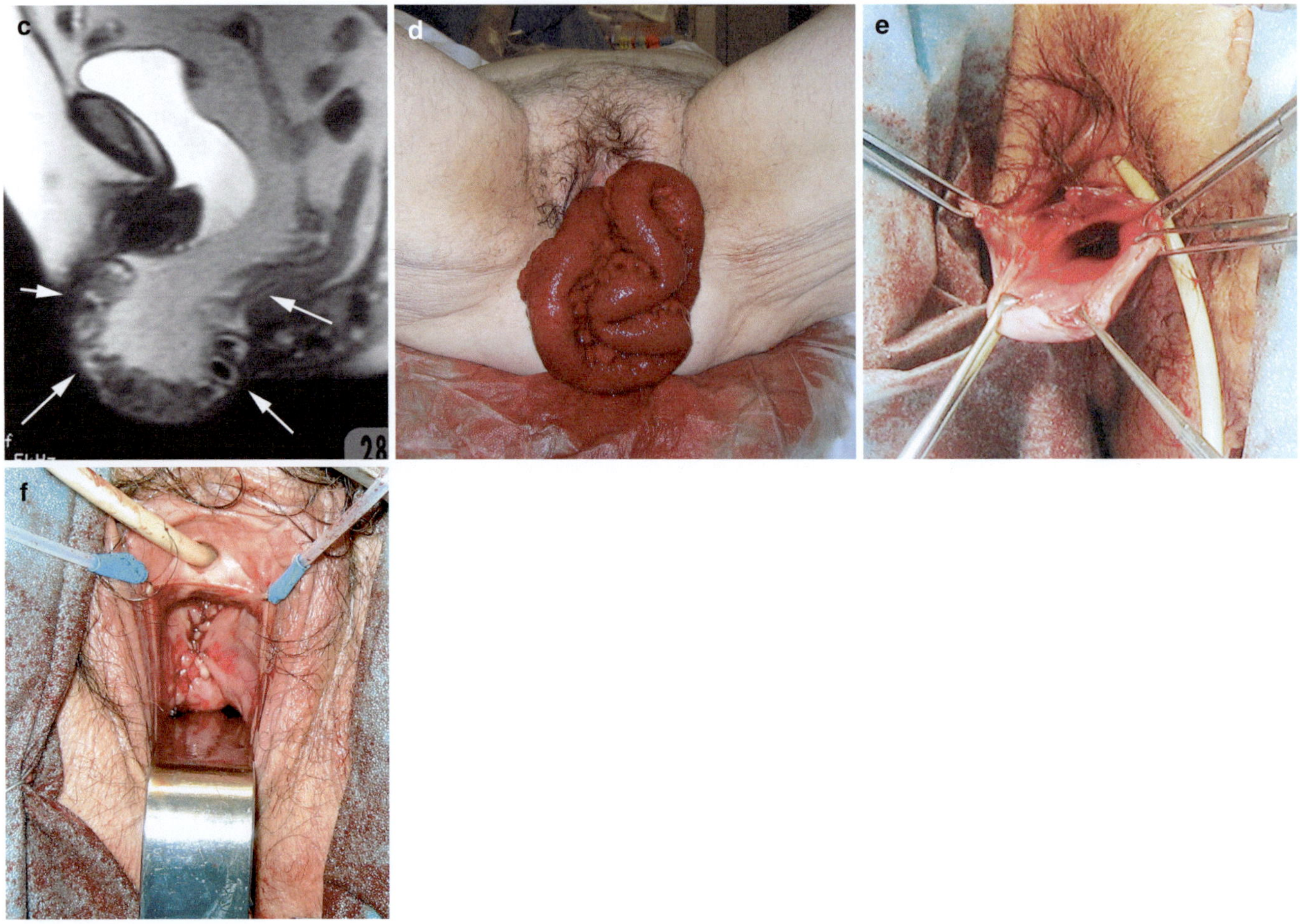

Fig. 9.27 (continued)

9.10 De Novo Urgency Incontinence

De novo bladder overactivity with urgency incontinence is a well-known complication of anti-incontinence surgery. Most often, symptoms were present preoperatively but become more pronounced in the postoperative period, as the accompanying stress urinary incontinence has been treated. This condition is often temporary and resolves over time, but some patients do develop new-onset de novo bladder instability, causing them to be surgical failures. The reported incidence of this complication varies considerably but may be as high as 28 %. The etiology is unclear; it may be related to unrecognized preoperative detrusor overactivity masked by severe sphincteric incompetence or to the creation of subclinical bladder outlet obstruction. The treatment is primarily medical, including behavioral modification, cholinolytics, and rarely sacral neuromodulation. In isolated cases, augmentation cystoplasty can be considered.

9.11 Urinary Outlet Obstruction

Chapter 7 discussed in detail the treatment of urethral obstruction. Although all the anti-incontinence procedures being used are nonobstructive by design, the potential for postoperative bladder outlet obstruction exists and has been reported in the literature, even when procedures are well performed. Obstruction most often occurs in the setting of improper suture or mesh placement, as discussed above, or it may be due to overzealous elevation of the bladder neck and proximal urethra while adjusting the tension of a sling. Slings of any variety should never be elevated under tension. Doing so may create postoperative outlet obstruction resulting in urgency, frequency, large post-void residuals, and possibly even urinary retention. Interposition of a clamp between the urethra and the mesh while adjusting the mesh tension could prevent obstruction. Pulling up the sutures or mesh under tension is unnecessary to produce urinary continence. In suspension procedures, we place a cystoscope sheath per urethra and incline it to 45° to the horizontal prior to tying the suspending sutures. This angle reapproximates the native position of the vesicourethra, preventing excessive elevation of the proximal urethra during tying of the sutures.

The initial incision for the insertion of a midurethral sling can be accidentally done deep to the periurethral fascia so that the mesh may be placed into the urethral wall itself, causing obstruction.

Finally, in some cases, postoperative development of a cystocele may cause bladder outlet obstruction. Failure to recognize and correct coexistent pelvic prolapse during an anti-incontinence operation may result in an enlarging postoperative cystocele, which kinks at the level of the bladder outlet in the location of the suspension sutures. If adequate bladder outlet support was attained at the time of bladder neck suspension, simple repair of the cystocele will result in the return of normal voiding function and the maintenance of urinary continence.

Outlet obstruction in women is a difficult diagnosis. The most helpful finding is a postoperative change in voiding symptoms in the setting of an increased post-void residual. These patients may present with the postoperative onset of new irritative voiding symptoms including urgency, frequency, and urge incontinence. These women should be differentiated from patients with some preoperative baseline irritative symptoms that remain after the surgery or perhaps are somewhat exacerbated by it. The vast majority of these patients will have resolution of their irritative symptoms with time. It is also common for patients with pure stress incontinence preoperatively to have some degree of urgency and frequency postoperatively owing to the inherent nature of pelvic surgery and perivesical inflammation. These patients are treated symptomatically with anticholinergic agents until the symptoms resolve, usually within 1–2 months.

Commonly, female patients with outlet obstruction do not exhibit the "high pressure, low flow" findings on urodynamics that are commonly seen in the obstructed male. Voiding cystourethrography may demonstrate urethral kinking or perhaps an oversuspended urethra and bladder neck, with the bladder neck elevated to an unphysiologically high retropubic position. Conversely, an obstructed urethra may be in good anatomic position but is fixed and is unable to funnel and open during a bladder contraction. Translabial ultrasound will help in the diagnosis of obstruction and deep placement of mesh into the urethral wall.

Treatment of these patients includes intermittent catheterization and cholinolytics initially. After a short period of observation, only the mesh or the suspension suture should be incised. In cases appearing late (more than 4 months) after the surgical procedure, a more extensive urethrolysis may be required to free up the urethra.

9.12 Vaginal Narrowing/Stenosis

Excessive excision of the vaginal wall may lead to narrowing of the vagina and stenosis. Additionally, excessive plication of tissue may lead to the development of ridges, which often become painful and tender. We use several steps to prevent these very avoidable complications. During cystocele, rectocele, or enterocele repairs, when excess vaginal tissue is excised, one must be cognizant of the amount of tissue to be removed. We use a Haney retractor to facilitate the identification of vaginal depth, adjacent structures, and avoidance of overexcision. Minimal tissue excision will help avoid narrowing, yet similarly, approximation of tissues too widely can cause the same result. One can avoid painful ridges by creating a smooth repair in a symmetric fashion. During rectocele repairs in particular, we find it necessary to continuously reassess the location of the sutures to prevent asymmetry. Placement of sutures too laterally in the distal phase of a rectocele repair can cause pain from levator spasm and tenderness; one should avoid any sutures through the levators.

In a patient with significant vaginal stenosis, a rotational flap of the inner thigh is performed (Fig. 9.28). This procedure is described in detail in Chap. 5.

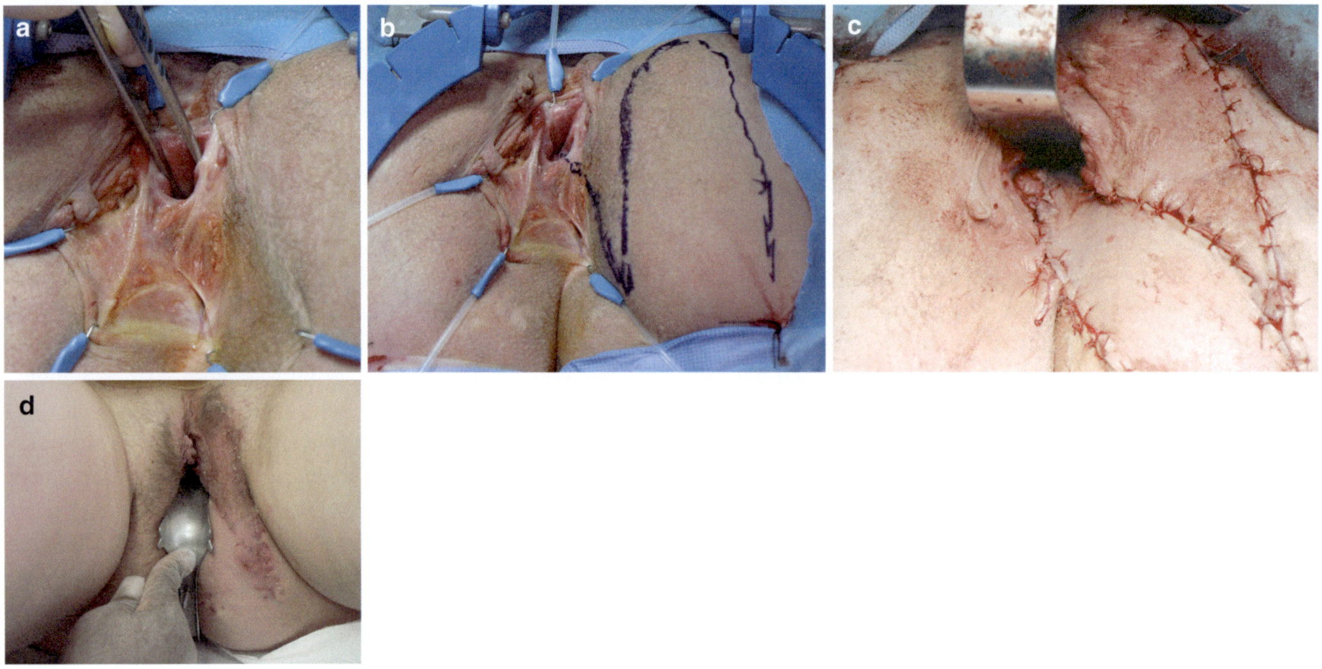

Fig. 9.28 (**a**) This patient had multiple anterior and posterior vaginal reconstructions for prolapse, resulting in severe stenosis of the vaginal introitus and proximal vagina. The vaginal examination showed severe stenosis, requiring a Hegar dilator for the initial exploration. (**b**) An inverted U inner thigh flap will be created and rotated medially, the labium will be mobilized and rotated laterally, and a 5 o'clock episiotomy will be performed to allow transfer of the inner thigh flap toward the vagina. (**c**) The inner thigh flap has been rotated to the vagina and anastomosed to the medial and lateral margins of the episiotomy. The labial flap is displaced laterally and anastomosed to the donor site at the inner thigh. (**d**) Three months after surgery, the size of the introitus and the vaginal depth are normal. The patient was able to resume sexual relations without complications

9.13 Recurrent Stress Incontinence

The treatment of primary or secondary stress incontinence is discussed in Chap. 2. Continued incontinence postoperatively is considered a surgical complication. The most common situation is that the patient has persistent stress incontinence after a sling procedure, either immediately or a few months later. The sling never provided adequate urethral compression or support and the patient continues to lose urine with stress. The anatomical position of the urethra does not correlate with the degree of incontinence.

If the patient complains of continued stress incontinence postoperatively or has recurrence of stress incontinence shortly after surgery, the surgeon must evaluate for any technical issues that may have led to the surgical failure. These include improper diagnosis, detachment of the anchors from the obturator fascia, lack of adequate urethral compression and support, malpositioning of the sling, deep urethral penetration creating fixation of the urethral wall, and surgical complications like urethral perforation or fistula. Physical examination or video-urodynamic studies will demonstrate continued bladder neck funneling and urethral leakage with stress.

Proper placement of a sling is important. The ideal position of a sling is at the midurethra, but in more than 50 % of the patients cured by a sling, the mesh is not found at the midurethra. Placement of sutures or mesh too proximal relative to the bladder neck will not adequately support the bladder outlet. The mesh or the sutures will, in effect, fix the bladder neck into an open position, creating loss of the proximal sphincteric mechanism at the level of the bladder neck. Very distal placement of a sling adequate support at the level of the urethra will lead to an inadequate urethral compensation during stress of the urethra, and the impact of the sling on the sphincteric unit will not be effective.

Patients may have recurrent incontinence due to damage to the sphincteric unit itself. Sutures or mesh placed into the urethral wall may damage the periurethral envelope (intrinsic smooth and skeletal musculature) with fibrosis, scarring, and atrophy of the urethral spongy tissue. Loss of the urethral spongy tissue will often result in poor urethral coaptation, loss of the mucosal seal mechanism, and the development of intrinsic sphincteric deficiency. A well-supported but "pipestem"-type urethra with no inherent resistance is the long-term surgical result.

Suggested Reading

Abbott S, Unger CA, Evans JM, Jallad K, Mishra K, Karram MM, et al. Evaluation and management of complications from synthetic mesh after pelvic reconstructive surgery: a multicenter study. Am J Obstet Gynecol. 2014;210(2):163.e1–8.

Abouassaly R, Steinberg JR, Lemieux M, Marois C, Gilchrist LI, Bourque JL, et al. Complications of tension-free vaginal tape surgery: a multi-institutional review. BJU Int. 2004;94:110–3.

Ashok K, Petri E. Failures and complications in pelvic floor surgery. World J Urol. 2012;30(4):487–94.

Blaivas JG, Sandhu J. Urethral reconstruction after erosion of slings in women. Curr Opin Urol. 2004;14:335–8.

Bontje HF, van de Pol G, van der Zaag-Loonen HJ, Spaans WA. Follow-up of mesh complications using the IUGA/ICS category-time-site coding classification. Int Urogynecol J. 2014;25(6):817–22.

Crosby EC, Abernethy M, Berger MB, DeLancey JO, Fenner DE, Morgan DM. Symptom resolution after operative management of complications from transvaginal mesh. Obstet Gynecol. 2014;123(1):134–9.

de Tayrac R, Sentilhes L. Complications of pelvic organ prolapse surgery and methods of prevention. Int Urogynecol J. 2013;24(11):1859–72.

Ellington DR, Richter HE. The role of vaginal mesh procedures in pelvic organ prolapse surgery in view of complication risk. Obstet Gynecol Int. 2013;2013:356960.

Khan ZA, Thomas L, Emery SJ. Outcomes and complications of transvaginal mesh repair using the Prolift™ kit for pelvic organ prolapse at 4 years median follow-up in a tertiary referral centre. Arch Gynecol Obstet. 2014;290(6):1151–7.

Klutke C, Siegel S, Carlin B, Paszkiewicz E, Kirkemo A, Klutke J. Urinary retention after tension-free vaginal tape procedure: incidence and treatment. Urology. 2001;58:697–701.

Kuuva N, Nilsson C. A nationwide analysis of complications associated with the tension-free vaginal tape (TVT) procedure. Acta Obstet Gynecol Scand. 2002;81:72–7.

Laurikainen E, Killholma P. A nationwide analysis of transvaginal tape release for urinary retention after tension-free vaginal tape procedure. Int Urogynecol J. 2006;17:111–9.

Marks BK, Goldman HB. Controversies in the management of mesh-based complications: a urology perspective. Urol Clin North Am. 2012;39(3):419–28.

Mothes AR, Mothes HK, Radosa MP, Runnebaum IB. Systematic assessment of surgical complications in 438 cases of vaginal native tissue repair for pelvic organ prolapse adopting Clavien-Dindo classification. Arch Gynecol Obstet. 2015;291:1297–301.

Muffly T, Barber MD. Insertion and removal of vaginal mesh for pelvic organ prolapse. Clin Obstet Gynecol. 2010;53(1):99–114.

Rice NT, Hu Y, Slaughter JC, Ward RM. Pelvic mesh complications in women before and after the 2011 FDA public health notification. Female Pelvic Med Reconstr Surg. 2013;19(6):333–8.

Sokol AI, Jelovsek JE, Walters MD, Paraiso MF, Barber MD. Incidence and predictors of prolonged urinary retention after TVT with and without concurrent prolapse surgery. Am J Obstet Gynecol. 2005;192:1537–43.

Unger CA, Walters MD, Ridgeway B, Jelovsek JE, Barber MD, Paraiso MF. Incidence of adverse events after uterosacral colpopexy for uterovaginal and posthysterectomy vault prolapse. Am J Obstet Gynecol. 2015;212(5):603.e1–7.

Wong KS, Nguyen JN, White T, Menefee SA, Walter AJ, Krulewitch CJ, et al. Adverse events associated with pelvic organ prolapse surgeries that use implants. Obstet Gynecol. 2013;122(6):1239–45.

Index

A
Abdominal autologous fascial slings
indications, 57
omega-shaped fascial sling, 55
cystoscopy, 63, 65
double-pronged passer, 63, 64
fascial strip, 63
punctures, 63, 64
tunnel, 63
spiral fascial sling, 55, 56
U-shaped pubovaginal sling, 55
delayed absorbable sutures, 57, 59
double-pronged passer, 57, 61
fascial strip, 57, 60
Foley catheter, 57
multiple interrupted absorbable sutures, 57, 62
oblique incisions, 57
right-angle clamp, 57–59
skin and subcutaneous exposure, 57, 58
small suprapubic puncture, 57, 60
suprapubic exposure, 57, 58
Anal sphincter reconstruction
anterior anal sphincter repair
ischial fossa and perirectal area exposure, 215
perineal skin flap, 214
perineum, vaginal area and rectum exposure, 214
ring retractor and hooks, incision, 214
skin flap, 214
sutures, 215–216
anterior and posterior anal sphincter repair
antibiotic solution, 218
semicircular inverted U incision, 217
transverse semicircular incision, 218
wide-open anal sphincter, 217
diagnosis, 212
indications, 211–212
intraoperative complications, 217
postoperative care, 217
postoperative complications, 217
Anterior vaginal wall repair. *See* Cystocele repair
Arcus tendineus fascia pelvis (ATFP), 14, 34

B
Bartholin's gland cyst
cystic lesion, 262
cyst marsupialization, 263
sexual stimulation, 262
vaginal examination, 263
Bladder neck closure
anterior inverted U vaginal flap, 219
anterior pubic bone dissection, 220
anterior vaginal wall exposure, 219
circular incision, 220
diagnosis, 219
indications, 219
intraoperative complications, 225
Martius flap, 224
postoperative care, 225
postoperative complications, 225
sharp and blunt dissection, 220
superior pedicle flap, 223
two-layer closure, 222
urethral necrosis and radiation, 223
Bladder neck suspension (BNS)
indications, 42–43
intraoperative complications, 49
postoperative care, 49
postoperative complications, 49
preoperative considerations, 43
surgical technique
Allis clamps, 44
cystoscope, 43, 48
double-pronged ligature carrier, 43, 47
lateral dissection, 43, 44
medial traction, 43
monofilament nonabsorbable suture, 43, 45
oblique incisions, 43, 44
placement of suspension sutures, 43, 45
retropubic space, finger in, 43, 45
small puncture, 43, 47
traction of sutures, 43, 47
Burch procedure, 40, 42, 241–242

C
Cadaveric dissection, 11
Cardinal ligament, 2, 19, 100
CRISP procedure. *See* Cystocele repair using interlocking sutures of polypropylene (CRISP) procedure
Cystocele repair
central and lateral defect repair, combination of
curved Mayo scissors, 92, 94
cystoscopy, 92, 96
delayed absorbable sutures, 92, 94, 95
double-pronged passer, 92, 95
four sutures, 92, 95
intraoperative complications, 92
monofilament nonabsorbable sutures, 92, 95
oblique incisions, 92, 94
PDS, 92, 93
postoperative care, 92
postoperative complications, 92–93

S. Raz, *Atlas of Vaginal Reconstructive Surgery*, DOI 10.1007/978-1-4939-2941-2

Cystocele repair (*cont.*)
central defect, repair of
anterior vaginal wall exposure, 80
cardinal–sacrouterine complex, 80, 81
central sutures, 80, 82
figure-of-eight sutures, 80–82
incision, 80, 81
delayed absorbable sutures, 80, 83
lateral dissection, 80, 81
periurethral fascia, 80, 81
perivesical fascia, 80, 82
scissors/coagulation knife, 80, 82
CRISP procedure
central and lateral suture placement, 83, 86
figure-of-eight suture, 83–85
four lateral sutures, 83, 85
lateral sutures, 83, 86
lateral vaginal flap and right flap, 83, 87
vertical incision, 83, 84
diagnosis
cystoscopy, 79
physical examination, 77, 78
straining, 77, 78
ureter, dilatation of, 77, 78
fascia lata lateral and central defect repair, recurrent cystocele
Crawford fascial stripper, 96, 97
cystoscopy, 96, 99
delayed absorbable sutures, 96, 99
mesh removal, 96, 97
scissors, 96, 98
small punctures, 96, 98
vertical incision, 96, 98
four-corner bladder neck and bladder suspension
advantage of, 87
curved scissors, 87, 88
cystoscopy, 87, 92
delayed absorbable sutures, 87, 92
four sutures, 87, 90, 91
long forceps, 87, 89
nonabsorbable monofilament suture, 87–89
oblique incision, 87, 90
retropubic space, finger in, 87, 88
small puncture, 87, 91
indications, 77
vaginal hysterectomy (*see* Vaginal hysterectomy)
Cystocele repair using interlocking sutures of polypropylene (CRISP) procedure
central and lateral suture placement, 83, 86
figure-of-eight suture, 83–85
lateral sutures, 83, 85, 86
lateral vaginal flap and right flap, 83, 87
vertical incision, 83, 84

D

Delayed absorbable sutures (DAS), 52, 54, 59, 63, 66–69, 75, 79, 83, 92–95, 97, 99, 121, 142–144, 156, 157, 167, 172, 176, 177, 180, 182, 184, 185, 196, 201, 206–208, 215, 216, 218, 222, 228, 230, 246, 253, 256, 257, 259, 315
Distal urethral polypropylene sling (DUPS)
indications, 49
postoperative complications, 55
surgical technique
absorbable sutures, 49, 53
Allis clamps, 49, 50, 54
cystourethroscopy, 49, 53
double-pronged ligature carrier, 49, 52, 53
hemostatic clamp, 49, 52
oblique incisions, 49, 50
puncture, 49, 51
right-angle clamp, 49, 51
small incision, 49, 52
soft polypropylene mesh, 49, 51

E

Ectopic ureterocele, 266–267
Enterocele repair
complex enterocele, 109
diagnosis, 110–112
indications, 110
intraoperative complications, 122
postoperative care, 122
postoperative complications, 122
preoperative considerations, 110
surgical technique for
anchoring sutures, 113, 116
closed cuff, 113, 121
delayed absorbable suture, 113, 116
Heaney posterior retractor, 113, 118
laparotomy pads, 113, 115
lateral peritoneal sutures, 113, 120
needle, transfer of, 113, 117, 119
PDS suture, 113, 118, 119
purse-string sutures, 113, 120
sharp dissection, 113, 114
vertical incision, 113, 114

F

Fascia lata autologous fascial sling, 66
postoperative care, 67
surgical technique
anchoring effect, 67, 68
Crawford fascial stripper, 67, 69
cystoscopy, 67, 71
double-pronged passer, 67, 70
fascial retrieval, 67, 68
figure-of-eight sutures, 67, 70
Foley catheter, 67, 70
oblique incisions, 67, 70, 71
right-angle clamp, 67, 68
sharp and blunt dissection, 67, 68

H

Haney retractors, 127, 133, 322
Heaney retractor, 113, 115, 118, 142
Hegar dilator, 142, 143, 322
Heineke–Mikulicz technique, 254–256

L

Labioplasty, excess labia majora
complications, 236
indications, 232
postoperative care, 236
surgical procedure, 232
labium, 233, 234
lateral labial skin incision, 233
medial and lateral labial incision, 235
oblique incision, 233
sutures, 234
Lateral cystogram, 241, 319
cystocele, 78, 240
high vesicovaginal fistula, 162

retropubic sling, 305
sling procedures, 39, 40
urethral mobility, 38, 39
Lowsley retractor, 163

M
Mackenrodt's ligaments. *See* Cardinal ligament
Mesonephric–Wolffian Gartner's duct cysts, 274–275
Mucosal sphincter, 27

O
Obturator membrane, 2, 3, 313
Omentocele, 110, 112

P
Pelvic anatomy, 1
bladder support, 15–18
bones and ligaments
fascial structures, 4
obturator membrane, 2, 3
osseous structures, 3
sacrospinous ligament, 2
sacrotuberous ligament, 2
innervation and vascular supply
hypogastric sympathetic plexus, 25
internal iliac artery, 24
sensory innervation, 26
pararectal fascia, 2
pelvic musculature, 5–7
perineal anatomy, 8
posterior vaginal wall and rectum support, 20–23
prerectal space, 10
presacral space, 9
pubocervical fascia, 9, 10
rectovaginal space, 9, 10
retropubic space, 9, 10
retrorectal space, 10
urethral support
pubourethral ligaments/fascia, 11–12
urethropelvic fascia, 13–14
vesicovaginal space, 9, 10
Pelvic floor relaxation (PFR), 123, 125
Perineal anatomy, 8
Perineal hernia repair
indications, 137–138
postoperative care, 139
postoperative complications, 139
preoperative considerations, 137
surgical technique
figure-of-eight sutures, 139, 140
ischiorectal fossa, 139, 140
levator musculature, 139, 140
perineal sutures, 139, 140
delay absorbable sutures, 139, 141
vertical incision, 139
Polydioxanone (PDS), 79, 93, 106, 113, 116, 118, 119
Posterior vaginal wall repair
classification, 125
diagnosis, 125–127
indications, 123–124
postoperative care, 51
postoperative complications, 51
preoperative considerations, 125
surgical technique
Allis clamps, 127, 129, 130
distal sutures, 127, 135
figure-of-eight sutures, 127, 134
Foley catheter, 127, 128
Haney/right-angle retractors, 127, 133
oblique incision, 127, 130
scissors, 127, 130, 131
delay absorbable sutures, 127, 132, 135, 136
straight incision, 127, 128
strip, excision of, 127, 132
triangular excision, 127, 128
V-shaped incision, 127–129
Puborectalis muscle, 5, 21, 212
Pubourethral ligaments, 11–12, 30, 38, 247, 282

R
Raz procedure. *See* Bladder neck suspension (BNS)
Rectal prolapse
indications, 141
postoperative care, 142
preoperative considerations, 141
surgical technique
delayed absorbable sutures, 142, 144
Heaney retractor, 142
Hegar dilator, 142, 143
levator sutures, 142, 143
medial retraction, 142, 143
postoperative defecogram, 142, 144
Rectoceles. *See* Posterior vaginal wall repair
Rectoperineal fistula
and anal sphincter reconstruction, 207–208
diagnosis, 199
intraoperative complications, 209
postoperative care, 209
postoperative complications, 209
preoperative considerations, 199
surgical technique
circular incision, 200
delayed absorbable sutures, 201
labia majora, 202
mattress sutures, 201
perineal examination, 202
perineal fat flap, 201
subcutaneous tissue, 202
superficial skin, 202
trans-anal fistulous tract, 200
Rectovaginal fistula
anal sphincter reconstruction, 203–206
diagnosis, 194
indications, 194
intraoperative complications, 199
postoperative care, 199
postoperative complications, 199
preoperative considerations, 194
surgical technique
fibro-fatty tissue, 198
fistulous tract and anterior rectal wall exposure, 195
Foley catheter, 195
Martius flap, 196
perineum exposure, 198
posterior vaginal wall flap, 198
prerectal flap, 196
U incision, 195
vertical incision, 196

S
Sacrocolpopexy, 15, 113, 123
Sacrospinous ligament (SPL), 2, 3, 6, 24, 106, 115–118, 142, 143, 306–308, 315–317
Sacrotuberous ligament (STL), 2, 3
Sacrouterine ligament, 2, 9, 19, 103, 104, 106, 109, 116, 118
Sigmoidocele, 110, 112
Skene's gland cyst, 243, 264–265
Sphincteric unit, 13, 27–29, 34, 37, 38, 151, 323
Spiral slings
  indications, 72
  postoperative complications, 72
  surgical technique
    absorbable sutures, 72, 75
    curved clamp, 72
    cystoscopy, 72, 75
    delayed absorbable suture, 72, 73
    finger control, 72, 73
    oblique incisions, 72
    small suprapubic puncture, 72, 75
    suprapubic incision, 72, 75
    tunnel, 72, 74
Stress incontinence
  abdominal autologous fascial slings
    indications, 57
    omega-shaped fascial sling, 55, 63–65
    spiral fascial sling, 55, 56
    U-shaped pubovaginal sling, 55, 57–62
  bladder neck suspension procedure
    Allis clamps, 44
    cystoscope, 43, 48
    double-pronged ligature carrier, 43, 47
    indications, 42–43
    intraoperative complications, 49
    lateral dissection, 43, 44
    medial traction, 43
    monofilament nonabsorbable suture, 43, 45
    oblique incisions, 43, 44
    periurethral and perivesical fasciae, 43, 46
    placement of suspension sutures, 43, 45
    postoperative care, 49
    postoperative complications, 49
    preoperative considerations, 43
    retropubic space, finger in, 43, 45
    small puncture, 43, 47
    traction of sutures, 43, 47
  clinical correlation
    pubourethral ligaments, 38
    sling procedures, 38–40
    suburethral support, impact of, 39, 41
    urethral mobility, 38, 39
  DUPS procedure
    absorbable sutures, 49, 53
    Allis clamps, 49, 50, 54
    double-pronged ligature carrier, 49, 52, 53
    hemostatic clamp, 49, 52
    indications, 49
    oblique incisions, 49, 50
    postoperative complications, 55
    puncture, 49, 51
    right-angle clamp, 49, 51
    small incision, 49, 52
    soft polypropylene mesh, 49, 51
  fascia lata autologous fascial sling
    anchoring effect, 67, 68
    Crawford fascial stripper, 67, 69
    cystoscopy, 67, 71
    double-pronged passer, 67, 70
    fascial retrieval, 66–68
    figure-of-eight sutures, 67, 70
    Foley catheter, 67, 70
    oblique incisions, 67, 70, 71
    right-angle clamp, 67, 68
    sharp and blunt dissection, 67, 68
  normal continence, mechanisms of
    anatomical support of urethra, 30–35
    closing function of urethra, 27–29
    urethral changes, 36–37
    urethral length, 30
  skeletal musculature, 28
  spiral slings
    absorbable sutures, 72, 75
    curved clamp, 72
    cystoscopy, 72, 75
    delayed absorbable suture, 72, 73
    fascial segment, 72, 74
    finger control, 72, 73
    indications, 72
    oblique incisions, 72
    postoperative complications, 72
    small suprapubic puncture, 72, 75
    suprapubic incision, 72, 75
    tunnel, 72, 74
  surgical correlation, 42
  treatment of, 42

T
Transvaginal enterocele repair. *See* Enterocele repair
Transvaginal pararectal repair, rectal prolapse. *See* Rectal prolapse

U
Urethral diverticula excision
  diagnosis
    cystic/soft mass, 148
    direct injection, 148, 150
    double-balloon positive-pressure urethrogram, 148, 150
    urethral sphincteric unit, 148, 151
    urethroscopy, 148, 149
    voiding cystogram, 148, 149
  intraoperative complications, 159
  postoperative care, 159
  postoperative complications, 159
  surgical indications and procedures, 147
  surgical technique
    anterior vaginal wall flap, 151, 153
    diluted indigo carmine, 151, 154
    figure-of-eight delayed absorbable sutures, 151, 157
    Foley catheter, 151, 155, 156
    inverted U flap, 151, 152
    large cystic mass, 151
    lines of sutures, 151, 158
    periurethral fascia sutures, 151, 157
    sharp dissection, 151, 155
    transverse closure, 151, 158
    transverse incision, 151, 153
    vaginal flap, 151, 158
Urethral obstruction
  diagnosis of, 237–238
  etiology of, 237
  preoperative considerations, 238

surgical techniques
bladder neck obstruction, 249
Burch procedure, 241–242
distal urethral diverticulum, 243
distal urethral stricture, 252–253
labial flap, 256–259
midurethral stricture, Heineke–Mikulicz technique, 254–256
periurethral abscess, 250–251
secondary cystocele, 240
suprameatal urethrolysis and retropubic Martius flap, 246–249
urethral erosion, 240
urethrolysis and retropubic Martius flap, 244–246
urinary retention, 239
Urethral reconstruction
anterior vaginal wall, 229, 231
fatty tissue, 230
in situ Martius flap, 228, 230
in situ vaginal wall, 227
labial and distal vaginal tissue, 228
labial margins, 231
longitudinal incisions, 229
Martius flap, 226
medial margins incision, 230
sutures, 231
U flap, 226
urethral defect, 227
urethral margins, 228
voiding cystogram, 229
Urethropelvic fascia, 11, 13–14, 16, 30–32, 34, 37, 39, 42, 43, 46, 51, 89, 90, 95, 156, 220, 225, 247
Urethrovaginal fistula
after anterior repair
anterior vaginal flap, 175
anterior vaginal wall exposure, 175
distal vaginal wall, 175
Foley catheter, 175
inverted U incision, 175
Martius flap, 178
midurethral fistula, 174
periurethral fascia, 177
transverse incision, 176
after mesh erosion
anterior vaginal wall exposure, 179
anterior vaginal wall flap, 181
circular defect, 180
end-to-end anastomosis, 180
Foley catheter, 180
in situ Martius flap, 181
inverted U anterior vaginal flap, 179
obturator fossa, 180
hymeneal excision
anterior vaginal flap, 183
anterior vaginal wall, 182
in situ Martius flap, 183
inverted U flap, 182
mucosa and urethral wall, 182
intraoperative complications, 193
postoperative care, 194
postoperative complications, 194
radiation
anterior vaginal wall, 174
circular incision, 172
fibro-fatty tissue, 173
Foley catheter, 172
left labia majora, 173
Martius flap, 173
perivesical fascia, sutures, 172
sutures, 172

V

Vaginal cyst and masses
Bartholin's gland cyst, 262–263
ectopic ureterocele, 266–267
endometrioma, 270
inclusion cysts, anterior vaginal wall, 268–269
inferior pubic rami, 280
leiomyoma (fibroid), 270–272
Mesonephric–Wolffian Gartner's duct cysts, 274–275
Müllerian cyst, 276
perineal leiomyoma, 278–279
posterior vaginal wall, 278–279
Skene's gland cyst, 264–265
urethra, fibroadenoma of, 273
urethral mucosa, distal thrombosis of, 277
urethral obstruction
anterior vaginal wall reconstruction, 284
distal and proximal urethras, 282
Foley catheter, 283
inverted U flap, 281
neourethra reconstruction, 283
periurethral fascia, 283
urethral replacement and displacement, 281
Vaginal hysterectomy, 123, 302, 303, 319
curved clamp, 19
for uterine prolapse
anterior retractor, 101, 105
circumferential incision, 101, 102
coagulation knife, 101, 102
diagnosis, 100
indications, 100
lateral traction, 101, 104
Metzenbaum scissors, 101, 102
Phaneuf clamp, 101, 104
posterior dissection, 101, 103
purse-string sutures, 101, 106–108
right-angle clamp, 101, 104
sacrouterine–cardinal complex, 101, 103
delay absorbable sutures, 101, 105, 106
urethral catheter, 101
uterine pedicle, isolation of, 101, 104
vault suspension suture, 101, 106
Vaginal surgery complications
anterior mesh exposure, 307
anterior mesh, removal of
cystocele repair with four arms, 316
cystocele repair without arms, 315
bladder injury (perforation)
absorbable sutures, 290
anterior vaginal wall exposure, 293
anterior vaginal wall flap, 293
bladder calcification, 291
cystoscopy, 290
fibro-fatty labial flap, 290
retropubic mesh, 292
suprapubic exploration, 293
suture perforation, 290
translabial ultrasound, 293
transvaginal and open bladder removal, 292
transvaginal exploration, 293
urethral Foley, 290

Vaginal surgery complications (*cont.*)
bleeding, 288
bowel and rectal injury, 304–305
de novo urgency incontinence, 321
infection, 289
neurologic injury, 306
obturator sling, removal of, 313–314
pelvic mesh, removal of, 307–308
posterior mesh removal of, 317–318
recurrent prolapse, 319–320
recurrent stress incontinence, 323
retropubic mesh, removal of, 311–312
suburethral segment, removal of, 310
ureteric injury, 301–303
urethral injury
anterior vaginal flap, 299, 300
end-to-end anastomosis, 300
fistulous tract, 299
in situ Martius flap, 299, 300
Martius flap, 296, 300
periurethral fascia, 300
sling erosions, 295
superior and inferior flap, 299
surgical finding, 300
urethral erosion, 296
urinary outlet obstruction, 321
vaginal narrowing/stenosis, 322
Vault prolapse
sacrocolpopexy, 15
and transvaginal enterocele repair
(*see* Enterocele repair)
Vesicopelvic fascia, 15–18, 81, 83, 84, 88–90, 95
Vesicovaginal fistula
colpocleisis, recurrent radiation
anterior vaginal wall exposure, 183
catheter insertion, 184
labial flap, 184
rotational flap transfer, 184
vaginal wall exposure, 185
voiding cystogram, 183
cystoscopic finding, 162
diagnosis, 161
inner thigh flap
absorbable sutures, 191
adductor fascia, 186
detached gracilis muscle, 192
distal flap, 187
incision area, 186
interrupted sutures, 187
inverted U flap, 189
labial flap, 190
lateral 5 o'clock episiotomy, 189
location area, 185
myocutaneous gracilis flap, 192
Penrose drain, 186
rectangular flap, 187
size and location, donor site, 192
skin defect, 188
subcutaneous tissue, 192
tight flap, 190
vaginal area exposure, 189, 192
vaginal examination, 192
vaginal sutures, 188
vascular supply, 187
voiding cystogram, 188
patient emotional distress, 161
preoperative considerations
abdominal/vaginal approach, 163
adjuvant measures, 163
estrogens and antibiotics, 163
fistulous tract excision, 163
timing of surgery, 162–163
surgery indications, 162
surgical techniques
anatomical location, 169
anterior vaginal wall flap, 171
distal vaginal flap, 171
fistulous tract exposure, 166
inverted "J"-shaped incision, 164
Lowsley retractor, 163
omentum, 168
peritoneal flap, 170
perivesical fascia, 167–169
sutures, 167
U-shaped anterior vaginal wall flap, 165
wide posterior vaginal flap, 166

MIX
Papier aus verantwortungsvollen Quellen
Paper from responsible sources
FSC® C105338

If you have any concerns about our products,
you can contact us on
ProductSafety@springernature.com

In case Publisher is established outside the EU,
the EU authorized representative is:
Springer Nature Customer Service Center GmbH
Europaplatz 3, 69115 Heidelberg, Germany

Printed by Libri Plureos GmbH
in Hamburg, Germany